W9-DGJ-815

PREGNANCY DAY BY DAY

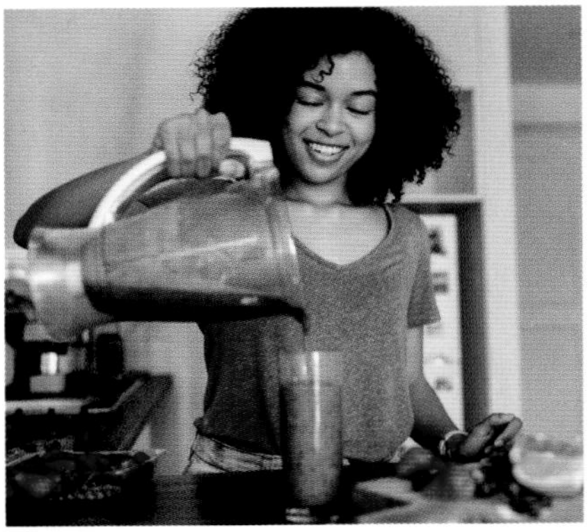
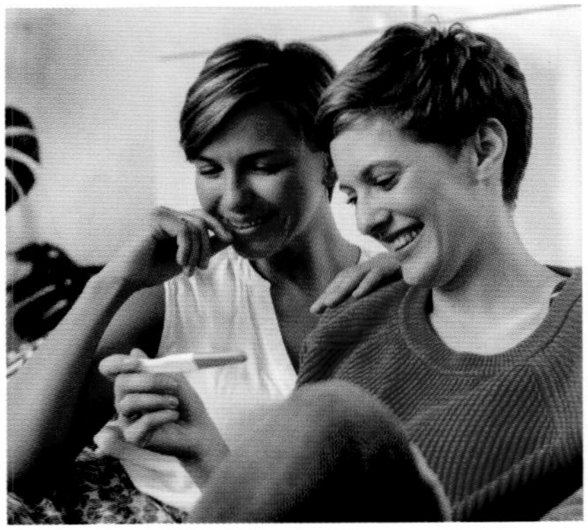
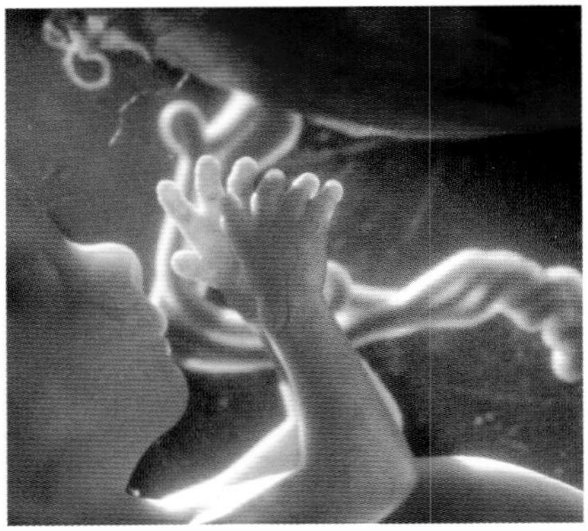
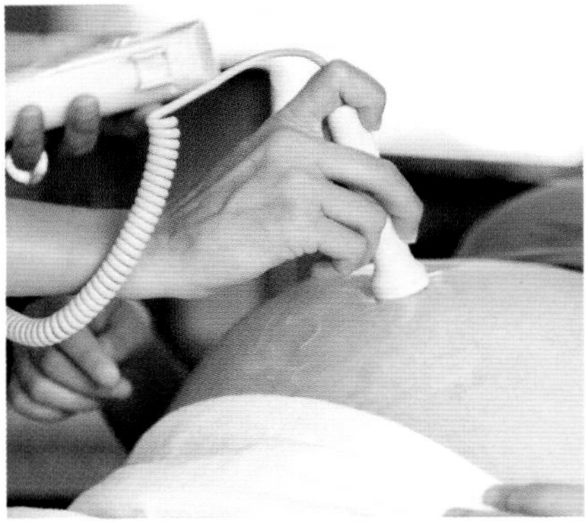
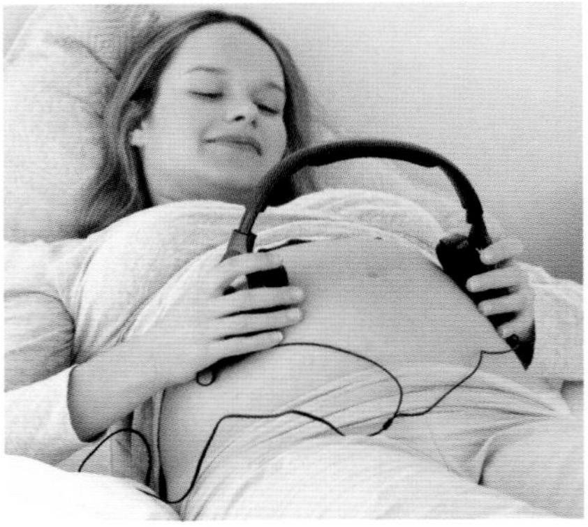
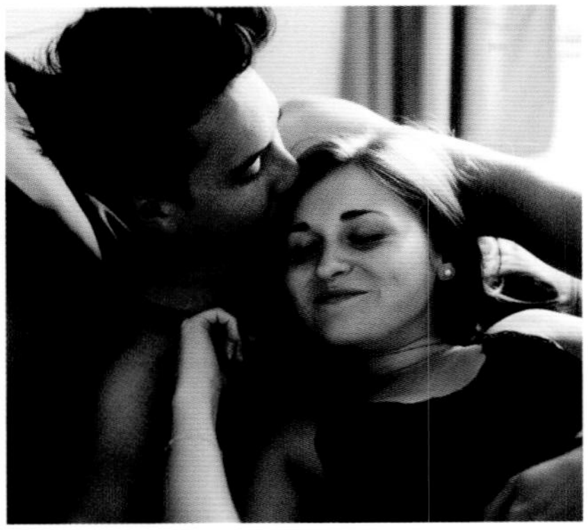
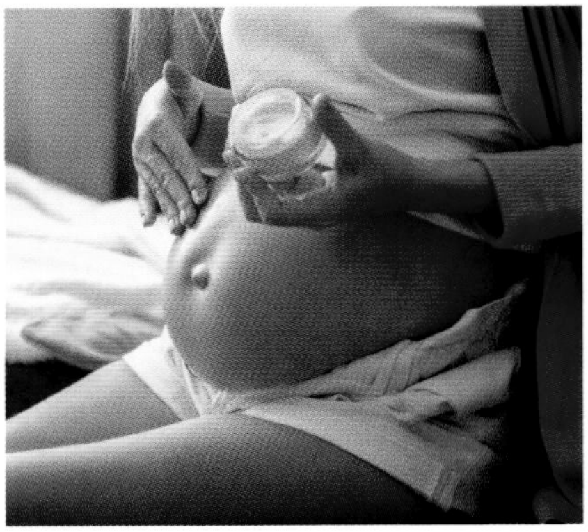
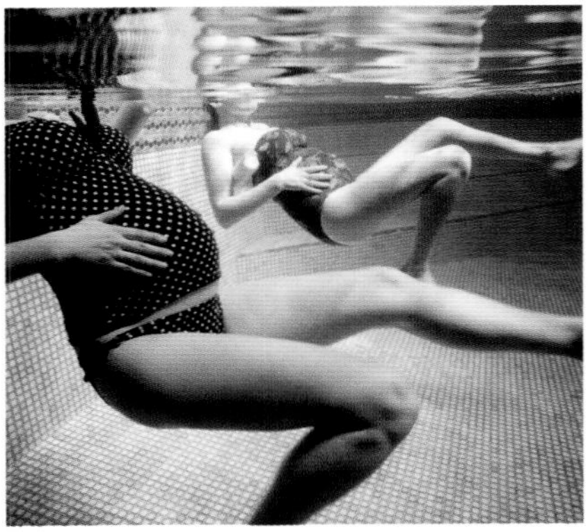
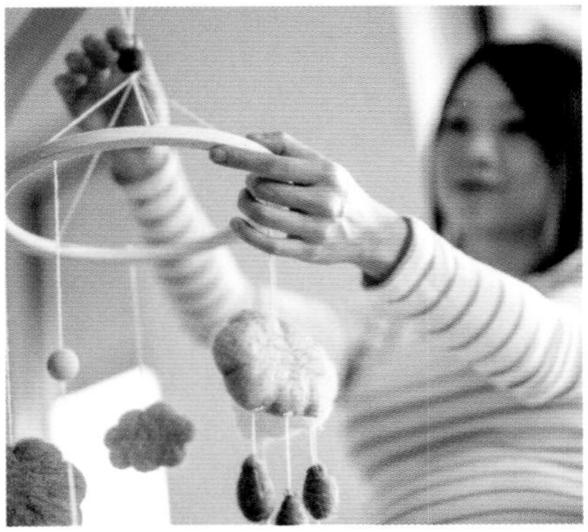
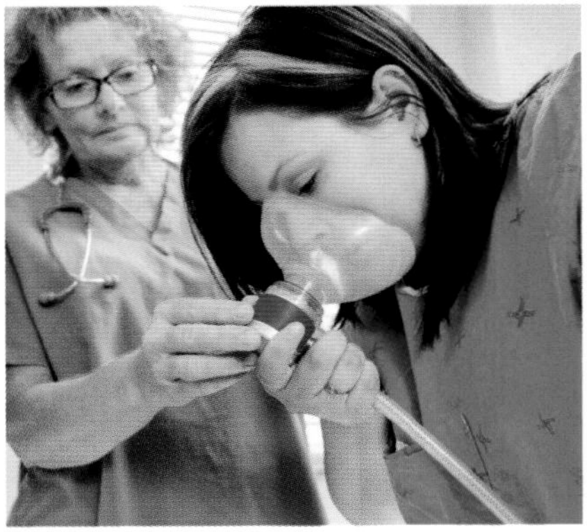
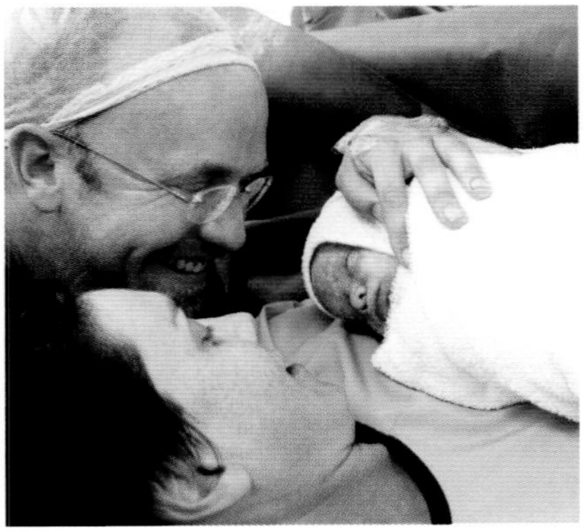
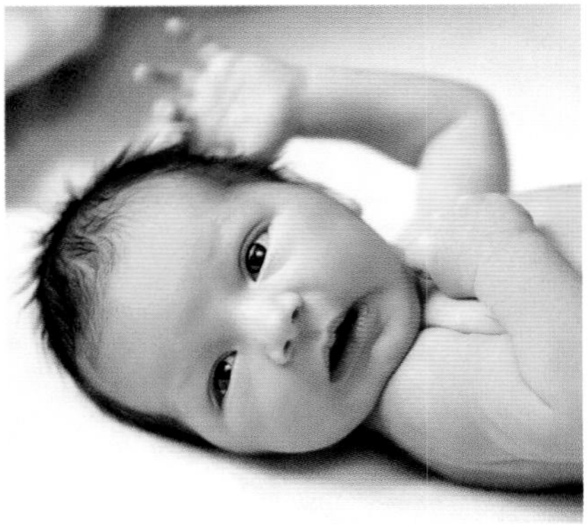

PREGNANCY DAY BY DAY

Count down your pregnancy day by day
with advice from a team of experts

CONSULTING EDITOR
Paula Amato, MD, Department
of Obstetrics & Gynecology
Oregon Health & Science University

EDITOR IN CHIEF
Dr. Maggie Blott, MBBS,
Consultant Obstetrician

Contents

[redacted]

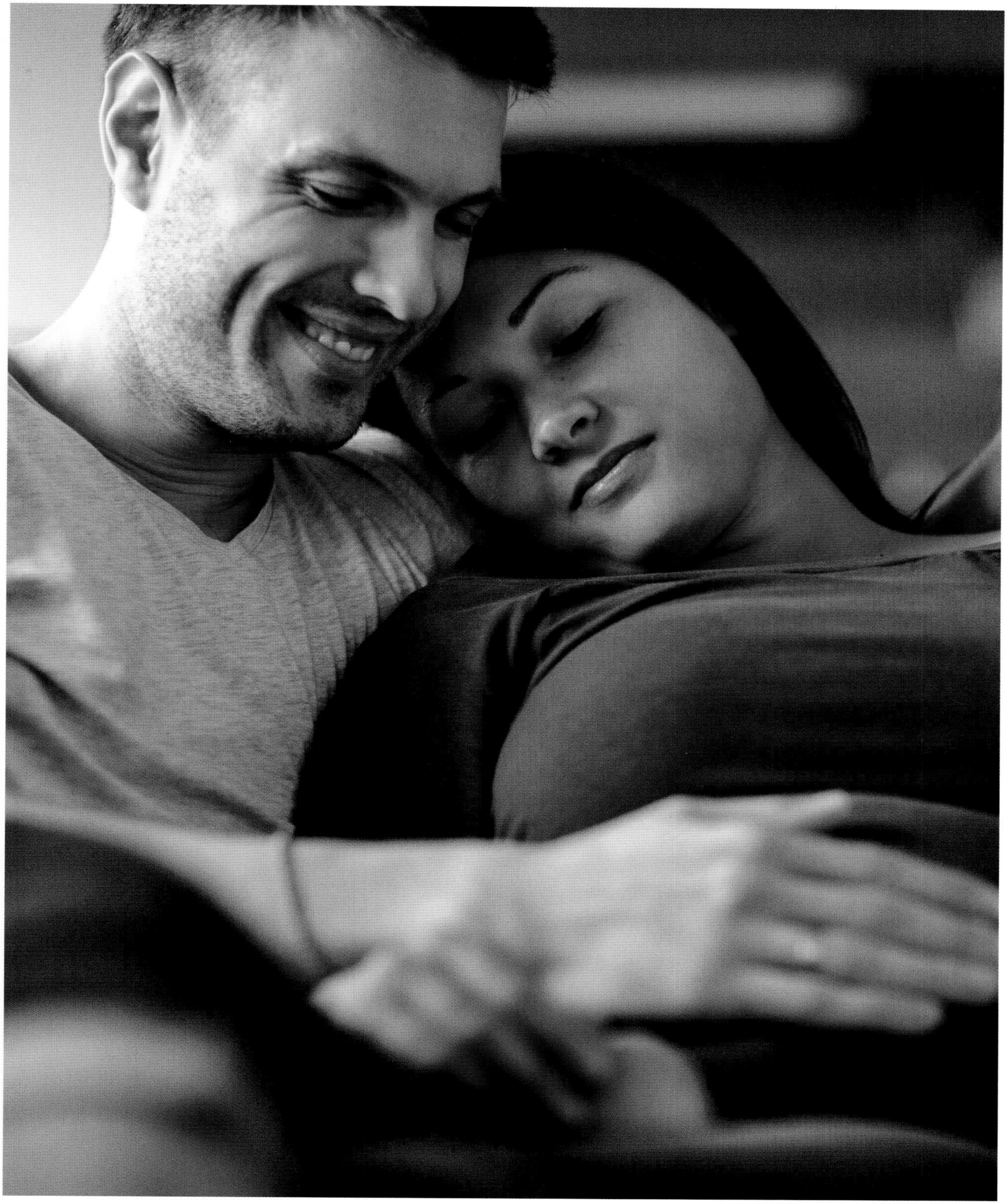

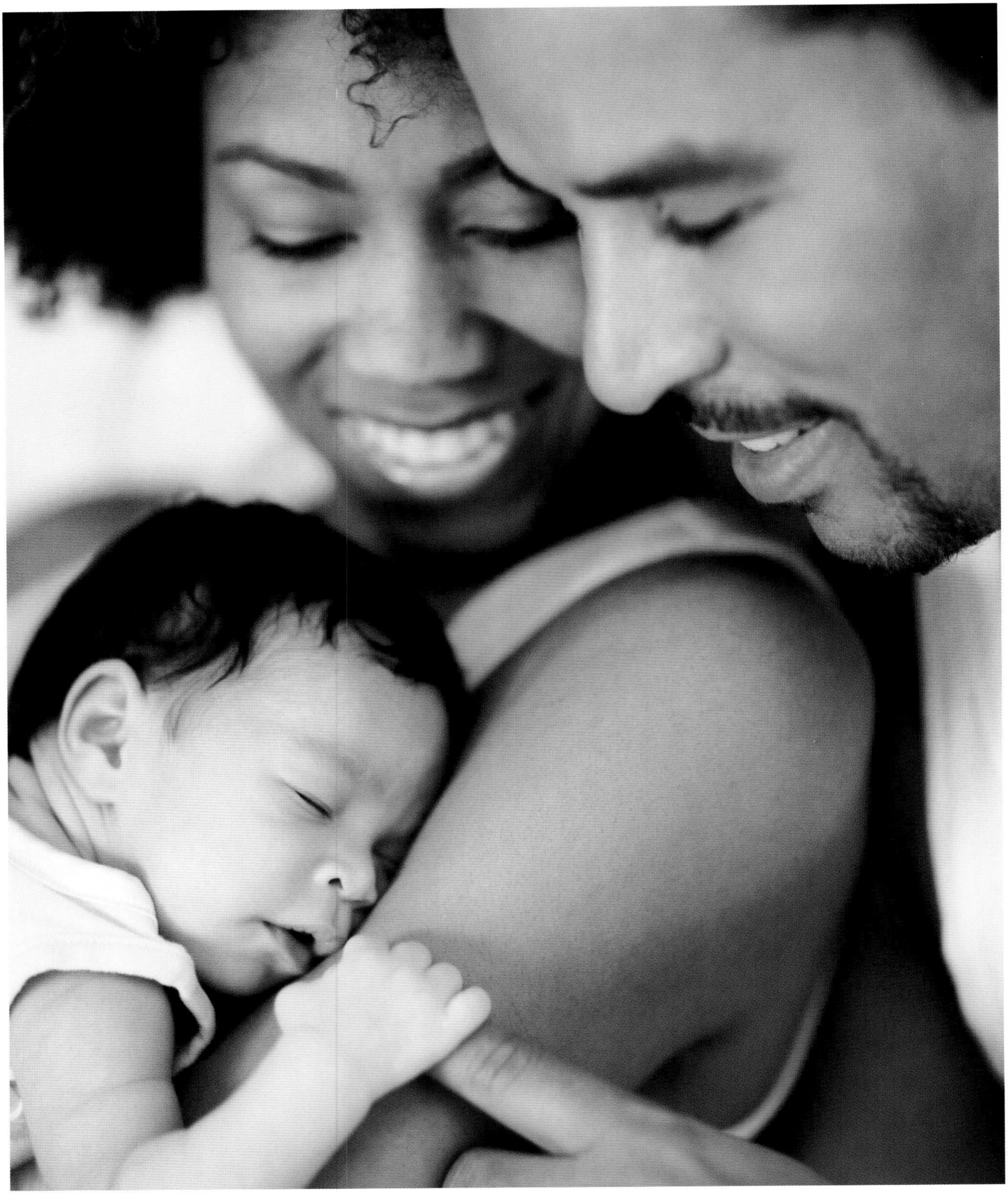

Labor and birth

Life with your new baby

Concerns and complications

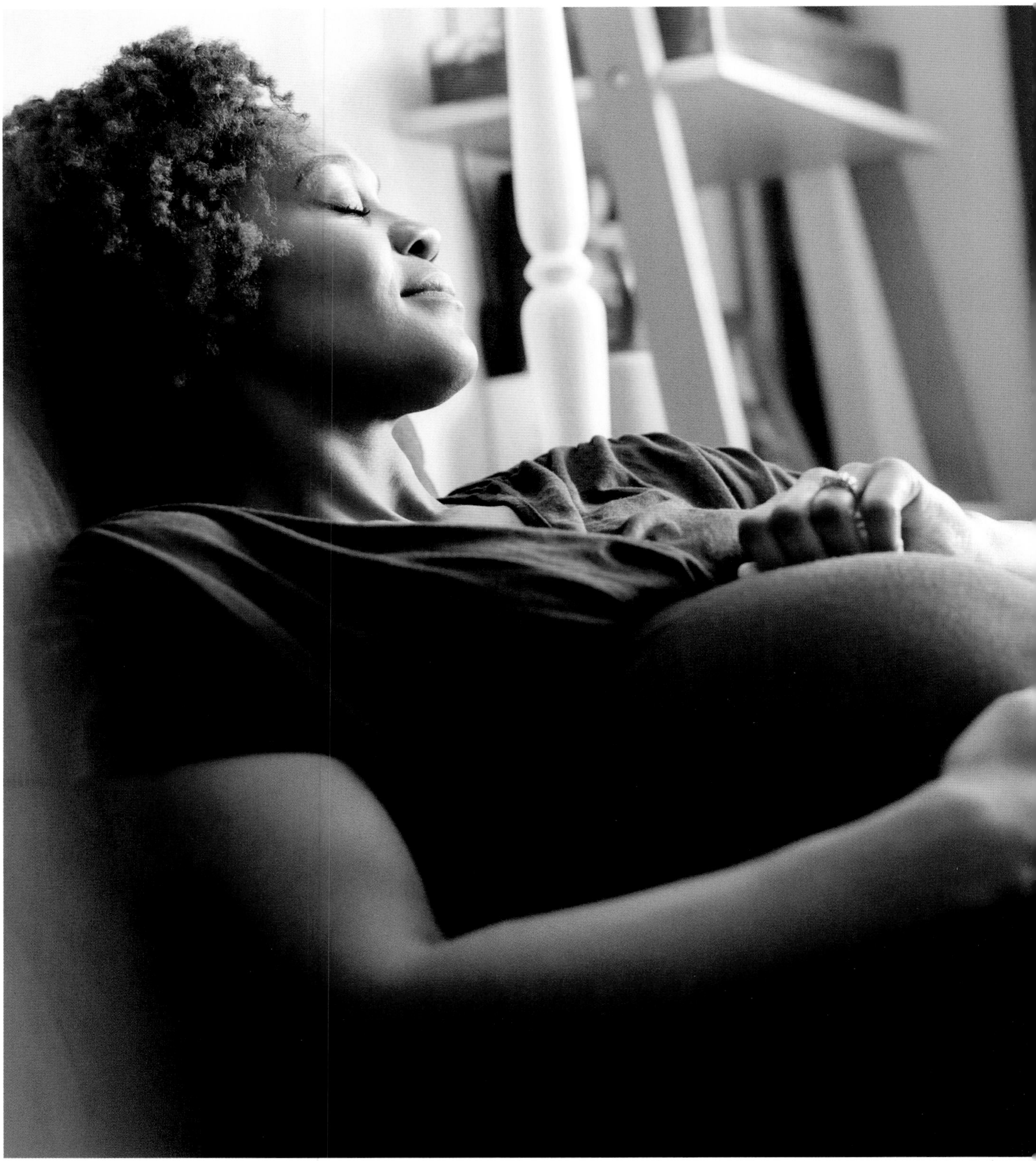

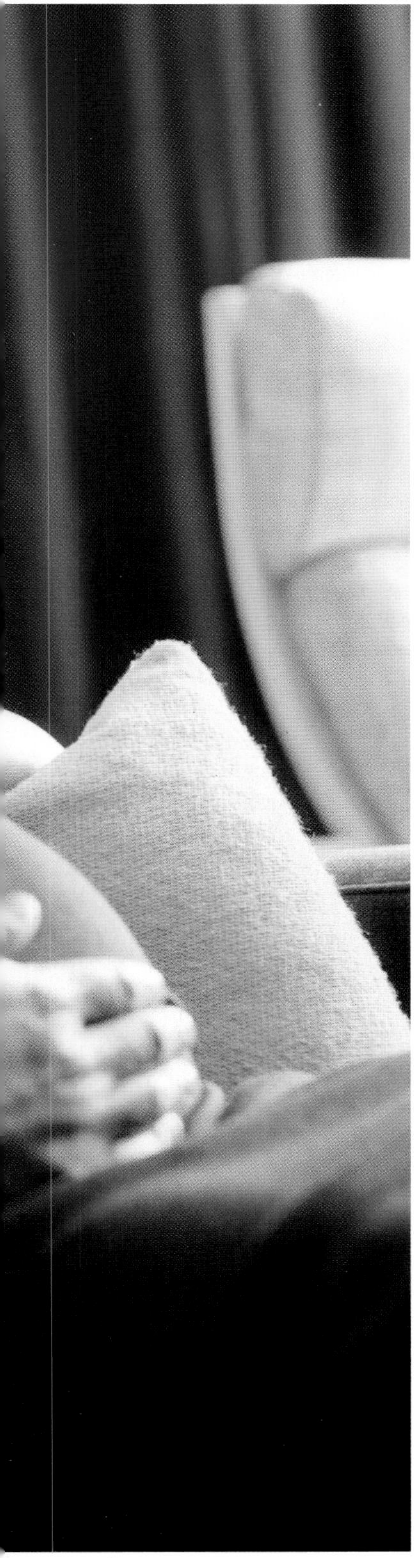

Introduction

When you find out that you are pregnant, you may feel excited and a little fearful of the unknown. Rest assured that most women have straightforward pregnancies, have uncomplicated births, and deliver a healthy baby. This book provides clear, unbiased, and, where possible, evidence-based advice to support you through the journey. The information has been written by a variety of health-care professionals, all of whom have contributed to the safe care of women in pregnancy and during birth, as well as taking care of newborn infants over many years. I thank them for their contributions.

This book gives guidance when planning a pregnancy and discusses the normal symptoms that many, if not all, women experience. Straightforward advice is given on the many practical aspects of pregnancy, such as how to choose a place of birth and issues to consider to ensure the safety of mother and baby.

Some women, in particular circumstances, may need additional information and knowledge. In this new edition, the existing text has been supplemented by descriptions of the new tests available in pregnancy. There is also information on the additional monitoring and interventions that are now performed if there are any complications that may impact on the health of the mother or her unborn baby.

Over 30 percent of women now give birth either by a planned or an emergency Cesarean section, so there is updated information on why a woman might need a Cesarean, what the process involves, a description of any complications, and a more detailed section on the recovery. Induction of labor rates continue to increase, so more information has been provided on why a woman might need to be induced and a description of the steps involved.

Also in this new edition, we have introduced an emphasis on the monitoring of fetal movements and screening for poor growth in the unborn baby, which can help to reduce the risk of stillbirth. There is also additional guidance provided on the situations in which women should seek urgent help.

I hope this book helps you to navigate one of the most exciting journeys that any woman can undertake.

Maggie Blott

Dr. Maggie Blott

How to use this book

This book starts with guidance on how to enjoy a healthy and safe pregnancy, with lifestyle advice that often applies to the preconceptual period too. The core section of the book gives a day-by-day account of pregnancy with detailed explanations of the physical and emotional changes that take place in your body along with fascinating insights into how your baby develops within the uterus. A labor and birth chapter takes you through the delivery of your baby, followed by a summary of the first two weeks with your newborn. A final chapter deals with concerns and complications in the mother and baby in pregnancy, labor, and the postpartum period.

A healthy pregnancy

This chapter provides the information you need to make lifestyle choices that will maximize your own health throughout pregnancy and give your baby the best possible start in life. It includes guidelines for exercising safely, eating healthily, avoiding hazards, and dealing with illnesses. It also addresses concerns you may have about how the emotional and physical changes of pregnancy may impact your relationships.

Pregnancy day by day

Here, the book takes you day by day through the extraordinary story of conception and pregnancy, counting down each of the 280 days until the onset of labor. Each day reveals how your baby is developing and the changes that are occurring in your body. The 280 days, or 40 weeks, of pregnancy are divided into three trimesters, each of which comprises around a third of the pregnancy. Beyond being a simple measure of time, each trimester represents a distinct phase in the development of the baby and in the pregnancy.

The first trimester The definition of the first trimester is given here as weeks 1–12, though you may also see weeks 13 and 14 included elsewhere. This trimester covers the time from the beginning of the menstrual period to the moment of conception, which is usually around two weeks. Because the exact moment of conception is unknown, pregnancy is counted from the one definite date, the beginning of the menstrual cycle. Although technically your pregnancy may not begin until two weeks into your menstrual cycle, these two weeks are

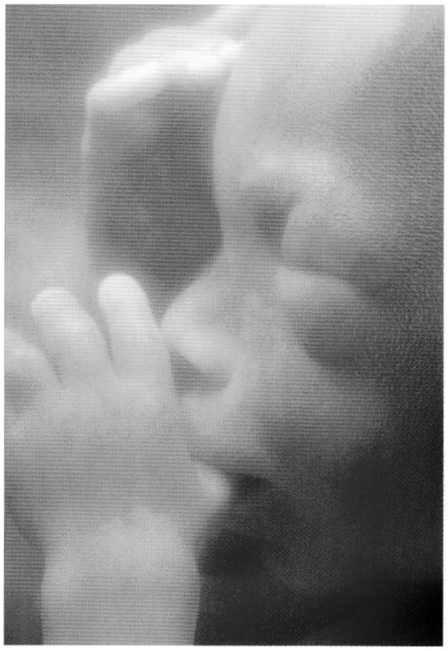

With amazing fetal images and fascinating facts, you can follow your baby's development throughout your pregnancy.

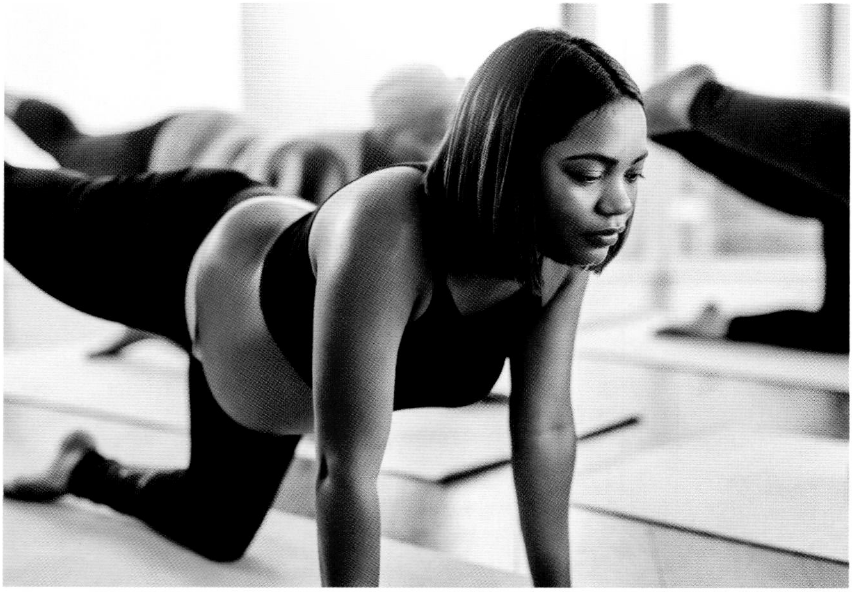

Learn simple ways to relax and tune in to your body. As well as being essential to your physical and mental well-being, exercise or physical activity will help you prepare for labor and birth.

very important in helping your body achieve a healthy pregnancy. In this section, we explain day by day the changes that take place in your uterus to prepare it for conception and implantation of the early embryo. There is dietary advice and recommendations from fertility experts to boost your chances of conceiving. The first trimester is a period of extraordinary development, when all your baby's major organs form, and they will grow faster than at any other period in life. A day-by-day account is given of the changes that you and your baby undergo, and advice offered on how to cope with the exhausting changes that occur in early pregnancy. There's also an honest appraisal of the emotional feelings you're likely to experience, reassuring you that negative as well as positive emotions are normal. Practical information on accessing prenatal care and detailed explanations of the choices that are available help you begin to plan your pregnancy and think about your options for the birth.

The second trimester In the second trimester, which is designated as weeks 13–25, your baby's organs mature further and growth continues. This is an exciting time as your body starts to change shape to accommodate your growing baby and you feel your baby move for the first time. However, it is also a time when women can experience symptoms that are often due to quite normal pregnancy changes but that can occasionally indicate a problem. For example, abdominal pain can be due to ligaments being stretched or to constipation; however, it could also indicate a problem with the placenta. Symptoms such as these are discussed at the relevant point in pregnancy, with detailed explanations that will provide reassurance or alert you to the possibility of something more serious that should be brought to the attention of your doctor.

The third trimester In the third trimester, designated as weeks 26–40, your baby continues to grow and mature and, if born early, could survive life outside the uterus. During this time, your body starts to prepare itself for labor. We describe the changes taking place and explain why they occur, as well as providing pointers to what is normal and which symptoms need to be reported to your doctor. Women recount their experiences, and questions that are presented daily to doctors are reproduced to provide a bank of vital knowledge. Practical guidance on all matters, from maternity leave entitlement information to reassurance that having sex won't harm the growing baby, helps you navigate your way through the final weeks of pregnancy.

Labor and birth

One of the best ways to cope with labor is to understand its stages. In the labor and birth chapter, a team of professionals covers in detail the progress of labor, each providing their own expert insight. A doctor writes about normal births and discusses natural pain relief. An anesthesiologist gives the options available for medical pain relief, including detailed descriptions of how epidurals are given and their pros and cons. While most women have a normal birth without complications, on average in the US over 30 percent have a Cesarean section, and less than 1 in 20 women have an assisted delivery, with either forceps or vacuum extraction. An obstetrician writes about difficult births, describing complications and the medical interventions that may be required.

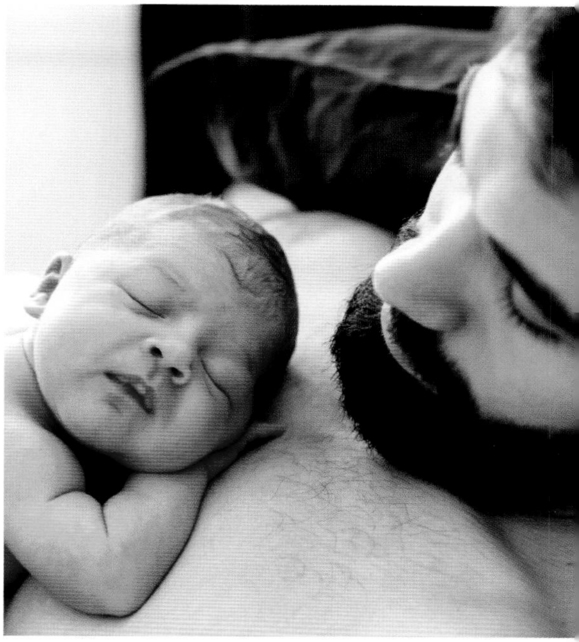

Discover how to make the most of those precious early days with your newborn baby. Amidst the constant newborn care and interrupted sleep, take time to strengthen your bond and just enjoy being together.

The first two weeks

Here, the early days as you adjust to life with your new baby are charted in the day-by-day format. A pediatrician addresses the practical issues of baby care. Also discussed are the emotional and physical renewal you undergo as your body recovers and you begin the new tasks of nurturing and feeding your baby.

Concerns and complications

This section is a concise guide to conditions in pregnancy and labor, and postpartum concerns in the mother and baby. Clear explanations enable you to digest medical information, understand which symptoms are not of concern, and feel reassured about how more serious conditions are managed in pregnancy, labor, and the postpartum period.

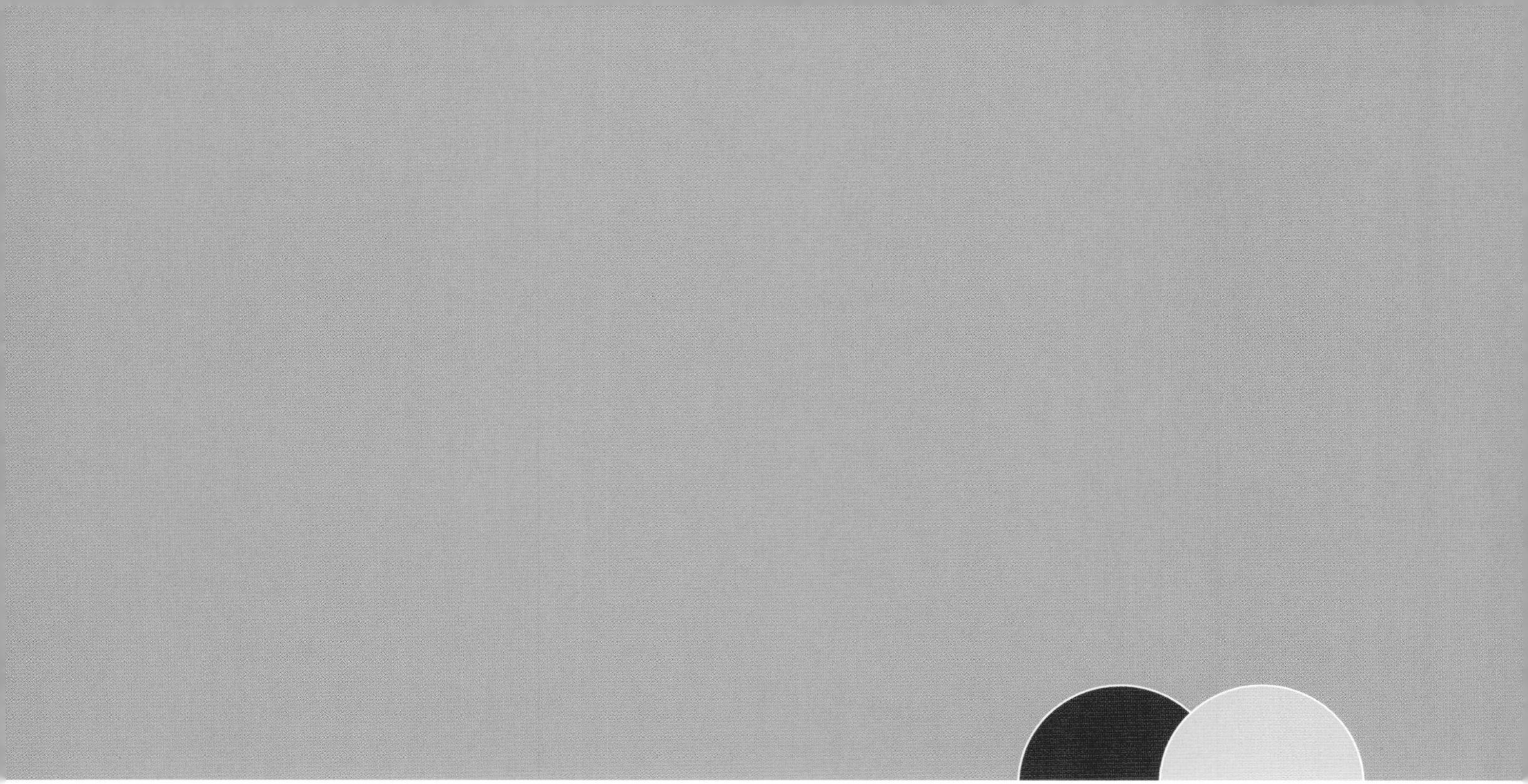

A HEALTHY PREGNANCY

With an ever-growing body of knowledge on how a mother's behavior in pregnancy impacts her baby's immediate and long-term health, you have the opportunity to ensure that your lifestyle choices positively benefit your baby. Eating healthily, exercising regularly, and avoiding hazards will all help give your baby the best possible start in life.

Your pregnancy diet

You can optimize your own health and your baby's future health by eating a nutritious, balanced diet throughout pregnancy.

In recent years, much has been learned about what constitutes a healthy diet in pregnancy. In addition to the importance of nutrients such as folic acid (see p.17), evidence is mounting that a person's health may be influenced by the mother's diet, including whether particular nutrients were received at certain times. Good nutrition in pregnancy may reduce a baby's future risk of obesity, diabetes, and heart disease, as well as help you deal with the demands of pregnancy.

A healthy diet

Getting the right balance of protein, carbohydrates, and fats in pregnancy is simple, since the ratios are the same in pregnancy as at other times: 45–65 percent of your calories should come from carbohydrates; 20–35 percent from fats; and 10–35 percent from protein over the course of a week. A diet with plenty of vegetables, fruits, whole grains, and good proteins and fats automatically contains the proper mix of nutrients.

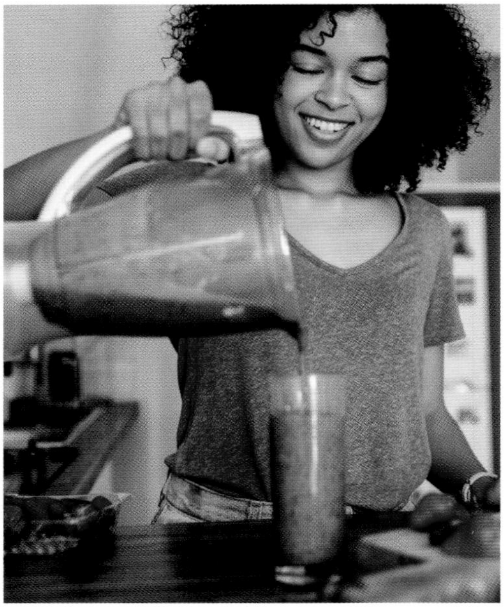

Eating regular nutritious food, such as smoothies, is vital during pregnancy to keep your energy levels up, and to provide your growing baby with all he needs to develop well.

Carbohydrates are an important source of fuel for you and for your baby since they are broken down into glucose, which passes easily across the placenta. Try to get six servings a day, a serving being equivalent to a slice of bread, 2 oz (60 g) of cereal, or five crackers.

Carbohydrates are divided into two subgroups: refined and unrefined. Refined foods such as white rice and white breads are rapidly broken down and enter the bloodstream as a glucose spike that could produce larger babies with a future obesity risk. Unrefined carbohydrates such as in whole-wheat bread and pasta, and brown rice, break down more slowly and release glucose steadily, and are a good source of fiber. At least half of your carbohydrates should come from unrefined sources.

Protein is essential for the growth of the baby and the placenta, as well as for your health. Pregnant women need around 2 oz (60 g) each day. Aim for two to three servings of protein-rich foods a day, a typical serving being 3 oz (85 g) red meat, or 5 oz (150 g) fish. Since most adults get about 3½ oz (100 g) of protein daily, there is usually no need to increase your intake, especially if you have protein at each meal. If you're vegetarian, in addition to protein at each meal, you should have a snack that contains protein. If you're having twins or more, ask your doctor how much protein to consume. When breast-feeding you'll need 2½ oz (70 g) daily.

Choose protein sources that contain less saturated fat, such as skinless chicken, lean beef and pork, tofu, low-fat cheese and yogurt, and skim milk. Fish, nuts, and seeds contain healthier unsaturated fats (see below), although your intake of some fish should be limited since they contain mercury, which could be harmful to your baby.

Fats contain vitamins and contribute to the healthy development of cells. However, although fats make a useful contribution to overall nutrition, their intake needs to be limited. Choose healthier unsaturated fats, found in foods such as fish and some types of oil, over unhealthy saturated fats found in whole-milk dairy products, meat, or trans fats found in processed foods.

Studies suggest that the development of the baby's nervous system may be boosted by omega-3 fatty acids, the richest source of which is found in fatty fish. Avoid fish high in mercury (see p.96); opt instead for fish such as salmon and anchovies, which are good, safe sources of omega-3 fatty acids. Wild salmon is very rich in omega-3, but farm-raised salmon is also a good source. Other sources include omega-3–enriched eggs, flaxseed, flaxseed oil, walnuts, canola oil, and omega-3 supplements and prenatal vitamins containing omega-3 fatty acids.

Dairy products are an important component of the diet since they provide a good supply of proteins and fats, as well as calcium and some vitamins. Calcium is essential for the healthy development of bones and teeth. Opt for low-fat dairy products and low-fat or skim milk. Aim for 2–3 servings each day, a typical serving being 1 oz (30 g) of hard cheese, or 1 cup (200 ml) milk.

Vitamins and minerals support the healthy functioning of body systems and provide antioxidants, which protect the body against harmful free radicals. See the table on p.17 for more.

A vegetarian diet, and vegan diets where dairy products are excluded, can be safe and healthy during pregnancy as long as you ensure a good balance of nutrients and sufficient protein (see p.126). Babies born to vegetarians are in a healthy weight range, although vegans need to be vigilant in getting adequate protein, as well as reliable sources of B12 and zinc. Vegans can discuss with their doctors whether they can meet

YOUR RECOMMENDED DAILY INTAKE

A healthy, balanced diet is essential for dealing with the additional demands on your body and providing your baby with needed nutrients. Eating a wide variety of healthy foods ensures that you both receive the correct balance of nutrients. Include foods from each of the major food groups each day.

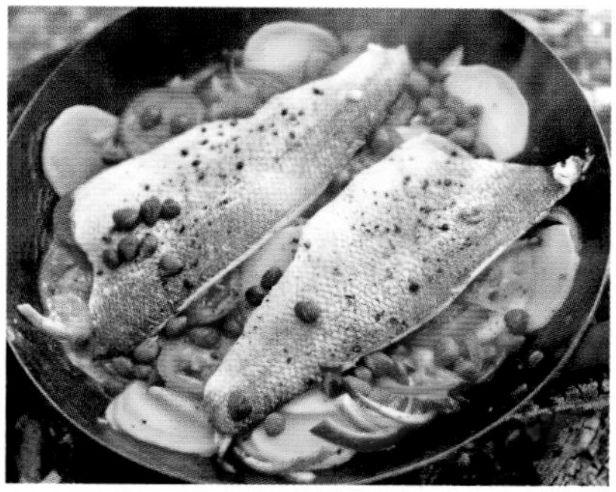

Include 2–3 portions each day of protein-rich foods, such as fish, lean meat, chicken, legumes, hard cheeses, and nuts to ensure that body structures grow in a healthy way and that you have fuel to keep you going.

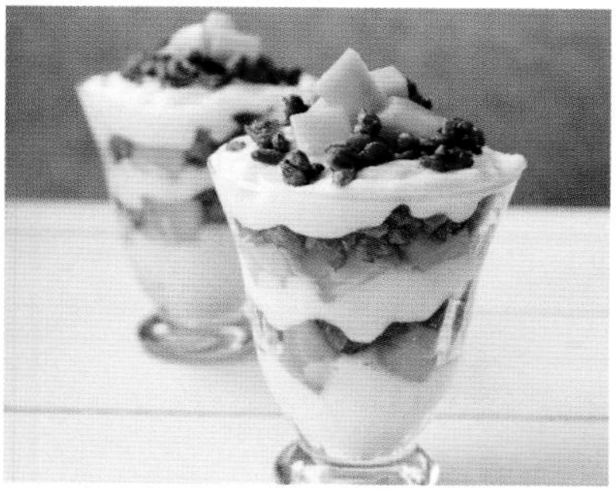

Try to include 3 servings of dairy products in your diet each day. Ideally, your choices should be low-fat products, such as low-fat milk, low-fat cheese, and low-fat yogurt.

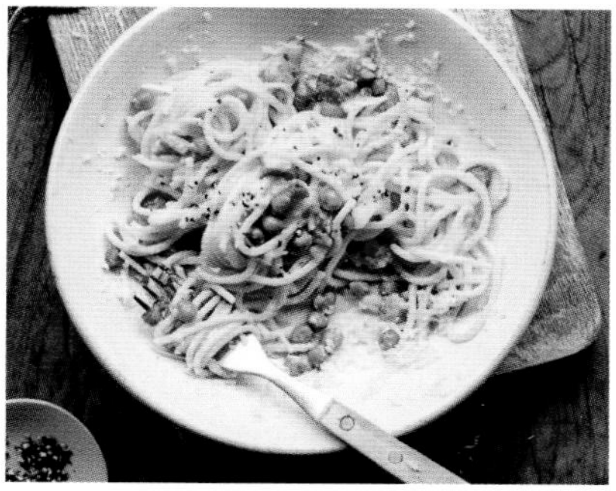

Have 3 servings of whole-grain carbohydrates, such as brown rice and whole-wheat breads and pasta, to keep up energy levels and ensure a supply of fiber, which helps relieve constipation.

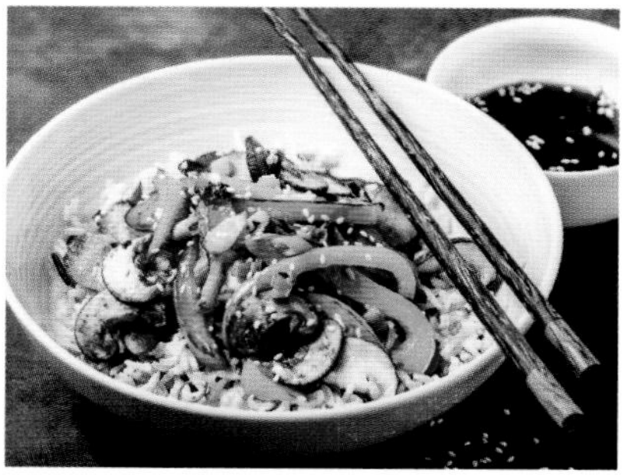

4–5 servings of vegetables each day will ensure a good supply of essential vitamins and minerals. Try to eat produce from all colors of the rainbow and don't overcook your vegetables.

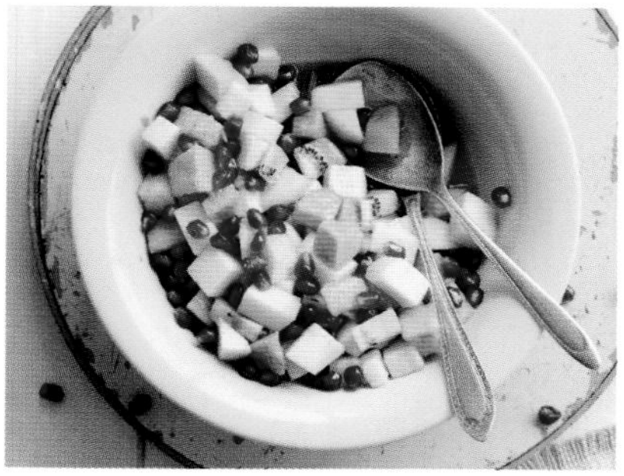

3–4 portions of fresh fruit every day will also provide a wide range of vitamins and minerals, many of which contain important protective antioxidants.

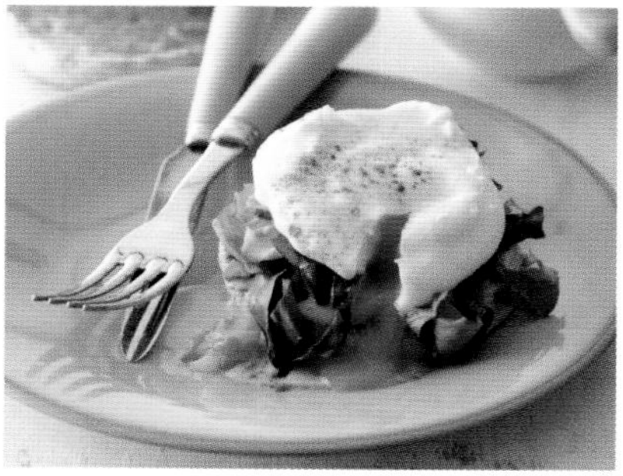

1–2 servings daily of iron-rich foods such as eggs or dark leafy green vegetables will help maintain healthy iron levels during pregnancy when demands are increased.

DIETARY PRECAUTIONS

Certain foods should be avoided or their intake limited since they may pose a risk to your unborn baby. Simple cooking and hygiene measures are also important to limit the risks.

Listeria is a food-borne bacteria to which pregnant women are more susceptible. It is found in unpasteurized dairy products, as well as refrigerated, ready-to-eat foods like meat, poultry, and seafood. To avoid it, thoroughly reheat hot dogs, lunch meats, or prepared deli foods and avoid unpasteurized dairy products; check labels of soft cheeses to be sure they're made with pasteurized milk.

Nearly all seafood contains at least trace amounts of mercury, which can affect the development of the fetal nervous system. Pregnant women should avoid swordfish, shark, king mackerel, and tilefish. To stay within safe limits, eat up to 12 ounces per week of lower-mercury seafood like shrimp, salmon, pollock, catfish, and canned light tuna.

Toxoplasmosis is a parasite spread through cat feces or undercooked beef, pork, or lamb that can harm the fetus. Avoid changing cat litter and practice careful hygiene in the kitchen when preparing raw meat, being careful not to contaminate other foods such as lettuce or vegetables. Beef, pork, and lamb all need to be well cooked.

Salmonella bacteria are found in chicken and eggs. Infection with salmonella can cause severe vomiting, but doesn't directly affect the baby. Avoid any products containing raw or undercooked eggs, and make sure all poultry is thoroughly cooked through, since cooking kills the bacteria.

their B12 needs through diet alone. Since B12 is found primarily in animal sources, a supplement may be required. Non-animal sources may be unreliable.

A low-GI diet· Glucose, the product of carbohydrates, serves as the primary fuel for your growing baby. A newer concept in nutrition is the glycemic index (GI), which looks at how much a food will raise the level of glucose in the bloodstream. Foods that release glucose gradually, such as unrefined carbohydrates (see p.14), and thus have a low GI, appear to be healthier.

Evidence suggests that a low-GI diet has health benefits for both the mother and baby. Maternal carbohydrate intake can affect glucose levels in the bloodstream, which in turn can affect the baby's growth. Higher glucose levels, even those in the normal range, can make for a bigger baby—above the 90th percentile (the top end of a baby's growth chart, see p.284). There are health risks later in life linked to a high birth weight, such as obesity, diabetes, and heart disease. One study found that women who consumed a low-GI diet had infants that were a normal size, but had less body fat than those from women who consumed a high-GI diet.

A low-GI diet can also help control glucose levels in mothers with gestational diabetes (see p.475), in turn reducing complications of labor and birth associated with this condition.

Your calorie intake· During pregnancy, most women need to increase their calorie intake by 100–300 calories a day for proper nutrition and weight gain. Your energy needs may vary depending on your pre-pregnancy weight and your activity levels.

HOW MUCH CAFFEINE?

Recent research indicates that there is no absolute safe level of caffeine, so current advice is to limit caffeine consumption to less than 200mg a day, which is equivalent to 2½ cups of instant coffee. High levels of caffeine is associated with an increased chance of having a miscarriage or a small baby. Be aware of how much caffeine drinks and chocolate contain:

- 7fl oz (200ml) instant coffee: 75mg
- 7fl oz (200ml) filter coffee: 140mg
- 8fl oz (225ml) latte: 75mg
- 8fl oz (225ml) flat white: 150mg
- 7fl oz (200ml) black tea: 33–50mg
- 11½fl oz (330ml) regular cola: 32mg
- 11½fl oz (330ml) diet cola: 42mg
- 9fl oz (250ml) energy drink: 80mg
- 1¾oz (50g) bar of plain (dark) chocolate: less than 25mg or milk chocolate: less than 10mg

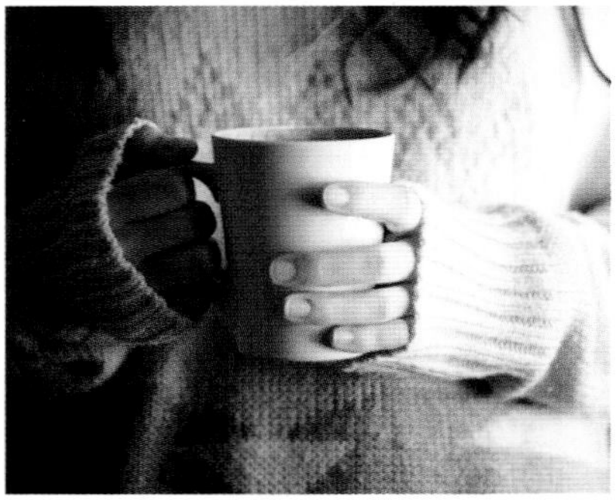

VITAMINS AND MINERALS

This table shows why you and your baby need vitamins and minerals and the top dietary sources.

VITAMIN	HEALTH BENEFITS	GOOD DIETARY SOURCES	SEE ALSO
Vitamin A	Cells and organ development; immune system; eyes, skin, and hair	Apricots, peppers, carrots, tomatoes	pp.46, 131
Vitamin B1	Helps release energy from what you eat for your baby	Pork, peas, brown rice	p.288
Vitamin B2	Energy release, protects DNA, helps metabolize iron	Milk, poultry, beef	p.131
Vitamin B3	Energy release, helps reduce tiredness; may help reduce risk of cleft palate in baby	Potatoes, turkey, pulses	
Vitamin B6	Development of central nervous system and brain; immune defense	Pulses, wheat germ, breakfast cereals	
Folate (folic acid) (Vitamin B9)	Protects against neural tube defects	Brussels sprouts, beets, oranges, asparagus	p.35
Vitamin B12	Protects against neural tube defects	Milk, meat, fish, eggs, algal sources	pp.66, 121
Vitamin C	Antioxidant; helps placenta work efficiently; increases iron absorption; fights infection	Citrus fruits, kiwis, peppers, broccoli, spinach	pp.135, 164
Vitamin D	Development of bones and teeth; acts as a hormone helping calcium to be used	Eggs, dark green leafy vegetables	pp.40, 79, 332
Vitamin K	For blood clotting	Green leafy vegetables	

MINERAL	HEALTH BENEFITS	GOOD DIETARY SOURCES	SEE ALSO
Iron	New blood cells, hemoglobin production, placenta formation, baby's cells and organs	Red meat, poultry, beans, tofu, lentils	pp.84, 126, 154, 191
Calcium	Development of bones, muscles, teeth, heart	Dairy, eggs, cereals, greens	pp.114, 131, 332
Magnesium	Development of proteins including DNA; forms part of baby's bones	Bread, potatoes, leafy green vegetables, seeds	
Zinc	Cell development; helps to prevent preterm delivery	Seafood, nuts	p.44
Iodine	Cell development; helps to prevent preterm delivery	Milk, fish	pp.80, 131
Selenium	Antioxidant, protecting cells against damage; helps prevent preeclampsia	Fish, lentils, sunflower seeds, Brazil nuts	pp.44, 165
Copper	Brain development; heart and immune system; cells	Nuts, lentils, shellfish	p.165
Potassium	Fluid balance in your blood and lymph system reduces risk of hypertension (high blood pressure)	Vegetables, plums, dried fruit, bananas, potatoes	

Exercising safely

Staying fit in pregnancy has many benefits for you and your baby and increases your stamina for labor and birth.

If you had an exercise program before you became pregnant, you can continue with this in the first trimester as long as you have the all clear from your doctor. As your pregnancy goes on, you may need to adapt your program.

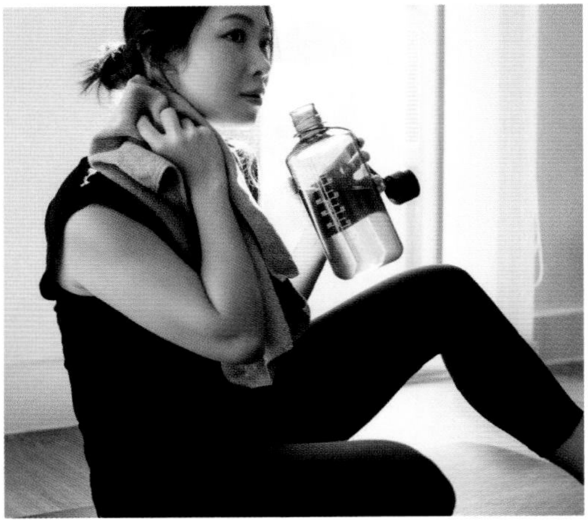

If you didn't have a regular exercise program before, now is the ideal time to adopt a new, healthier way of life from which you will reap the rewards for years to come. If you do start exercising now, build up gently; listen to your body and do only what feels comfortable.

Regular gentle exercise is much better than intense irregular bouts of exercise (which aren't advisable in pregnancy), since your body responds more positively to consistent, moderate exercise.

How exercise helps

In addition to increasing your energy levels, exercise helps you maintain a positive outlook and feel confident about your changing body image. Exercise can also ease common pregnancy discomforts such as nausea, leg cramps, swollen feet, varicose veins, constipation, insomnia, and back pain. By keeping muscles strong and toned, exercise makes it easier for your body to deal with changes in posture during pregnancy. There is also evidence that increased fitness helps shorten labor and your postpartum recovery time and lessens your overall anxiety about the birth.

Stay well hydrated by sipping water before, during, and after your workout.

Food for fuel

A nutritious, balanced diet is vital in pregnancy, and even more important when you're exercising too. By drinking water and taking a snack such as nuts, fruit, or a yogurt with you when exercising, you'll avoid being tempted by sugary snacks and drinks.

EXERCISE GUIDELINES

Follow these guidelines to exercise safely in pregnancy.

Do:

- Warm up and cool down for at least 5–7 minutes before and after exercise.
- Drink enough water before, during, and after exercising.
- Wear loose, comfortable clothes that don't restrict your rib cage.
- Try to exercise regularly for about 30 minutes, 2–3 times a week.
- Adjust your expectations; pregnancy is not a time to go for personal bests.
- Build your strength gradually. Do Kegel exercises (see p.69). Breathe properly while exercising, especially when lifting weights.
- Protect your back when getting up from a lying position: roll onto your left side and sit up using your legs.
- Avoid exercises that feel awkward or uncomfortable or that make you feel unstable on your feet.
- Focus on posture and alignment when doing any exercise.
- Stop immediately and seek advice if you feel severe localized pain, especially in your abdomen; experience vaginal bleeding or dizziness; or if you just feel unwell.
- Eat frequent small meals and snacks to maintain energy and avoid having your blood-sugar levels fall.

Don't:

- Exercise in heat or humidity.
- Do jerky or bouncy moves and stretches or twist or rotate your abdomen.
- Lift weights that are too heavy. You should be able to lift weights easily for at least 10 repetitions.
- Do sports where you risk falling, such as skiing or horseback riding, or any high-impact movement.
- Overstretch: the pregnancy hormone relaxin can make you feel more supple than you are.
- Exhaust yourself. Decrease the intensity or duration and rest for an hour for each hour of exercise daily.

Sex and relationships

You may find that you and your partner need to adapt to the emotional and physical changes that accompany pregnancy.

In a low-risk pregnancy, sex is perfectly safe, although your levels of desire may fluctuate. Most women report that their interest in sex is the same or slightly reduced in the first trimester. In the second trimester, it varies from woman to woman, and in the third trimester libido often falls.

Sex during pregnancy

During the first trimester, the hormonal changes that cause nausea, vomiting, and fatigue can naturally result in a reduced interest in sex. However, other pregnancy changes may increase your desire, such as an increased blood flow, which produces swelling in the clitoris and labia, and extra vaginal secretions. In the second trimester especially, vaginal lubrication and intensity of orgasm can increase. This may be accompanied by gentle contractions; these are normal and are nothing to worry about. Many women find that their libido falls toward the end of pregnancy since a bigger belly makes sex more awkward and uncomfortable, and they may also feel increasingly anxious about the birth.

How your partner feels

Your partner may have a range of feelings towards sex in pregnancy. While some may find their partner's new, fuller shape particularly sensuous, others may feel apprehensive about sex, fearing that they may harm the baby. Some men may feel a combination of these emotions. Unless there are concerns about your pregnancy (see right), it's generally thought that sex won't cause harm, since your baby is well protected by the amniotic fluid and your uterus.

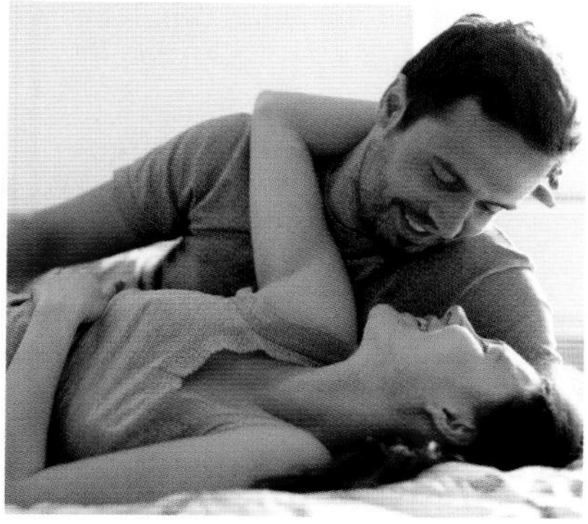

You may both feel differently about having sex during pregnancy, so keep communicating.

When to seek advice

Some women experience vaginal bleeding after sex in pregnancy. This is most likely to be harmless and is often caused by the increased blood flow to the cervix in pregnancy, which can cause it to bleed on contact with the penis. If this is the cause, the bleeding should resolve after the birth. However, since there are other possible causes, report any bleeding to your doctor.

In addition to the size of your belly causing discomfort during sex, some women experience pain during sex toward the end of pregnancy as the baby moves farther into the pelvis; or they may find that the contractions during an orgasm cause discomfort. These symptoms are unlikely to be a cause for concern, but speak to your doctor if you need reassurance.

AN INTIMATE PREGNANCY

During pregnancy, fatigue, feelings of insecurity about your new shape, and concerns about the safety of sex can all take their toll on your relationship. Allowing yourself time to adjust and keeping the channels of communication open will help you and your partner enjoy this new stage in your relationship.

Talk to each other about your feelings and be aware that, for both of you, levels of interest may fluctuate.

If your belly makes some positions uncomfortable, experiment with alternative ones that accommodate your size, such as side-by-side, rear entry, or woman-on-top positions.

Enjoy other ways to maintain intimacy besides intercourse, such as touching and massage.

Intercourse in late pregnancy may not be safe if you've had a previous premature labor or risk factors for premature labor, such as a weak cervix, or if you have placenta previa (see p.473), or leakage of amniotic fluid. If you have any concerns, don't be afraid to ask your doctor for advice.

Being able to enjoy sex in pregnancy will help you and your partner feel close. Psychologists have found that couples who enjoy sex in pregnancy are more tender toward each other and communicate better after the birth.

Illnesses and medication

Knowing how to manage illness and what medications are safe to take is important to protect your own and your baby's health.

If you have an existing medical condition, seek advice from your doctor before you conceive as some medications may need to be changed before becoming pregnant.

Preexisting conditions

If you have a condition such as high blood pressure, asthma, epilepsy, or diabetes, your pregnancy will be classified as high risk and you'll need to be monitored carefully. Women with high blood pressure, kidney disease, diabetes, systemic lupus erythematosus, previous preeclampsia, a BMI greater than 35, or a maternal age over 40 may be advised to start taking low-dose aspirin between 12 and 16 weeks of pregnancy. If you become pregnant while taking medication for a condition, don't stop taking the medication; consult your doctor as soon as possible. Your medication may be safe, or you may need to change to another type of medication. The most important thing is to control your condition during pregnancy to minimize the risks to you and your baby, which will usually mean continuing with medication.

Diabetes If you have diabetes and are planning to conceive, discuss with doctor the best way to control your blood sugar levels and how you will manage diabetes in pregnancy. Women with diabetes are advised to take a prenatal vitamin with folic acid before trying to conceive and for the first three months of pregnancy. Diabetic women who are overweight may be advised to lose weight before getting pregnant, and they'll likely be told to monitor their blood sugar more frequently and take their medications on time during their pregnancy. Babies born to diabetic women also have a greater risk of higher birth weight, respiratory problems at birth, jaundice, and low blood sugar at birth.

As soon as you're pregnant, you should be referred to an obstetrician who specializes in pregnancy and diabetes, where you'll receive extra care. You will have more frequent prenatal visits, additional scans, and extra blood tests to monitor your blood sugars. You may need diabetes medication and/or insulin injections each day; the dose usually changes throughout pregnancy and needs to be monitored. The better your blood sugar control, the less likely you or your baby is to experience problems during pregnancy.

Since diabetic women have an increased risk of late pregnancy problems such as preeclampsia (see p.476) and premature labor (see p.431), you may be advised to have an induction of labor before your due date (see p.432). The exact timing will depend on factors such as your blood-sugar control during pregnancy and the size of the baby. Once in labor, your blood sugar levels will be closely monitored, and you will probably be given an insulin and glucose IV. After the birth, your baby's blood sugar levels will be closely monitored, too, for 24 hours. If you're planning to breastfeed, your insulin dose may need to be changed after the birth.

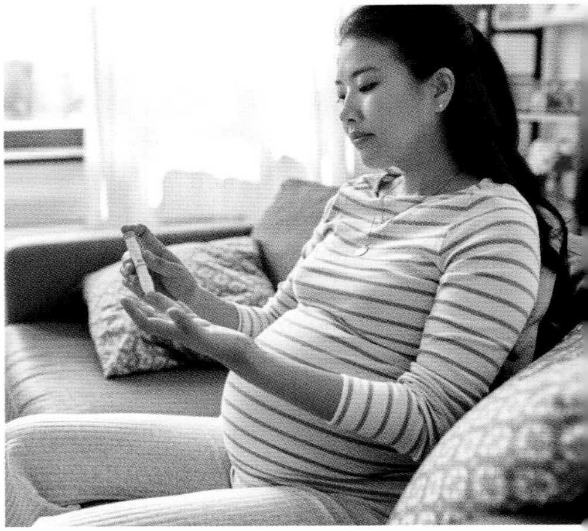

If you have diabetes and become pregnant, talk to your doctor about how to best monitor your blood sugar levels and manage medications.

Epilepsy If you have epilepsy, it's very important to discuss pregnancy with your doctor before you conceive, as certain drugs carry a small risk of causing harm to the developing baby. Nonetheless, it's also important that your epilepsy be controlled. Your doctor will ensure that you are on the lowest possible effective dose of medication before you get pregnant. Women with epilepsy are advised to take 5mg of folic acid for three months prior to conception and for the first 12 weeks of pregnancy. Most maternity units will assign a specialist team to look after women with epilepsy in pregnancy and you will have regular scans to confirm the baby is growing normally. The anomaly scan (see p.214) will check for problems such as cleft palate, which are slightly more common with certain medications. Most women with epilepsy have an uncomplicated pregnancy. If you have concerns, contact your maternity unit.

Systemic lupus erythematosus This is an autoimmune disorder that can affect many parts of the body, including the kidneys, joints, skin, nervous system, heart, and lungs. The condition is more common in women, and particularly in those of childbearing age. Some women find that the symptoms for this condition ease during pregnancy; however, for some, they can worsen. It's important to control the condition during pregnancy since it can affect the developing baby, with an increased risk of miscarriage, poor growth, premature labor, and stillbirth. Most medications for lupus are safe to use during pregnancy, but some aren't, so you need to check with your doctor about whether you need to change your current medication. From around 32 weeks, your baby will be closely monitored and their growth and well-being will be checked. If there are concerns about you or your baby, labor may be induced early, or you may have a planned Cesarean.

ASK A DOCTOR

I'm asthmatic. Can I use my inhalers during pregnancy?
It's essential that you keep asthma under control in pregnancy, which means continuing to use your inhalers, since the risks from uncontrolled asthma are greater than any risk from taking asthma medication. If asthma is uncontrolled, it can mean that not enough oxygen gets to the baby, leading to a low birth weight or other problems. One of the best ways to control asthma, in addition to taking medication, is to avoid asthma triggers such as pet fur and dust mites. Use air filters, vacuum often, and damp dust; and use duvet, mattress, and pillow protectors. Sometimes, pregnancy reduces the severity of asthma, but if you feel wheezier than usual, talk to your doctor about reviewing your medication.

Homeopathy seems to be a popular form of therapy. How effective is it and is it safe?
Homeopathy works on the principle of treating like with like to stimulate the body's natural healing mechanisms. There has been debate about the efficacy of homeopathy, and the scientific opinion is that there is insufficient evidence to show that it has any effect beyond that of a placebo. But talk to your doctor before using any homeopathic products or remedies during pregnancy, since homeopathy is an area of complementary and alternative medicine that's associated with much debate and scientific controversy. If your doctor gives you the okay, a certified homeopath may be able to provide treatment.

What's the verdict on taking herbal remedies and teas during pregnancy?
The US Food and Drug Administration does not regulate herbs and other dietary supplements, and there's not much research about the health effects of many herbs on pregnant women, so it's best to avoid them while you're pregnant, including herbal teas. Decaffeinated black teas are your best bet, but if you want a fruit or ginger tea, read the ingredient label on the package carefully to be sure that no herbs are present. If you want to use an herbal remedy, talk to your doctor first.

High blood pressure Check with your doctor that the medication you are on is safe to use during pregnancy. It's important to continue your medication so that your blood pressure is controlled, because high blood pressure can be dangerous for both you and your baby. Your doctor will frequently check your blood pressure, and will test your urine for protein, because high blood pressure and protein in the urine are symptoms of preeclampsia. Your doctor may also recommend additional scans to check that your baby is growing well.

Thyroid problems If you have an underactive thyroid gland for which you are taking thyroxine, you'll need to have a blood test to ensure that your thyroid is functioning well and that the dose is correct, as thyroxine requirement can increase in pregnancy. It's important that you are not lacking in thyroxine, because this may affect the baby. If you are being treated for an overactive thyroid gland, check with your doctor that you're taking a thyroid medication that is safe in pregnancy. Your thyroid function will be monitored to check that your medication doesn't need to change.

Bowel disease Women with inflammatory bowel conditions, such as ulcerative colitis or Crohn's disease, usually find that their condition improves during pregnancy, although you may relapse after the baby is born. Although it's unusual for bowel conditions to cause major problems during pregnancy, it is important to check that you are not anemic, which can be a side effect of some bowel conditions, and your doctor may recommend extra scans to check that the baby is growing well.

Infections during pregnancy

When you're pregnant, your immune system is slightly suppressed. This is necessary to stop you from rejecting the baby. This means that you may be slightly more susceptible to colds, coughs, sore throat, or food poisoning, and the illness may last longer.

Colds and coughs Most pregnant women get a cold at some stage. However, cold medications can contain ingredients not safe in pregnancy, so avoid taking them, especially in the first trimester (see opposite). Steam inhalations and saline nasal sprays can ease congestion, and hot honey drinks help soothe a sore throat.

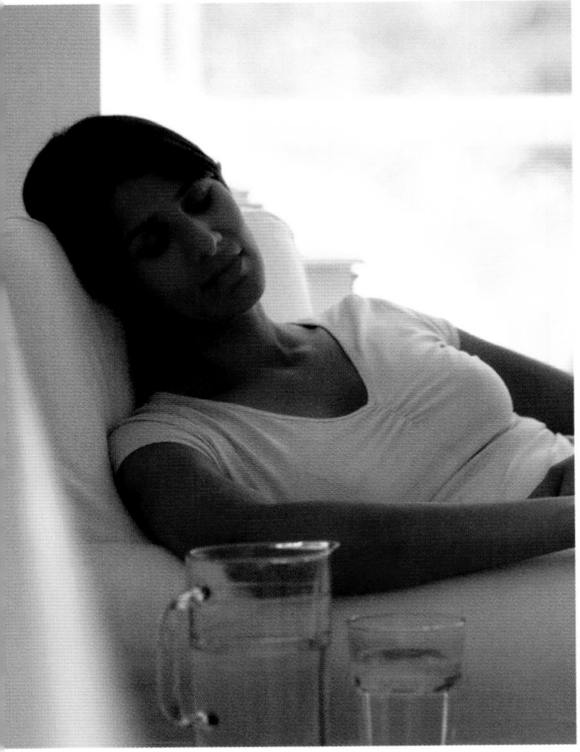

If you're laid low with an illness during pregnancy, take time to rest and recuperate since pregnancy can exacerbate everyday symptoms.

Flu If you get the flu during pregnancy, call your doctor. Drink lots of liquids and get plenty of rest. Don't take any flu or medications without talking to your doctor first. Flu complications can include dehydration and pneumonia and are more common in pregnant women. The US Centers for Disease Control and Prevention (CDC) recommends that all pregnant women get flu vaccinations. However, the nasal-spray flu vaccine is not approved for pregnant women.

Food poisoning and stomach upsets It's vital to practice good kitchen hygiene (see p.104) to avoid getting food poisoning. If you do develop food poisoning or a stomach upset during pregnancy, try to drink plenty of fluids, and if it continues for more than 24 hours, see your doctor (see also Gastroenteritis, p.470).

Yeast If you have a thick, white discharge and itching inside or outside the vagina, it is likely that you have yeast (candidiasis). This is common in pregnancy and nothing to be concerned about, but since the itching can be intense, it is worth a trip to your doctor. A swab may be taken to confirm the diagnosis, and an appropriate local antifungal treatment prescribed (see opposite). Eating plain yogurt may help restore the bacterial balance in your vagina. Wearing cotton underwear and avoiding tight clothing is also recommended.

Urinary-tract infections (UTIs) Many pregnant women get UTIs because the hormone progesterone relaxes all the smooth muscle, allowing the bacteria that normally live in your vagina to travel up the urethra (the tube that leads to the bladder) where they may cause an infection. The symptoms may be slightly different in pregnancy. Classic symptoms include burning when urinating and frequent urination; back pain, lower abdominal pain, nausea, or vomiting. These are usually easily treated with antibiotics, most of which are safe in pregnancy.

COVID-19 While there is still a lot of research to be done regarding the effects of COVID-19 in pregnancy and the virus is rapidly evolving, pregnant women are at increased risk of complications from infection. The best way to protect yourself, and your baby, from COVID-19 infection is to get vaccinated. If you test positive for COVID-19 during pregnancy, discuss your symptoms with your doctor. Current treatments including monoclonal antibodies and antiviral medications can be used in pregnancy and may be offered to you.

EXPOSURE TO CHICKENPOX OR RUBELLA

Chickenpox in pregnancy can be severe, possibly leading to pneumonia, and can cause problems both for you and for your baby. If you contract rubella for the first time in early pregnancy, it can cause miscarriage or severe problems in the fetus.

If you encounter chickenpox, contact your doctor who can check your immunity. If you aren't immune, your doctor may advise an injection to protect you from severe chickenpox.

Your rubella status is checked at the start of pregnancy. If you aren't immune, you can be vaccinated after the birth. Meanwhile you need to be extra careful.

If you develop chickenpox or suspect rubella because of a rash, contact your doctor immediately, but don't go to the doctor's office, where you may spread the infection to other pregnant women.

TAKING MEDICATIONS DURING PREGNANCY

During the first three months of pregnancy, it's best to avoid all over-the-counter medications. Take the lowest possible dose. After the first trimester, some other medications are considered safe, but consult your doctor if in doubt. The following provides guidance on medications used for treating common pregnancy complaints and minor illnesses.

Antacids Heartburn and indigestion are common, particularly during the third trimester when the increased size of the baby puts pressure on your stomach. Some antacids are safe to use during pregnancy, although you should avoid sodium bicarbonate because it may increase fluid retention. Consult your doctor or pharmacist about which ones are recommended.

Antibiotics Many antibiotics used to treat infection are safe for use during pregnancy. These include antibiotics containing penicillin, although there are safe alternatives if you're allergic to penicillin. The following antibiotics should be avoided during pregnancy:
- Streptomycin. This can damage the ears of the fetus as it develops and may result in hearing loss in the baby.
- Sulfonamides. These can cause jaundice in the newborn baby.
- Tetracyclines. These drugs shouldn't be taken because they can affect the development of the baby's bone and teeth and can cause discoloration in the teeth.

Antiemetics If you have severe nausea and vomiting and natural remedies such as gingersnaps or ginger tea don't relieve the problem, your doctor may recommend an antiemetic medication that is safe to use during pregnancy.

Antifungal remedies You should avoid over-the-counter antifungal remedies, including oral and local remedies, for treating yeast. Consult your doctor, who can recommend an antifungal medication that is appropriate for use in pregnancy.

Cold remedies Remedies for coughs and colds often contain a range of ingredients, such as caffeine, antihistamines, and other decongestants, many of which aren't safe in pregnancy. Ideally, avoid all cold remedies and instead have steam inhalations and hot caffeine-free drinks. If you need relief, talk to your doctor before using any over-the-counter treatments.

Diuretics It's normal to experience some swelling in the hands and feet during pregnancy, and you shouldn't attempt to deal with this by taking diuretics, including herbal diuretics. If you have sudden swelling in the face, hands, or feet, you should consult your doctor immediately because this can be a sign of preeclampsia (see p.476).

Laxatives The first step in dealing with constipation is to take dietary measures by increasing your intake of fiber and drinking plenty of fluids. If this isn't enough to ease constipation, then some over-the-counter laxatives may be safe to take during pregnancy, including laxatives that contain bulking agents. Those containing castor oil may cause uterine contractions. Check with your doctor before taking any laxatives.

Analgesics The general advice is to avoid all analgesics during pregnancy, especially during the first trimester. Before using pain medication for a common problem, such as a headache or backache, first try natural remedies; massage or a warm bath are often effective in relieving aches and pains. If these aren't sufficient, call your doctor for advice. High-dose aspirin and anti-inflammatories such as ibuprofen should be avoided throughout pregnancy.

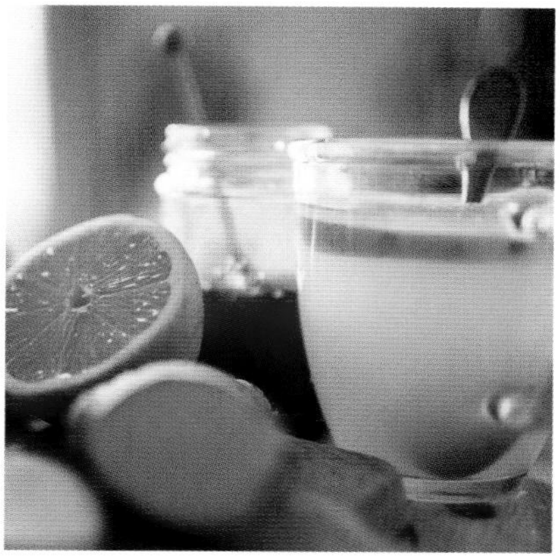

Making your own natural cold remedies from honey and lemon is preferable to taking over-the-counter remedies.

The pain medicine codeine can sometimes be used for a short period to treat specific pain, but should only be taken on the advice of a doctor.

Rehydration solutions If you have a stomach upset resulting in a severe bout of diarrhea that lasts for an extended period, your doctor may recommend a rehydration solution that is safe to use in pregnancy.

Steroids If you have eczema, or find that this condition develops or worsens during pregnancy, your doctor may prescribe a steroid cream such as hydrocortisone. Corticosteroids, which are used to treat eczema, aren't associated with birth defects, but they are known to cross the placenta, so both topical and oral corticosteroids aren't recommended during pregnancy. Your doctor will provide advice and guidance on safe usage.

Steroid inhalers used to treat asthma are safe in pregnancy, and it's important to control your asthma while you're pregnant.

Oral steroids may also be prescribed for certain other conditions, and these may be safe to continue with under the guidance of your doctor. Anabolic steroids should not be taken during pregnancy.

Lifestyle hazards

Pregnancy can be beset with anxiety about potential hazards. Being aware of exactly what to avoid will help to allay fears.

Whether you're pregnant or are planning to conceive, now is the time to do a safety check on your social habits and home and work environment. Anything that could affect your well-being could affect your baby too, especially in the first trimester. Don't become overanxious, but arm yourself with the facts so that you can avoid hazards and enjoy your pregnancy.

Your social habits

The decision to have a baby may inspire you to review your social habits and, if necessary, make changes.

Alcohol consumption You should stop drinking alcohol while trying to get pregnant and once you're pregnant according to the US Surgeon General. There is no known safe consumption level for pregnant women, so abstaining from drinking is the safest option. What isn't in doubt is the damage caused to the fetus by excessive alcohol intake and could lead to fetal alcohol syndrome (see p.216). The effects include retarded growth, facial and joint abnormalities, and heart problems.

If you drank in the weeks before you knew you were pregnant, try not to worry, but stop now. Many women also decide to give up alcohol while they're trying to conceive to optimize fertility.

Smoking Ideally, stop smoking before you get pregnant. If you're still smoking once you conceive, stop right away. If your partner or friends smoke, ask them not to smoke in your home or near you. Inhaled cigarette smoke interferes with the supply of oxygen to the baby, which can lead to a low birthweight and increases the risk of stillbirth or the death of a baby in the first month of life. If you smoke in pregnancy, you will be advised to take low-dose aspirin and offered smoking cessation classes. The doctor will also monitor your carbon monoxide levels, which is especially dangerous as it reduces the amount of oxygen available to the baby and may affect the baby's growth.

Recreational drug use In addition to damaging your own health, recreational drugs are not advised in pregnancy since some pose dangers for the fetus and other hazards.

Heroin and cocaine are damaging to both a pregnant woman and her unborn baby. These drugs stunt fetal growth, affect the placenta, and can cause miscarriage or premature birth, as well as health problems in the newborn. Babies born to women who use heroin often show drug withdrawal symptoms. A report on ecstasy linked the use of this in pregnancy to a rise in birth defects. The specific effects of amphetamines and LSD are unclear, but it's safest to avoid them.

Although marijuana may be legal in some states, use of marijauna in pregnancy and breastfeeding is not safe for your baby. Using marijuana, in any of its forms, can cause problems with your baby's developing brain as well as low birthweight.

Hazards at home

Many people use chemicals daily in and around the home, contained in toiletries and cleaning products. When products are used in accordance with the manufacturers' instructions, there is little chance of them causing harm in pregnancy. However, minute traces of chemicals can enter the bloodstream, either through the skin or by inhalation, and cross the placenta. No hard evidence shows that this has an ill effect, but it makes sense to minimize the chances of chemicals reaching the baby.

When using products, wear rubber gloves to prevent skin contact and ventilate rooms. To avoid inhaling

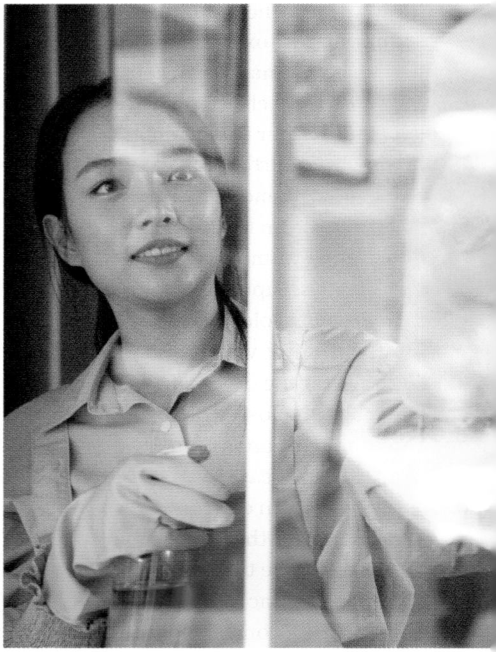

Wearing rubber gloves when using household cleaning products will reduce your exposure to chemicals.

mists or vapors, choose nonaerosol products. Also, choose products recommended for their low environmental impact, which contain fewer chemicals. Where possible, use natural alternatives to chemicals.

Painting and decorating Don't climb up ladders or stand on tables to reach high places since your belly alters your center of gravity. Also avoid skin contact or inhalation if you use oil-based paints, spray paints, paint strippers, floor varnishes, and sealant adhesives. Make sure rooms are well ventilated while decorating. Ideally, get someone else to do the decorating.

Pets and infections Certain infections that could harm the fetus can be picked up from pets. The parasitic infection toxoplasmosis is spread through contact with cat feces. It may produce flulike symptoms, or no symptoms at all, and many unknowingly acquire immunity through previous exposure. However, although it rarely happens, contracting toxoplasmosis for the first time in pregnancy can cause serious problems, such as miscarriage or birth defects. Other pets, such as dogs, caged birds, and turtles, can carry salmonella bacteria. Salmonella infection doesn't directly harm the baby, but can make a pregnant woman ill.

Being scrupulous about hygiene helps you avoid such infections. Wear rubber gloves when handling a cat litter box, cleaning cages where animals are kept, or disposing of dog feces, then wash your hands (and the gloves) afterward. Wear gloves also for digging or weeding in case animals have defecated in the garden. Or get someone else to do these tasks.

Toxoplasmosis and salmonella can also be contracted from eating undercooked or raw meat or eggs, so be careful with kitchen hygiene and cooking (see p.17).

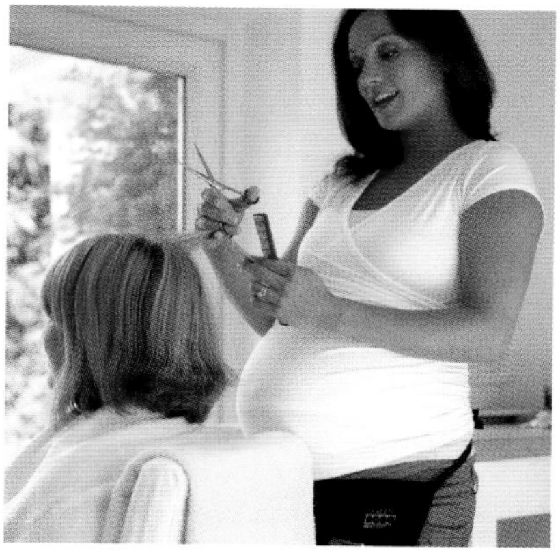

If your job involves handling chemicals, ensure that a risk assessment is done and that you are able to avoid harmful substances.

Workplace hazards

It's the legal responsibility of your employer to provide a safe environment. Being aware of your rights can help protect you and your baby.

In recent decades, women worried about whether working at a computer screen put their babies at risk. It's now clear that using a VDT (as well as photocopiers and printers) is safe. Some environments do pose possible dangers. If you work in a health-care setting with ionizing radiation or cancer-treatment drugs, inform your department that you're pregnant. Hospital regulations will ensure that you are given alternative duties.

Women employed in places such as hairdressers, manicure salons, labs, and craft workshops may be exposed to toxic chemicals. Working around some dry cleaning solvents has been linked to miscarriage. It's up to employers to ensure protection from hazards. Talk to your boss or HR manager.

Standing on your feet all day and physical work that involves heavy lifting can be exhausting in pregnancy. Ask if it's possible to switch to less tiring tasks.

ASK AN EXPERT

Is it safe to use a cell phone during pregnancy? I've read that phones emit radiation.

The radiation emitted by cell phones is "non-ionizing." This is not the same as the radiation received from X-rays, which can be harmful in large doses. There is no evidence to show that using a cell phone is a health risk to either you or your baby.

I go swimming twice a week and love it, but is the chlorine in the pool bad for my baby?

In the past there has been some debate about whether it's safe to swim in chlorinated pools during pregnancy. However, now most experts believe that swimming in chlorinated water does not pose any health risks for pregnant women and their developing babies. You may find that the smell of chlorine might add to your nausea if you are suffering from morning sickness, although this is less of a problem in an outdoor pool. Try not to swallow the water. If you do, drink fresh water after your swim. Shower thoroughly afterward. Swimming has great benefits during pregnancy. It has a low risk of injury while providing a good cardiovascular workout and improving muscle tone, so don't be put off by unnecessary worries.

Is it OK to use nicotine patches or gum while I'm pregnant?

Nicotine is known to decrease the blood supply to the fetus. This could affect the baby's growth, especially in early pregnancy. Although tobacco substitutes such as patches, gum, and lozenges deliver less nicotine to your body than smoking, you should never use them without a doctor's advice. Ask your doctor for information on safer ways to beat cigarette and nicotine cravings.

Skin, hair, and teeth

In addition to affecting what happens to you internally, hormonal changes in pregnancy can also affect your external appearance.

Many women look and feel better than ever during pregnancy, while those less fortunate report that there is a downturn in their appearance. However pregnancy affects you, the changes will be temporary and you'll be back to your normal self soon after the birth.

Skin

You may find that your skin looks better in pregnancy due to hormonal changes, mild fluid retention, and increased blood flow. These can all result in smoother skin and are responsible for the famous "pregnancy glow." On the other hand, you may find that your skin gets drier and more pimply and you may need to take extra care of it during pregnancy.

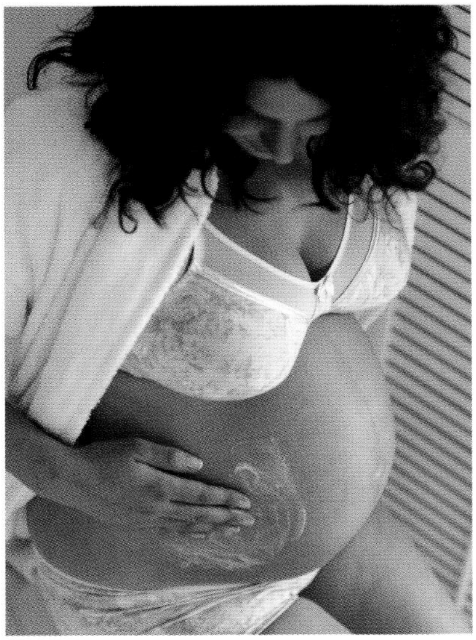

Applying moisturizing creams to relieve dry, itchy skin, or ones recommended to reduce stretch marks, is safe during pregnancy.

Skin also tends to darken during pregnancy. The reason for this is unknown, but may be explained by the increased levels estrogen and melanocyte-stimulating hormone, which stimulate skin pigmentation.

Stretch marks (striae gravidarum) Many women develop stretch marks during pregnancy, which can occur on bellies, breasts, hips, or legs. These initially appear as pink or purple lines and may be quite itchy. After pregnancy they fade into pale wrinkles. Nobody knows for sure why these occur, but they probably result from a combination of pregnancy hormones and your skin stretching. You're more likely to get stretch marks if you're very young, if you gain a lot of weight in pregnancy, or if you have a very big baby. There is less agreement about the role of other factors such as a family history, being very overweight before pregnancy or belonging to a particular ethnic group.

Many creams, lotions, and oils have been marketed for the prevention or treatment of stretch marks but none has been proven to work. Studies performed on such products are inconclusive. Commercially produced creams, lotions, and oils are safe to use and may help to minimize stretch marks by maintaining the elasticity of the skin; unfortunately, however, there is no guarantee that they will prevent them.

Chloasma This describes the increased pigmentation of the cheeks, nose, and chin that affects around 50–70 percent of pregnant women. Using a protective sunscreen and avoiding the use of any photosensitizing skin-care products may reduce chloasma. A recent study found that using a highly protective sunscreen (SPF 50 and UVA-PF 28) prevented most pregnant women from developing chloasma.

Hair and nails

Hair stays longer in the growth phase during pregnancy, meaning that your scalp hair is likely to grow and thicken. Not so welcome is the fact that facial and body hair may also increase. After the birth, many women find that they suddenly lose a lot of hair as the growth phase stops. You should find that your hair is back to normal within six months.

Fingernails may also change, often becoming stronger, although some find that they become softer and brittle. Nails may develop white spots or transverse grooves, but these are rarely anything to worry about and don't mean that you're lacking in vitamins.

Teeth

Pregnant women are more prone to tooth decay (dental caries), bleeding gums, and chronic gum infection (periodontal disease). Poor dental health not only affects you but can also have an impact on your baby. Studies have linked infection of the gums in pregnant women to premature birth, and if a woman has ongoing tooth decay after the birth, her baby may acquire bacteria directly from her saliva, leading to tooth decay in the child later on. It's therefore important that you take care of your teeth during pregnancy and visit your dentist and dental hygienist regularly.

To keep your mouth healthy during pregnancy, brush twice a day with fluoride toothpaste and floss every day. Routine dental treatment and some local anesthetics are safe in pregnancy, although it's better to postpone elective dental treatments until after pregnancy or take care of them before pregnancy. Many women worry about having their teeth X-rayed in pregnancy. The radiation exposure from dental X-rays is minimal and the risk to your baby probably negligible. However, dentists will take every precaution to minimize your radiation exposure, covering you with a leaded apron before the X-rays.

ASK AN EXPERT

I am 18 weeks' pregnant and due to go on a beach vacation. I have become uncomfortable with my facial and body hair. How can I safely remove it?
You can safely tweeze, wax, and shave new stray hair. Skin bleaching and hair removal creams are probably safe during pregnancy, but there has been insufficient research to clear them since they can be absorbed through the skin and their effects on the baby are unknown. Permanent hair-removal techniques, such as laser and electrolysis, are thought to be safe in pregnancy. Both techniques penetrate the skin no deeper than a few millimeters. Consult your doctor to see if this is okay.

I've been using topical cream to treat acne and I've just found out that I'm pregnant. Will it harm my baby?
Tretinoin belongs to a group of medications called retinoids that contain vitamin A and may be associated with birth defects. Studies have looked at the effects of this cream in pregnancy and have found that babies whose mothers used it, even in the first trimester, had no increase in birth defects. However doctors recommend avoiding tretinoin cream in pregnancy. Another similar medication, isotretinoin, which is taken orally, may increase the risk of birth defects and is therefore contraindicated in pregnancy.

I'm in the first trimester and will be going to my sister's wedding. Can I have highlights put in my hair?
Although the research into the safety of hair dyes if used in the first trimester may seem conflicting, the amount of chemicals used is small and it's unlikely that hair dyes cause harm. Also, if your hairdresser uses foil, the dye is kept off your skin.

I've heard that nail polish needs to be removed if you have a cesarean. Why is this?
Previously, women were encouraged to remove nail polish before surgery. One of the reasons was that the "pulse oximeter," a device attached to your finger to measure the oxygen in your blood during surgery, may give lower readings if placed over nail polish. However the device works as intended with nail polish or long nails if it's mounted sideways on a finger. Therefore there's no need to remove your polish.

BEAUTY TREATMENTS AND COSMETICS

Hair and nail products Shampoos, conditioners, manicures, and pedicures are safe. Minute amounts of hair dye may be absorbed through the skin, but there's no evidence that this affects the baby. Chemical hair straighteners and curlers are also thought to be safe.

Piercing Facial piercing or piercing the belly button, nipples, or genitalia isn't advised since you're at a higher risk of infection. If you have a navel piercing already, you can change a metallic ring for a flexible plastic retainer made from PTFE (polytetrafluoroethylene). Nipple rings can affect breast-feeding, so remove a ring before birth so the skin can heal. Vaginal or vulval piercings are best removed to avoid damage at birth.

Tanning Tanning beds aren't advised because of harmful UV rays. Tanning beds can cause your body to overheat, which can harm your baby, and UV rays may break down folic acid. Tanning lotions are safe.

Body wraps/ Hot tubs These raise body temperature, which is unsafe for you and your baby. Heat exposure from a hot tub in the first three months can increase the risk of a baby developing spina bifida.

Facials The cosmetics used for facials are thought to be safe.

Botox The Food and Drug Administration recommends that women who are pregnant or breastfeeding should not use Botox. Although it's used for cosmetic reasons, it is a drug and should be considered as such. Doctors also advise against having Botox during pregnancy.

Traveling in pregnancy

Your growing belly shouldn't put a stop to travel plans. Just a bit of extra planning is required to help your vacation run smoothly.

Provided your pregnancy is normal, going to faraway places is perfectly possible. However, discomforts such as extreme heat, high altitude, and makeshift accommodations may be less tolerable and, in some cases, may compromise the safety of your baby.

The best time to travel

In the first trimester, you may find that morning sickness and fatigue lessen your enthusiasm for travel. Most women feel at their best in the second trimester, and this is also seen as the safest time to travel since your risk of miscarriage is low, energy levels are increased, and your due date is still some way off. After 28 weeks, the size of your belly, fatigue, and the looming birth date are likely to make home seem the best place to be.

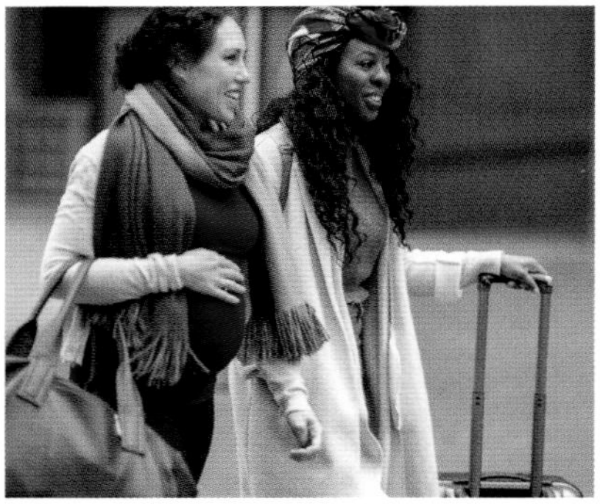

The best time to travel is often during the second trimester when nausea has abated and your belly size is not yet uncomfortable.

Making plans

A little extra planning is the key to successful travel in pregnancy. Think carefully before you book. How will you get there and how long will it take? Pregnancy adds to the stress of a long-haul trip. If you want to fly, check with the airline about its policy. Some require a current letter from your doctor confirming your due date and your fitness to fly after 36 weeks, largely because of the possibility of going into labor.

Find out about the medical facilities in case you have any health problems while on vacation. Unless you have no choice, avoid visiting countries where disease is a high risk factor. Many doctors agree that protective drugs, such as certain vaccines and antimalarial pills, are not advisable in pregnancy or when trying to conceive. Check

ADVANCE PLANNING

You've found your passport and put the tickets in your bag. However, when you're pregnant, you may also need to take the following items:

• A note from your doctor stating your due date and giving you the all-clear to travel (helpful if you're over 28 weeks).

• Any special medical records regarding your pregnancy or general health.

• A list of numbers for health-care facilities at your destination.

• Remedies for heartburn or other minor pregnancy problems, such as hemorrhoids. You may not be able to buy your usual products abroad.

TRIMESTER-BY-TRIMESTER TRAVEL GUIDE

Think about the implications of traveling at different times in your pregnancy when planning a trip.

1st trimester (weeks 1–12)

• Period of highest risk for miscarriage and development problems in the baby. Be extra careful to avoid extremes of temperature and overly vigorous activities.

• Motion sickness could make morning sickness worse.

• Flying is allowed, provided you have no pregnancy complications.

• Insurance is unlikely to be a problem.

2nd trimester (weeks 13–25)

• You are likely to be feeling your best, and the chances of miscarriage or fetal development problems are greatly reduced.

• Flying is allowed, but check to see whether you need to carry a doctor's letter stating your due date.

• Check with individual travel insurance companies to see if you can get coverage—policies vary.

3rd trimester (weeks 26–40)

• Your belly is huge and travel may be very uncomfortable now.

• Some airlines may not allow you to fly after 36 weeks without a letter from your doctor written within 72 hours of your flight that includes your due date and confirms your fitness to fly.

the internet for information about an area's health hazards and local hospitals. If you have a condition such as diabetes that could cause complications, make sure you can get treatment while away.

Take out travel insurance. Some companies consider pregnancy a preexisting condition and won't provide coverage for your trip.

Avoiding bugs

Pregnancy reduces the efficiency of your immune system, increasing your risk of an infection. When you're traveling, "stomach bugs" caused by contaminated food and water are more likely to strike.

If you're unsure about local tap water, buy bottled water (make sure the seal is unbroken) and use it when brushing your teeth as well as for drinking. Avoid drinks with ice and don't eat salads or fruit you can't peel since they may have been washed in contaminated water. A less obvious danger is fruit such as melon, which may have been injected with water to increase its weight.

Avoid outdoor stalls or cafés where food might have been prepared hours in advance. Try to find restaurants where food is freshly cooked and standards seem high. Be scrupulous about hygiene, and carry moist wipes in case hand-washing facilities are inadequate.

On the trip

If you're traveling by car, stop regularly to stretch your legs, have a snack, or find a bathroom. On a train or plane, keep your circulation moving with foot and ankle exercises, and every so often walk down the aisle. Stay hydrated by drinking lots of water or juice. Carry a bag of dried fruit or nuts with you on trips. Comforts, such as a cushion and a cooling water spritzer, can make a trip more bearable.

Vacation activities

Forego water skiing and horseback riding, as a fall could harm your baby. Scuba diving is dangerous because of the risk of air bubbles forming in the bloodstream and the potential lack of oxygen. Avoid going on white-knuckle theme park rides.

If you're used to exercising, there is no reason not to go swimming or walking, just don't overdo it—hiking up hills under a blazing sun could send your temperature soaring, In the first trimester especially, extreme heat can affect fetal development. You might also become dehydrated, which, later on, can increase the risk of premature labor.

Hot tubs and saunas should be avoided since the heat could make you feel faint and may be harmful to your baby. Some aromatherapy oils may be toxic to the baby, especially in the early months. Look for spas with treatments for pregnant moms and always seek a qualified pre- and postpartum therapist, if possible.

In pregnancy, your skin becomes more sensitive to the sun so be careful to protect against overexposure.

ASK AN EXPERT

I am five months pregnant and about to go on a beach vacation. Is it safe for me to sunbathe while I'm pregnant?
It is safe to do a little sunbathing in pregnancy. However, it is important to avoid getting overheated since this will make you feel very unwell. It is generally best to sit in the shade and make sure you have plenty of cool drinks to avoid becoming dehydrated. Remember to use a strong sunscreen because your skin may be more sensitive than usual while you are pregnant.

I'm worried about flying to my vacation destination because someone told me there is a high risk of DVT in pregnancy. Is this true?
Deep vein thrombosis (DVT), the formation of a blood clot in a vein (often in a leg), is sometimes caused by long periods of immobility, such as sitting on a plane (see p.186). Although the risk factor may be slightly increased in pregnant women, because their blood tends to clot more easily, the chance of your developing DVT is still very low. To minimize the risk even more, you could wear some special support socks, which are designed to improve blood flow in the legs.

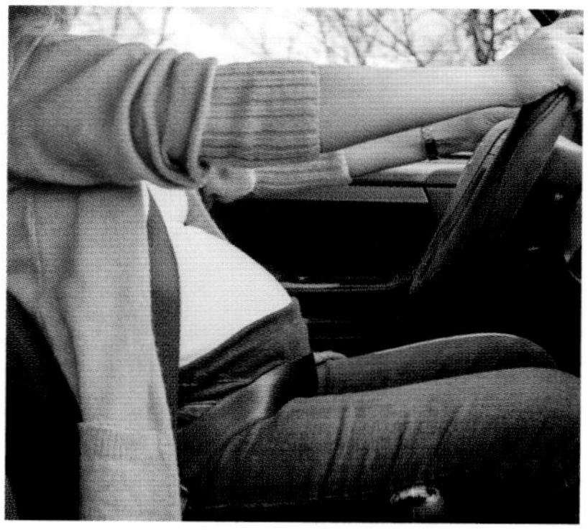

The position of your seat belt may need adjusting to accommodate your bump.

Are car seat belts and airbags safe to use in pregnancy?
In the event of an accident, these appliances are far more likely to prevent injury than cause it—never travel without fastening your seatbelt. For comfort, position the straps above and below your belly rather than across it. Being hit by an inflated airbag will not hurt you or the baby, but to lessen the impact, you should position your seat as far back as possible.

1ST TRIMESTER

2ND TRIMESTER

3RD TRIMESTER

PREGNANCY
DAY BY DAY

The 9 months of pregnancy are a time of constant change as your body continually adapts to accommodate the new life growing inside you. This extensive chapter guides you through the physical and emotional changes you'll experience and offers reassurance, advice, and practical tips. Your baby's progress is charted in fascinating detail with scans and day-by-day insights into how your baby grows and develops within your uterus.

Welcome to your first trimester

WEEK 1

WEEK 2

WEEK 3

WEEK 4

WEEK 5

WEEK 6

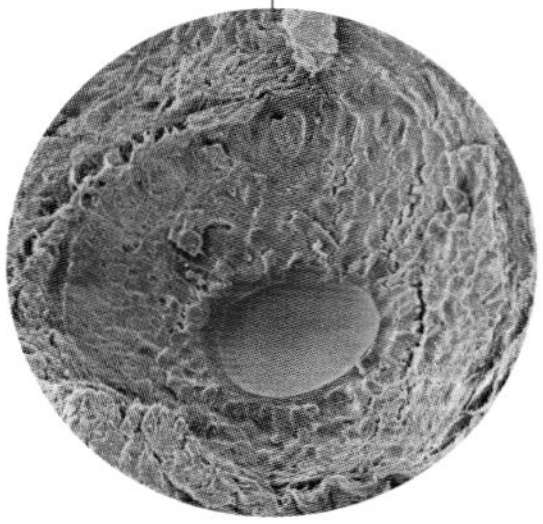

An egg has developed in the ovary. It will be **released** around day 14—ovulation.

WEEK 1: NOTE THE DAY YOUR PERIOD STARTS

This date becomes highly significant once you conceive because your pregnancy will be dated from the first day of your last menstrual period. Your estimated due date will be based on that date.

WEEK 4: DO A HOME PREGNANCY TEST

If by the end of week 4, the 28th day of your menstrual cycle, your period hasn't started, take a home pregnancy test. It will give you a highly accurate result within minutes. Hopefully congratulations are in order!

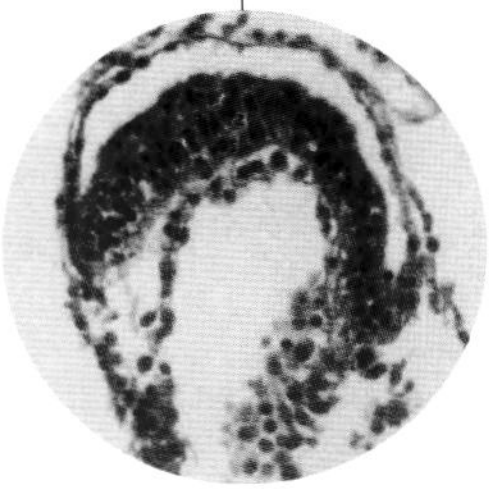

The cells that will become your baby will **divide** and **multiply**. Soon the **embryo** will transform from two layers of cells to three.

> "You may not look pregnant in the first 12 weeks, but your baby will grow at a faster rate than at any other stage."

WEEK 7

WEEK 8

WEEK 9

WEEK 10

WEEK 11

WEEK 12

WEEK 8: PREPARE FOR YOUR FIRST PRENATAL APPOINTMENT

At anytime from around week 8 to week 10, you will have an appointment to confirm your pregnancy and then start your prenatal care. Some basic health checks will be carried out and you will be asked about your medical history. There is always opportunity for you to ask questions, too, so prepare in advance if you can.

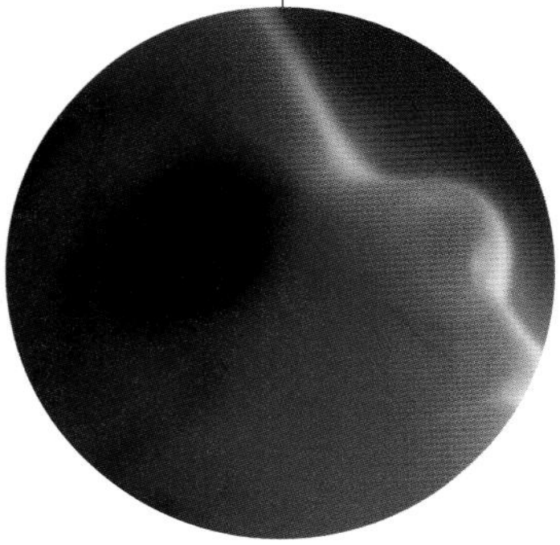

The **facial features** are growing distinctive around now. The **eyelids** have fused over the developing eye.

YOU AND YOUR BABY **AT 12 WEEKS**

Your baby has developed from a ball of cells to an active fetus that can already yawn and swallow. As your uterus rises out of the pelvis, your bump may begin to show. By the end of this first trimester, symptoms of early pregnancy, such as nausea and fatigue, begin to settle down for many women.

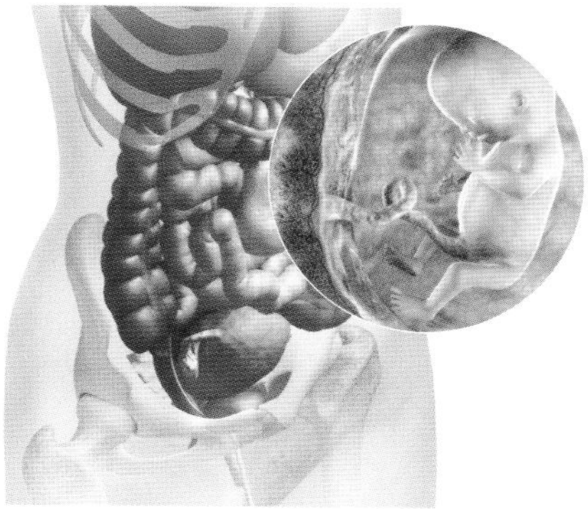

Your 1st week

THE 280-DAY COUNTDOWN BEGINS HERE—EVEN THOUGH YOU HAVEN'T YET CONCEIVED

It's business as usual for your body this week. You're having a period, so you know you're not pregnant. But if you conceive during this menstrual cycle, the first day of your period will count as the first day of pregnancy. It's a good idea to review your lifestyle and to make sure that you understand how everything works "inside." Knowing the facts may help increase your chances of conceiving.

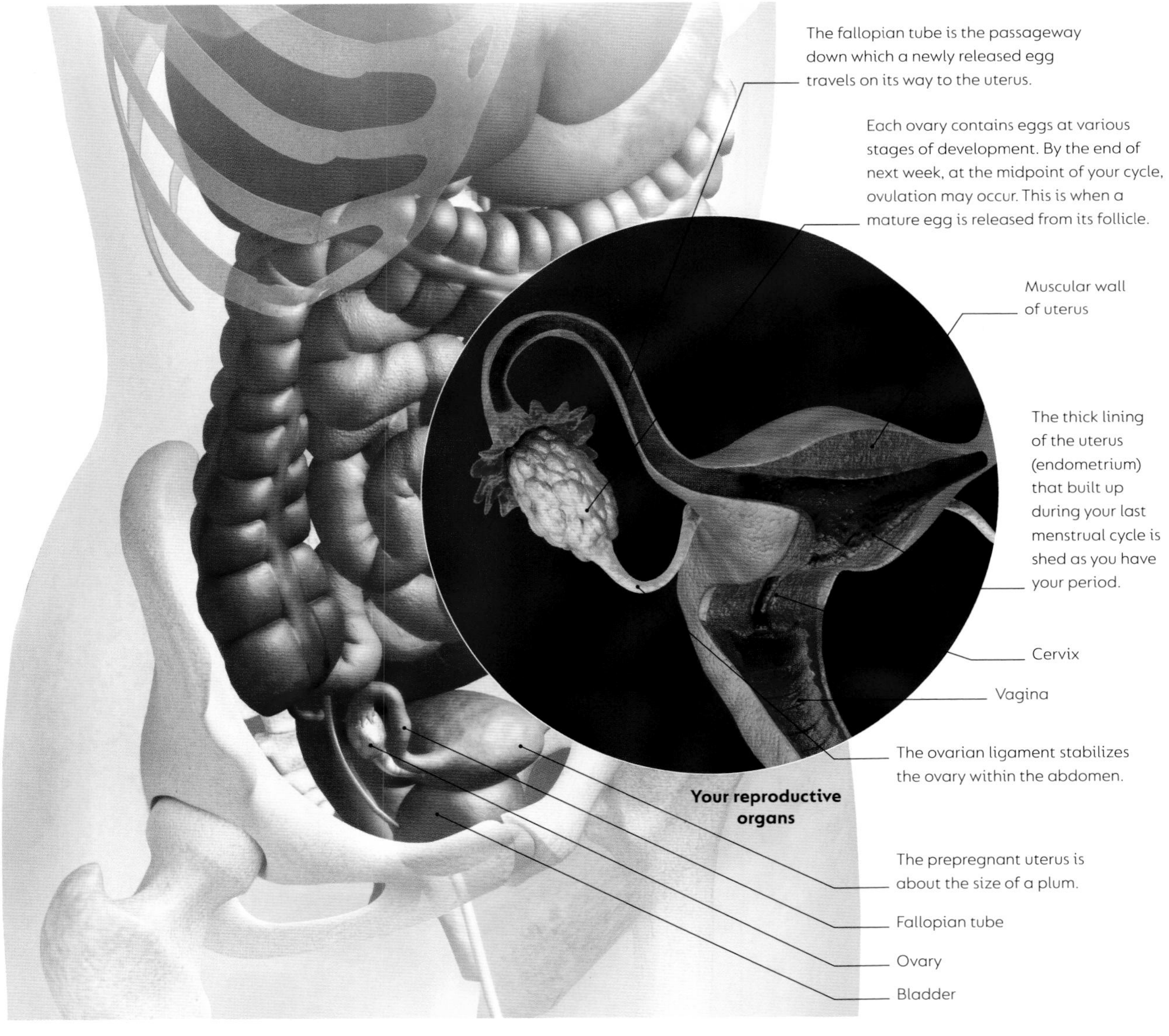
The fallopian tube is the passageway down which a newly released egg travels on its way to the uterus.
Each ovary contains eggs at various stages of development. By the end of next week, at the midpoint of your cycle, ovulation may occur. This is when a mature egg is released from its follicle.
Muscular wall of uterus
The thick lining of the uterus (endometrium) that built up during your last menstrual cycle is shed as you have your period.
Cervix
Vagina
The ovarian ligament stabilizes the ovary within the abdomen.
The prepregnant uterus is about the size of a plum.
Fallopian tube
Ovary
Bladder

Your reproductive organs

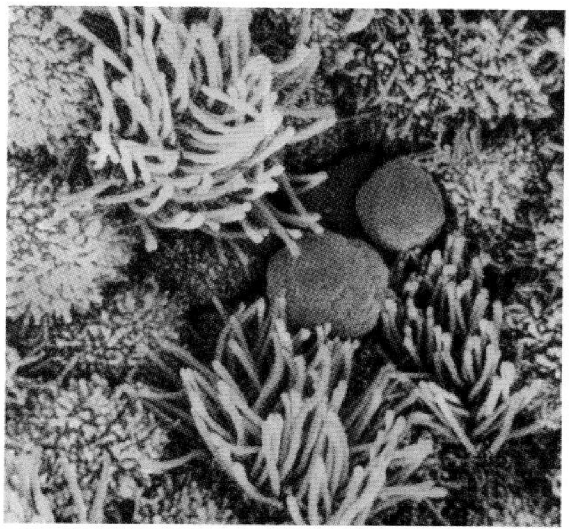

THIS IS **DAY 1 OF YOUR MENSTRUAL CYCLE**

279 days to go

WHAT'S HAPPENING INSIDE

The lining of the uterus builds up in the first two weeks of the menstrual cycle to prepare for pregnancy. The yellow and blue areas seen here are cells and the pink area, secretions. If no pregnancy occurs, the lining breaks down and menstruation occurs.

> "This is day one of your period. If you are trying to conceive during this menstrual cycle, keep a note of this highly significant date."

Although this is officially the first day of your pregnancy, you won't conceive until around two weeks from now. This is classified as "day one" because once you conceive your pregnancy will be dated from the first day of your menstrual period. It would be more logical to date a pregnancy from the day of ovulation or conception, but, like most women, you're unlikely to know the day on which you ovulate, let alone conceive. You are, however, far more likely to remember when your last period started, especially if you're hoping to get pregnant and are keeping a record of your menstrual cycle.

While dating a pregnancy in this way is a handy, if slightly baffling, convention, it does mean that your body is getting geared up for pregnancy from today. In around 280 days, or nine months' time, you could be holding your newborn baby in your arms. Good luck and enjoy the journey!

Be patient and try not to get too stressed if you don't conceive right away. Keep in mind that just 20 percent of couples actively trying to conceive become pregnant in any monthly cycle. For 80 percent of couples, it takes up to a year to conceive.

DECIDING TO HAVE A BABY

There's no perfect time to become parents, but you might want to bear in mind the following:

- **While practical matters** such as the state of your finances and the size of your house are considerations, remember that being parents is about more than what you are able to offer your baby materially.
- **This is a decision** only you and your partner can make. Don't act on the advice of family members and friends.
- **You might conceive** immediately or it could take several months, so relax and don't have a set date in mind.

FOLIC ACID

Take this vital vitamin now, from day one, if you haven't already because it will be essential to your baby's development in early pregnancy (see p.17). Taking 400 mcg folic acid a day is recommended, but women who have a BMI over 30, have diabetes, or have already had a baby with neural tube defects (see p.83) need to take 5 mg daily. You may need to take more for a twin pregnancy. Eat folate-rich foods such as oranges, broccoli, brussels sprouts, beets, and black-eyed peas as well as fortified foods such as breakfast cereals and spinach.

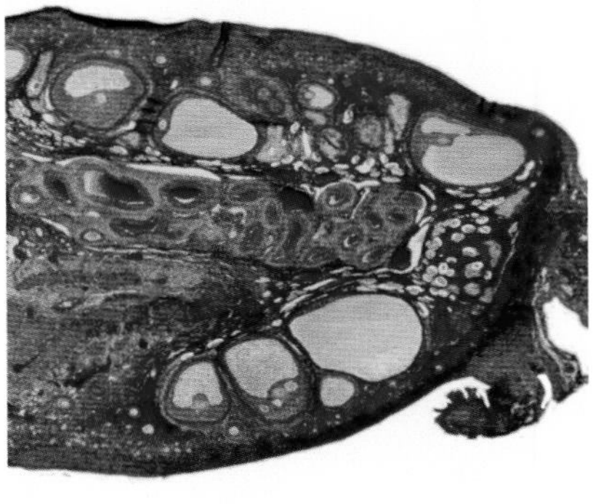

THIS IS **DAY 2 OF YOUR MENSTRUAL CYCLE**

278 days to go

WHAT'S HAPPENING INSIDE

Your eggs are already developing, as can be seen in this color-enhanced ovary. The small white structures are the immature follicles that contain the eggs at different stages of development. Once one of the follicles matures, the egg will burst out.

> "By tracking your menstrual cycle and understanding how it works, you may increase your chances of conceiving."

This is day two of your period and day two of your complete menstrual cycle, which starts on the first day of your period and ends on the first day of your next period. A full cycle is, on average, 28 days, but many women have a shorter or longer cycle.

This may be the time when your period is at its heaviest, since the tissue and blood that make up the lining of the uterus (the endometrium) is shed. The average blood loss during menstruation is around 2 tablespoons (30 ml). While the lining is being sloughed off, the blood vessels in the uterus constrict, which can cause cramplike period pains. As soon as your period has finished, an egg begins to mature within its follicle in one of your ovaries, ready to be released around midcycle. This is called ovulation (see p.49).

Meanwhile, the lining of the uterus starts to build up again under the influence of the hormones progesterone and estrogen, ready to receive a fertilized egg. If the egg is not fertilized, hormone levels fall, the lining sheds, and the cycle begins again.

CHANGES DURING THE MENSTRUAL CYCLE

The monthly cycle of an egg as it grows to maturity inside an ovary is shown at the top of the chart. It is released from its follicle around day 14. The bottom of the chart shows the corresponding development of the lining of the uterus—shedding at the start of a period, then rebuilding in preparation for the fertilized egg.

The empty egg follicle (called the corpus luteum) secretes progesterone, which is a hormone that helps the endometrium reach a thickness of about 0.2 in (6 mm) over the 28 days of the menstrual cycle, ready to receive a fertilized egg.

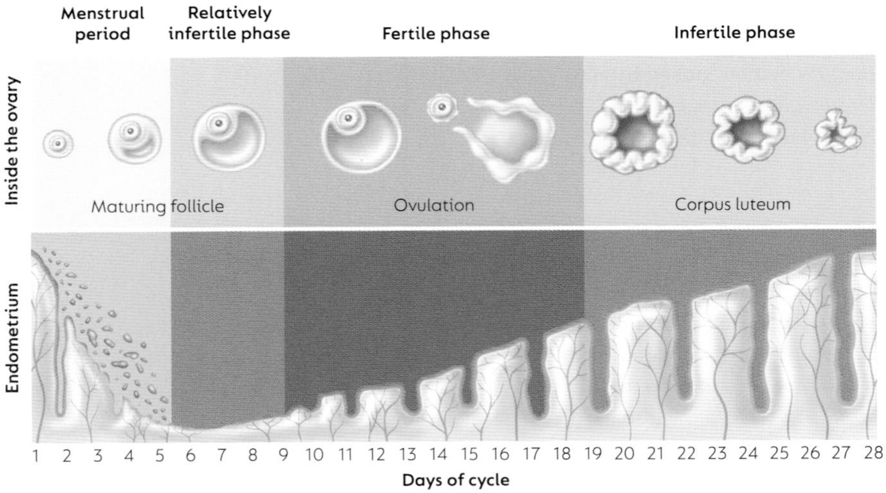

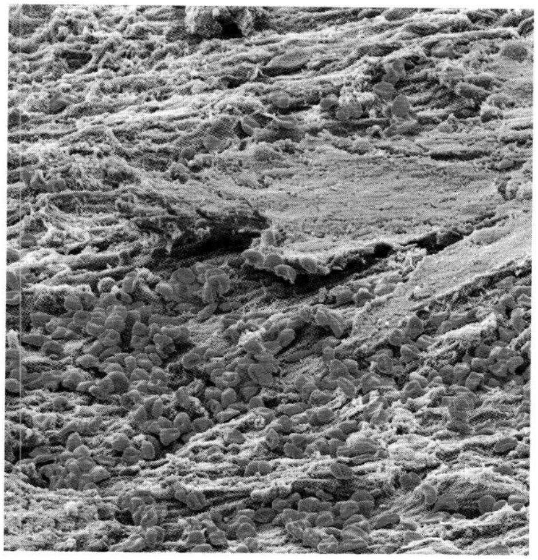

THIS IS **DAY 3 OF YOUR MENSTRUAL CYCLE**

277 days to go

WHAT'S HAPPENING INSIDE

The lining of the uterus, known as the endometrium, can be seen here (pink structure) shedding during menstruation. This happens if a fertilized egg does not implant. The red dots are red blood cells, released when the blood vessels break down.

You may notice the timing, frequency, and volume of your period differs. Your menstrual cycle can be affected by stress as well as by medical conditions, such as an overactive thyroid. In both these cases, periods can become lighter or less frequent. If your periods are erratic, it can be difficult to predict when you might ovulate. Irregular or missed periods may mean that ovulation isn't occurring at all, such as in polycystic ovary syndrome. If you know this is the case because you're monitoring your ovulation or using predictor tests (see p.43), seek medical advice.

You may be able to become pregnant naturally and easily despite problems related to your period, but some conditions that cause long, irregular, or heavy periods are linked to lower fertility. Heavy periods can be caused by conditions such as fibroids (see p.218), which can affect fertility. A higher than average level of blood loss can also make you anemic, which is not the best start for pregnancy for you or your baby, so you may want to look at boosting your iron intake (see p.154).

Painful periods can affect fertility. Endometriosis is a common disorder that can make periods painful and cause discomfort during sex. If you have these symptoms, you may be referred to a specialist. In endometriosis, cells resembling those that line the uterus come to lie outside the uterus on structures such as the ovaries, fallopian tubes, and walls of the pelvis. This condition can sometimes be treated by surgery, especially severe cases, which may boost a woman's chance of conceiving.

> " When you're trying to get pregnant, it helps to be aware of lifestyle and medical factors that can affect your menstrual cycle. "

STIMULATING EGG FOLLICLES

IVF (in vitro fertilization) may be an option if you are having trouble conceiving. The first stage with this procedure is to stimulate the ovaries to produce several follicles, so that multiple eggs can be fertilized outside the body. Starting on around day two of your cycle, you will be given drugs to stimulate your ovaries. You will need to inject yourself or sometimes use a nasal spray to suppress the normal cycle, followed by injections of a follicle-stimulating (and sometimes lutenizing) hormone. Egg retrieval will then take place (see p.57).

ASK A DOCTOR

Should I monitor my menstrual cycle?

Yes, this is an important part of planning for pregnancy because it can help you to roughly figure out which day you're ovulating on (see p.49). You can then ensure that you have sexual intercourse around the right time to improve your chances of conceiving.

If you have regular monthly periods, it is likely you are ovulating. It's helpful to note the length of your cycle, which may vary. Note that from ovulation to the start of your next period is around 14 days, so when you get your next period you can figure out roughly when you ovulated.

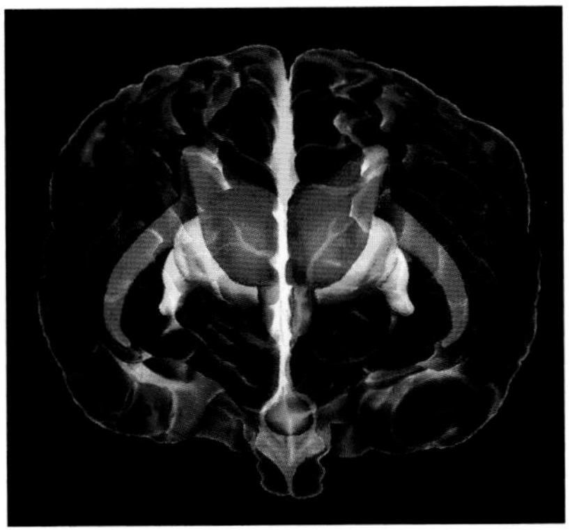

THIS IS **DAY 4 OF YOUR MENSTRUAL CYCLE**

276 days to go

WHAT'S HAPPENING INSIDE

In this 3-D scan of the brain, the green central structure is the hypothalamus. This controls emotions and body temperature, and releases chemicals that regulate the release of hormones from the pituitary gland (green circle at bottom).

> "Like many women, you may sometimes feel ruled by your hormones, and it helps to understand why they fluctuate."

ASK A DOCTOR

Will our chances of conceiving be affected by my partner being overweight and having high cholesterol? These two conditions, along with a resistance to insulin, high triglycerides, and high blood pressure, can reduce fertility. Advise your partner to have some checks done by their doctor if you are struggling to conceive, and seek the advice of a nutritionist.

The hormone buildup to ovulation starts right now in week one of your menstrual cycle. Your pituitary gland, which lies in the base of your brain, produces the follicle-stimulating hormone (FSH). During your period, the level of FSH rises steadily, triggering the development of the follicles (around 15–20 each month) in each ovary. In addition to containing an egg, the follicles produce estrogen.

The hormone estrogen circulates, affecting the pituitary gland and causing it to produce luteinizing hormone (LH)—this triggers ovulation (see p.49). This week your estrogen levels are low and steady, but will rise dramatically later in your cycle.

Progesterone levels are low during your period, but start to rise several days afterward and stay high for the second part of the cycle. Under the influence of progesterone, the muscles in the cervix relax, easing open the cervical canal. Changes also affect the mucus, which becomes more fluid, so sperm find it easier to swim through. It is progesterone that enables the lining of the uterus to thicken in preparation for implantation of the fertilized egg.

Premenstrual syndrome (PMS) is one of the many symptoms women can get when their hormones fluctuate, but did you know that men get PMS too? Scientists have confirmed there's a male version of PMS—Irritable Male Syndrome. Mood swings, temper tantrums, and loss of libido in men were found to be caused by falling levels of testosterone due to stress.

CHANGES DURING THE MENSTRUAL CYCLE

There are four hormones at work during the menstrual cycle: FSH (follicle-stimulating hormone) causes the egg follicles to start developing in the ovary; oestrogen is produced by the developing egg and peaks just before ovulation; LH (luteinizing hormone) triggers ovulation; and progesterone thickens the lining of the uterus.

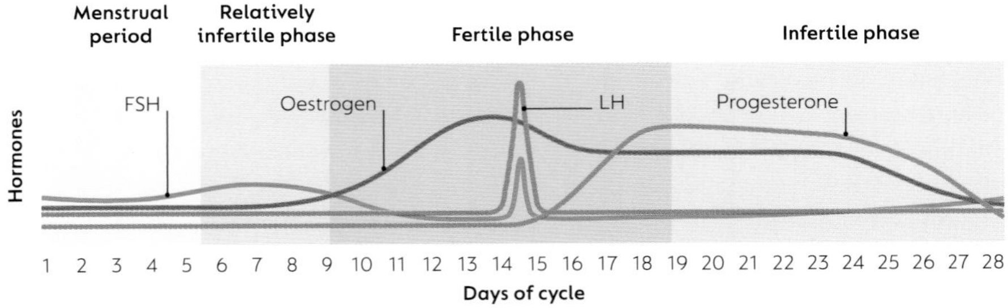

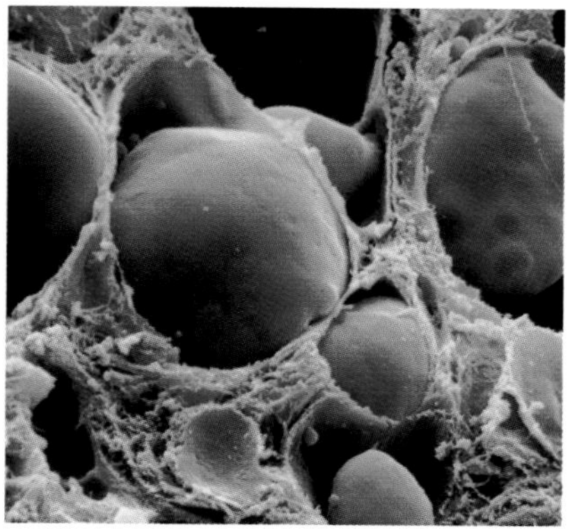

THIS IS **DAY 5 OF YOUR MENSTRUAL CYCLE**

275 days to go

WHAT'S HAPPENING INSIDE

This cross section through the ovary shows several ovarian follicles. Between each follicle, the connective tissue can be seen. Each month about 15–20 follicles mature, but it is usually only one that will fully mature and release an egg.

Try to ensure you're in the best possible health to maximize fertility. One way is to cut down or stop your alcohol intake and, if you take drugs, seek help to stop.

Heavy drinking can reduce the chances of conceiving and, if you do get pregnant, it can also harm your unborn baby's development. There is plenty of evidence that drinking beyond the recommended amounts is harmful. What's lacking is evidence of the effects on conception and pregnancy of the occasional alcoholic drink. There is no known safe level of alcohol consumption for pregnant women. However, many women decide to err on the side of caution and stop drinking alcohol entirely while trying to conceive and in early pregnancy. Some find that morning sickness naturally puts them off alcohol. Alcohol also affects male fertility. It has adverse effects on the quantity and quality of sperm. Drinking large amounts sometimes causes impotence.

You may find alcohol helps you and your partner relax and puts you in the mood for sex, thereby increasing your chances of conception, but you may want to rethink having the very occasional glass of your favorite cocktail.

Illicit or recreational drugs can harm your baby so stop using them before you conceive. Get medical support to stop. Ask your doctor for advice and a referral to a support group.

> "Making some lifestyle changes is essential when you're trying to get pregnant and cutting down on alcohol is a good start."

HAVING MEDICAL CHECKS

Before you try to conceive, speak to your doctor about the following tests:

- **Rubella:** have a blood test to check that you have antibodies against rubella (German measles). Being infected by the rubella virus for the first time in early pregnancy is associated with an increased risk of the baby developing hearing or sight problems, as well as increasing the risk of miscarriage. If you were vaccinated against rubella as a child, your antibody level may be high enough to protect your baby. If not, you will be offered two MMR injections three months apart. You must wait one month after the second vaccine before conceiving.
- **Screening for infectious disease:** Talk to your doctor about screening for gonorrhea, chlamydia, syphilis, HIV, and hepatitis B and C. If you have an increased risk for tuberculosis (TB), you should be screened and treated for TB before pregnancy.

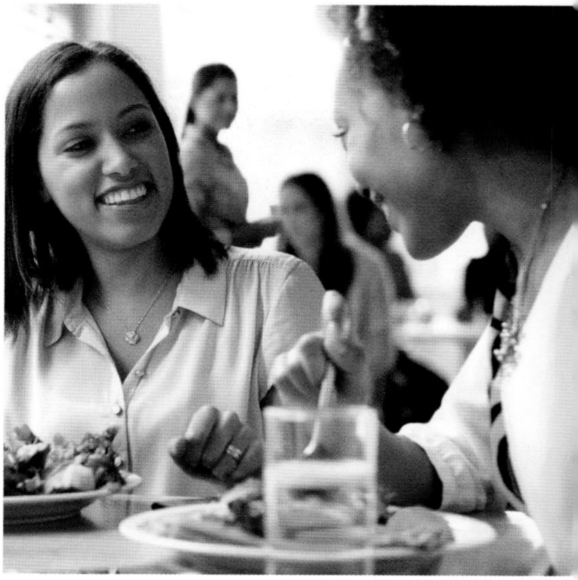

Opt for nonalcoholic drinks if you're trying to get pregnant. A high intake of alcohol can adversely affect your chances of conceiving.

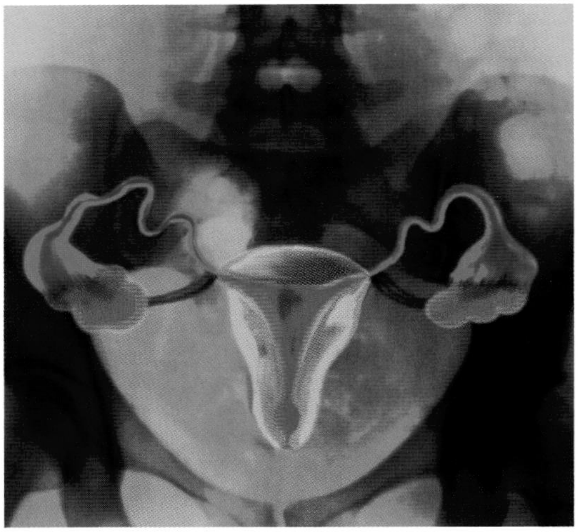

THIS IS **DAY 6 OF YOUR MENSTRUAL CYCLE**

274 days to go

WHAT'S HAPPENING INSIDE

In this artwork of the uterus, the green central structure is the pear-shaped uterus itself; the red part is the cavity of the uterus. The blue structures to either side are the fallopian tubes, which each have an ovary, seen in pink here, at the end.

“ Eating well is an essential part of conception and pregnancy so you and your partner should get into good habits now. ”

ESSENTIAL NUTRIENTS

You may need to top off your body's reserves of certain nutrients in preparation for pregnancy. Some nutrients such as iron, calcium, and vitamins A and D are stored by the body, but if you've had a restricted diet, your reserves may be low when you become pregnant. Make sure you eat fortified dairy alternatives (see p.15) if you avoid milk, and check out the sources of iodine you eat (p.80).

Take the time in these first two weeks of your cycle, before you ovulate, to look at what you eat on a daily basis. If you and your partner (see p.44) make some simple changes to your diet, it might just improve your chances of conception.

Use this opportunity to check your weight, i.e., your Body Mass Index (BMI; see p.16) since a BMI of under 19 or over 24 could adversely affect fertility.

If you're overweight, excess fat tissue may affect your metabolism and hormones and you may not ovulate as regularly, or at all. If you need fertility treatment, the chances of success are also lower if you're overweight, because you may respond less well to the drugs that stimulate ovulation. Once you're pregnant, being overweight can also cause an increased risk of complications, decreasing the chance of carrying the pregnancy to full term.

Weighing too little when you're trying to conceive isn't healthy either. Pregnancy takes its toll on a woman's reserves, so a little stored fat is a good thing for mother and baby. Being seriously underweight can affect ovulation and make periods irregular or absent, and conception unlikely.

Your BMI when you conceive is also a good indication of how much weight you should gain once you're pregnant (see p.99) so it's worth getting it checked at this point.

GET FIT AND FERTILE!

Regular exercise can increase your chances of conceiving by allowing your body to work at optimum levels. If you're fit and have a healthy lifestyle, you could limit the level of toxins in your body and be less stressed, which makes it easier to conceive. Exercise will also regulate your energy and your blood-sugar levels, which assists the body in regulating the hormonal cycle—a key player in the reproductive process. Conversely, overexercising can put more stress on your body, adversely affect the ovulation process, and make conception more difficult. The guidelines for exercising at this crucial time of conception are to continue weight-bearing exercise, such as walking, running, or aerobics, for at least 30 minutes five times a week at a moderate intensity. Moderate means where the exercise isn't too hard but is pushing your body enough to get the benefits. Afterward, you should feel energized, not fatigued.

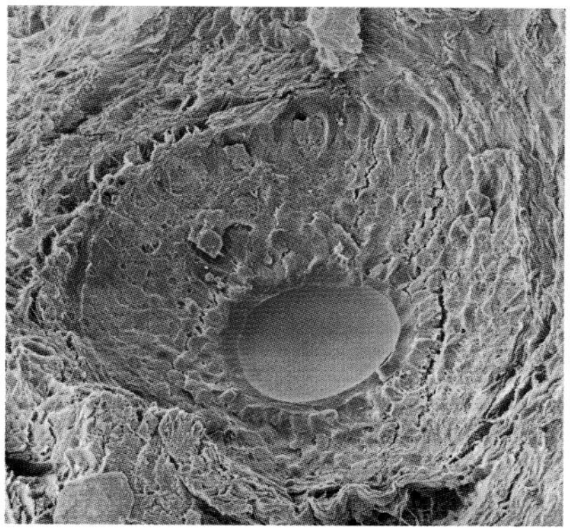

THIS IS **DAY 7 OF YOUR MENSTRUAL CYCLE**

273 days to go

WHAT'S HAPPENING INSIDE

Here an egg can be seen, in orange, developing in the ovary. The cells of the follicle, in which it is contained, can be seen surrounding the egg. At birth, baby girls have millions of follicles present in their ovaries.

In about a week's time, you are likely to ovulate. The ovaries are filled with follicles—fluid-filled structures in which the egg grows to maturity. Females are born with their lifetime supply of about 1 million eggs. They are not capable of making new eggs, and there is a continuous decline each month. By the time a girl enters puberty, only around 300,000 eggs remain. Of these, only 300–500 will ovulate over the 30–40 years of a woman's reproductive life. It is possible to conceive from puberty until menopause. Menopausal women are advised to use contraception for two years after their last period.

Women in their early 20s are considered at their most fertile, and although, for most women, periods continue until their early 50s, the rate of fertility gradually lowers in the 30s, 40s, and 50s, and the rate of chromosomal abnormalities and miscarriage increases. Nonetheless, every year thousands of babies are born to women in their late 30s and 40s.

Fertility begins to fall off sharply after the age of 35. Your age also affects the quality of your eggs. In women in their early 20s, around 17 percent of eggs have a chromosomal abnormality, but the figure rises to over 75 percent in women in their 40s. Chromosomal problems increase the chances of having a child with a disorder such as Down syndrome (see p.478). It is possible to have a blood test that can give an indication of your remaining ovary reserve so that you know how much reproductive time you have left. While some traditional tests are based on levels of FSH (see p.38) and estrogen, others use markers found in the blood, such as anti-Mullerian hormone (AMH) and inhibin B. Alternatively, a vaginal ultrasound procedure, called an antral follicle count, can assess the number of small follicles seen in the ovaries. But conceiving is about more than ovulation; the egg has to be fertilized, implanted, and then the pregnancy maintained.

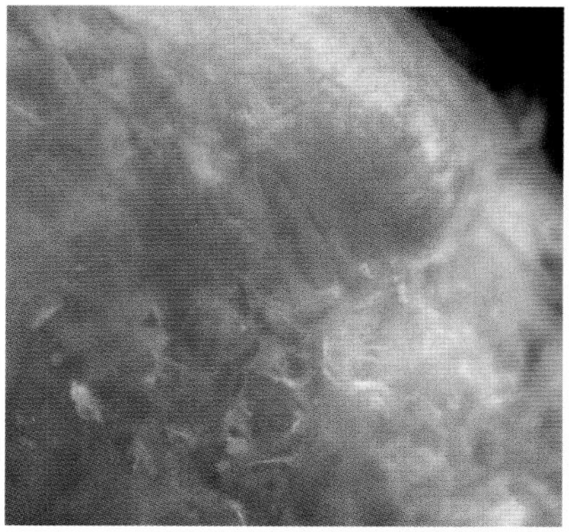

The follicle lies below the surface of the ovarian wall and protrudes just prior to ovulation. The follicle is most likely to rupture and release an egg midcycle.

> “When you're trying to get pregnant, you need to take your age into account because your fertility will decline as you get older.”

THE MALE BIOLOGICAL CLOCK?

Although men can continue to make sperm throughout their lifetime, changes in the amount and characteristic of sperm as men age does also result in decreased fertility. Although data is limited, advanced paternal age seems to be associated with an increased risk of Down Syndrome, autism spectrum disorder, as well as other psychiatric disorders and some birth defects.

Your 2nd week

YOUR "FERTILE WINDOW" IS APPROACHING AND THIS COULD BE THE TIME YOU CONCEIVE

Toward the end of this week, one of the eggs in your ovaries is likely to have reached full maturity. Ovulation occurs as the egg, under the influence of hormones, bursts out of its follicle. If it meets a sperm, you may become pregnant. Now is the time to enjoy lots of sex with your partner, so go for it—as often as you like. If you have any anxieties about fertility, try to put them aside and relax.

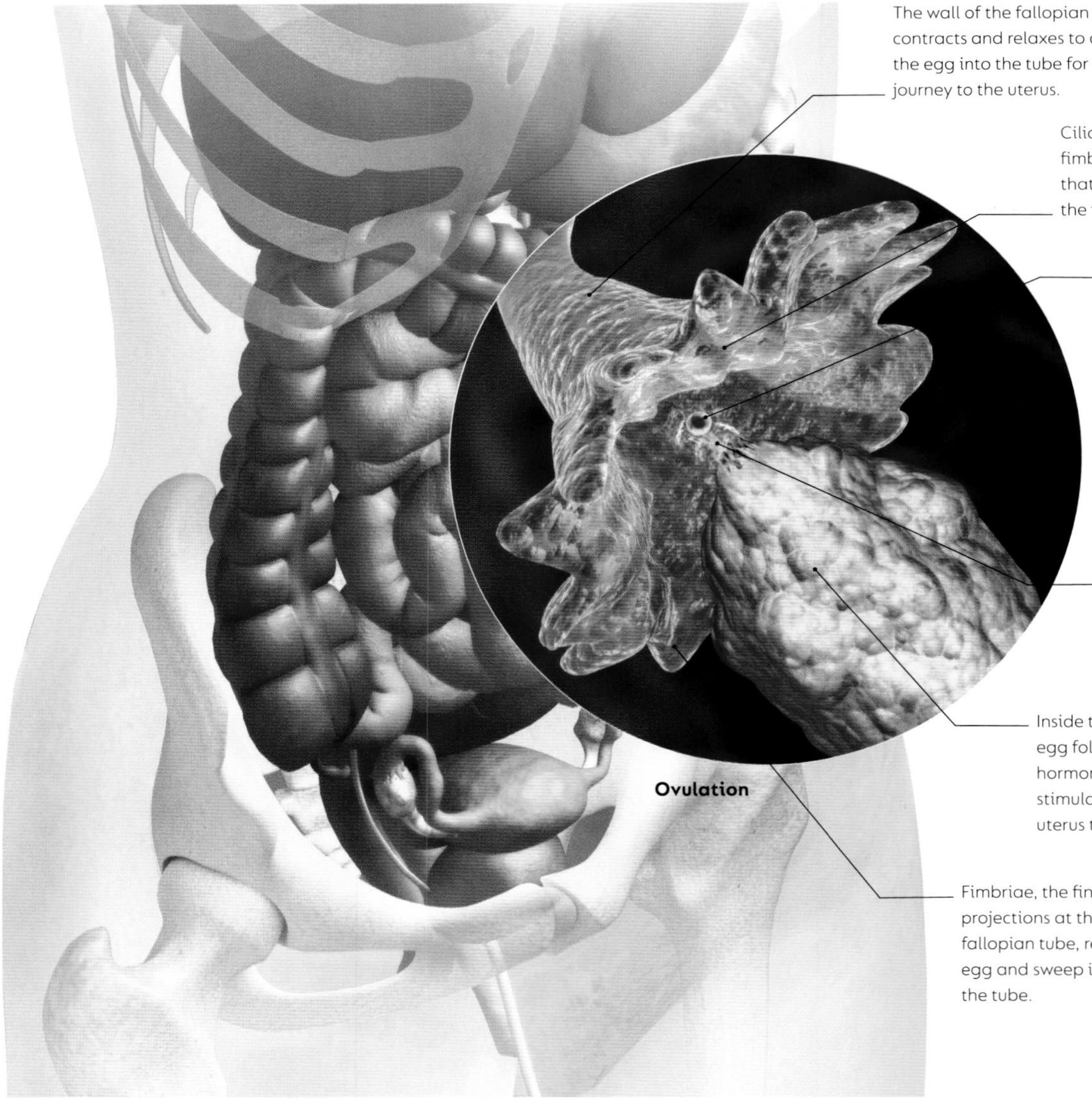
The wall of the fallopian tube contracts and relaxes to draw the egg into the tube for its journey to the uterus.
Cilia (small hairs) lining the fimbriae produce currents that help move the egg into the fallopian tube.
The mature egg is released from its follicle and breaks through the surface of the ovary. To meet a sperm, and be fertilized, it must enter the fallopian tube.
Fluid from the egg follicle is released with the mature egg.
Ovulation
Inside the ovary, the empty egg follicle produces the hormone progesterone, which stimulates the lining of the uterus to thicken.
Fimbriae, the fingerlike projections at the end of the fallopian tube, reach for the egg and sweep it gently into the tube.

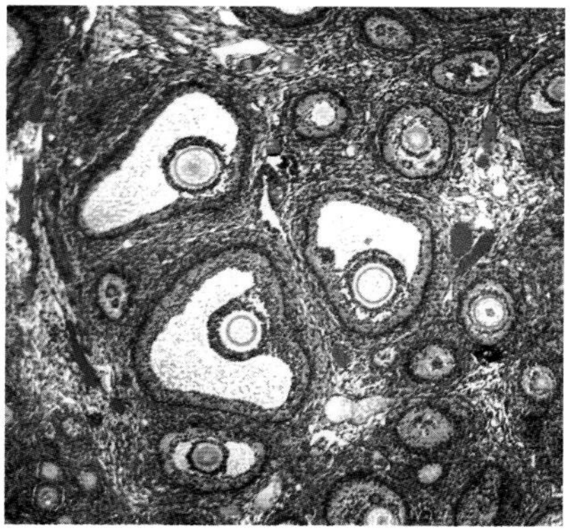

THIS IS **DAY 8 OF YOUR MENSTRUAL CYCLE**

272 days to go

WHAT'S HAPPENING INSIDE

Here, three developing ovarian follicles can be seen in white. The inner circle of each is the egg. Of the follicles shown, it is likely that only one will be fully mature at ovulation (see p.49) and release an egg.

> “By the end of this week you're likely to have ovulated. It's a good idea to know the signs that indicate you're at your most fertile.”

This is week two of your cycle. You will probably ovulate by the end of this week and will therefore be fertile. Since sperm can survive for three days inside you and an egg lives for 12-24 hours after ovulation, the window for an egg to be fertilized is 6 days. However, since the day of ovulation varies from day 12 to day 16, (approximately day 14 of a 28-day cycle), the fertile phase is regarded as spanning around 8 days. If you have regular periods,ovulation can be easier to track, but you may want to look for natural signs (see below) or use an ovulation kit. The kit tests urine to detect a surge in LH, the hormone that triggers egg release.

After a positive test you should ovulate 12–16 hours later. Results are about 99 percent accurate, but occasionally the result is a false positive or a false negative. If your result was negative, test the next day. Once you have a positive result, stop testing for that month.

While they are useful, testing kits are expensive and can be counterproductive because they make sex more clinical and less enjoyable. The best way to conceive is to have sex regularly.

CHANGES DURING THE MENSTRUAL CYCLE

Body temperature rises sharply after ovulation. Basal body temperature (when you first wake in the morning) rises slightly. **Cervical secretions** start off moist and sticky in the days leading up to ovulation, then become wetter and stretchy. **Lower abdominal pain** is experienced by some women.

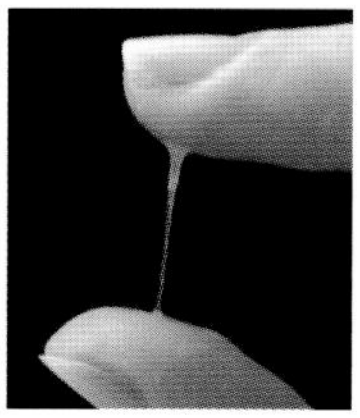

If you feel some of the cervical mucus with your fingers, you will find you can stretch it out. This is a sign that you are about to ovulate.

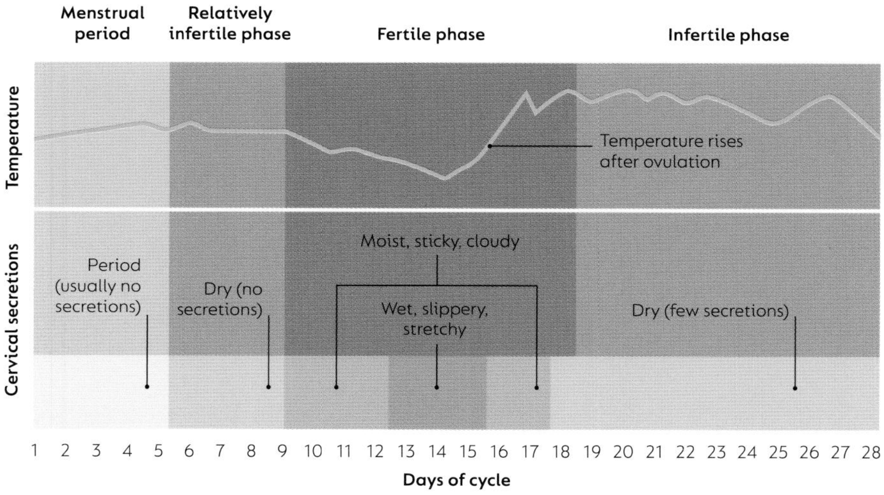

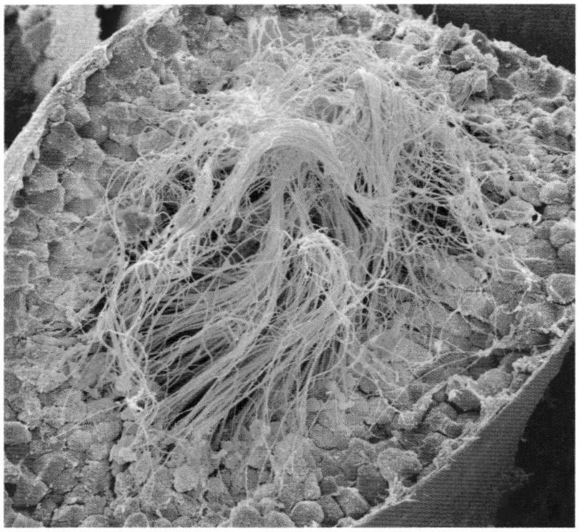

THIS IS **DAY 9 OF YOUR MENSTRUAL CYCLE**

271 days to go

WHAT'S HAPPENING INSIDE

In your partner's body, sperm is constantly being produced. Here the sperm cells can be seen: they consist of a head (green), which contains the genetic material, and fertilizes the egg, and a tail (blue), which propels the sperm along.

“While you wait to ovulate, fascinating changes are occurring in your ovaries as your follicles mature to release an egg.”

In the time leading up to ovulation, which will happen later this week, the most advanced follicle moves to the surface of the ovary, ready to release its precious cargo. While you were having your period, around 15–20 follicles were developing in your ovaries.

Both of your ovaries contribute to follicle growth, but in each cycle usually only one ovary brings a follicle to ovulation. This depends on chance since ovaries do not operate in a strict rotation. As the dominant follicle grows, it enlarges greatly, filling with fluid secreted inside the follicle. About 1 percent of women may release more than one egg some months (see p.49). If both are fertilized, nonidentical twins are conceived.

By the time of ovulation, the follicle will be about 1 in (2.5 cm) in diameter, while the egg is just about visible without a microscope.

To mature, follicles need FSH (follicle-stimulating hormone) produced by the brain's pituitary gland (see p.38), but their early growth doesn't appear to rely on it. It may, however, depend on other hormones and chemicals.

SPECIALIZED MEDICAL ADVICE

If you have an existing medical condition, it may affect your pregnancy, so seek medical advice before you conceive. If you are taking regular medication for diabetes, asthma, high blood pressure, heart trouble, deep vein thrombosis (DVT; see p.186), thyroid conditions, sickle-cell disease, epilepsy, or any other ongoing medical condition, consult your doctor before you conceive. If you conceive while you are on medication, do not stop the treatment, but see your doctor immediately.

BOOSTING MALE FERTILITY

Sperm take some weeks to mature, so if you want to become a dad, eat a healthy diet at least two to three months before conception. Being overweight can adversely affect male fertility, so exercise and try to improve your diet.

- **Antioxidants** including vitamins A, C, and E, selenium, and zinc, help prevent damage to sperm DNA.
- **Selenium** helps to make sperm, improve their motility, and protect against DNA damage. Increase the amount of oily fish you eat, such as mackerel and salmon, and snack on Brazil nuts—these are an unusually rich source of selenium.
- **Zinc** is present in large amounts in semen. Eat fish, lean meat, shellfish, turkey, chicken, eggs, whole grains, rye, and oats.
- **Essential fatty acids** may improve sperm motility, so again eat oily fish as well as seeds and nuts.
- **Use caution with soy** since soy products are high in isoflavones, plant chemicals that mimic estrogen hormones. A high intake may reduce sperm concentration.

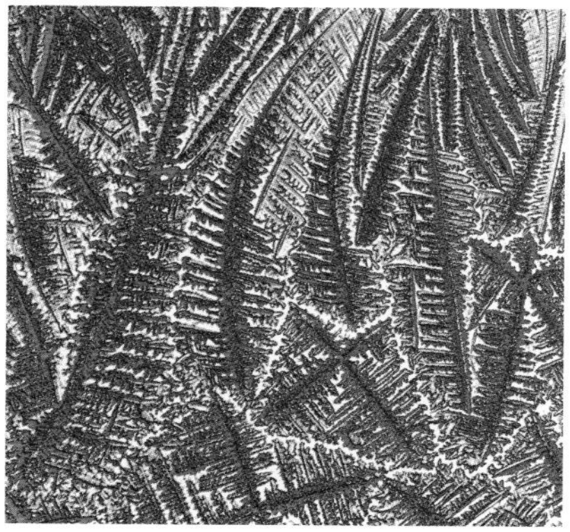

THIS IS **DAY 10 OF YOUR MENSTRUAL CYCLE**

270 days to go

WHAT'S HAPPENING INSIDE

As ovulation approaches, more cervical mucus is produced. Here it has crystallized to form a "fern leaf" pattern. Around the time of ovulation the mucus becomes clear, slippery, and stretchy, which makes it easier for sperm to swim through.

> " You may not care whether you have a boy or a girl, but according to some theories you can influence gender. "

Conceiving is all about having sex at the right time this week, but if you're hoping to have a child of a specific gender, the timing could be even more important. Some experts claim there is a link between when you have sex and the baby's gender (see below).

Recent research suggests that women who have a high calorie intake (especially if they eat bananas) are marginally more likely to bear a boy. Those who skip breakfast or have a low calorie intake are more likely to have a girl. One reason for this is thought to be that the extra calories consumed affect vaginal secretions help to give the Y sperm that makes baby boys a vital boost.

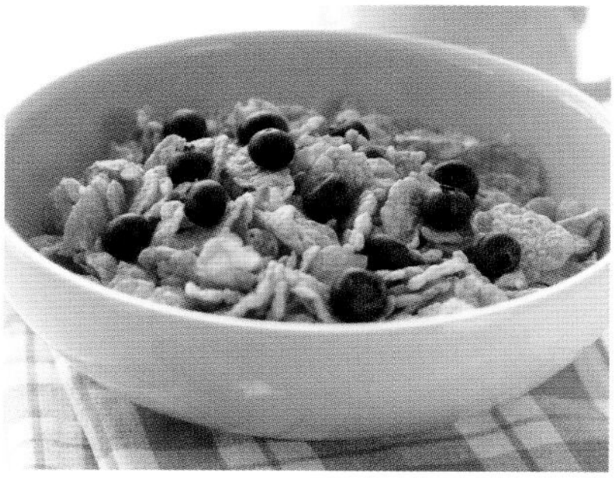

Research has found that women with high glucose levels, achieved by eating normally and not skipping breakfast, were more likely to conceive a boy.

CONCEIVING BOYS AND GIRLS

The Shettles method, devised by Dr. Landrum Shettles, is based on the fact that Y sperm (for boys) are smaller, faster, and less resilient than X sperm (for girls), and are less able to withstand an acidic environment in the vagina.

To conceive a boy, the Shettles method advises:

- Timing sex as close to ovulation as possible and adopting positions such as rear-entry that promote deep penetration.
- The woman should orgasm, ideally at the same time as the man to make the vagina less acidic and favor Y sperm.
- Drinking a cup or two or strong coffee just before sex to give Y-sperm an added kick.

The Whelan method, devised by Dr. Elizabeth Whelan, suggests that having sex earlier on in the cycle, some four to six days before ovulation, is more likely to result in a boy. Sex nearer the time of ovulation is more likely to result in a girl. This is more or less the opposite of the advice given by Shettles.

But what works? The mainstream medical view, supported by reports in journals such as the *New England Journal of Medicine*, is that the timing of sex has little or no bearing on gender. The possible exception is that having sex two days before ovulation may be slightly more likely to favor a girl.

If you already have two same-sex children, you're 75 percent more likely to conceive a child of that sex again. Although the sex of the baby conceived is random, conceiving children of the same sex could be down to the fact that some men produce better quality X sperm, which makes baby girls, or Y sperm, which makes baby boys. Statistically, couples who have two children of different sexes are less likely to try for a third child.

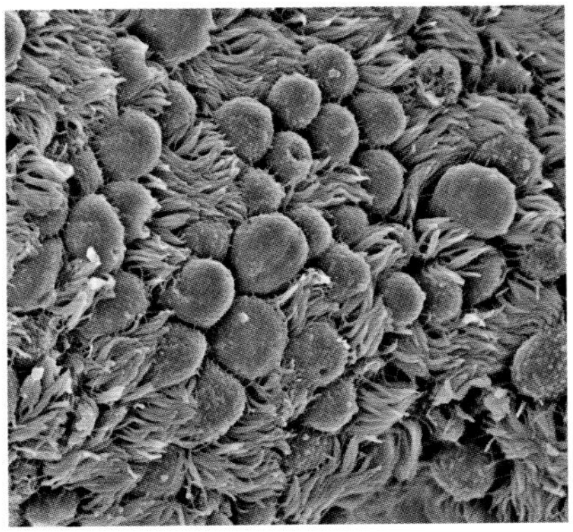

THIS IS **DAY 11 OF YOUR MENSTRUAL CYCLE**

269 days to go

WHAT'S HAPPENING INSIDE

The lining of the fallopian tube, seen here, has a moist mucous membrane. This contains cells (brown) that protect the tube's surface. The hairlike cilia (blue) move the eggs along the tubes following ovulation.

> " If this isn't the first month you've been trying to conceive, don't be too disappointed. It's normal for it to take some time. "

Have you been trying for a baby for some time? Not being able to conceive when you want to can be difficult to handle, especially if you're someone who has achieved in other areas of your life.

With reproduction, there's a large element of chance. Even for young women at their peak of fertility, the odds of conceiving in any one cycle are 20–30 percent. It's not unusual to try for six months, or even 12 months, without success. Around 10–15 percent of couples can take over a year to achieve a pregnancy or find it difficult to conceive. So plan for conception over a longer time frame, say 12 months, unless you have any specific reasons to be concerned about your fertility or your health in general.

The main exceptions are if you are over 35 or have a known fertility problem or gynecological issue. In this case, see your doctor after trying for about six months. The first step is likely to be a blood test for you, and a semen analysis for your partner. Rest assured that you may still get pregnant the old-fashioned way, but you have to be more proactive if you are in this older age group. The hitch is that if you do end up needing assisted fertility techniques, it all takes time.

ASK A NUTRITIONIST

Why can't I take supplements that contain vitamin A? The plant version of vitamin A, called beta-carotene, is safe to eat. It is found in orange, yellow, red, and dark green vegetables and fruits. The animal form, retinol, is found in eggs, butter, and meats, and it is six times more potent. A healthy diet should contain all the vitamin A you need in pregnancy. Too high doses have been associated with abnormalities developing in the brain and heart of the baby and linked to miscarriage. Take only multivitamin preparations recommended for pregnancy. These contain carotenoids, which are the precursor to vitamin A and can be converted into vitamin A by the body as needed.

STOPPING CONTRACEPTION

You can get pregnant as soon as you stop using some contraception.

- **IUD (coil):** you can get pregnant if you have sex in the week before it's removed since sperm can live three to five days.
- **Pill:** assume you're fertile immediately.
- **Implants:** fertility can return immediately after removal of the implant, but some women find it takes longer. Occasionally periods can take three to nine months to become regular. This suggests that the effects of the hormone are still lingering, but you may still conceive.
- **Injections:** irregular bleeding can continue for months, and you may not be able to conceive for several months either. However, as with implants, it's possible to get pregnant before your periods return properly.
- **IUD or IUS:** you could get pregnant if you have sex in the week before removal of the IUS system, but because the system contains progesterone, conception is less likely than if you have a regular coil fitted (see left).

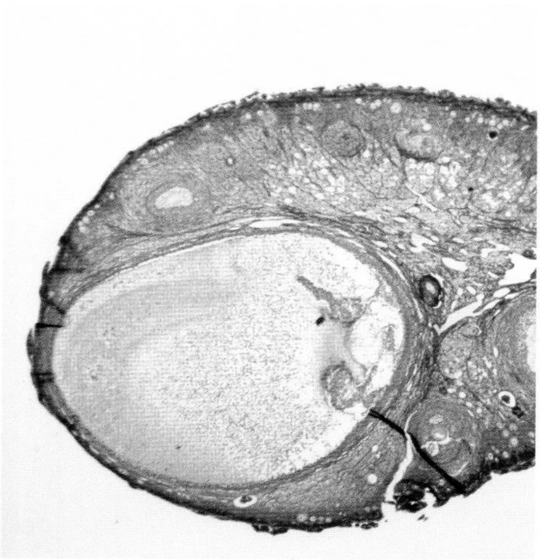

THIS IS **DAY 12 OF YOUR MENSTRUAL CYCLE**

268 days to go

WHAT'S HAPPENING INSIDE

This mature ovarian follicle contains a fluid-filled cavity (pale pink) known as the follicular antrum. At this stage, just prior to ovulation, one follicle has become much larger than the others, and it is this follicle that will rupture to release an egg.

“As your hormone level rises around this stage of your cycle, so might your libido—it seems nature takes care of everything!”

Estrogen levels are rising and reach their peak today, based on a 28-day menstrual cycle. The rise in estrogen from the follicles is what stimulates the release of the LH hormone (see p.38), which surges about 24 hours before ovulation. FSH (see p.38) from the pituitary gland starts rising later this week. Progesterone levels are low. There's no call for this hormone until the uterus lining needs to thicken. In fact, high levels would make the cervix hostile to sperm, so they would have trouble getting through to the uterus and the fallopian tubes to fertilize the egg.

Women also produce testosterone, which reaches a peak around ovulation. This male hormone is responsible for libido in both sexes so both you and your partner may be in the mood for making babies.

Try to stay as relaxed as you can, because being stressed can affect your ability to conceive. One reason might be that it reduces the ovary's response to the luteinizing hormone surge at midcycle. There is also a link between stress and the failure of fertility treatments.

ASK A DOCTOR

I had a miscarriage four weeks ago. Can I try for another baby right away? As a general guide, wait until you've had one period. This will help date the pregnancy if you conceive quickly. However, your doctor may advise waiting longer, especially if your miscarriage was linked with an infection or a known medical problem or was recurrent. It makes sense to have any tests first. You and your partner may also need time to grieve. Rest assured that the vast majority of women who have a single miscarriage go on to have a baby.

There is some recent evidence from a Scottish study that women who conceived again within six months were significantly less likely to have another miscarriage.

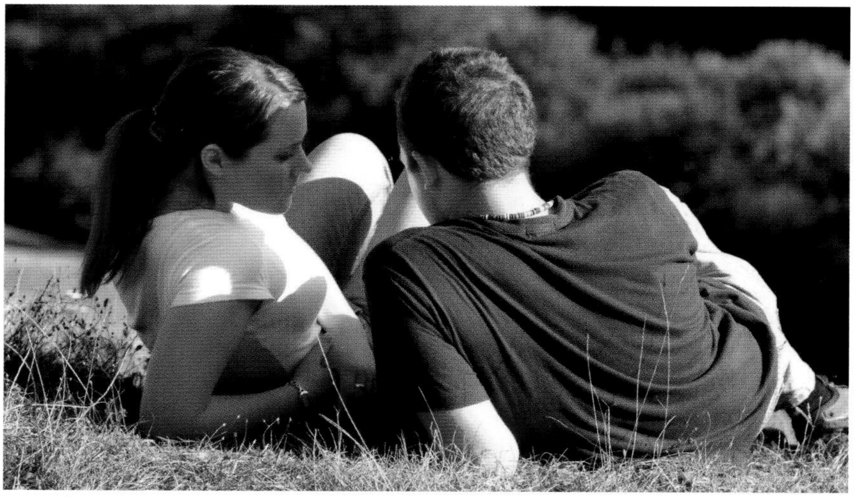

It's a good idea to talk about and work through your grief together before trying to get pregnant again. Miscarrying can be extremely tough and may put a strain on your relationship.

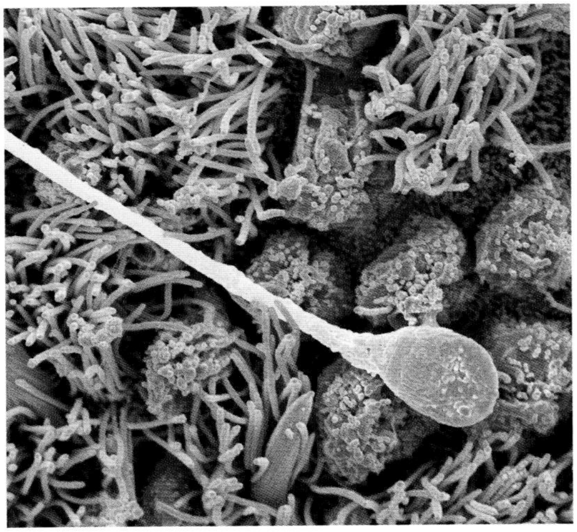

THIS IS **DAY 13 OF YOUR MENSTRUAL CYCLE**

267 days to go

WHAT'S HAPPENING INSIDE

The sperm cell can be seen here inside the fallopian tube. Since sperm can stay active and alive inside you for up to three to five days, it's possible to get pregnant even if you don't ovulate until several days from now.

> "This is an optimum time to conceive, but try not to think too much about when you might be ovulating and just enjoy having sex!"

SEXUAL POSITIONS

It seems that how you have sex can help conception. Sexual positions that maximize penetration, such as rear entry, may work best since sperm is deposited as close to the cervix as possible. If the man is on top, the woman could try placing a pillow under her buttocks to raise her pelvis and help the movement of sperm toward the cervix. Woman-on-top positions may lead to leakage of sperm. Avoid using lubricants because they can adversely affect sperm.

Use the time around ovulation to put some excitement and spontaneity back into your sex life. With all the recommendations and restrictions, not to mention old wives' tales, that supposedly maximize conception rates, it's easy to forget that sex is meant to be enjoyable. If you're hell bent on conceiving, then the fun can get forgotten. You might want to try different positions, times, or places for sex. If you and your partner aren't usually that adventurous, this is a good opportunity to try varying things a little.

Try to have sex every 48–72 hours. If your partner ejaculates regularly, it will encourage the production of quality sperm. The benefits of abstaining have been greatly overstated in the past. It is true that not having sex for up to seven days can boost the number of sperm, but research now shows that abstinence can impair the motility (swimming ability) of sperm, especially if the sperm were already borderline. The longer the period of abstinence, the more marked the effect will be. So have fun and if you conceive, that's a bonus! If the woman has an orgasm, it can boost the chances of conception. One theory is that the female orgasm is an evolutionary device designed to convey semen into the cervix as the uterus contracts. If the woman climaxes before her partner, or she doesn't orgasm, she will retain less semen than if she comes at the same time or after him.

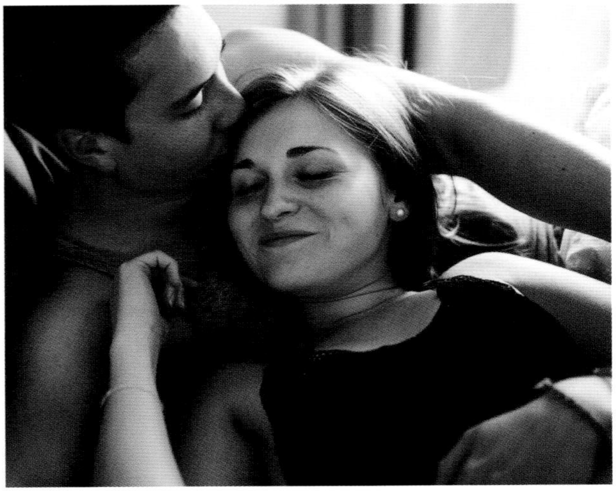

Although your goal is to conceive, try to stay relaxed and make sure sex remains a pleasure and not a chore.

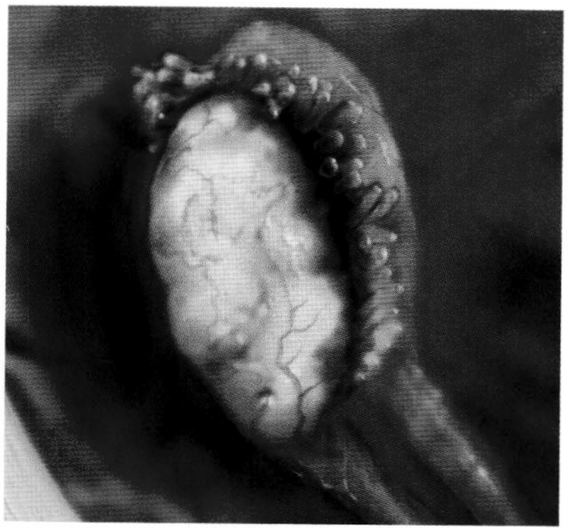

THIS IS **DAY 14 OF YOUR MENSTRUAL CYCLE**

266 days to go

WHAT'S HAPPENING INSIDE

The ovary can be seen here at the end of the fallopian tube. At around this time of the menstrual cycle, a follicle at the surface of the ovary releases an egg, which is swept down the tube by clearly visible fingerlike projections called fimbriae.

> "You're highly likely to ovulate today, if you haven't already, and if egg meets sperm you may soon be pregnant."

Typically ovulation occurs around day 14 but it can occur earlier or later. Ovulation is when an egg is released from your ovaries (sometimes two eggs are released—see box, below). LH rises thanks to estrogen output from the growing follicles (see p.47), and it is this rise that triggers the events that now take place in the follicle. LH makes the egg inside the follicle become fully mature, ready for release and fertilization. This is the point at which the egg reduces its number of chromosomes (see p.54) from 46 to 23.

The follicle is rich with fluid by now. Just before ovulation, it is some 1 in (2.5 cm) or more in diameter. In position, it lies just below the surface of the ovary. If you could see the follicle, it would look like a blister about to burst.

Next the follicle produces enzymes that digest its outer layer, releasing the egg on to the surface of the ovary.

Once the egg has been released from the follicle, it is soon swept into the nearest fallopian tube by the fingerlike projections that form the end of the tube, where it will hopefully be fertilized.

MULTIPLE TWIN PREGNANCIES

If you've had nonidentical twins already, your chance of having another set quadruples. Nonidentical twins occur when more than one follicle ripens completely and the two eggs released at ovulation are both fertilized. The chance of having another set of twins is increased because most women who conceive nonidentical twins (without fertility drugs) show a pattern of releasing more than one egg per cycle. Your chance of having a second set of twins is about 1 in 3,000.

PRESSURE TO CONCEIVE

If you're trying to conceive, you may have little else on your mind and this can put a strain on your relationship. With the goal of pregnancy in mind, it's easy to become clinical about sex. At this point, you and your partner may be regarding each other not so much as sex objects, but as components of a baby-making machine. Enjoyment can so easily get lost.

Understandably, you may find that your partner becomes aggrieved if he feels pressure to provide sperm; the distress may have an adverse effect on a man's willingness and even ability to have sex. If this happens, it can lead to a downward spiral, which naturally makes conception less likely, and may cause discord.

Make an effort to be loving and work together rather than against each other. Consider taking a break; couples often conceive when they're away on vacation and more relaxed. Make sure you also enjoy some stress-free sex outside of your fertile window.

Conception

Pregnancy begins with conception, a complex process that involves the release of one or more eggs from the ovary, successful fertilization by a sperm in a fallopian tube, and implantation in the lining of the uterus.

The release of an egg

Each woman is born with her full quota of follicles that contain immature eggs, some of which will mature and be released in her lifetime. Every month, follicle-stimulating hormone (FSH), released from the pituitary gland, encourages a number of the follicles to ripen. These follicles in turn produce the hormone estrogen, rising levels of which encourage the uterus to thicken to prepare for the implantation of a fertilized egg. As the eggs mature, the level of estrogen rises and the pituitary gland receives a message to produce luteinizing hormone (LH). Every month, this surge in LH triggers one follicle (and sometimes more than one) to release a mature egg—the moment of ovulation.

Once the egg leaves the ovary, it enters the fallopian tube, which lies close by, and starts to travel through the tube to the uterus. The fallopian tube is just 4 in (10 cm) long and its lining has many tiny fronds that literally brush the egg in the direction of the uterus. Even so, the journey takes five days or more. In the course of this voyage, the fertilization of the egg takes place.

The journey of the sperm

During sex, the man releases an abundance of sperm—around 250 million at each ejaculation—into the

THE EGG AND SPERM

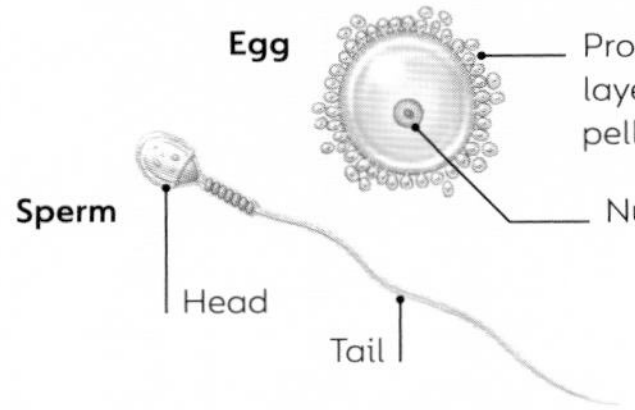

The mature egg has a diameter of 0.1 mm and is surrounded by a protective outer layer known as the zona pellucida. The far smaller sperm consists of a head, which contains the male genetic material and enzymes to help break down the egg's outer layer, and a tail that propels the sperm up the vagina and uterus to the fallopian tube.

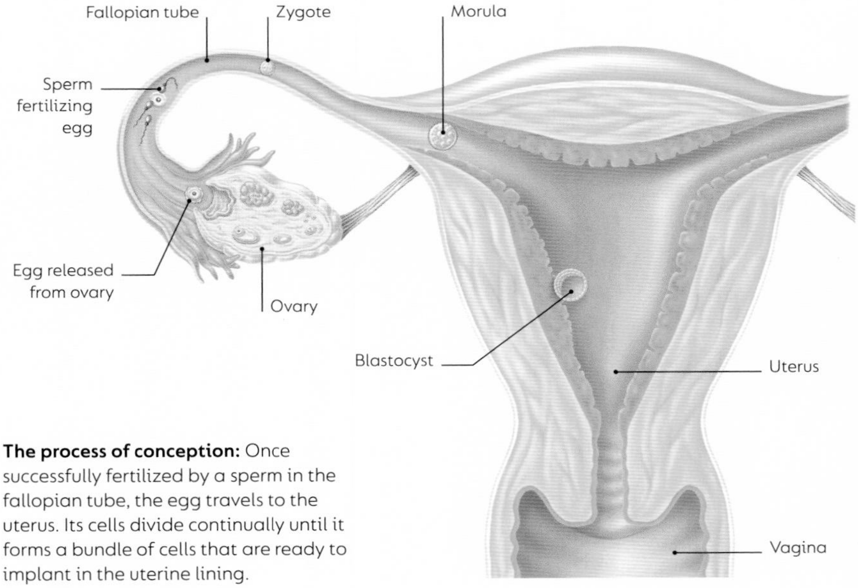

The process of conception: Once successfully fertilized by a sperm in the fallopian tube, the egg travels to the uterus. Its cells divide continually until it forms a bundle of cells that are ready to implant in the uterine lining.

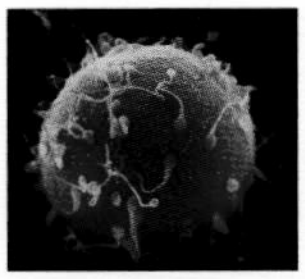

At fertilization, one sperm penetrates the egg. Once the egg and sperm have merged, they form a single cell called a zygote.

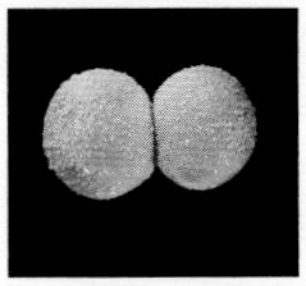

The zygote divides into two identical cells, and continues to divide as it travels down through the fallopian tube.

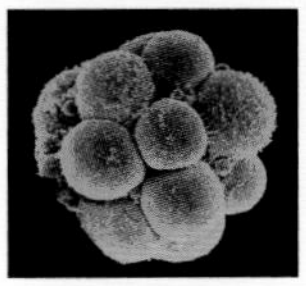

A morula—a bundle of around 16 cells—has formed by around three to four days after fertilization of the egg.

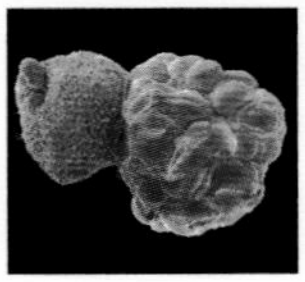

A blastocyst, a mass of up to 100 cells, hatches out of the egg's protective layer and prepares to implant in the uterus.

vagina. Each sperm has a long tail to propel it, so it's well equipped to swim up to the fallopian tube, where fertilization of the egg takes place. The whole distance, from the vagina through the uterus and up into the fallopian tube can be accomplished in hours. However, the sperm can survive in the vagina and the uterus for three to five days, meaning there is a window of around six days in which fertilization can take place (an egg lives 12–24 hours after ovulation). Not all of the millions of sperm make it as far as the fallopian tube; in fact, most of them die, seep out of the vagina, or get lost along the way. Around just 200 sperm, only a tiny fraction of the number originally released, arrive at the site of the egg.

The moment of fertilization

Although many sperm cluster around the egg and try to penetrate its outer layer, only one of them will manage to burrow its way through the surface and fertilize the egg. Once this happens, the egg's outer layer thickens quickly to keep out other competing sperm, so that each egg can be fertilized by only one sperm.

Implantation in the uterus

By the time the fertilized egg reaches the uterus, it has grown from a single cell into a compact cluster of cells, called a blastocyst. This cluster attaches to the uterine lining loosely, then more deeply and permanently.

At this early stage, the blob of cells, which is more than just a fertilized egg, but not quite an embryo, is sometimes referred to as a "conceptus." Although its sex is already determined, it's not remotely baby-shaped yet. The cells produce enzymes that allow it to digest its way into the uterus lining, and lie snugly below the surface.

Assisting conception

If you haven't become pregnant after a year of trying, your doctor may suggest tests and then you may be advised to embark on fertility treatment. The most popular is in vitro fertilization (IVF). This involves taking medication to stimulate your ovary to grow more eggs in this cycle. The eggs are harvested and fertilized with your partner's sperm, and you're given hormone treatments to prepare the uterus to receive the embryos 2–5 days later. If the sperm quality is poor, a procedure called intra-cytoplasmic sperm injection (ICSI) may be used—a single sperm is injected directly into an egg and the fertilized egg is transferred to the uterus.

In intrauterine insemination (IUI), sperm that have been sorted for viability are put directly into the uterus. This is used if semen analysis reveals mild abnormality, or there are ovulation or intercourse problems.

You should be made aware of all risks of assisted conception, such as an under- or over-response of the ovaries and a multiple pregnancy.

HOW TWINS ARE CONCEIVED

Today in the US, one in every 31 births is a twin birth. Twins are conceived in two ways that result in either identical or nonidentical twins.

Identical twins occur when one fertilized egg splits into two separate cells. This type of twin is half as common as nonidentical twins. Identical twins have the same genes and are the same sex, so they are very alike, although subtle differences in their environment can mean they're not always identical in every way. Identical twins are known as "monozygotic" twins, since they come from one "zygote," or fertilized egg. Triplets, quads, and higher multiples can be monozygotic too. However, triplets and more can arise from more complex combinations. For example, there may have been two fertilized eggs, one of which split into two.

Nonidentical twins occur when two eggs are released at ovulation. Each twin's genes come from the parents, but the twins don't share the same mix of genes. Nonidentical twins are also called "fraternal" twins, since they're no more alike than other siblings and can be of a different sex. They're also referred to as "dizygotic" twins, because they come from two separate "zygotes," or fertilized eggs. Nonidentical triplets arise when three eggs are released instead of one. This is more likely to occur when ovulation is induced with fertility drugs (see below).

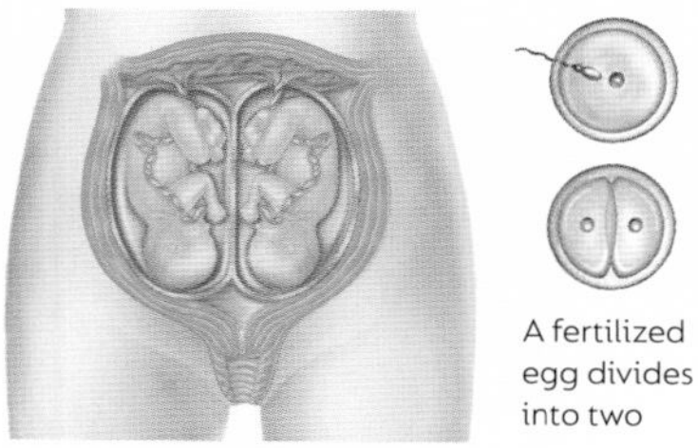

Identical twins that result from the division of one fertilized egg may share a placenta in the uterus. Occasionally, they also share an amniotic sac.

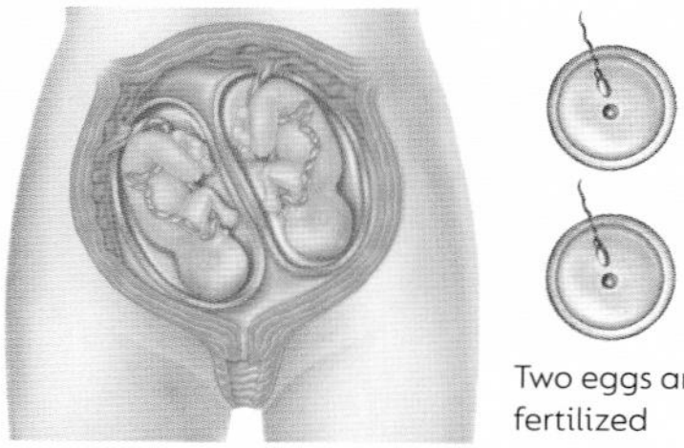

When two eggs are fertilized at the same time, nonidentical twins are formed, each with its own placenta and amniotic sac.

Your 3rd week

THIS IS THE WEEK A MIRACLE TAKES PLACE—YOUR BABY IS CONCEIVED If you ovulated and the egg met a sperm, amazing things will happen fast. It takes just four days from fertilization for a single egg to divide into a ball of 58 cells. By the end of the week, this ball, called the blastocyst, will have reached the uterus, where it will start to implant in the lining. It will be a couple of weeks before you know whether you've conceived, but special hormones kick in now to help maintain the pregnancy.

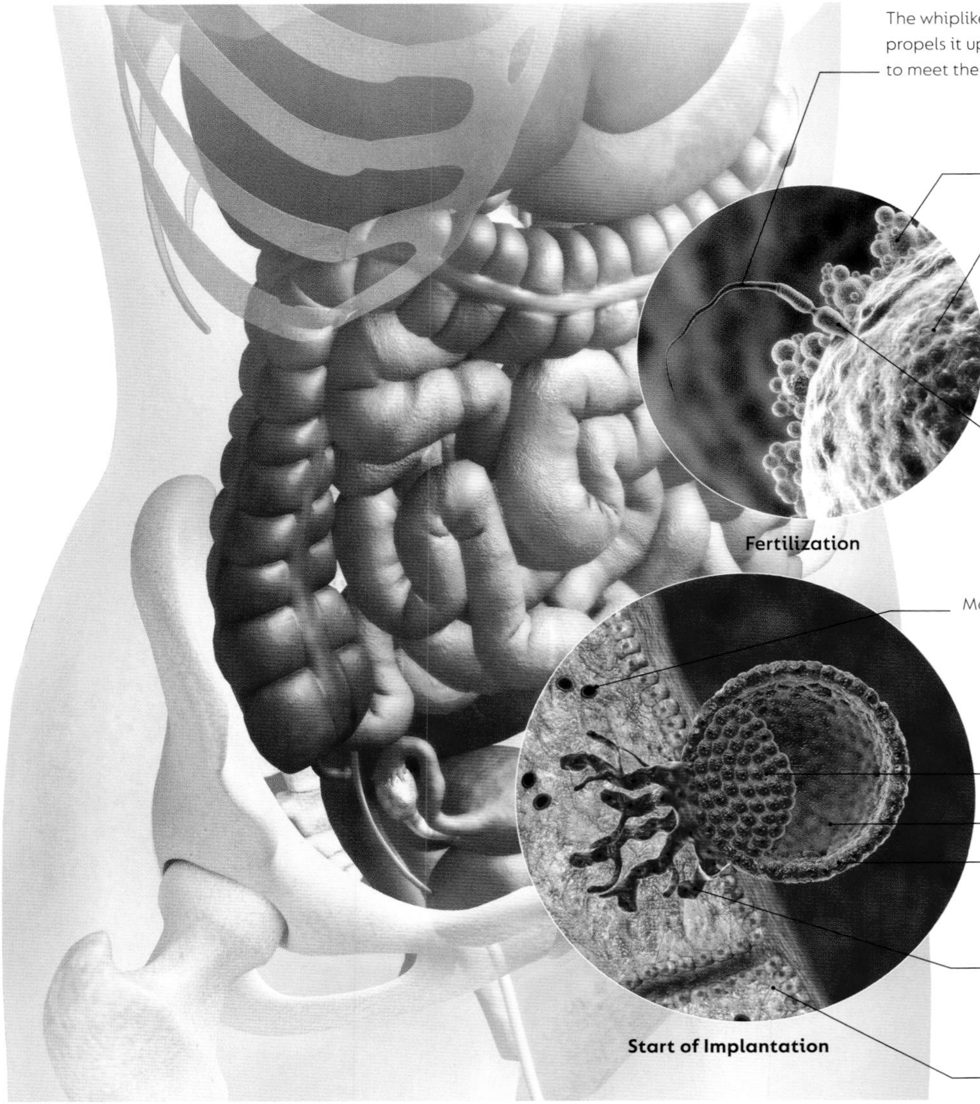
The whiplike tail of the sperm propels it up the fallopian tube to meet the egg.
Cells surrounding the egg secrete chemicals that aid egg development.
Egg
The sperm's head carries genetic material along with enzymes that enable the sperm to penetrate the egg's tough outer layer.
Fertilization
Maternal blood vessels
Cell cluster within the blastocyst's fluid-filled cavity forms the beginnings of the embryo.
Fluid-filled cavity
Blastocyst
The outer cells of the blastocyst anchor into the lining of the uterus.
Start of Implantation
Lining of uterus

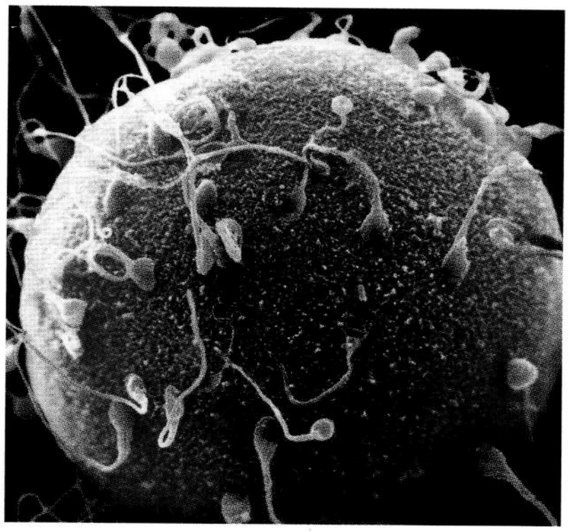

YOU ARE **2 WEEKS AND 1 DAY**

265 days to go

WHAT'S HAPPENING INSIDE

Here the egg is shown surrounded by sperm. Although only one sperm will fertilize the egg, several hundred are thought to be necessary to break down its defensive layers and enable fertilization to take place.

You are likely to have ovulated and your unfertilized egg now begins its journey. Once it has been released by the ovary, the egg is swept up by one of your fallopian tubes and, moving in the direction of the uterus, comes to rest in the widest portion of the tube, awaiting fertilization.

It is no exaggeration to say that for each sperm released the chance of even reaching the site of fertilization is in the order of one in a million. Around 300 sperm reach the tube but only one will fertilize the egg. Once the sperm has penetrated, it triggers a reaction that makes the surface impenetrable. Each sperm and egg contain 23 chromosomes, half of the total genetic material required. The egg will always contain an X chromosome but the sperm will carry either an X or Y chromosome and therefore determines the sex of the embryo. The sperm and egg chromosomes combine forming the "zygote" and fertilization is complete.

The hormones responsible for the production of sperm are released every 60 to 90 minutes. So a man is constantly producing sperm cells. In theory, this means that a male is always fertile, but it takes sperm a 72-day period to fully develop. So leading an unhealthy lifestyle during that time will impinge on the quality. For this reason, if you're trying to conceive, your partner should embark on a healthy lifestyle for two to three months to produce good sperm.

> "Your newly released egg will only survive 24 hours, but hopefully in that time it will meet sperm and be fertilized."

MALE FERTILITY

If you want to become a dad, there are many reasons why you should ensure you're in good shape, not least to support your partner as she prepares for pregnancy. However, while a couch potato lifestyle isn't desirable for men who want to conceive, it seems that pulling out all the stops at the gym might not be the best course of action either.

Researchers asked a group of fit young men to exercise intensively four times a week for two weeks. Afterward, their semen was tested and found to contain fewer sperm and lower levels of the hormones essential for conception. These hormonal changes were temporary and returned to near normal within a few days of the men resuming previous levels of activity.

The concern is that recovery might not be so fast among older men, or in those who have poor sperm counts and/or low hormone levels. So stay in shape but don't overdo it.

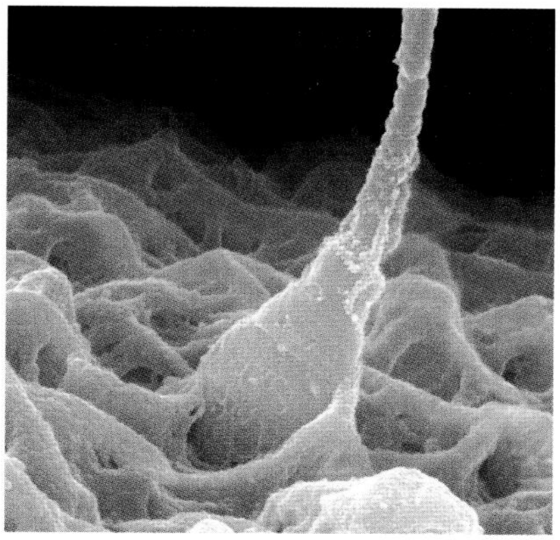

A few hundred sperm survive the journey and encounter the egg in the fallopian tube, but it is just one sperm that actually fertilizes the egg.

Genes and inheritance

The genes that parents pass on to their children at least partly determine their children's physical and mental characteristics. In some cases, an abnormal gene may be passed on, resulting in an inherited genetic disorder.

What are genes?

Genes are located on rodlike structures called chromosomes that are found in the nucleus of every cell in the body. Each gene occupies a specific position on a chromosome. Because genes provide instructions for making proteins, and proteins determine the structure and function of each cell in the body, it follows that genes are responsible for all the characteristics you inherit.

The full genetic instructions for each person, known as the human genome, is carried by 23 pairs of chromosomes, and consists of around 20,000–25,000 genes.

How inheritance works

At conception, the embryo receives 23 chromosomes from the mother's egg and 23 chromosomes from the father's sperm. These pair up to make a total of 46 chromosomes. Pairs 1 to 22 are identical or nearly identical; the 23rd pair consist of the sex chromosomes, which are either X or Y. Each egg and sperm contains a different combination of genes. This is because when egg and sperm cells form, chromosomes join together and randomly exchange genes between each other before the cell divides. This means that, with the exception of identical twins (see p.51), each person has unique characteristics.

How gender is determined Of the 23 pairs of chromosomes that are inherited, one pair determines gender. This pair is composed either of two X (female) chromosomes, in which case the baby will be a girl, or of one X and one Y (male) chromosome, in which case the baby will be a boy.

An egg always contains one X chromosome, while a sperm can carry an X or a Y chromosome. Whether your baby is a boy or a girl will therefore always be determined by the father. If a

GENES THROUGH THE GENERATIONS

Through each generation, genes are shuffled and reshuffled. Half of a baby's genes come from its father and half from its mother. The baby's parents in turn inherited half each of their genes from each of their own parents. One quarter of each person's genes therefore come from the grandparents. So how does this happen? Instead of containing the full complement of 46 chromosomes, each egg and each sperm has just half, or 23, chromosomes each. When they meet at conception the chromosomes pair up to again make up the full complement that now forms the genetic blueprint for the new individual. One of the 23 pairs of chromosomes are sex chromosomes, so sex is also determined at conception. Each egg carries an X chromosome and each sperm either an X or Y. If two X chromosomes combine, the baby will be a girl; if an X and Y chromosome combine, the baby will be a boy (see right).

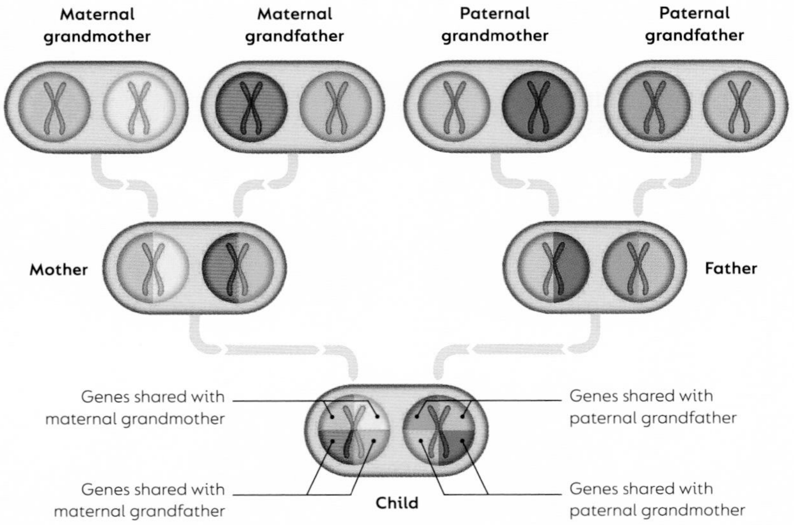

Maternal grandmother
Maternal grandfather
Paternal grandmother
Paternal grandfather
Mother
Father
Genes shared with maternal grandmother
Genes shared with maternal grandfather
Genes shared with paternal grandfather
Genes shared with paternal grandmother
Child

sperm carrying an X chromosome fertilizes the egg, the resulting embryo will be a girl. If a sperm with a Y chromosome fertilizes the egg, the resulting embryo will be a boy. In the male, both the X and Y chromosomes are active. In females, however one of the two X chromosomes is deactivated early in development of the embryo in order to prevent duplicate instructions. This could be the X chromosome from either the mother or the father.

Gene variations Each gene within a cell exists in two versions, one inherited from each parent. Often they are identical, but some paired genes occur in slightly different versions, called alleles. There may be two to several hundred alleles of a gene, although each person can only have two. This variation in alleles accounts for the differences between individuals, such as eye color and ear shape. A dominant allele may "overpower" a recessive one (see right).

Why genetic disorders occur

Sometimes a gene is faulty. Genetic disorders arise either when an abnormal gene is inherited or when a gene changes, or mutates. Genetic disorders may follow a dominant or recessive pattern of inheritance (see right). They can also be passed on via the X chromosome. Such sex-linked disorders are usually recessive, which means that a woman can carry the faulty gene without being affected, because she has another healthy X chromosome to compensate. If a boy receives an affected X chromosome, he will be affected; a girl will be a healthy carrier like her mother. An affected male could pass on the affected gene only to his daughters.

DOMINANT AND RECESSIVE GENES

Genes come in pairs, and each gene in a pair may differ slightly. One gene may be dominant, and override the other gene, which is recessive. A recessive gene only has an effect if both genes in a pair are recessive. An example is eye color, although this is not as simple as depicted here.

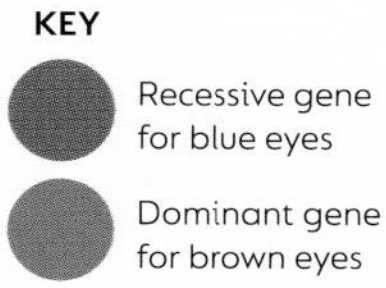
KEY
Recessive gene for blue eyes
Dominant gene for brown eyes

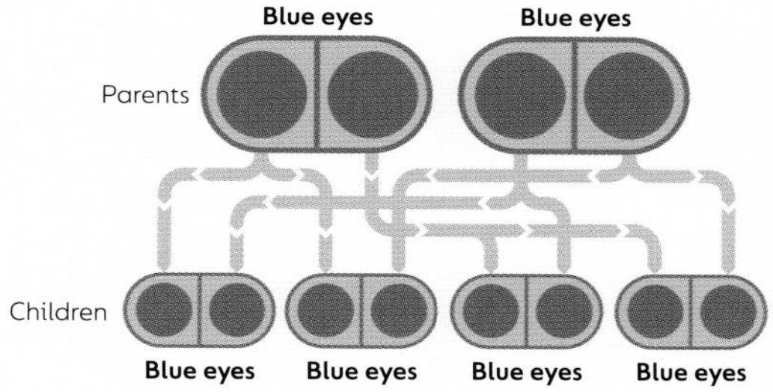
Blue eyes
Blue eyes
Parents
Children
Blue eyes
Blue eyes
Blue eyes
Blue eyes

Two pairs of recessive genes When both parents have blue eyes, as shown here, they will both have a pair of recessive genes for blue eye color. All of the children will therefore have blue eyes since there is no dominant gene present to mask the recessive gene.

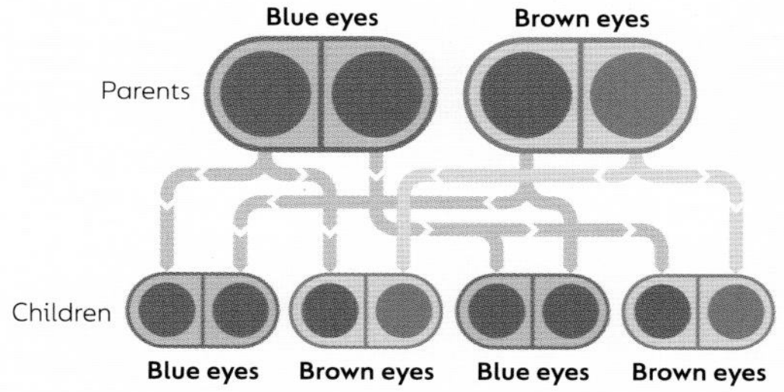
Blue eyes
Brown eyes
Parents
Children
Blue eyes
Brown eyes
Blue eyes
Brown eyes

Recessive and mixed genes In this example, each child will inherit at least one recessive blue eye gene from the parents. Depending on whether the other gene is dominant or recessive, the couple's offspring have a 1 in 2 chance of inheriting blue eyes, and a 1 in 2 chance of inheriting brown eyes.

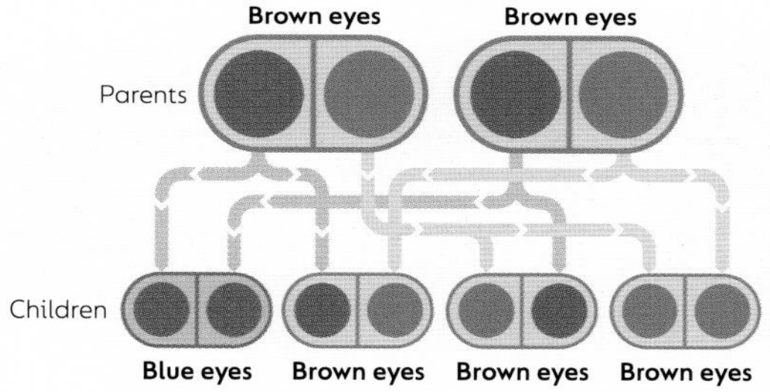
Brown eyes
Brown eyes
Parents
Children
Blue eyes
Brown eyes
Brown eyes
Brown eyes

Two pairs of mixed genes Here, each child has a 1 in 4 chance of inheriting two recessive genes and having blue eyes, and a 3 in 4 chance of inheriting a dominant gene for brown eyes. The brown-eyed offspring may have either a pair of dominant genes, or mixed genes.

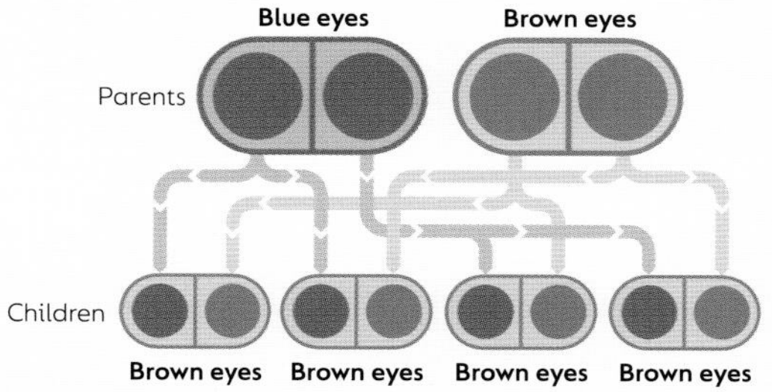
Blue eyes
Brown eyes
Parents
Children
Brown eyes
Brown eyes
Brown eyes
Brown eyes

Recessive and dominant genes In this example, all of the children will have brown eyes. This is because each child receives a recessive gene from one parent and a dominant gene from the other parent. The dominant gene will override the recessive gene on each occasion.

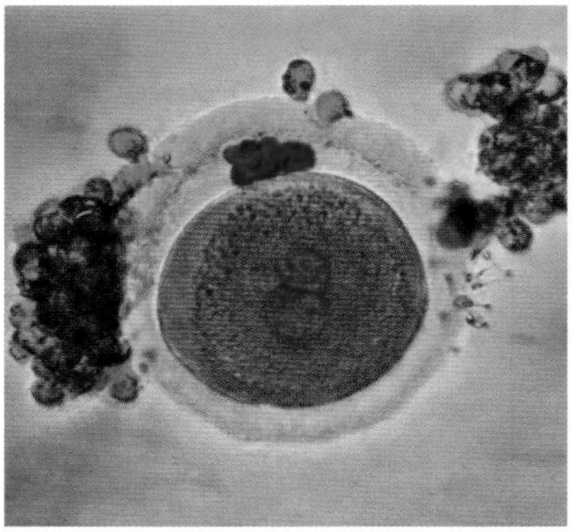

YOU ARE **2 WEEKS AND 2 DAYS**

264 days to go

WHAT'S HAPPENING INSIDE

Here a human egg cell 24 hours after fertilization is artificially colored purple. Around the egg is a thick layer (yellow) that has now become impenetrable. The two red areas, or pro-nuclei, contain genetic material from the mother and father before it has fused.

" When your egg has been fertilized, hormonal changes naturally occur to stop your normal menstrual cycle. "

At this early stage following fertilization of your egg, the developing embryo will signal its existence to the pituitary gland in your brain and switch off your menstrual cycle. It does this by producing a new hormone, called human chorionic gonadotropin (hCG). This hormone overrides your usual monthly cycle and maintains the high progesterone levels that are essential for your pregnancy. The hormone progesterone (see p.38) is essential to an embryo's survival in the uterus, and therefore to your baby's well-being and development before birth.

Later, starting around weeks four to five, your embryo will make all the hormones needed to maintain its own life. Of course its nourishment and shelter come from you, but even in the very early weeks of pregnancy the embryo behaves like an independent human, at least as far as its hormones and genes are concerned.

HEALTHY CONCEPTION

When you're trying to conceive, you'll find you are more aware of your general health. Colds, flu, and other common infections are unlikely to affect your fertility or your baby if you have conceived. Some infections and viruses, however, can have a more serious impact:

Shingles and chickenpox (both caused by the same virus) are best avoided around the time of conception if you haven't had chickenpox before.
Food poisoning, for example caused by listeria bacteria, can be harmful (see p.16).
Toxoplasmosis can be contracted from handling cat feces (see p.101).

In low levels, testosterone may aid fertility, but too much can affect the menstrual cycle and lead to infertility. Small quantities of testosterone are secreted from the adrenal gland and the ovaries.

ASK A DOCTOR

I've been doing ovulation tests, but they've all been negative. Does this mean I haven't ovulated this month? Even if you don't appear to have ovulated this month, you may still have. It's possible to miss the LH surge just by chance. This is more likely if you don't test at the same time each day, or you drink a lot of water. Remember too that ovulation tests are imperfect, and it's possible to get a false negative. If you had other symptoms of ovulation, such as pain, or changes in your mucus (see p.43), it's likely that you ovulated anyway. However if you have gone two or three months with consistently negative tests, then you might not be ovulating regularly. In that case, it's worth seeking medical advice.

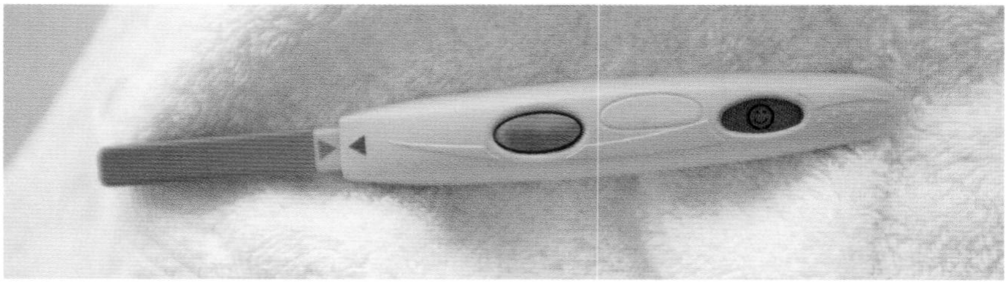

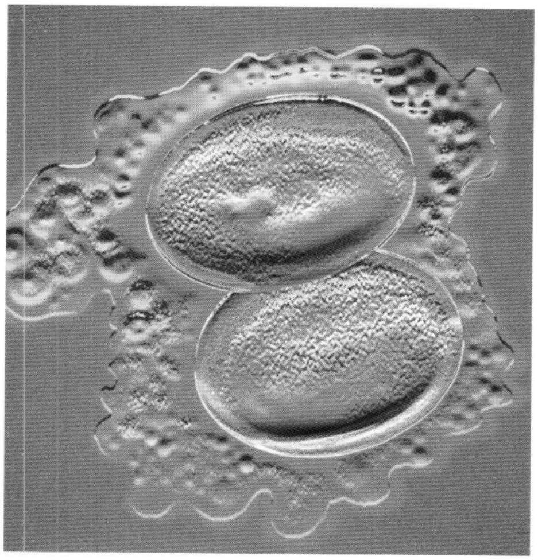

YOU ARE **2 WEEKS AND 3 DAYS**

263 days to go

WHAT'S HAPPENING INSIDE

When the two nuclei have pooled their genetic material to create a cell containing its full complement of 46 chromosomes—23 each from the mother and father—the cell can start dividing, shown here at the first division creating a two-celled body.

> "Vital cell divisions are now taking place as the fertilized egg begins its journey toward implantation."

The chromosomes from the sperm and egg joined over 24 hours ago. It takes around 30 hours for the resulting zygote to complete its first cell division. The zygote, at only 0.1 mm in diameter goes on to divide into 16 cells, forming a compact ball.

Cell division is such that the ball of cells is hardly any larger than the original zygote. The ball of 16 cells, now known as a "morula" (as it resembles a mulberry), travels toward the uterus, entering on day three to four after fertilization. Every cell within the morula is totipotent, meaning it is able to form any type of cell. From this point onward the cells will lose this function as they start to specialize.

ASK A DOCTOR

I'm fairly sure I've ovulated. Do we need to keep having sex to make sure I conceive? Even if you've been tracking your ovulation by monitoring your temperature or cervical mucus, or by using an ovulation kit, you can't be sure exactly when it occurred.

Since the fertile window is several days, continue having sex for at least a couple of days after what you think is your most fertile time. Also, it's good to stay intimate at the times you're not trying to conceive.

Remember also that abstention doesn't usually have the hoped-for effect of banking up and improving the quantity and quality of sperm. In fact, the opposite may happen (see p.48).

FROM EGGS TO EMBRYOS

Egg collection will be scheduled following the first stage of IVF (see p.37). Not all follicles that were stimulated will contain eggs. Two days after, you will be given progesterone to thicken the uterus lining. Two to five days after fertilization, the most promising embryos are chosen to be transferred. A pregnancy test is performed about two weeks later. If you are under 40, you will usually have only two to three embryos transferred. Over the age of 40, you may have up to four embryos transferred. Any leftover good-quality embryos can be frozen for future treatment cycles. Research suggests that frozen embryos give comparable pregnancy rates to fresh ones since only the best are selected.

The outcome depends largely on age, but on average each cycle has a 20–40 percent success rate.

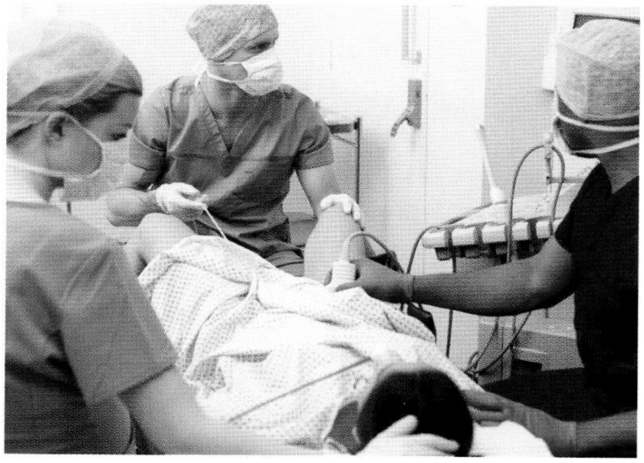

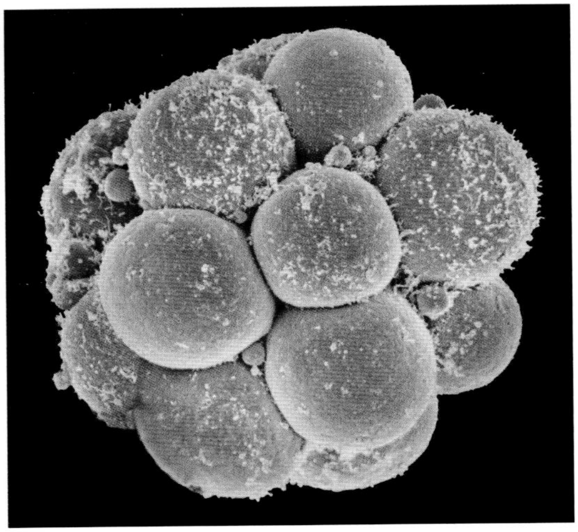

YOU ARE **2 WEEKS AND 4 DAYS**

262 days to go

WHAT'S HAPPENING INSIDE

This is an embryo at the 16-cell stage, when it has changed from a zygote into a morula. It is in the process of dividing into a hollow ball of cells, the blastocyst, which will eventually implant in the lining of the uterus.

> “ Significant changes are taking place daily within your uterus and within just 72 hours from now, the fertilized egg will implant. ”

Around four days following fertilization, fluid begins to collect within the morula (see p.57). This creates a separate outer cell layer, one cell thick that encapsulates an inner mass of cells. The inner layer will become the embryo, and the outer layer the placenta (see p.76). The whole structure now consists of approximately 58 cells and is termed the “blastocyst.”

The blastocyst spends several days within the cavity of the uterus before implanting. The morula had an impenetrable outer surface as it traveled, but this disappears as the blastocyst prepares for implantation in the lining of the uterus.

ASK A MOM

How can I stop people asking me whether or not I've conceived? I certainly found that once I'd told people I was trying to have a baby, they were inordinately interested in the process. It was difficult, especially in the week when I was waiting to find out if I'd conceived. The best way to deal with it is to respond by saying that you'll let people know if there's news. If you're struggling to conceive, telling people you're having difficulties should help stop them from asking.

THE ALTERNATIVE APPROACH TO FERTILITY

If you're having difficulty conceiving, or just want to improve your chances, consider using a complementary therapy. Always inform the practitioner that you might be pregnant.

- **Reflexology** works by manipulating pressure points in the feet to improve energy flow to specific parts of the body. While there is plenty of anecdotal evidence that reflexology helps conception, this isn't currently backed up by scientific research. However, it may help relieve stress, which can be a factor in couples who have problems conceiving.
- **Acupuncture** (see right) works on the principle that problems such as infertility are caused by blockages in the body's energy flow or “qi.” By inserting tiny needles into energy points that are linked to the reproductive organs, the flow is restored. The recent scientific evidence is debatable—some studies suggest a beneficial effect while others do not. However, if it relaxes you while undergoing fertility treatment then go for it, since it certainly won't be harmful.

Acupuncture is thought to boost male fertility by improving sperm health and reducing stress, a factor that can impede the chances of conception.

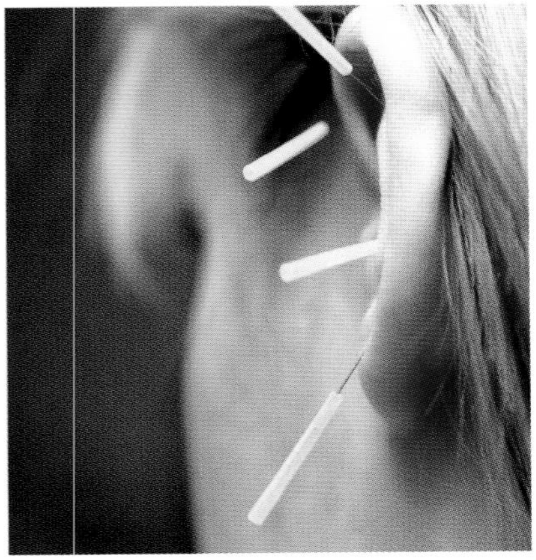

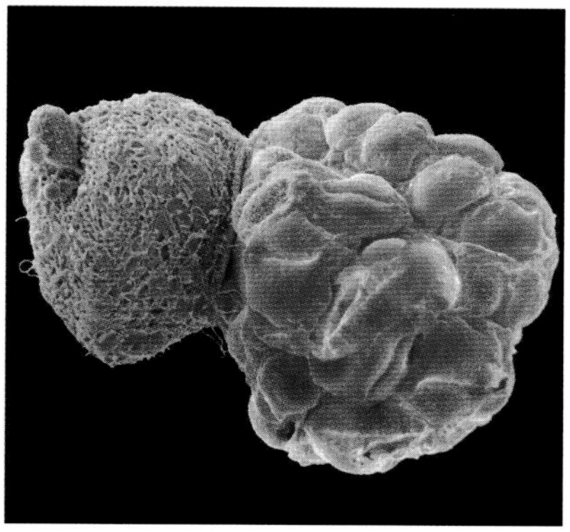

YOU ARE **2 WEEKS AND 5 DAYS**

261 days to go

WHAT'S HAPPENING INSIDE

This is an embryo at the blastocyst stage, five days after fertilization. It is seen hatching from the shell that originally surrounded the unfertilized egg. At this stage, the blastocyst has moved into the uterus and is preparing to implant.

> "While playing the waiting game, you may want to consider how you'd feel if there are two fertilized embryos waiting to implant!"

Have you conceived, and might it be twins? Twins can be nonidentical or identical and each type of twins is conceived differently.

Nonidentical (dizygotic) twins are the result of two separate eggs being fertilized by separate sperm. They may also occur as a result of IVF (see p.37) if two embryos are placed in the uterus. Some estimate that the chances of having twins after fertility-enhancing treatment is as high as 1 in 38.

Identical (monozygotic) twins occur when a single egg is fertilized by a single sperm and divides into two embryos. This split can occur at any stage up to nine days after fertilization and its timing is critical to the way the placenta(s) and amniotic sac(s) are formed. If the zygote (see p.57) splits within the first three days, two separate placentas and amniotic sacs develop. If the split occurs at blastocyst stage, four to nine days after fertilization, the fetuses will share a placenta but have separate sacs; when the split occurs after day nine, the fetuses will share a placenta and a sac. The odds of having identical twins are about 3.5 in 1,000.

Having nonidentical (fraternal) twins depends a lot on family history. Your chances of having twins are simply higher if you have a close relative with twins, but twins never become inevitable.

Family history is most relevant when the nonidentical twins are on the mother's side as they rely on a woman releasing two eggs in any one cycle, which may be hereditary. However, a family history of twins on the male side can be important too. It may be that the man carries a gene that makes his daughter release more than one egg at a time at ovulation.

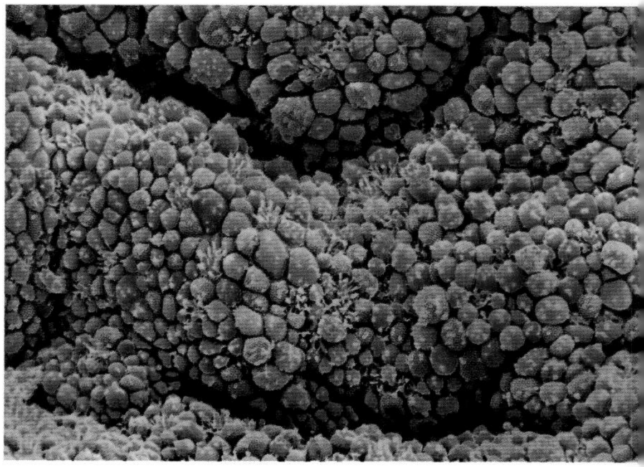

The lining of the uterus, when fertilization occurs, becomes secretory to nourish an embryo. The lining prepares itself in the same way, no matter how many embryos implant.

THE LOST TWIN

Twin conceptions may be more common than they appear. Without knowing it, some women miscarry one twin in early pregnancy. It is sometimes possible to have symptoms of a miscarriage, yet, confusingly, the pregnancy then appears to continue until term, culminating in the birth of a completely normal singleton baby.

Nobody is quite sure how often this happens, or why. While one in every 31 births in the US today is a twin birth, research using scans in very early pregnancy suggests that at conception the figure is much higher. Some experts believe that 15 percent of all births may start off as twins. Their loss could simply be nature's way of dealing with imperfections.

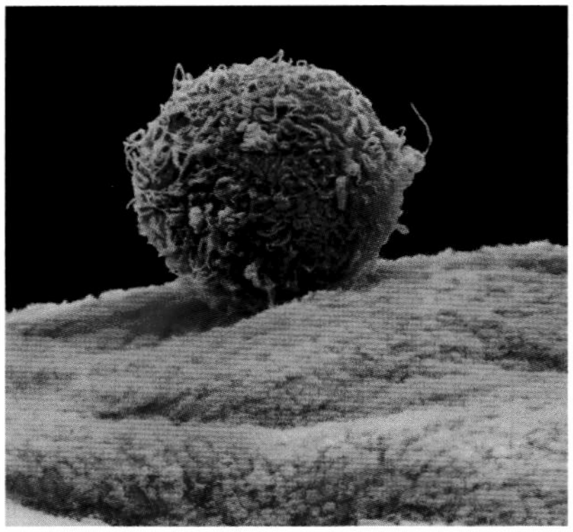

YOU ARE **2 WEEKS AND 6 DAYS**

260 days to go

WHAT'S HAPPENING INSIDE

The blastocyst prepares to embed itself in the lining of the uterus—the endometrium. Once it is completely implanted—usually around seven days after fertilization—the pregnancy will become established.

> "Your reproductive organs undergo complex processes that will enable your body to maintain the pregnancy."

If you have conceived, the ball of cells known as the blastocyst that will eventually form the fetus will now be preparing to embed in the lining of your uterus, and the placenta will be starting to form.

Before this happens, however, there is another important change going on. After you ovulate, the empty ovarian follicle develops into a structure called the corpus luteum (which means, literally, "yellow body"). This small, fluid-filled sac becomes increasingly "vascular," developing blood vessels and beginning to produce the hormone progesterone. This is required to create mucus to allow your fertilized egg to survive, and build up the lining of your uterus, in which the blastocyst will soon embed (see opposite).

The corpus luteum also produces a little estrogen. By about 8–12 weeks of pregnancy, your placenta will take over the production of progesterone, but the corpus luteum continues to play a small role in hormone production until about six months, when it usually shrinks away.

ASK A DOCTOR

Should I stop taking medication in case I've conceived? Many medicines are safe to take, but some are not, or have not been fully evaluated. This last group includes many antihistamines for allergies, over-the-counter sleeping pills, and many analgesics (see p.23).

If you've accidentally taken an over-the-counter medicine that's not considered appropriate for use in pregnancy, you're unlikely to have done any harm with just one dose. However, seek medical advice if you're concerned.

If you need to continue using a medicine in pregnancy, ask if it's safe to do so. While pharmacists are well-informed on all medicines, your doctor is the best person to consult on prescription-only drugs. Talk to your doctor before stopping any prescription drugs.

THE MIRACLE OF CONCEPTION

When you consider the multitude of events that have to fall neatly into place before a baby is conceived, it's hard to believe that anyone can become pregnant. No wonder they talk about the miracle of life!

To become pregnant the following have to happen:

- **Your hormone balance** must be correct for the egg to develop.
- **Ovulation must take place:** if you don't release an egg, there is no way for fertilization to occur.
- **You need to have sex** at the right time in your menstrual cycle; sperm can last about three days in healthy cervical mucus, but if your timing is off, egg and sperm are unlikely to meet. In some cases there may be only two or three days each month when you can conceive.
- **Your partner needs to produce** plenty of good, healthy sperm that can penetrate your cervical mucus to reach the egg.
- **When the egg has been fertilized,** the blastocyst has to implant securely in the lining of the uterus.
- **The right levels of the hormone** progesterone must be produced by the corpus luteum to maintain the pregnancy.

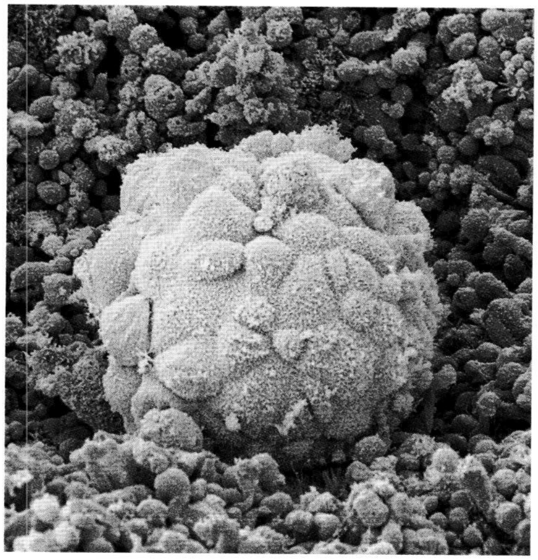

YOU ARE **3 WEEKS EXACTLY**

259 days to go

WHAT'S HAPPENING INSIDE

The blastocyst is firmly embedded in the lining of the uterus. Once this has happened, the placenta (the temporary organ that supplies the growing embryo with oxygen and nutrients) will begin to develop.

Around seven days after fertilization, the blastocyst implants in the lining of the uterus. The outer cell layer, no longer protected, is able to attach to the lining of the uterus. The lining is now more receptive and has undergone changes that make it more "sticky" to aid attachment. The blastocyst erodes cells to sink beneath the surface.

What was originally a single outer layer of cells now transforms into two layers. The outermost layer of cells creates space by eroding the lining, and it secretes hormones. These hormones inform your body that you're pregnant and stimulate the uterus to support the pregnancy rather than shed its lining in what would normally be your period.

The innermost cell layer of the blastocyst will become the placenta and the amniotic sac that encloses the embryo. Within the blastocyst there is an inner cell mass of cells that will eventually form the embryo.

> "It's a week since the egg was fertilized and it now implants in your uterus, where it will soon develop into an embryo."

STRETCH AND UNWIND

It can help to relax in this interim period, before you do a pregnancy test. Fill some time by getting in shape with these simple stretches. Getting into the habit of doing these exercises now will help your body deal with the increased demands once you know you're pregnant. Stretch before and after exercising to prevent muscle strain.

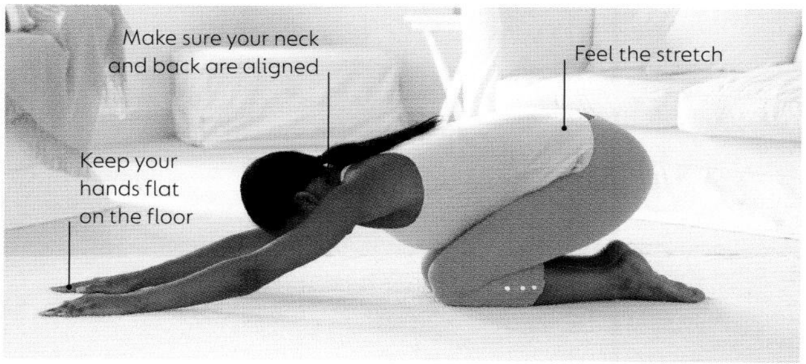
Make sure your neck and back are aligned
Feel the stretch
Keep your hands flat on the floor

Back stretch: get on all fours and lower your bottom toward your feet while stretching your arms in front of you. Lower your forehead, keeping your neck and back aligned, and stretch your arms. Inhale slowly and then relax your back and arms as you exhale. Inhale and exhale 10 times.

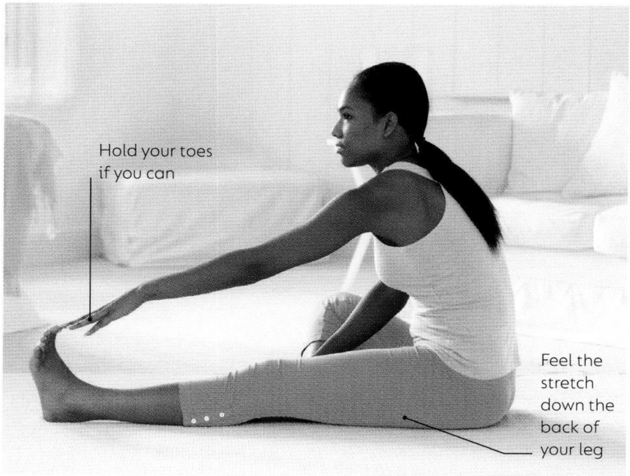
Hold your toes if you can
Feel the stretch down the back of your leg

Leg stretch: sit on the floor and stretch your left leg in front of you. Using your left hand, take hold of your left foot for a few seconds. If you can't reach your toes, don't worry. Inhale to begin and exhale as you stretch. Repeat with your right leg.

Your 4th week

THIS WEEK, YOU'LL NEED A LITTLE PATIENCE AS YOU WAIT, WONDER, AND HOPE

The embryo-to-be, now securely implanted in the lining of your uterus, is starting to develop. Although you could do a home pregnancy test this week, you may end up disappointed or uncertain because at this stage a definite result is unlikely. It can be nerve racking, wondering if an unwanted period is about to arrive and dash your hopes. Talk to your partner and share your feelings with them—they may be anxious, too.

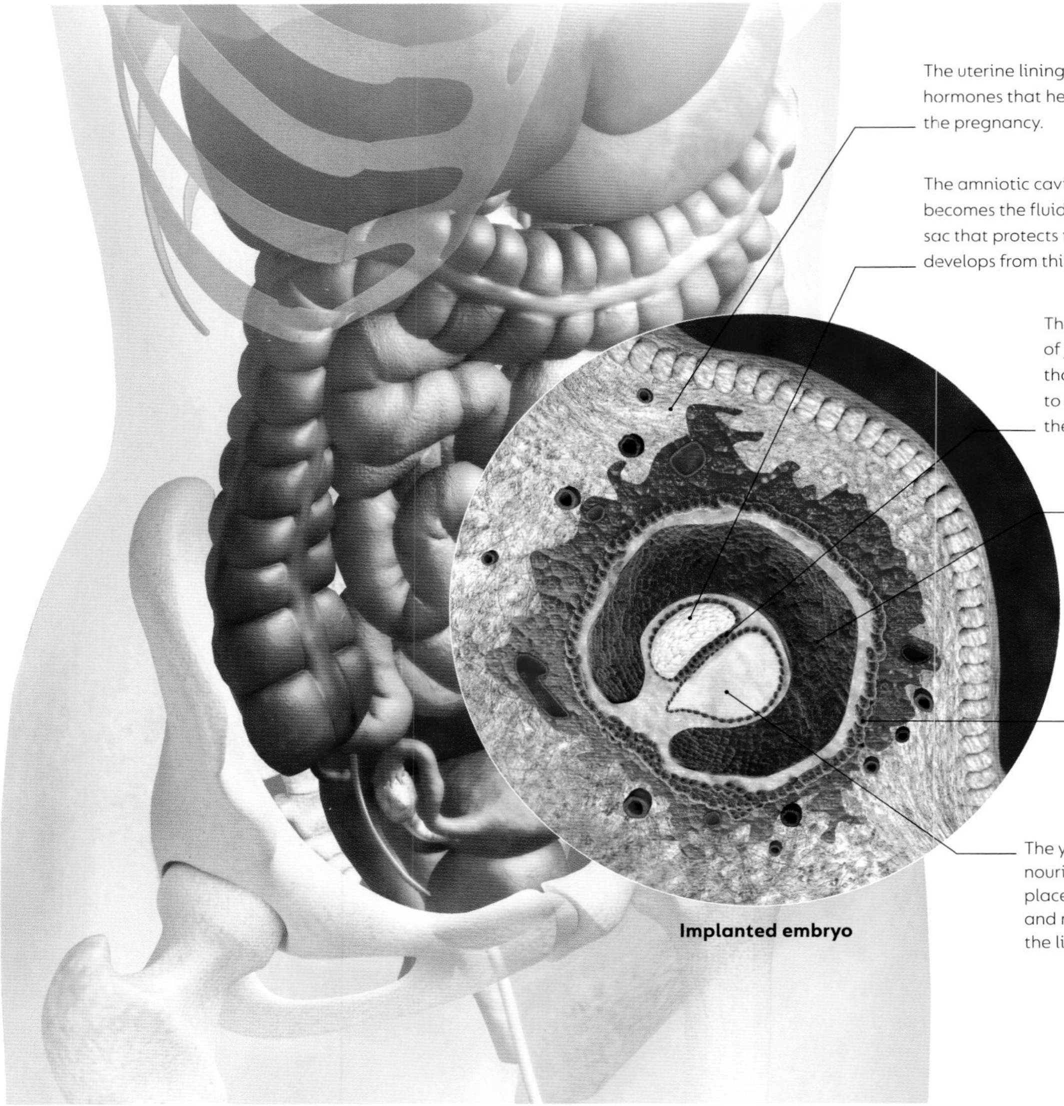

The uterine lining secretes hormones that help to support the pregnancy.
The amniotic cavity, which later becomes the fluid-filled amniotic sac that protects the baby, develops from this area.
The embryo consists of just two layers of cells that will divide very rapidly to form the beginnings of the baby's body.
Chorionic cavity
The placenta starts to develop here. Soon the cells will penetrate the lining of the uterus.
The yolk sac is forming. It will nourish the embryo until the placenta starts functioning and make blood cells until the liver can do this.

Implanted embryo

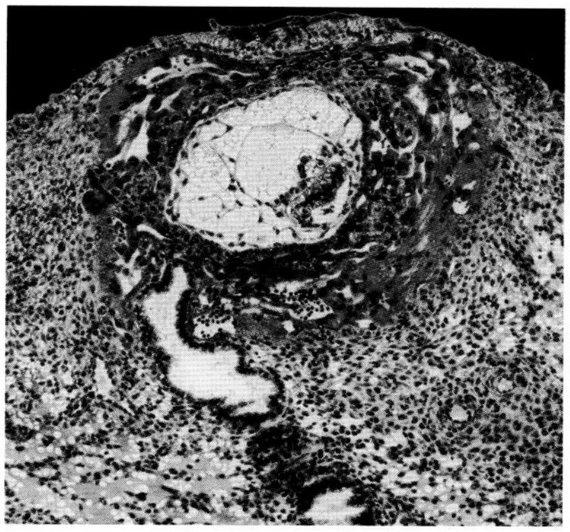

YOU ARE **3 WEEKS AND 1 DAY**

258 days to go

YOUR BABY TODAY

This is a cross section of the ball of cells embedded in the uterus at this early stage of pregnancy. It contains fluid in the center and two areas of white cells with a darker streak of cells between them—these will form the embryo, now less than 0.5 mm long.

> “ Pregnancy hormones are being produced, but it may be difficult to detect them accurately, so it's best to wait before you do a test. ”

You might be eager to do a pregnancy test as you enter the fourth week of your cycle. Most women use over-the-counter home pregnancy tests (see p.71). These are simple to use and work by detecting the levels of hCG in your urine—this is the hormone that is produced as soon as the embryo implants in the lining of the uterus (see p.61).

There are home pregnancy tests that claim to detect a pregnancy six days before your period is due. But if you use one of these and test this early, your hCG levels (see above) may not be high enough to give a positive result, even though you might be pregnant.

ASK A DOCTOR

I'm worried about doing a pregnancy test because I think my partner is going to be disappointed if I'm not pregnant. Feeling pressured to conceive is stressful, and this can affect the hypothalamus (see p.38)—the structure in your brain that governs your menstrual cycle. So your partner's avid interest may actually be counterproductive.

Be honest with your partner about how you feel. Explain to him that you share his enthusiasm for having a baby, but that you're feeling pressured, and that you're worried it will affect your ability to conceive. Conversely, if you aren't entirely sure that you are ready for a baby, now is the time to discuss this, too. Pregnancy is a life-changing event, and both you and your partner need to be fully committed, and also aware that it can, in itself, be stressful. Have fun together and make sure the pressure to conceive doesn't take the fun and spontaneity out of your lovemaking (see p.49).

YOUR PREGNANCY DIARY

Trying to get pregnant is an exciting experience, so why not keep a written record—it's a good way to pass time in this interim period while you're waiting to take a pregnancy test. Rather than just noting down the dates of your period and signs of ovulation, use it to record the highs and lows so far.

Once you're pregnant, you can continue to use the diary to record your feelings: for example, your emotions when you saw the positive symbol on the pregnancy testing kit; how you broke the news to your partner and their response; what your baby's first kick felt like; the best and worst aspects of being pregnant. You may also find that letting off steam about your partner's quirks or your mother-in-law's idiosyncrasies, for example, is surprisingly therapeutic!

Besides providing a unique record of your pregnancy, keeping a journal can also help you in subsequent pregnancies: for example, you may find it reassuring to look back and find that morning sickness was just a phase.

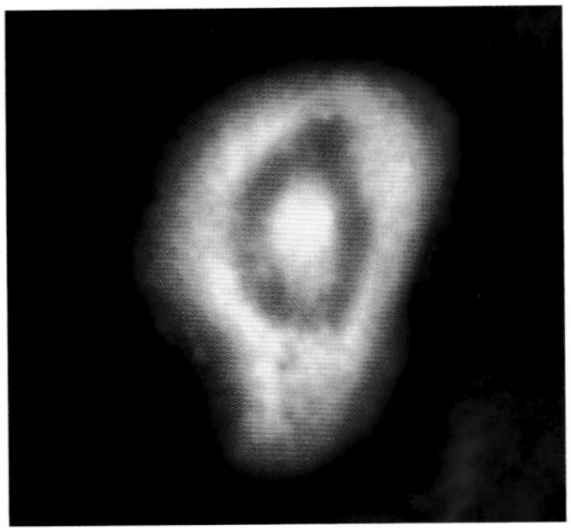

YOU ARE **3 WEEKS AND 2 DAYS**

257 days to go

YOUR BABY TODAY

In this computer-generated image the entire blastocyst can be seen embedded in the lining of the uterus. The cells that will develop into the embryo are seen as the dark area in the 12 o'clock position.

Once your pregnancy is confirmed in the next week or so, you'll find you're bombarded with more health information than ever. Is your diet well balanced? Do you need to look at the amount of salt, sugar, and fast food you eat? Have you started taking your folic acid supplements (see p.35) and your vitamin D too (see p.79)? Are you exercising enough and safely? Even though you don't know you're pregnant yet, it's worth being aware of the recommended advice and making some basic dietary and lifestyle changes. Turn to the section on pages 14–29 for some up-to-date information. It's also worth being aware of the early signs of pregnancy so you know what's normal.

If you have a preexisting medical condition or are taking medication, seek medical advice.

> "Adopting a healthy lifestyle and improving your well-being are sensible measures now that you might be pregnant."

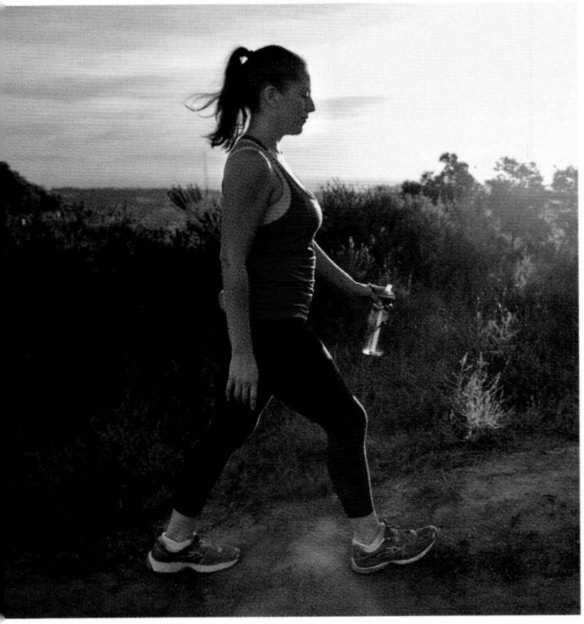

Get gentle exercise, such as walking or swimming, which are ideal before, during, and after pregnancy.

LIFESTYLE CHANGES

If you smoke, you should quit (so should your partner) for health reasons. Once you're pregnant, not smoking will reduce the risk of miscarriage, stillbirth, premature birth, low birth weight, and sudden infant death.

There are at least 30 chemicals in cigarette smoke that can adversely affect fertility. Because smoking reduces the rate at which cells replicate, it may cause most damage during the first days and weeks of pregnancy. Smoking can also have negative effects on sperm and reduce testosterone in men.

Because smoking reduces the rate at which cells replicate, it may cause most damage during the first days and weeks of pregnancy. In addition to causing fertility problems in women, smoking can have negative effects on sperm and reduce testosterone in men.

CULTURAL BELIEFS

In some countries, there is great emphasis placed on protecting the unborn baby:

- Hindu fathers part the hair on their partner's head three times upward from the front to the back to boost the development of the growing baby.
- In Thailand, the pregnant woman's abdomen may be painted to ward off evil spirits. It is also believed that giving gifts before the birth will attract evil spirits.

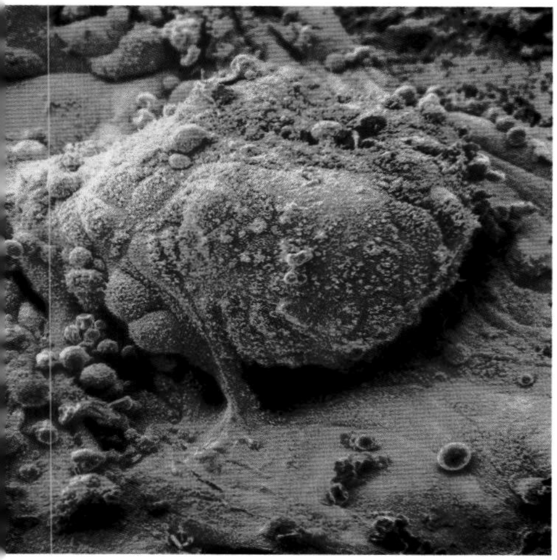

YOU ARE **3 WEEKS AND 3 DAYS**

256 days to go

YOUR BABY TODAY

The embryo is implanted and is 10 days old. The entry point at which the embryo buried into the lining of the uterus is now covered by a clot, and this prevents blood loss and protects the embryo.

> “ Try to stay busy to distract yourself from constantly wondering whether you're pregnant, and think positively. ”

Waiting for your period to start—or better yet, not start—can be quite stressful when you're trying to conceive. If your menstrual cycle is irregular you may not know when your period is due and therefore may not know if you're late and potentially pregnant or not. The uncertainty is likely to make you anxious and every time you go to the bathroom you dread seeing that your period has started.

Whether or not you know you have fertility problems, the wait can be difficult. If you do get your period, the disappointment can be hard. The cycle of having your period, waiting for ovulation, hoping you're pregnant, and then finding out you're not can become very wearing month after month.

If you have been trying to conceive for a year with no luck then you should go to your doctor for tests. Or go at six months if you are over 35 or know that you may have fertility problems, such as blocked fallopian tubes. Try confiding in a good friend about your problems so that you have someone to talk to, but try not to become obsessive and let it dominate all your relationships.

If you've only just started trying, remember there is only a 1 in 4 or 5 chance that you will conceive each month, so you're unlikely to get pregnant in the first month of trying!

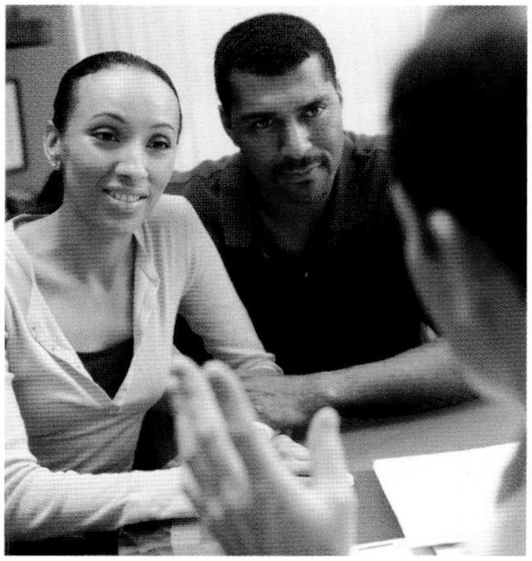

If you're over 35 and have been trying to conceive for six months, speak to your doctor about fertility tests. You should both go for checkups because your partner's sperm will need to be tested too.

ASK A DOCTOR

I did an early pregnancy test and have failed to conceive again, for the sixth month. Could it be because I have irregular periods? Menstrual cycles that vary significantly in length from month to month are considered irregular. An irregular cycle can be troublesome when trying to conceive, but being aware of the signs of ovulation (see p.43) may help you determine when you are approaching your short window of fertility.

Irregular ovulation and menstruation account for around 30–40 percent of fertility problems. Many factors determine how fertile a woman is, such as her age, whether her cervical fluid is wet enough to sustain sperm, or whether her fallopian tubes are open, but the most important factor is whether she ovulates regularly. Sometimes, a condition called anovulation occurs, in which there is irregular menstrual bleeding with no ovulation. If you don't release an egg each month, you won't have as many chances to conceive. To improve your chances of conceiving, you may be given medication to stimulate egg production and boost ovulation.

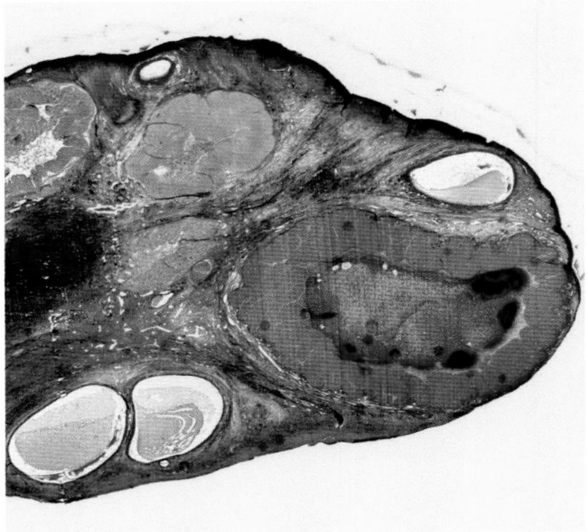

YOU ARE **3 WEEKS AND 4 DAYS**

255 days to go

YOUR BABY TODAY

To embed itself in the lining of the uterus, the embryo-to-be needs the help of progesterone, secreted after ovulation by the empty egg follicle, the corpus luteum (shown in pink in this cross section of an ovary). Progesterone helps the lining thicken.

" Do you feel different? You'll find yourself analyzing every twinge in your body as you look for signs that you're pregnant. "

It's still very early and you're unlikely to have pregnancy symptoms yet—although you may have some light spotting (see opposite). Some women claim to "feel" pregnant, even before changes to their breasts are noticeable or before they start feeling sick. Some women say that they just "know." You may be very in tune with your body and may notice that your body is changing even before you are able to take a test. Unfortunately, sometimes our minds can play tricks on us: you may want to be pregnant so much that you can sometimes convince yourself that you're feeling different. If you don't feel any different, don't worry, this is also completely normal.

Either way the only definitive way to know whether or not you are pregnant is to take a pregnancy test (see p.71). You don't need to go to your doctor to confirm your pregnancy. If the test is positive, you're pregnant!

DIET BAN

Don't diet! Restricting your food intake during pregnancy may mean your unborn baby misses out on valuable nutrients and increases risk of complications.

The doctor will weigh you and measure your height at your first visit to calculate your BMI and give you dietary advice if necessary. Eat normally and do not eat for two. Sensible weight gain in pregnancy will reduce the risk of gestational diabetes and preeclampsia.

If you are already on a restricted diet due to advice from a health professional, seek advice on how to adapt your diet for pregnancy. If you have been following food trends that limit eating particular foods or food groups, such as clean eating, dairy-free, or gluten-free (see right), seek advice to make sure your diet is not lacking in essential nutrients.

ASK A NUTRITIONIST

Can I eat a gluten-free diet during pregnancy? If you have celiac disease, it's important to keep your diet gluten-free in pregnancy to reduce your risk of complications. Or you may use gluten-free foods if you are intolerant of gluten. In either case, additional calcium, iron, and vitamin B12 may be needed, so make sure you have at least three portions of dairy products or alternatives a day, and eat lean red meat for iron and vitamin B12, or take supplements. In the US, almost 95 percent of flour is enriched with iron and four of the B vitamins including folic acid. Since gluten-free bread is not made with wheat, these nutrients need to be supplied elsewhere.

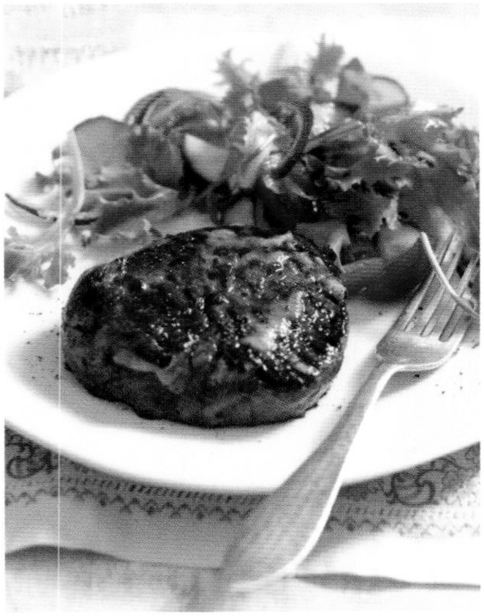

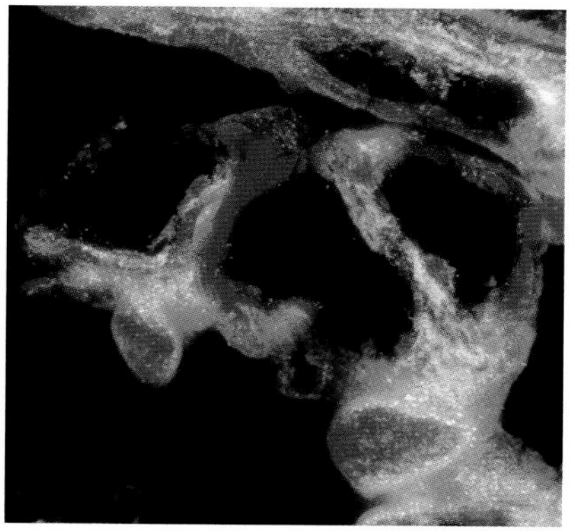

YOU ARE **3 WEEKS AND 5 DAYS**

254 days to go

YOUR BABY TODAY

The first stage of placental development—your baby's life support system—is shown here. The image shows nuclei (blue) within a continuous network of cells that will become the placental villi. At first the tiny villi are solid; later, they will contain blood vessels.

The ball of cells, known as the blastocyst, that will form the embryo has now completely embedded within the lining of the uterus and the lining has regenerated over it. Only about half of all fertilized eggs progress to become a blastocyst and only about half of these successfully implant.

When the blastocyst embeds, there may be some bleeding, known as "spotting." This can lead to confusion when dating the pregnancy as it can occur around the time that you would normally start your period. In most cases, the blood is pinkish, although bright red blood (fresh blood) can occur, as can brownish, old blood. As long as it is not profuse, the color really doesn't matter. If the bleeding lasts for a short period, and you don't experience discomfort, it's likely that things are just fine, but do see your doctor for a checkup.

Around 25 percent of women will bleed in early pregnancy, but most go on to full-term. However, in some cases of bleeding, especially if there is also period-like pain, it does mean a miscarriage is occurring, so always report it to your doctor. Up to a third of pregnancies miscarry up to the fifth week and around a quarter between the fifth and seventh weeks. The risk becomes much lower as the weeks go by, decreasing dramatically after the 12th week of pregnancy.

> " As the fertilized egg becomes completely embedded in your uterus, it may cause some light bleeding. "

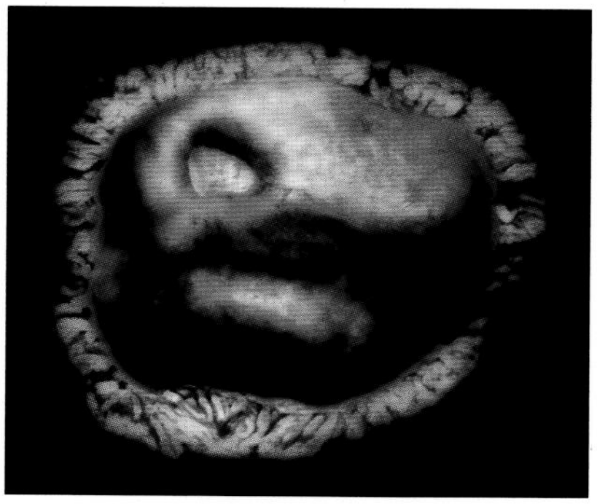

This computer-generated image shows the ball of cells—the blastocyst—as it appears situated within the uterus. The outer ring of interconnected cells that will eventually form the placenta are clearly seen.

DOUBLING UP

As with many parents, you probably thought long and hard about trying to conceive your second child. There's no ideal age gap, but consider:

The pros of a small age gap:

- **You are in "baby mode"** and will be used to the routine and all aspects of baby care. You will have all the equipment you need from bottles to a stroller and crib.
- **A two-year-old** might find it easier to accept his new sibling than a four-year-old who is much more conscious of having the sole attention of his parents.
- There will be squabbles, but children close in age tend to play better together.

The cons of a small age gap:

- **It's tiring** caring for a one- or two-year-old while pregnant.
- **It can put a strain on your body** to have pregnancies close together.
- If you have a second baby before the first one can walk, you will be doing a lot of carrying, increasing the risk of backache.
- **You won't have as much time** to get to know your first child before your second is on the scene.

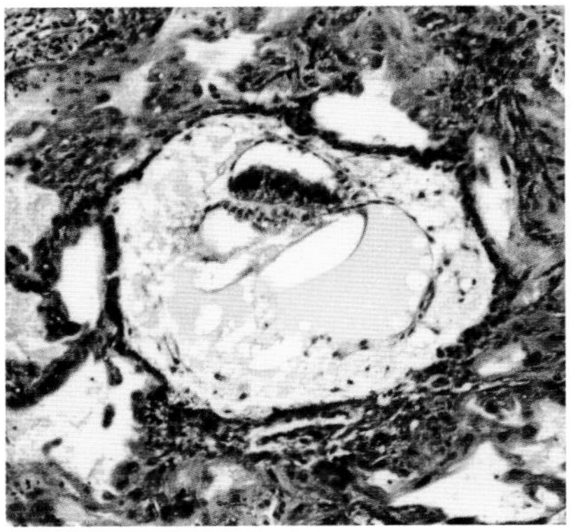

YOU ARE **3 WEEKS AND 6 DAYS**

253 days to go

YOUR BABY TODAY

This microscope view of an embedded blastocyst shows the amniotic cavity (semcircular white area at top), with the cells that will develop into the baby just below (dark oval at the 12 o'clock position). The yolk sac is the pink area below.

" Complex changes are taking place inside your uterus to create a safe and nourishing environment for your unborn baby. "

The ball of cells embedded in the uterus is already laying down the foundations for its future life as an embryo. At two layers thick, the germ cells form a flat disk that divides the fluid-filled inner part of the ball of cells into two chambers. The smaller of these fluid-filled chambers will become the amniotic sac. The larger chamber, lying closest to the future placenta, will become the yolk sac that supports the early embryo.

The umbilical cord will eventually develop close to the smaller chamber. The inner germ cells have been developing at a slower rate than the rapidly expanding outer cell layers.

At first the umbilical cord is a simple stalk, containing no blood vessels but simply anchoring the embryo to the future placenta (see p.76), which will eventually become your unborn baby's lifeline.

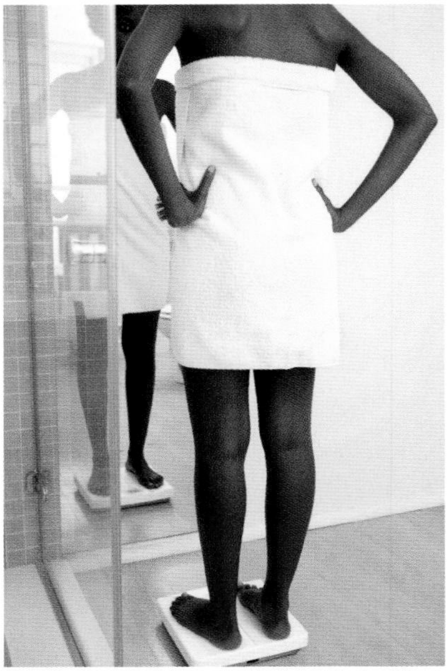

You'll gain weight, but not necessarily an excessive amount. Try not to become obsessive about weighing yourself.

ASK A NUTRITIONIST

I'm hoping I'm pregnant, but I'm already worrying about the amount of weight I might put on. These days, it is almost impossible to avoid seeing the latest celebrity who has not only fit right back into her clothes after having her baby, but who actually weighs less than she did before pregnancy. However, this is concerning for health professionals, since a dramatic weight loss after the birth is not good for mother or baby.

The recommended weight gain during pregnancy is 25–35 lb, have a BMI (see p.16) within the normal range. Your baby and her support system will make up a good proportion of this, as will the increased pregnancy fluids, fats, and an enlarged uterus (see p.99). Be reassured that much of this extra weight will be lost as soon as your baby is born.

Also, after the birth, some of this extra weight provides nutrients for breast-feeding, which uses up to 500 calories a day.

The most sensible approach to controlling your weight during pregnancy is to eat a healthy diet and get gentle exercise to ensure that weight gain is not too dramatic. You only need additional calories in the last trimester of pregnancy. Aim for an additional 200 calories a day, which is the equivalent of a banana and a glass of milk.

Newborns are getting heavier mostly due to improved diet and living standards. However, obesity in the mother is another factor—if the mother is overweight, there is an increased risk of diabetes (see p.475), which can increase the baby's weight.

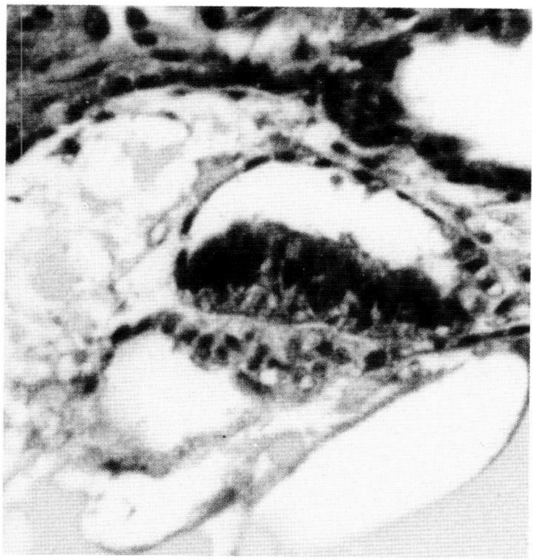

YOU ARE **4 WEEKS EXACTLY**

252 days to go

YOUR BABY TODAY

This highly magnified image shows that the embryo consists of two layers of cells. Those of the upper darker layer are more rectangular in shape and lie on the side of the amniotic cavity, and those of the lower layer lie on the side of the yolk sac.

Nature has a strange way of working. You might feel low if you have your usual PMS symptoms and think it means that you haven't conceived, but in fact, there are many similarities between PMS symptoms and those of early pregnancy. This is because the hormones that cause PMS are raised in pregnancy and so can cause the same symptoms. In addition to this, you might be irritable and emotional even without having PMS, just due to the anxiety of wanting to be pregnant and waiting to see whether or not your period arrives.

While you are in the middle of this storm of hormones and raging emotions, it can be difficult to remain calm. Talk to your partner about your emotions and anxieties—just expressing that you're finding things stressful can help you get through this tense time. Alternatively, confide in a female relative or friend, who might be able to relate to how you're feeling.

Frustratingly, at this point it is still a waiting game; all you can do is try to be patient until you take your pregnancy test. If your period was due today—day 28 of your cycle—and hasn't made an appearance, you can take a test as early as today or tomorrow. Good luck!

> **" Are you feeling irritable and tired, and are your breasts tender? Well, you might just be pregnant! "**

PELVIC FLOOR EXERCISES

It's never too early to start Kegel exercises and you'll be glad you did once you become pregnant. The pelvic floor is a broad sling of muscles that stretches between your legs and extends from the pubic bone in front to the spine at the rear. It holds and supports your bladder, uterus, and bowel in place and controls the muscles that hold closed the anus, urethra, and vagina.

Try these simple steps to tone your pelvic floor:

First try to locate your pelvic floor; close your eyes—now visualize the sling of muscles stretching right across your body holding your uterus and bladder.

Next contract your pelvic floor muscles pulling inward and upward, hold for a count of five, then release. Repeat this exercise at least 10 times a day.

Test: if you're having trouble identifying the muscles, imagine that you are trying to stop the flow of urine; the muscles you feel contracting are those of the pelvic floor.

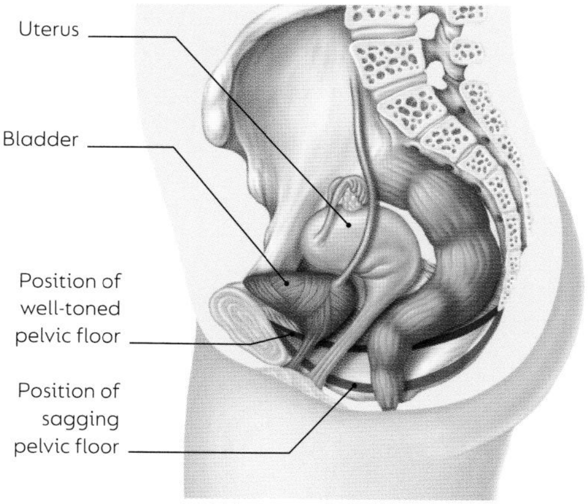
Uterus
Bladder
Position of well-toned pelvic floor
Position of sagging pelvic floor

Your 5th week

IF YOU HAVE NO PERIOD AND A POSITIVE TEST RESULT, YOU'RE GOING TO HAVE A BABY! When your pregnancy is confirmed, it's natural to experience a mixed bag of emotions—excitement, disbelief, joy, and anxiety. Everything is about to change forever for you and your partner. Give yourselves time to take in the big news. You may not feel pregnant yet, but momentous changes are taking place in the hidden world of your uterus. Step by step, the building blocks of life are being set in place.

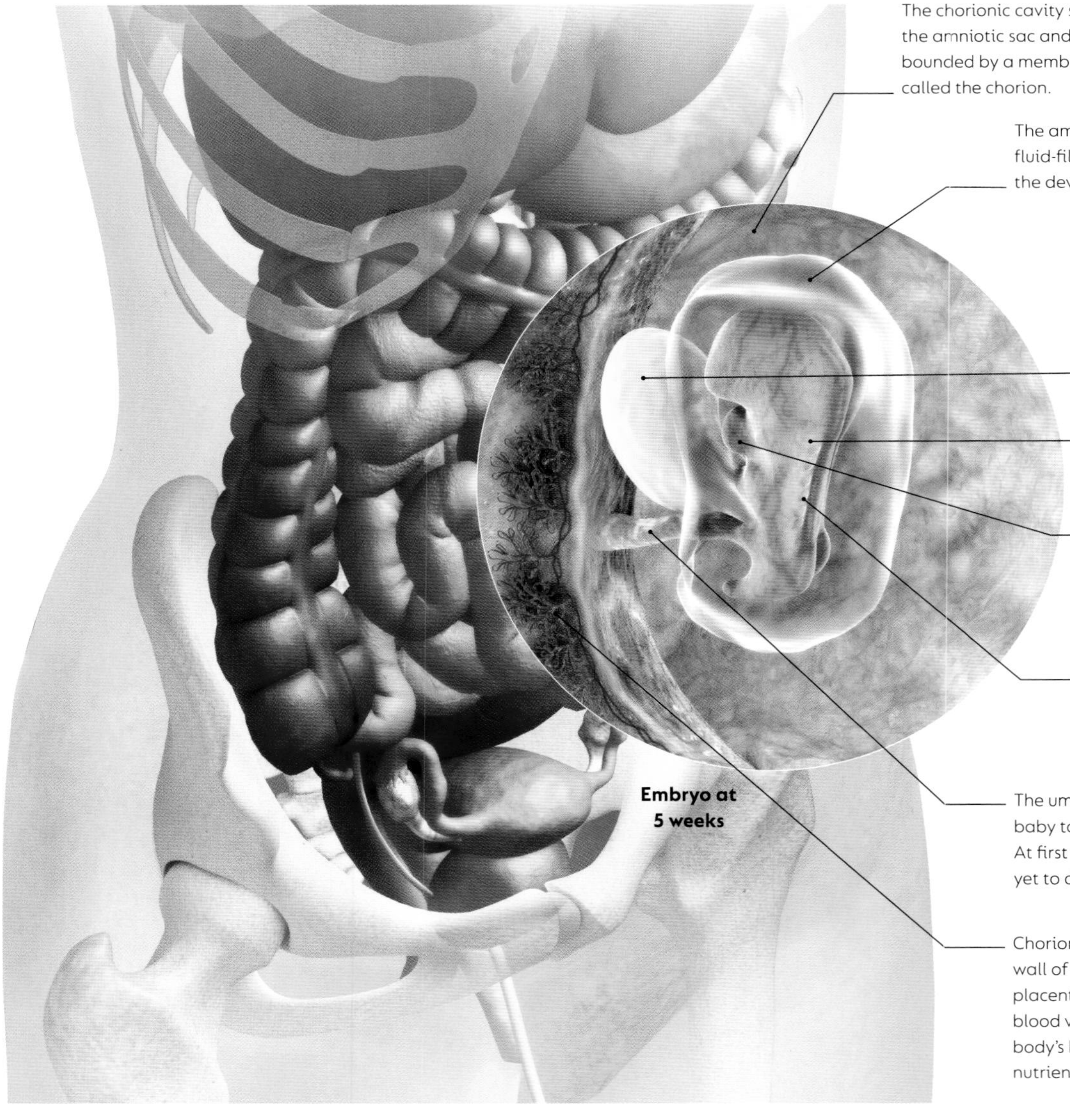

The chorionic cavity surrounds the amniotic sac and is bounded by a membrane called the chorion.

The amniotic sac is a fluid-filled sac that cocoons the developing embryo.

The yolk sac nourishes the embryo until the placenta is established and can provide nutrients through its blood supply.

The embryo now measures 0.09 in (2.5 mm).

Embryonic tissues are already forming into a structure that will become the heart.

A fold down the back of the embryo marks the beginnings of the spine.

The umbilical cord connects the baby to the developing placenta. At first it is rather short and has yet to develop any coils.

Chorionic villi reach into the wall of the uterus to form the placenta. The villi contain blood vessels that tap into your body's blood supply to access nutrients for the baby.

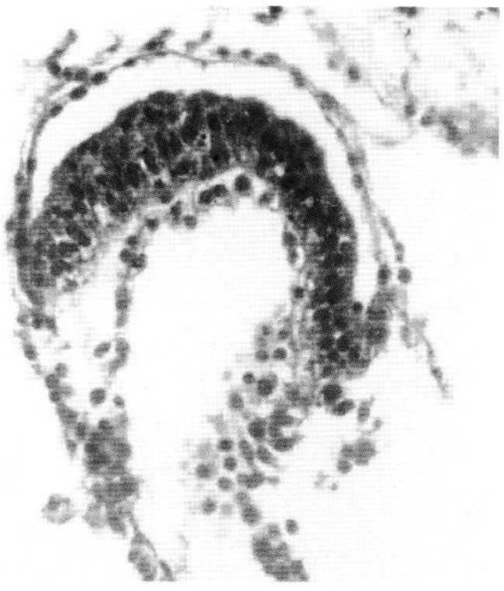

YOU ARE **4 WEEKS AND 1 DAY**

251 days to go

YOUR BABY TODAY

This is a microscope view of the amniotic cavity with the cells that will become the baby in close-up. These cells will repeatedly divide and multiply, becoming more and more specialized at each stage of their development.

“ The waiting is over. If your period hasn’t started, take a home pregnancy test to find out whether you’ve conceived. ”

If you’ve missed your period (if your normal cycle is no more than 28 days and that your period is therefore late), you may want to do a home pregnancy test today.

A home pregnancy test, available at pharmacists and most supermarkets, contains a chemical that reacts if your urine contains the hormone hCG (human chorionic gonadotropin). This is produced by an implanting embryo and will be found in your urine if you are pregnant. Levels of hCG are likely to be over 50 mIU/ml on the day your period is due. With between 97 and 99 percent accuracy, the majority of over-the-counter tests are sensitive enough to detect this amount, so they can be used on the first day of your missed period; some can be used earlier (see p.63).

The tests turn positive once there is a certain level of the hCG hormone present in your urine: if you test too early, the result might be negative even though you’re pregnant. Therefore, if you don’t get your period but had a negative result, test again after two to three days. If you are pregnant, the levels of hCG will have risen, giving a positive result. If you get a positive result but your period starts anyway, it may be that you have suffered a very early miscarriage.

HOW TO USE A HOME PREGNANCY TEST

Always read the instructions, but most tests work as follows:

- **You urinate on the stick** and leave it for a specified number of minutes.
- **A symbol will appear** in the control window to indicate the test is working (if this does not appear, the test is faulty). If a symbol then appears in the results window, you are pregnant.
- **It is advisable to do the test** first thing in the morning when your urine is most concentrated. By doing this, the hCG levels are likely to be detected more easily.
- **The results symbol** gradually fades, so read it after the specified time, not later. Do another test the next morning if you’re unsure of the result.

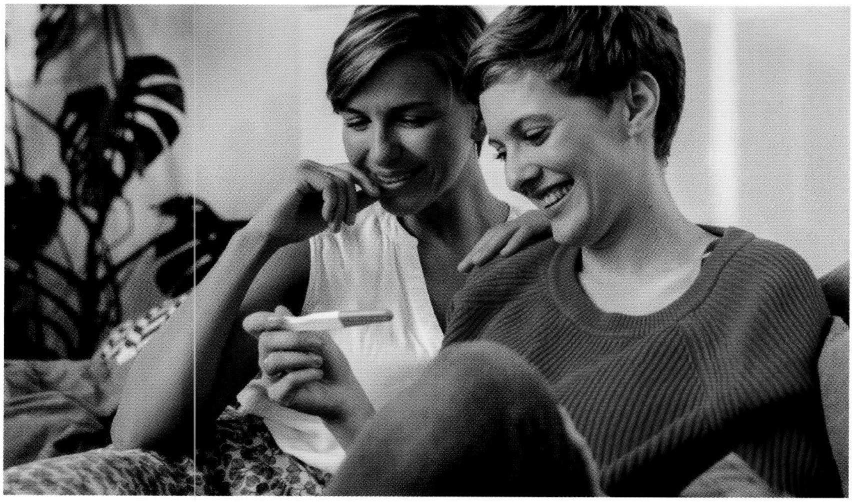

You can find out within minutes whether or not you are expecting a baby, but as you await this life-changing result, it can seem like a lifetime before the symbol appears.

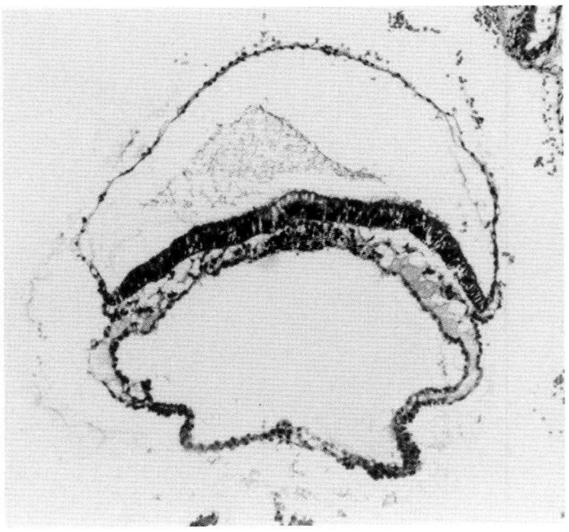

YOU ARE **4 WEEKS AND 2 DAYS**

250 days to go

YOUR BABY TODAY

The embryo until this stage of development has consisted of two layers of cells. Now, a third layer starts to become visible as a "bulge" between the two—this bulge can be seen in the center of this image.

> " In this third week since conception, the cells that will become the embryo move to form the basis of the central nervous system. "

While you're busy coming to terms with being pregnant, there are incredible changes taking place inside you. The group of cells, that will become your baby is currently shaped as a flat disk and undergoing significant development. A narrow groove begins to form down the middle of the cells. The leading edge of the groove is slightly wider, forming a circular "node." The outer edges of the node and groove are slightly raised. The cells move from the rolled edges of these structures downward into the groove to lie between the original two layers of cells. This creates three layers of cells, those on each outer disk surface and those sandwiched between them. The node and groove do not extend along the entire length of the disk.

At the head end, a separate groove forms. Called the neural groove, this ultimately forms the brain and spinal cord (the central nervous system). In four days' time, the disk will lengthen and widen at the end that will form your baby's head. In six days' time, the neural groove has folds on either side that will later meet to form the neural tube.

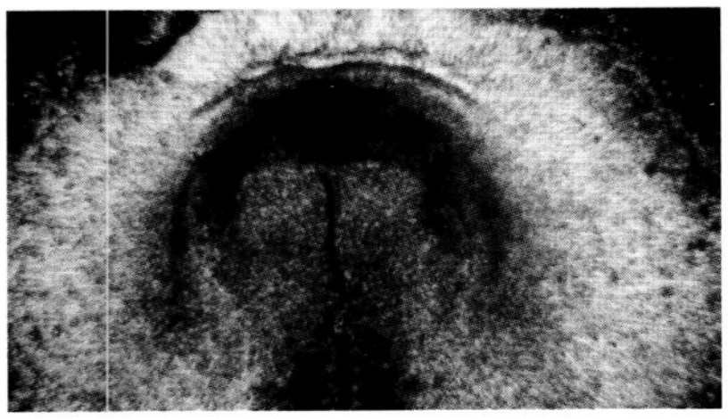

Shown here is the neural tube of an embryo in the early stages of pregnancy. The brain and spinal cord will develop from the neural tube. If the tube does not fully close, it can lead to birth defects, most commonly spina bifida.

ASK A DOCTOR

I've been having difficulty getting pregnant and have now been diagnosed with polycystic ovary syndrome. What is this? This condition causes the ovaries to be bigger than normal and they produce a large number of small follicles that never grow to full maturity. Therefore an egg is not released to be fertilized and periods are very irregular.

The condition is a common cause of fertility problems. Treatments are aimed at stimulating ovulation and reducing some of the symptoms such as increased body hair and acne. Polycystic ovary syndrome appears to run in families.

FOCUS ON RELATIONSHIPS

It's the positive result you've been waiting for—hopefully!—but how do you share it with your partner? You could present them with an envelope containing your positive pregnancy test, or explain that you have a "special gift" but it won't be ready until about, oh, nine months. It shouldn't take them long to figure it out! Ideally, choose a time when you are both alone and feeling relaxed so that it can be a special moment. You may want to do another test with your partner just to make sure and also so that they feel involved.

Even if you're excited, and even if you can't get in touch with your partner for a day, don't be tempted to tell your mom and close friends first. Your partner may be upset if others know they're going to be a parent before they do.

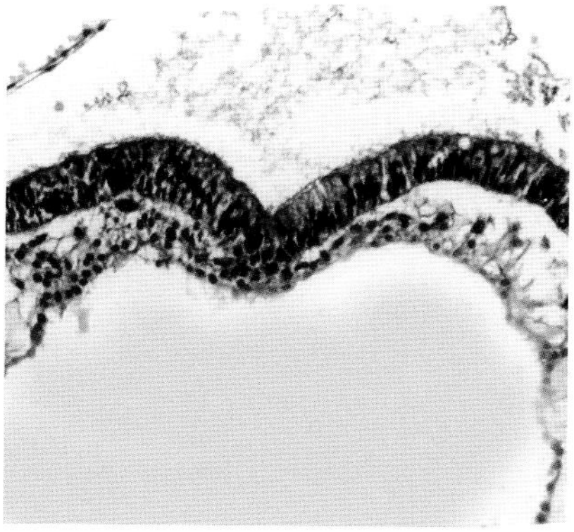

YOU ARE **4 WEEKS AND 3 DAYS**

249 days to go

YOUR BABY TODAY

As the embryo transforms from two cell layers into three, a groove develops along the back of the embryo. This groove (the dark area in the center of this image) will develop into the embryo's neural tube—the forerunner of the brain and spinal cord.

> "Happy? Excited? But a little nervous? There is no greater life-changing event than finding out you're going to have a baby."

CONNECTING THROUGH DREAMS

Pregnant women often try to connect with their baby through dreams. You may find it difficult to bond fully with your baby and believe you're actually pregnant. A common dream in pregnancy is that you're swimming; it is thought to be a way of trying to "reach" the baby, who will soon be bathed in water (fluid) inside you.

In the few days since you conceived, you may have experienced a whole host of different feelings. Even if you planned to get pregnant, it's perfectly normal for the initial elation to be replaced with some anxiety as the reality hits you that you are going to have a baby. You might also doubt the result of the test you've taken and not actually believe it until you begin to have some of the early symptoms of pregnancy.

Your partner may react differently than you. If they don't appear as excited, don't interpret this as meaning that they are not happy about the news; not everyone deals with big events in the same way, and it might be some time before the reality of becoming a parent hits them. Withdrawing may be their way of processing the information. Conversely, you may find they are actually more excited about the news than you!

Handling your feelings might be made more difficult by trying to keep the pregnancy a secret, for the time being. Most couples decide not to tell people until after the 12-week scan when the miscarriage risk is significantly decreased, but you may find that confiding in a few close relatives and friends will give you a much-needed outlet to talk about your feelings.

SURPRISED TO BE PREGNANT?

If you become pregnant while using contraception, it is unlikely to have done your baby any harm, but here's what you should do:

- **Contraceptive pill:** stop taking it.
- **Contraceptive patch:** remove it.
- **Contraceptive implant:** see your doctor to have it removed.
- **IUD or IUS (intrauterine device or intrauterine system):** visit your doctor without delay if you're using either since there's a 6 percent risk that the pregnancy could be ectopic (see p.93). Even if a scan shows that the pregnancy is not ectopic, the IUD or IUS should be removed because there is a 50–60 percent chance of miscarriage. After 12 weeks of pregnancy, the device should not be removed since this could trigger a miscarriage.
- **Contraceptive injection (Depo-Provera):** see your doctor if you conceive while using this. Research indicates that it won't affect the unborn baby, but you should not have any more injections.
- **Morning-after pill:** once an egg has implanted, the morning-after pill has no effect. Do, however, see your doctor if you're concerned.

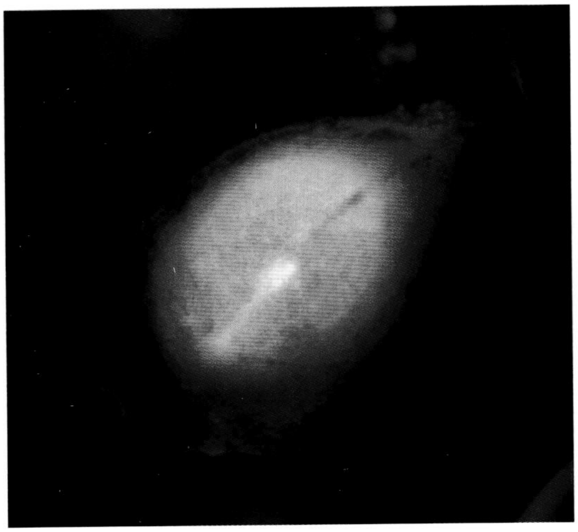

YOU ARE **4 WEEKS AND 4 DAYS**

248 days to go

YOUR BABY TODAY

The embryo seen from above now has a subtle groove (the primitive groove) and a small central depression (the primitive node), both seen here in white. These changes start at what will become the base of the spine and progress toward the head.

> **“ You’re probably eager to know when your baby will be born. The chart below will tell you the expected date of delivery. ”**

Until you have an ultrasound in a few weeks’ time, your baby’s due date will be calculated by counting 280 days from the first day of your last menstrual period—see chart, below. At the dating scan (see p.137), your baby will be measured and the age calculated. The scan date will then be used since it is considered to be accurate.

While you’re bound to want to know the due date, try not to get too fixated on it. Most babies are born within about two weeks of their due dates, but your baby will be considered to be born at term if you give birth between 37 and 42 weeks. So your estimated delivery date is just that—an estimate.

WHEN WILL YOUR BABY BE BORN?

To figure out your expected date of delivery (EDD)—also known as the due date—you need to know when you started your last menstrual period (LMP) (see p.35). Find your LMP date on the chart below to discover when your baby is expected. For example, if your last LMP was January 13, then your baby will be due on October 20.

January	**1**	**2**	**3**	**4**	**5**	**6**	**7**	**8**	**9**	**10**	**11**	**12**	**13**	**14**	**15**	**16**	**17**	**18**	**19**	**20**	**21**	**22**	**23**	**24**	**25**	**26**	**27**	**28**	**29**	**30**	**31**
Oct/Nov	8	9	10	11	12	13	14	15	16	17	18	19	20	21	22	23	24	25	26	27	28	29	30	31	1	2	3	4	5	6	7
February	**1**	**2**	**3**	**4**	**5**	**6**	**7**	**8**	**9**	**10**	**11**	**12**	**13**	**14**	**15**	**16**	**17**	**18**	**19**	**20**	**21**	**22**	**23**	**24**	**25**	**26**	**27**	**28**			
Nov/Dec	8	9	10	11	12	13	14	15	16	17	18	19	20	21	22	23	24	25	26	27	28	29	30	1	2	3	4	5			
March	**1**	**2**	**3**	**4**	**5**	**6**	**7**	**8**	**9**	**10**	**11**	**12**	**13**	**14**	**15**	**16**	**17**	**18**	**19**	**20**	**21**	**22**	**23**	**24**	**25**	**26**	**27**	**28**	**29**	**30**	**31**
Dec/Jan	6	7	8	9	10	11	12	13	14	15	16	17	18	19	20	21	22	23	24	25	26	27	28	29	30	31	1	2	3	4	5
April	**1**	**2**	**3**	**4**	**5**	**6**	**7**	**8**	**9**	**10**	**11**	**12**	**13**	**14**	**15**	**16**	**17**	**18**	**19**	**20**	**21**	**22**	**23**	**24**	**25**	**26**	**27**	**28**	**29**	**30**	
Jan/Feb	6	7	8	9	10	11	12	13	14	15	16	17	18	19	20	21	22	23	24	25	26	27	28	29	30	31	1	2	3	4	
May	**1**	**2**	**3**	**4**	**5**	**6**	**7**	**8**	**9**	**10**	**11**	**12**	**13**	**14**	**15**	**16**	**17**	**18**	**19**	**20**	**21**	**22**	**23**	**24**	**25**	**26**	**27**	**28**	**29**	**30**	**31**
Feb/Mar	5	6	7	8	9	10	11	12	13	14	15	16	17	18	19	20	21	22	23	24	25	26	27	28	1	2	3	4	5	6	7
June	**1**	**2**	**3**	**4**	**5**	**6**	**7**	**8**	**9**	**10**	**11**	**12**	**13**	**14**	**15**	**16**	**17**	**18**	**19**	**20**	**21**	**22**	**23**	**24**	**25**	**26**	**27**	**28**	**29**	**30**	
Mar/Apr	8	9	10	11	12	13	14	15	16	17	18	19	20	21	22	23	24	25	26	27	28	29	30	31	1	2	3	4	5	6	
July	**1**	**2**	**3**	**4**	**5**	**6**	**7**	**8**	**9**	**10**	**11**	**12**	**13**	**14**	**15**	**16**	**17**	**18**	**19**	**20**	**21**	**22**	**23**	**24**	**25**	**26**	**27**	**28**	**29**	**30**	**31**
Apr/May	7	8	9	10	11	12	13	14	15	16	17	18	19	20	21	22	23	24	25	26	27	28	29	30	1	2	3	4	5	6	7
August	**1**	**2**	**3**	**4**	**5**	**6**	**7**	**8**	**9**	**10**	**11**	**12**	**13**	**14**	**15**	**16**	**17**	**18**	**19**	**20**	**21**	**22**	**23**	**24**	**25**	**26**	**27**	**28**	**29**	**30**	**31**
May/June	8	9	10	11	12	13	14	15	16	17	18	19	20	21	22	23	24	25	26	27	28	29	30	31	1	2	3	4	5	6	7
September	**1**	**2**	**3**	**4**	**5**	**6**	**7**	**8**	**9**	**10**	**11**	**12**	**13**	**14**	**15**	**16**	**17**	**18**	**19**	**20**	**21**	**22**	**23**	**24**	**25**	**26**	**27**	**28**	**29**	**30**	
June/July	8	9	10	11	12	13	14	15	16	17	18	19	20	21	22	23	24	25	26	27	28	29	30	1	2	3	4	5	6	7	
October	**1**	**2**	**3**	**4**	**5**	**6**	**7**	**8**	**9**	**10**	**11**	**12**	**13**	**14**	**15**	**16**	**17**	**18**	**19**	**20**	**21**	**22**	**23**	**24**	**25**	**26**	**27**	**28**	**29**	**30**	**31**
July/Aug	8	9	10	11	12	13	14	15	16	17	18	19	20	21	22	23	24	25	26	27	28	29	30	31	1	2	3	4	5	6	7
November	**1**	**2**	**3**	**4**	**5**	**6**	**7**	**8**	**9**	**10**	**11**	**12**	**13**	**14**	**15**	**16**	**17**	**18**	**19**	**20**	**21**	**22**	**23**	**24**	**25**	**26**	**27**	**28**	**29**	**30**	
Aug/Sept	8	9	10	11	12	13	14	15	16	17	18	19	20	21	22	23	24	25	26	27	28	29	30	31	1	2	3	4	5	6	
December	**1**	**2**	**3**	**4**	**5**	**6**	**7**	**8**	**9**	**10**	**11**	**12**	**13**	**14**	**15**	**16**	**17**	**18**	**19**	**20**	**21**	**22**	**23**	**24**	**25**	**26**	**27**	**28**	**29**	**30**	**31**
Sept/Oct	7	8	9	10	11	12	13	14	15	16	17	18	19	20	21	22	23	24	25	26	27	28	29	30	1	2	3	4	5	6	7

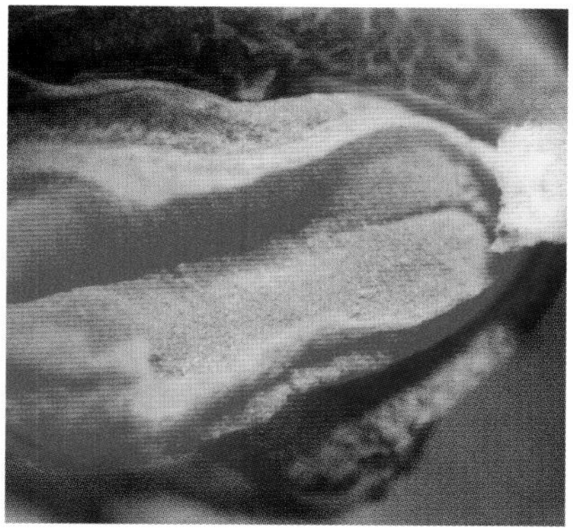

YOU ARE **4 WEEKS AND 5 DAYS**

247 days to go

YOUR BABY TODAY

The embryo, still less than 3 mm long, now has a deep and narrow groove extending along its entire length. This groove will soon become so deep and its edges will curl over so much that it forms into a tube running along the length of the embryo.

> “Although there’s lots of information to take in, try to enjoy this time and remember pregnancy is a natural process.”

No sooner than you found out you were pregnant, like most expectant women, you may have begun to worry about all aspects of your lifestyle and your unborn baby’s health. To put things in perspective, remember that in generations gone by pregnancy was considered to be a natural event, and few women made lifestyle changes to accommodate the condition. So in the past, pregnant women were likely to continue eating unhealthy foods, drinking alcohol, and smoking.

Furthermore, pregnancy tests tended to be much less accurate or sensitive, meaning that many pregnancies ended in early miscarriage without anyone being aware. For this reason, many of the problems now known to be risk factors for pregnancy complications or miscarriage were not analyzed or addressed, or worried about.

Today, with the benefit of a great deal of research, and precise monitoring of ovulation, conception, and pregnancy, women are very aware of what is happening inside their bodies, and are informed about the potential pitfalls. This is a mixed blessing: while it is important to avoid anything known to adversely affect your unborn baby, it is equally important to relax and enjoy the pregnancy, because stress is not good for you or your baby.

ORGANIC FOODS

Organic foods in the US can be fortified. Organic foods are usually preferable, but for dairy alternatives, such as soy milk, make sure that the minerals such as calcium and iodine that milk supplies have been added.

ASK A DOCTOR

I’m 40 and in great shape. Will the doctors still see my pregnancy as potentially high-risk? Women over age 40 are at higher risk in pregnancy from conditions such as diabetes, high blood pressure, problems with the placenta, and birth complications. They are also at an increased risk of having a baby with a chromosomal disorder.

For these reasons, you will be monitored to be sure that both you and your baby remain healthy. This way, any potential problems can be addressed and hopefully rectified early on. You will be offered increased monitoring and regular scans to check the growth of your baby.

You may be offered aspirin to start between 12 and 16 weeks to reduce the risk of preeclampsia (see p.474).

Due to a slight increase in late stillbirth you will also be offered induction of labor around your due date.

Try not to see the extra monitoring as an intrusion. It’s great that you’re in good shape, and if you continue to take care of your health and exercise regularly, you will reduce the risks of any complications occurring.

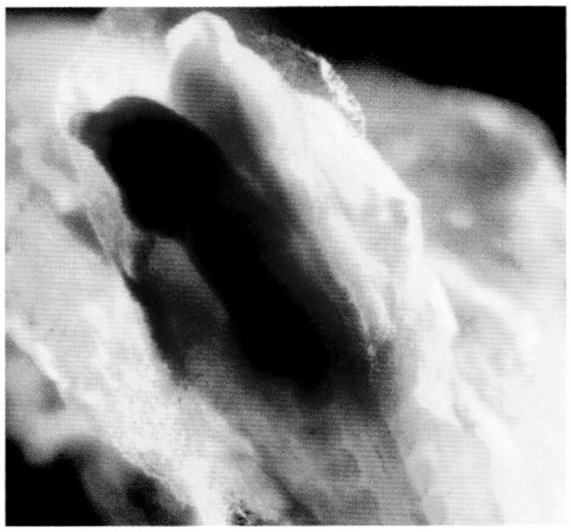

YOU ARE **4 WEEKS AND 6 DAYS**

246 days to go

YOUR BABY TODAY

The upper part of the embryo is shown. There is still a wide opening along the back of the embryo that will gradually close over the next few days. The head and lower spine portions are the last to close.

" The placenta—the structure that will become your unborn baby's lifeline—is forming. "

Your pregnancy test result may be the only sign that you're pregnant, but there are many fascinating changes taking place inside you. The basic structures that will form the placenta (see p.127) are now in place. The outer layer of cells that originally entered the lining of the uterus are now coated with projections of placental tissue. It is the outer cells that are in direct contact with small lakes of your blood. The inner placental projections or fronds are termed "villi." Some villi anchor the pregnancy to your tissues and, from these, smaller free-floating villi arise. Later, more branches will appear and ultimately resemble the branching pattern of a fern leaf. The villi are still immature and have not established a blood supply of their own. It will be several weeks before the placenta is mature enough to supply all the oxygen and nutrients that your developing baby needs.

ASK A MOM

I really wanted a baby, but now that I have a positive pregnancy test result, I'm suddenly not so sure. Is this normal?
I felt exactly the same at first and after talking to friends discovered that lots of them had mixed feelings, especially at the beginning. I found a good way to overcome this was to focus on the reasons why I wanted the baby. I wrote these down. Then I tried to figure out what I was really worrying about. Was it the thought of giving up some freedom? Financial worries? Concerns that I wouldn't be a good parent? This helped me get things in perspective and realize I really did want the baby.

SEEING YOUR DOCTOR

If you've had a positive pregnancy test, call your doctor's office to schedule your first prenatal visit, which will be between 8 and 12 weeks. The receptionist will likely ask the date of your last menstrual period to properly time the appointment.

- **At the appointment,** your doctor will confirm your home pregnancy test results with urine and blood tests and possibly an ultrasound, as well. She will also determine your estimated due date based on the date of your last menstrual period.
- **This first visit will typically be your longest appointment,** since the doctor will give you a thorough physical examination, take your family and personal health history, and answer any of your pregnancy-related questions or concerns.
- **You will be weighed** and have your blood pressure checked.
- **You'll also have blood drawn** for several tests, including your blood type, Rh status, and a variety of sexually transmitted diseases.

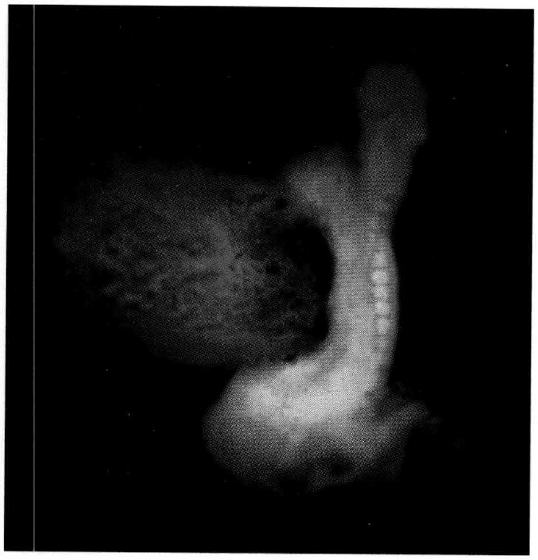

YOU ARE **5 WEEKS EXACTLY**

245 days to go

YOUR BABY TODAY

The bulge at the lower part of this image will eventually become the baby's head. Segments called somites (seen as bright, round areas running down one side of the embryo), which will form the baby's spine, have started to develop.

> “ At this important stage of development, the building blocks of your baby's spine are being laid down. ”

By the end of this 5th week, individual elements that will form the embryo have begun to develop.

Starting at what will become the head end, individual segments, called “somites,” form. Roughly three new pairs of somites appear every day and each forms part of your baby's spine as well as the muscles associated with each segment of the body. Eventually there will be four somites at the head, eight in the region of the neck, 12 at chest level, five in the lumbar region, and five in the pelvic area.

More somites develop in the baby below the pelvis but most disappear.

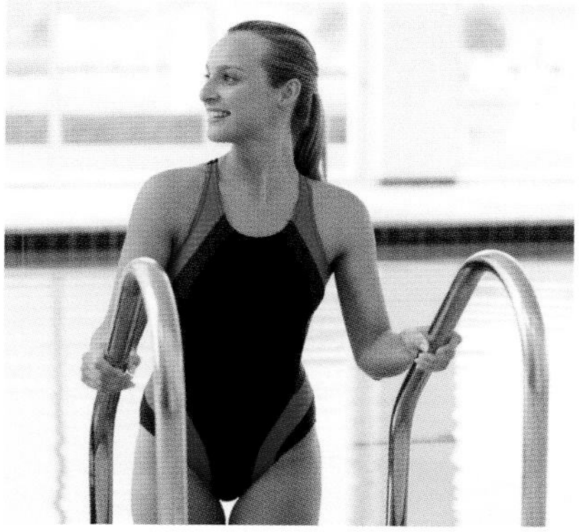

Getting regular moderate aerobic exercise during pregnancy—such as walking or swimming—will be highly beneficial to both you and your baby.

ACTUAL SIZE OF YOUR BABY

At 5 weeks of pregnancy, the embryo is 2.5mm long.

5 weeks

HEALTHY EATING AND EXERCISE

Eating regular meals and snacks that contain protein, complex carbohydrates, and unsaturated fats (see pp.14–16) will help you gain weight appropriate to your needs. Opt for nutrient- and calorie-dense foods such as avocados and whole-milk dairy products; as well as lean red meat, oily fish, nuts, and seeds, and drink plenty of milk and dairy-based smoothies.

Having a BMI (see p.16) of less than 18.5 increases the risk of nutritional deficiencies during pregnancy. These could cause your baby to be born prematurely, have a low birth weight, and be vulnerable to lifelong health problems.

If you have an eating disorder, it's essential to tell your doctor so that she can support you.

Regular exercise will increase your base metabolic rate, which is the rate at which your body burns calories. During pregnancy, your metabolism will already be slightly elevated. When you exercise, your body naturally uses energy stored in your organs and muscles, but your body will keep enough reserve energy to facilitate the growth of your baby. Exercise will also help your body regulate blood sugar (see p.92) and energy levels.

Your 6th week

THIS WEEK YOU MAY NOTICE THE FIRST SYMPTOMS OF PREGNANCY—IF NOT, DON'T WORRY

Not all women start to feel pregnant this early on. Some experience a twinge of nausea or breast tenderness, while others notice no changes. Of course, it's natural to long for "proof" that your pregnancy is progressing, even if that happens to be morning sickness. But a lack of symptoms doesn't mean something is wrong; it's all really happening and your baby is going through some critical stages of development.

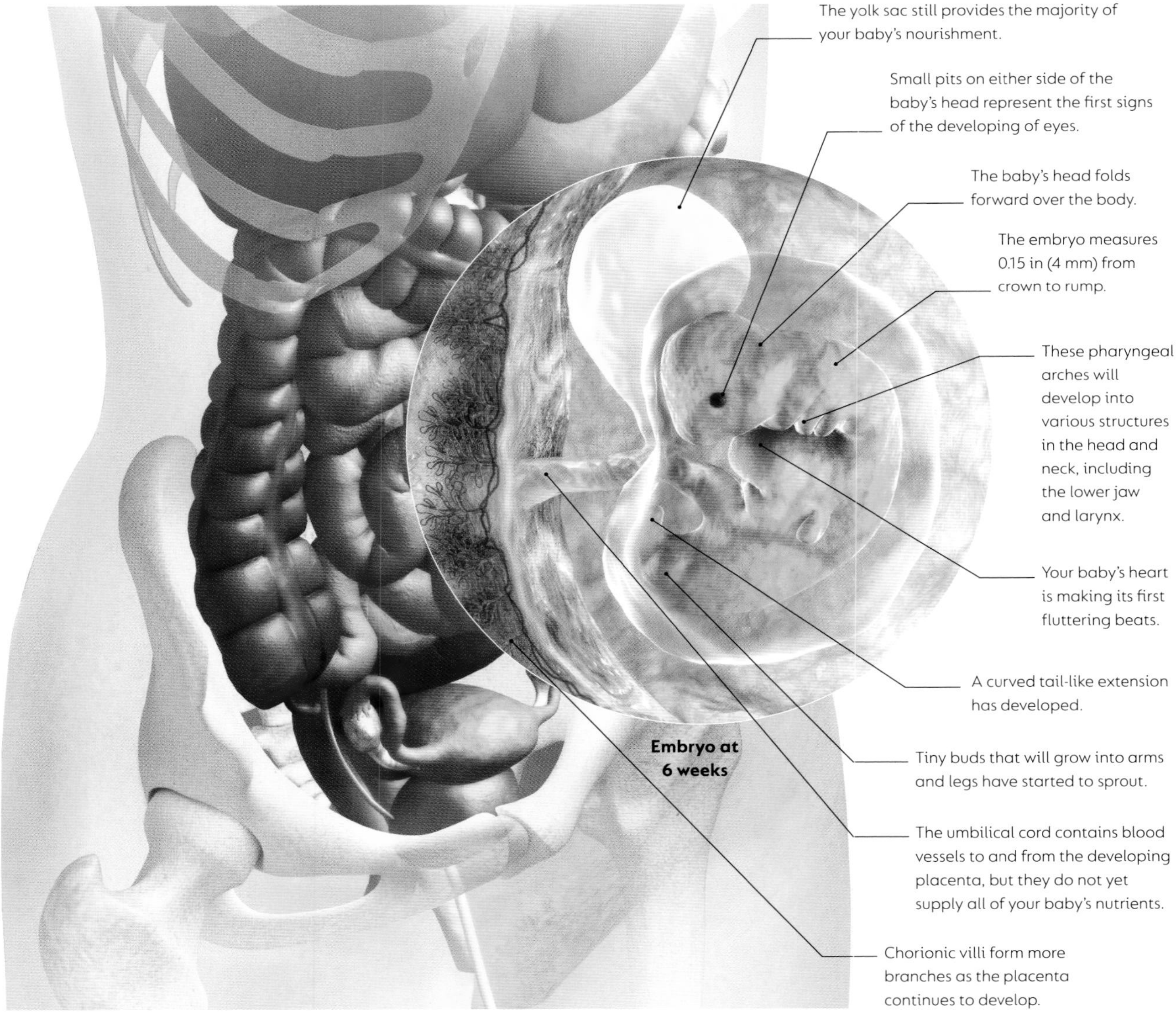
The yolk sac still provides the majority of your baby's nourishment.
Small pits on either side of the baby's head represent the first signs of the developing of eyes.
The baby's head folds forward over the body.
The embryo measures 0.15 in (4 mm) from crown to rump.
These pharyngeal arches will develop into various structures in the head and neck, including the lower jaw and larynx.
Your baby's heart is making its first fluttering beats.
A curved tail-like extension has developed.
Embryo at 6 weeks
Tiny buds that will grow into arms and legs have started to sprout.
The umbilical cord contains blood vessels to and from the developing placenta, but they do not yet supply all of your baby's nutrients.
Chorionic villi form more branches as the placenta continues to develop.

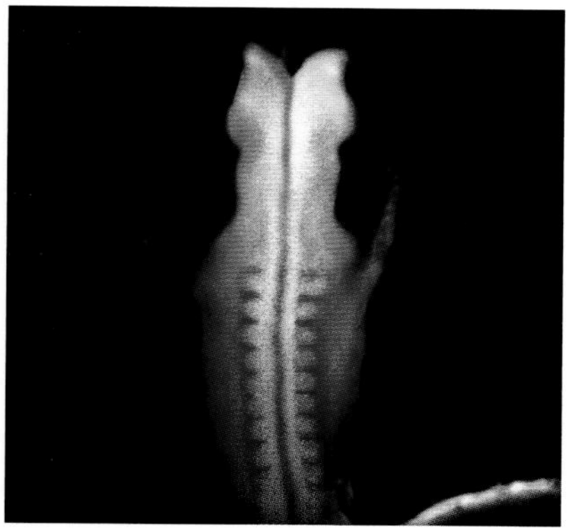

YOU ARE **5 WEEKS AND 1 DAY**

244 days to go

YOUR BABY TODAY

The embryo now has 14 somites—the building blocks of your baby's muscular system. The first nine pairs are shown here. The upper part of the image shows the head end of the neural tube, which has now nearly closed.

> "If you've had no symptoms as you enter your 6th week, you may be on the lookout for signs that you are in fact pregnant."

You and your partner are probably the only people who know you're pregnant, and you may still be wondering if it's real. At this stage you may not have any symptoms at all, despite the rapidly changing and growing embryo inside you. This absence of pregnancy signs is completely normal and is not a cause for concern. Try to remember that the majority of pregnancies are without any complications. It's normal for a healthy pregnant woman to have a wide range of side effects or none at all. So don't worry if you're feeling great—in fact count yourself lucky!

ASK A NUTRITIONIST

Since being pregnant, I don't have much of an appetite. Is this normal? It is common to not want to eat food, especially if you are suffering from morning sickness (see p.81). You may no longer be able to stomach your favorite foods, but it's important to eat when you can. Try eating smaller meals, perhaps cold options if cooking smells turn your stomach. Yogurt-based smoothies and chunky soups are nutritious. Always drink plenty.

Vitamin D helps your body absorb calcium, which is vital for the development of your unborn baby's skeleton. You can boost your vitamin D levels through exposure to the sun and by eating eggs, oily fish, and red meat. But it is also recommended that all pregnant women take a 400 IU vitamin D supplement daily.

EARLY ULTRASOUND SCANS

Some women will have an early ultrasound scan, but the majority of women will have one around the 12th week of pregnancy (see p.137). Early scans are usually done vaginally, with a scanning probe inserted gently into the vagina. They are performed for the following reasons:

- **If there is a history of multiple births** in your family (or you have used IVF or another form of assisted pregnancy), your doctor may want to check the number of fetuses.
- **If you've had a miscarriage in the past,** or show signs of cramping or spotting, or more profuse bleeding, a scan can be done to check that there is still a heartbeat.
- **To establish the cause of vaginal bleeding.** Your baby may be healthy, but fibroids or other conditions may be causing you to bleed. This will be addressed by your doctor.

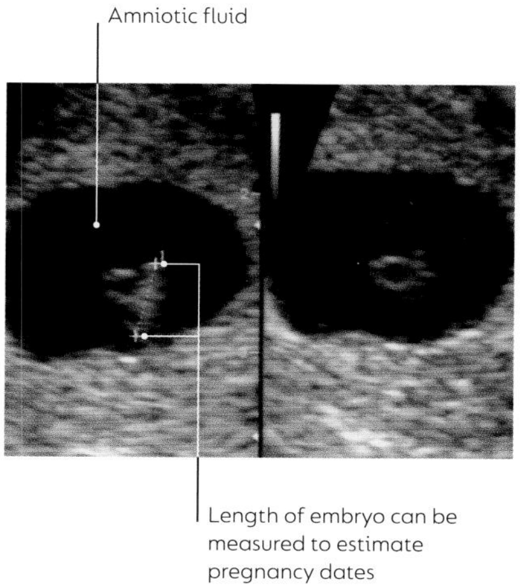
Amniotic fluid
Length of embryo can be measured to estimate pregnancy dates

Early vaginal scans do not show a great deal of detail. The sonographer waits until the embryo is in the correct position (left) to be measured.

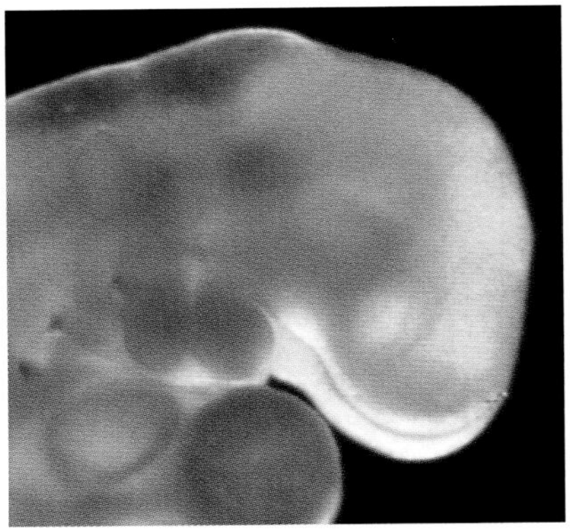

YOU ARE **5 WEEKS AND 2 DAYS**

243 days to go

YOUR BABY TODAY

The center of this image shows the baby's developing heart (darker gray), a very primitive structure at this stage. The baby's head is to the right of the image. The embryo is almost completely transparent.

> "There won't be any visible signs of pregnancy on the outside for some time, but there are many changes taking place inside."

At this early stage, all your unborn baby's needs will be met by the yolk sac. Attached to the embryo by a connecting stalk, this essential balloonlike structure indicates the site of your pregnancy and can usually be seen as early as this week as a sphere 0.1–0.2 in (3–4 mm) across. At first the yolk sac is as large as the disk of embryonic cells that will eventually become your baby.

Containing cells that perform a similar function to the liver, the yolk sac releases several pregnancy hormones and produces the embryo's first red blood cells. After week 9 the liver will take over these functions as the yolk sac gradually disappears and the placenta takes over, by around the 10th week of pregnancy.

Over the next seven days, a primitive circulatory system develops, well before any blood circulates to the placenta in the 10th week. And, by the end of this week, using the highest quality ultrasound equipment, it is just possible to see the embryo's heartbeat. At this early stage of pregnancy, the unborn baby's heart is simply a tube.

ASK A NUTRITIONIST

Should I be eating for two? Unfortunately, pregnancy is by no means a license to eat anything and everything you'd like. "Eating for two" is a myth, and if you do so, you'll end up consuming too many calories and gaining too much weight. The best advice is to use your common sense. Studies show that pregnant women who eat according to their appetite naturally eat the proper amount and gain a healthy amount of weight.

Caloric needs in pregnancy vary greatly from woman to woman, depending upon prepregnancy weight and physical activity. However, you only need to eat more calories in the last trimester of pregnancy, or if you are having twins or more. In the first trimester, when up to 80 percent of women are nauseous or vomiting, getting enough calories can sometimes be a challenge. Like many pregnant women, you may feel most nauseous when your stomach is empty. One good trick is snacking. Eating five small meals rather than three large ones can be soothing to a nauseous stomach, while at the same time giving you the energy and nutrients that you need.

In the US salt is the main source of iodine. But another good source is milk. Organic milk contains less, and some dairy alternatives contain none. Fish, especially white fish, and seaweed are great sources, but avoid eating kelp since it contains too much iodine.

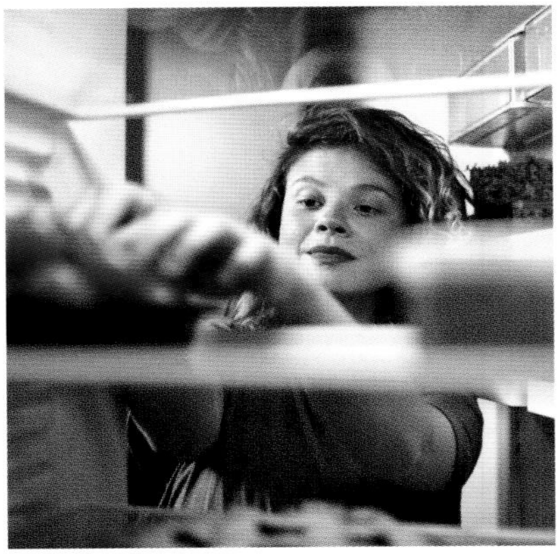

If you can't stomach big plates of food, try eating a combination of small portions at mealtimes and as snacks.

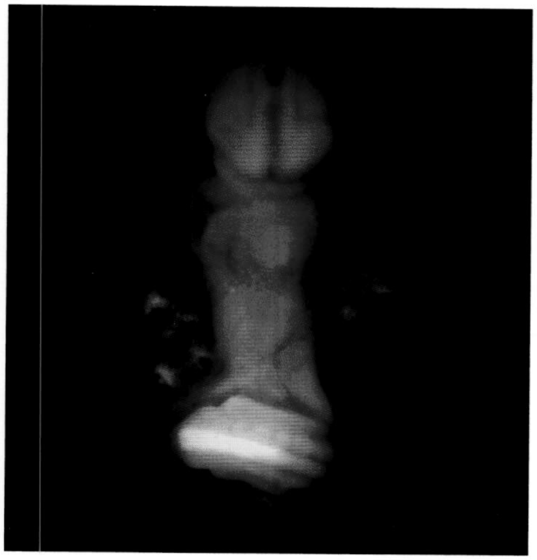

YOU ARE **5 WEEKS AND 3 DAYS**

242 days to go

YOUR BABY TODAY

A front view of the embryo: the head region is bent downward so that the central nervous system can be seen. The tubelike structure in the head region is the developing spinal cord. The tail of the embryo is curving upward.

> “Morning sickness is one of the most common and least welcome symptoms of pregnancy.”

Feeling sick and vomiting are common symptoms of early pregnancy. There are various theories to explain why morning sickness occurs; one is that it's due to the rising levels of hCG (human chorionic gonadotropin) hormone during the first trimester. Morning sickness, unfortunately, doesn't only happen before breakfast; in fact it can happen at any time of day and more than once in 24 hours.

One of the greatest challenges of early pregnancy is keeping it a secret from colleagues. If you have to keep rushing to the bathroom to vomit, people are likely to become suspicious. They may also notice that you look unwell or are more tired than usual. To help you handle this, you may want to tell one or two colleagues or your boss. You could ask them to keep it a secret for the time being. It's a good idea to keep some face wipes, toothpaste, and a toothbrush in your drawer, together with any snacks that you have found help to ease your nausea.

If you're finding it difficult to handle your vomiting, or are worried you are vomiting too much, seek advice from your doctor. Rarely, the sickness can become more serious and require medical treatment (see p.111).

EASE THE NAUSEA

Unfortunately there is no definitive cure-all for morning sickness, though you could try the following natural remedies:

- **Eat little and often**—having low blood-sugar levels may make the nausea worse so even if you feel sick, eating small snacks may help.
- **Try eating a plain cracker** first thing in the morning before you get out of bed.
- **Stick to bland foods** such as cereal, pasta, a baked potato, or toast. Avoid fatty and spicy foods.
- **Try having foods and drinks that contain ginger or peppermint**. One study found that the decrease in nausea happened four days after including ginger in the diet daily; so persevere with it. Put a slice of fresh ginger in a cup and pour in boiling water to make an infusion, or try crystallized ginger chews or a ginger cookie. Ginger ale doesn't usually contain real ginger, and you might not tolerate the carbonation

Drink plenty if you are vomiting, to avoid becoming dehydrated. Carry a bottle of water with you at all times and sip it gradually throughout the day. If your urine is getting very concentrated, it can be a sign of dehydration; you may need to see a doctor.

If the nausea or vomiting is too much to bear, then consult your doctor, who will be able to prescribe anti-nausea medications.

A changing world

The family unit is ever changing and has undergone some major shifts in the past few decades. Although times have changed, your role as a parent is the same as ever: to give your child consistent love, loyalty, and care.

Families today

There are many varieties of family life. Although studies report on the problems of modern childhood, children tend to be familiar with and tolerant of different cultures, and living and working practices.

Mature moms The number of births to women in the US between 35–39 has risen 52 percent since 1990; the birth rate in women 40–44 has risen 65 percent since 1990 and is at an all-time high. Benefits are that older women are more likely to be settled, financially stable, and mature.

Single parenting Approximately 23 percent of US children under the age of 18 live in a single-parent family, which is the highest rate in the world. There's no doubt that children in single-parent families can be disadvantaged, but it's thought that much of this is due to financial constraints and that those who have adequate socioeconomic resources do well.

Blended, or mixed, families This is when families combine, forming a blend of stepchildren, adopted or foster children, and biologic children. It is the fastest-growing household type.

Modern dads

Dads today are more involved in family life. Some 93 percent attend the birth (compared to 5 percent in 1965), and over 70 percent take time off after the birth. In the 1970s, dads of children under five devoted less than 15 minutes a day to child-related activities, compared to over two hours by the 1990s. Research shows that children whose dads spend considerable time with them do well educationally and at work.

Child care

Studies show that good care outside the family has a positive impact on social skills, intellect, and language. A good grandparent relationship provides stability and family values, and is thought to improve cognitive development. Grandparents care for about 30 percent of US babies.

Multiple cultures

Your baby will live in a multicultural society, affecting education and friendships. There's a strong chance a child will be cared for by someone from another culture at some point.

THE STATISTICS

Changing family life

The statistics below reveal how family life has changed over decades.

- In the US, 64 percent of moms with children under the age of six work; in the UK, 55 percent of mothers of children under five work (compared with around 25 percent in 1975).
- About 25 percent of children under five with working moms are cared for full-time by dad and 30 percent of working parents share child care.
- About 25 percent of married moms stay at home full time with the children.
- The number of single-parent families has been roughly stable since 2010, in which 27 percent of children lived with one parent and no other adult in the household. Nearly 80 percent of single-parent homes are headed by single mothers.
- In 2017, between 2 and 3.7 million children had an LGBTQ parent.

THE GENDER GAP

Boys versus girls Historically, about 106 boys have been born for every 100 girls—believed to be nature's way of compensating for the fact that males are more likely to be killed in conflicts. But ratios are changing. One factor may be increased stress (women under stress produce more girls than boys).

Research studies in the US and Sweden have also discovered that certain chemical pollutants in the environment can impact the human sex ratio at birth of babies..

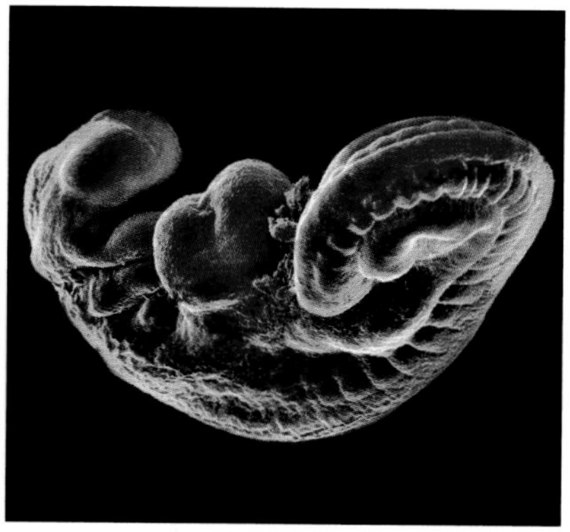

YOU ARE **5 WEEKS AND 4 DAYS**

241 days to go

YOUR BABY TODAY

This image shows just how curled up the embryo is at this stage. The head end of the embryo is on the left. The embryo now has 22 pairs of somites (building blocks of the musculoskeletal system) running along the back.

> “This is a crucial time for your developing baby as the neural tube, which will become the brain and spinal cord, is forming.”

This week your baby begins to grow rapidly and starts to become more recognizable as a fetus. There are three types of cells, each committed to a separate function. The first will form the skin and nervous system; the second forms blood vessels, muscles, and bones; the third forms the entire digestive system.

The cells responsible for the spine and nervous system are at work. Changing shape from a flat disk, the embryo starts to curl up. The edges of the groove that has already partially formed along the back gradually start to meet, closing and fusing to form a tube, which will become the brain and spinal cord. The last parts of the tube to close are at the very top of the head and then the base of the spine, two days later.

Being careful to get an adequate intake of folic acid (see p.35) in early pregnancy is essential to ensure the neural tube closes completely, with no gaps.

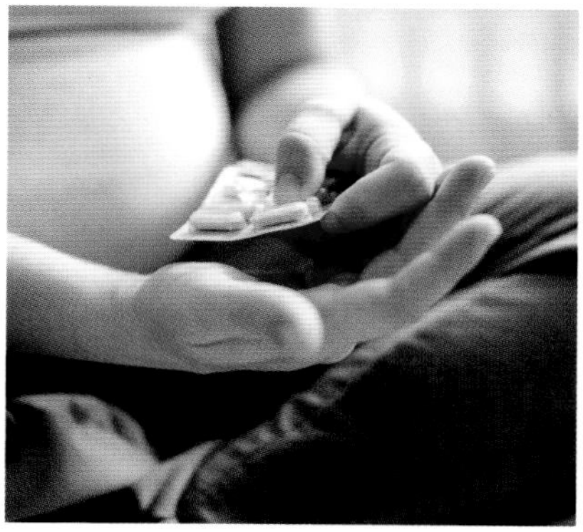

Although folic acid is found in foods, such as green leafy vegetables, taking a supplement in early pregnancy is recommended.

FOCUS ON PARTNERS

Your first reaction to finding out that your partner is pregnant might be to tell the world. After all, you may be excited or nervous and may want to confide in people who you can trust. Think twice before telling lots of people (see box, right) and don't do so without talking to your partner. Of course your partner may find it hard to hide some aspects of pregnancy, such as morning sickness.

Most importantly, make sure that you are both in agreement that it is the right time to tell others.

IS IT TIME TO TELL?

You're excited to be pregnant, but should you tell people yet?

- Most parents-to-be wait to share their exciting news until after week 12 when the risk of miscarriage falls. You may, however, decide you want to confide in family and close friends.
- Most women don't tell their employers yet, unless severe morning sickness interferes with their ability to keep up with work responsibilities. Most wait until after the first trimester or when they start to show. If you want time off for prenatal appointments before this, you'll need to explain why.
- Similarly, if your job involves anything that could be a health and safety risk (for example, heavy lifting or working with chemicals), you should inform your employer early so your role can be adapted. It's also sensible to tell your boss the good news before office gossip about your expanding girth snowballs.

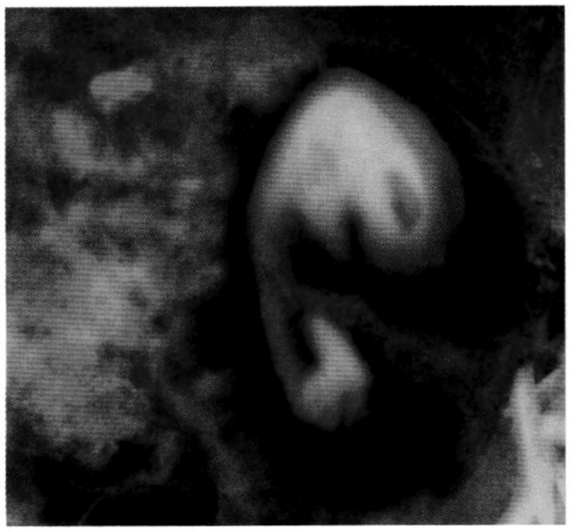

YOU ARE **5 WEEKS AND 5 DAYS**

240 days to go

YOUR BABY TODAY

This is a view of the right side of an embryo with the fronds of the chorionic villi in the background. The curled shape of the embryo is clearly demonstrated. The umbilical cord attachment to the early placenta can just be seen.

“ Are you feeling up one minute and down the next? Be reassured that this is a perfectly normal response to pregnancy hormones. ”

It may not happen quite yet, but be forewarned that you may become very emotional or irrational during pregnancy and suffer from mood swings. You may cry at things that had previously not affected you. This is due to a combination of your rapidly fluctuating hormones and the fact that pregnancy is a major life change.

Mood swings can be difficult for both you and your partner—try to keep communicating with each other and explain how you are feeling, no matter how irrational it may seem.

MORE VEGGIES PLEASE!

Be creative to stimulate your appetite and get fiber, vitamins, and minerals:

- **Make an easy vegetable soup** with prepared vegetables.
- **Throw in a few vegetables** when you make a smoothie (see p.135)— cucumber, celery, peppers, and carrots are mild in flavor, but nutritious.
- **Grate zucchini and carrots** into soups, pasta sauces, and stews, or throw a handful of squash, frozen peas, broccoli, asparagus, or green beans into a risotto.
- **Experiment with vegetable pasta** such as butternut squash noodles. Use half pasta and half vegetable pasta.
- **Top a pizza** with vitamin C-rich peppers—they're crunchy, colorful, and nutritious.
- **Try sauerkraut and kimchi** —fermented vegetables are good for your gut bacteria.

TACKLING FATIGUE

You might find you have a sudden loss of energy as your body adapts, but after about week 13, you should start to feel more energized.

One cause of tiredness is anemia. If you had a restricted diet when you started pregnancy, your iron reserves may be low. Your doctor may recommend a blood test and advise taking supplements.

Try to eat iron-rich foods. There are two types of iron: heme iron found in animal foods is easily absorbed—eat lean red meat, canned sardines, and eggs. Nonheme iron is less well absorbed. It's found in whole-grain cereals, legumes, green vegetables, and dried fruit. Vitamin C helps iron absorption, so have tomatoes with a meal or orange juice with breakfast. Tea and coffee inhibit absorption so avoid them at mealtimes.

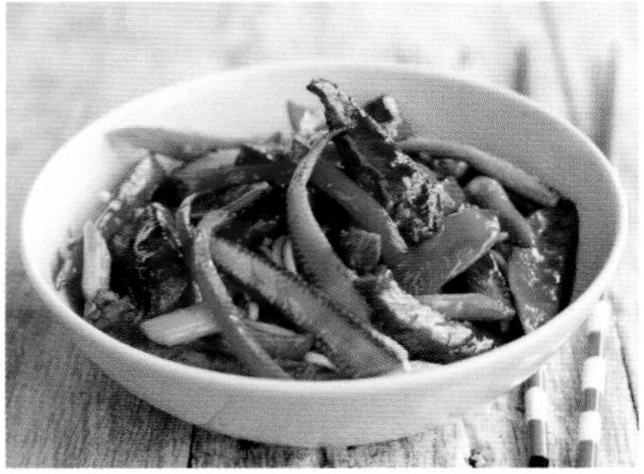

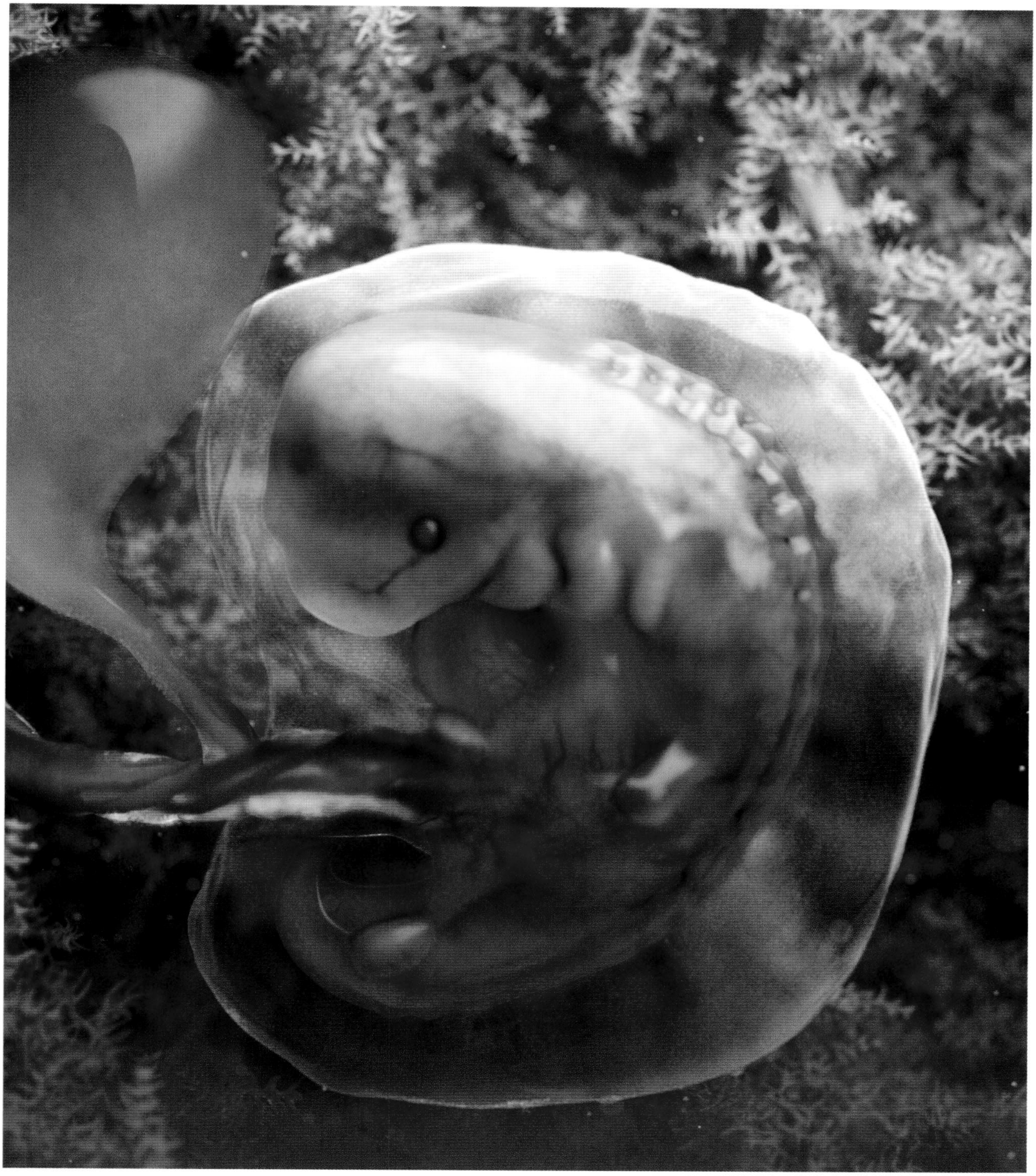

The embryo is developing rapidly, although still only 4 mm long. The spinal column is in place and the eyes have formed. The yellow yolk sac on the left is larger than the embryo which it is nourishing.

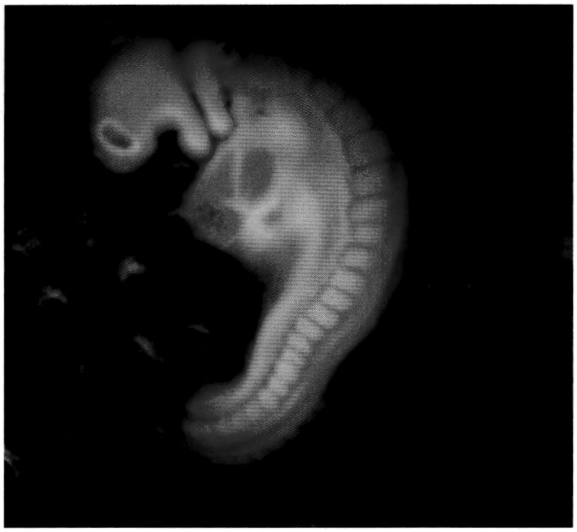

YOU ARE **5 WEEKS AND 6 DAYS**

239 days to go...

YOUR BABY TODAY

Development in the upper body usually precedes that in the lower body—this image shows the bulge containing the heart and liver, and the very earliest sign of development of the upper limb buds, but as yet there is no sign of the lower limb buds.

> “You may notice a marked increase in your breast size, even at this early stage of pregnancy.”

The first part of your body to change shape is likely to be your chest. Your breasts may increase in size quite rapidly, looking bigger and feeling heavier. They may become quite tender to touch.

Each breast will increase, on average, by 2in (5cm) and 3lb (1.4kg) during pregnancy. That is why it is important to wear the right bra, that fits you properly, even in the early stages of pregnancy.

Your nipples will also change: the areola (the darker skin around the nipple) may become darker in color and your nipples may tingle. As your breasts get bigger, you might notice blue veins appearing. All these breast changes are due to the hormone estrogen.

ASK A MIDWIFE

How can I ease the soreness in my breasts? Wearing a supportive bra can help with both the feelings of heaviness and soreness in your breasts, which are common in pregnancy. If your breasts are very tender at night, wearing a soft bra or bralette while you sleep may help. Try to avoid sleeping on your front if this causes discomfort. You may find that rubbing in a cream containing aloe vera is soothing.

ASK A NUTRITIONIST

I’m a bit of a coffee addict! Should I give it up now that I’m pregnant? The American College of Obstetricians and Gynecologists advises that pregnant women should drink no more than 200 mg of caffeine per day. Caffeine is mostly found in coffee, tea, chocolate, and cola drinks (see p.16).

If you drink a lot of coffee, then consider replacing it with decaffeinated varieties. There are various methods of decaffeination and, contrary to some popular belief, there is little evidence that the process of removing caffeine has a negative effect on health.

Many women can’t stomach the smell and taste of coffee in pregnancy, and this can be one of the first signs you are pregnant. Even if you can tolerate it, consider replacing some of your cups of coffee (or tea if you drink more than three or four mugs a day) with water, hot or cold, infused with lemon or ginger. Don’t forget that milk, soups, and broths provide valuable fluids and useful nutrients, too.

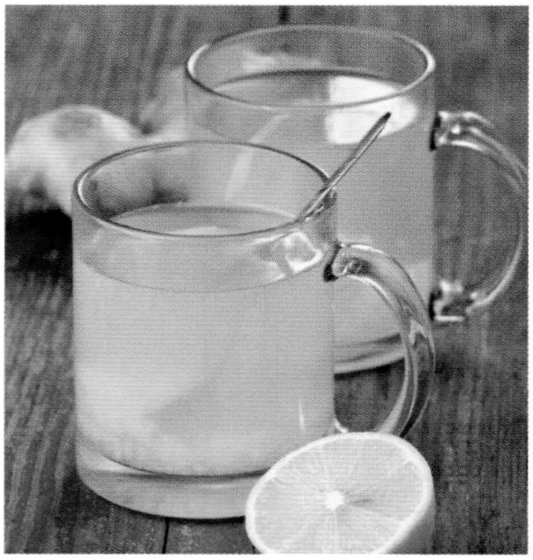

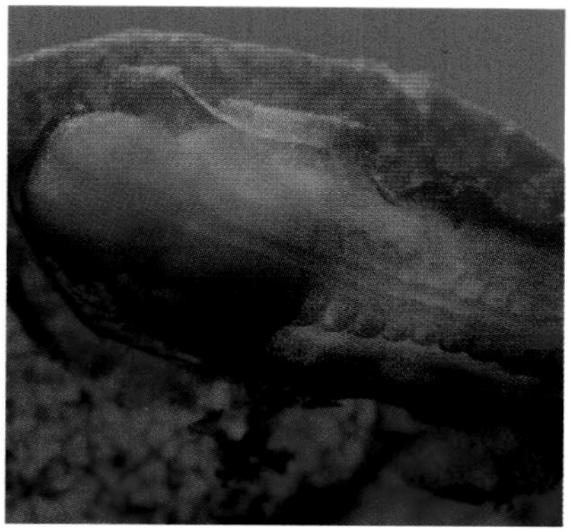

YOU ARE **6 WEEKS EXACTLY**

238 days to go...

YOUR BABY TODAY

Here the back of the embryo can be seen lying over the yolk sac. The opening overlying the developing brain has now closed (left side of image) and this will be followed two days later by closure of the opening at the base of the spine (out of view).

Your developing embryo may still be tiny,but is undergoing rapid and complex development.

The heartbeat is now more easily recognized on an ultrasound scan. The heart continues to form from a simple smooth tube which, as it becomes more muscular, loops, folds, and divides to form four chambers. On the left side the upper chamber (left atrium) takes in blood from the lungs. From here blood passes through a one-way valve (the mitral valve) into the main left pumping chamber (the left ventricle). This then pumps blood out of the heart to the body along the main artery (the aorta). On the right-hand side of the heart, the upper chamber (right atrium) collects blood returning from the body and passes it through a one-way valve (tricuspid valve) into the right main pumping chamber (right ventricle). This pumps blood to the lungs and the cycle continues.

At this stage of development, the circulation is very basic with the heart tube simply sending blood around the length of your baby. No blood travels from your baby's circulation to the placenta (see p.127).

" By the end of this sixth week, the baby's heart is rapidly developing and circulating blood. "

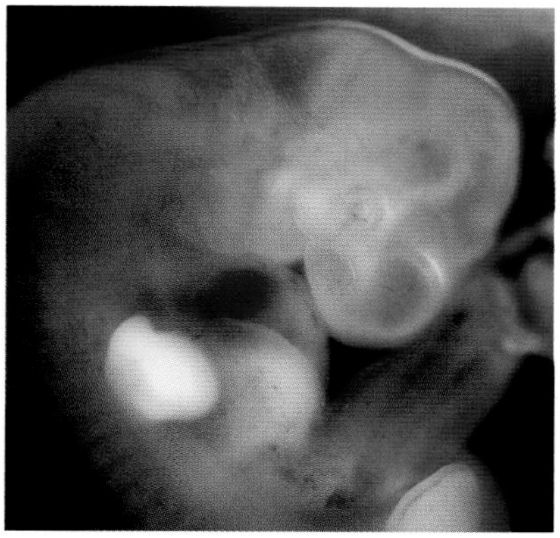

It's at an early stage of development, but the developing heart can be seen here as the dark red area. It lies just above the larger, slightly paler red area, which is the liver. Below the liver is the umbilical cord.

HAVING A MISCARRIAGE

At this early stage, a common concern is that the pregnancy will miscarry. A miscarriage is the spontaneous loss of a pregnancy at any time up until the 20th week.

After 20 weeks the loss is referred to as a stillbirth. The signs of a miscarriage are vaginal bleeding and period-like cramps.

Unfortunately, there is nothing that you can do to prevent a miscarriage. In around 60 percent of cases, it is caused by a one-time genetic problem. Bleeding does not always mean that the pregnancy is being miscarried. Since not all miscarriages follow the same pattern, there are various terms to describe what happens:

- **A threatened miscarriage** occurs when the pregnant woman experiences bleeding and possibly pain, but the baby survives.
- **An inevitable miscarriage** occurs when there is bleeding and pain due to the pregnant woman's uterus contracting. The cervix opens, and the fetus is expelled.
- **A missed miscarriage** is when the fetus dies but is not expelled. Surgery may be needed to remove it.

ACTUAL SIZE OF YOUR BABY

At 6 weeks, your baby's crown to rump length is 0.15 in (4 mm).

5 weeks

6 weeks

Your 7th week

SET YOURSELF SOME FITNESS STANDARDS TO SEE YOU THROUGH YOUR PREGNANCY Getting in shape now will stand you in good stead as your pregnancy continues. Keeping active is important, so work up a daily exercise routine to strengthen your muscles and reduce fatigue—but listen to your body and don't exhaust yourself. This week your baby's vital organs, including the lungs and gut, start to develop. Your baby's head already looks too big for his body as the brain rapidly enlarges.

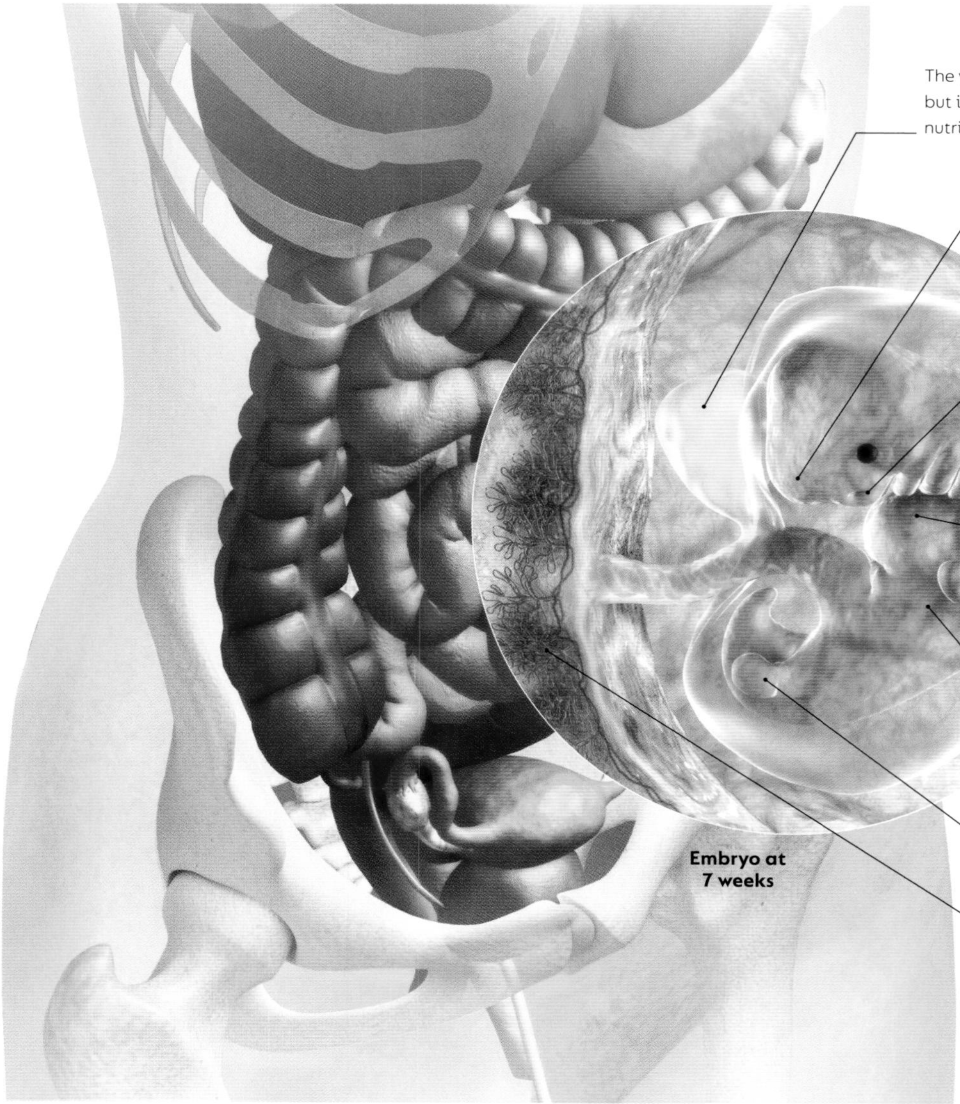
The yolk sac has shrunk but is still supplying nutrients to the embryo.
A prominent forehead bulges out as the brain develops.
Nostrils appear as shallow pits.
The embryo measures 0.31 in (8 mm) crown to rump.
The heart is now providing your baby with a simple circulation.
The liver is starting to make blood cells.
The arm and leg buds are lengthening.
The placenta is becoming well established, although it is not yet ready to function as a supply line.
Embryo at 7 weeks

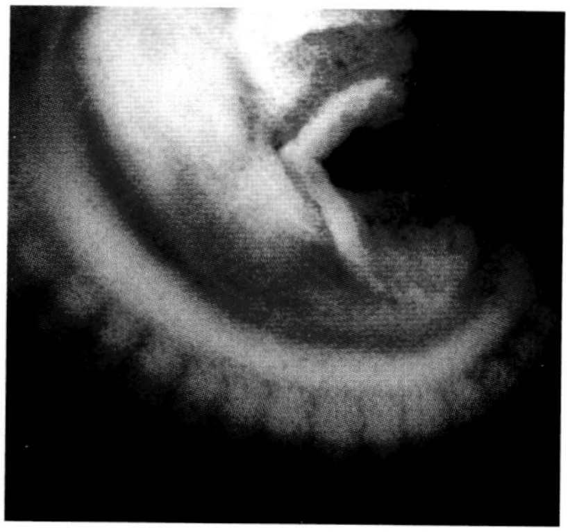

YOU ARE **6 WEEKS AND 1 DAY**

237 days to go

YOUR BABY TODAY

In this side view of the embryo the spinal cord is clearly curved as it begins to develop. The pale-yellow ridgelike structures along the back are somites—your baby's developing muscular system.

“You may be spending a lot of time in front of the mirror trying to spot your “bump,” but it could be weeks yet before you show.”

Like most newly pregnant women, you're probably on the lookout for a rounded belly, but it's unlikely to make an appearance just yet. On average, the fourth month marks the greatest period of growth, with your pregnancy most definitely appearing as a rounded abdomen.

If it's not your first pregnancy, you might show earlier, possibly as early as eight to 10 weeks, since your abdominal muscles will be more relaxed. Conversely, women who have firm abdominal muscles may show later. If you are expecting twins or triplets, you can expect to show even earlier.

ASK A DOCTOR

Can having sex in pregnancy harm the baby? Unless you have been told by your doctor to avoid sex because of specific problems, such as a history of miscarriage or unexplained bleeding, then sex is safe at any stage. Enjoying intimacy with your partner is beneficial to your relationship.

Your baby is cushioned in fluid in the amniotic sac inside your uterus and protected by a plug of mucus at the cervix. Even deep penetration isn't harmful.

STRENGTHEN YOUR ABDOMINALS

Toward the end of the first trimester, or when you start “showing” (see left), you should stop doing abdominal exercises on your back (see p.250). When you are doing abdominal exercises, it's important to breathe correctly—inhale to start and exhale on each effort.

The purpose of abdominal exercises is to strengthen core muscles. The deeper transverse abdominis muscle that runs horizontally across your body is vital for core stability and strength as your baby develops. The rectus abdominis muscle that runs vertically down your body will stretch during pregnancy and weaken, so it's vital to keep the transverse muscle and the back muscles strong to help your posture and support your spine.

The sooner you begin to strengthen the transverse abdominis, the better. Below is one of the exercises you can do during the first trimester to strengthen this muscle .

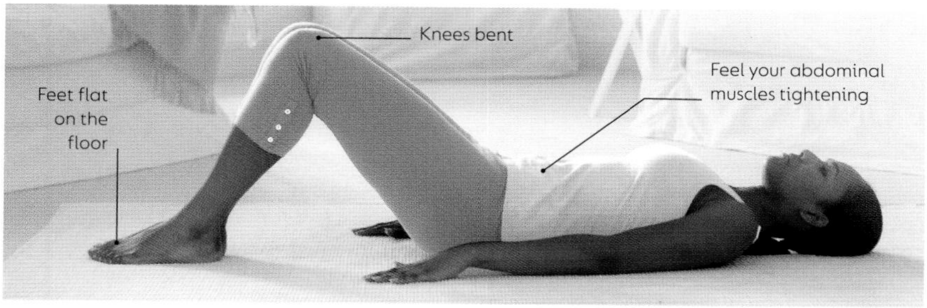

Knees bent
Feel your abdominal muscles tightening
Feet flat on the floor

Lie on your back, feet flat on the floor and arms at your sides. Inhale to begin and as you slowly exhale, push your lower back flat on to the floor. Hold this position for 3–5 seconds and repeat.

Strengthening and toning exercises

Exercises that strengthen your muscles will help you deal with the additional demands of pregnancy and to manage better during labor and birth.

The exercises shown are sometimes called "functional movement enhancers" because they increase the strength of the muscles that you use for everyday functions such as walking, carrying, lifting, sitting, and standing. The workout can be used alongside walking, swimming, or other cardiovascular exercises and should be done three to four times a week.

Warm up Walk in place, swinging your arms back and forth. Continue for 3–5 minutes until your muscles are warm.

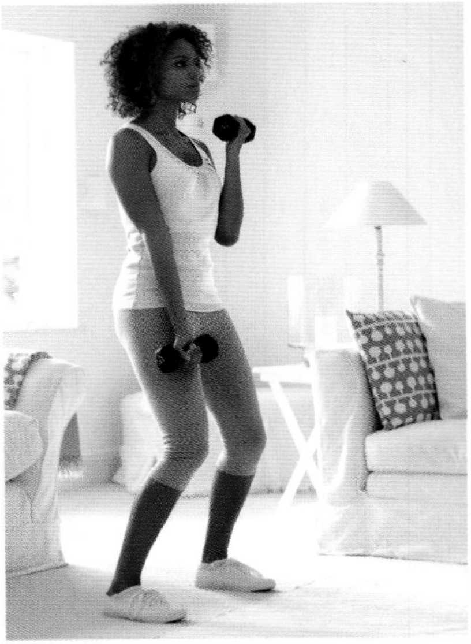

Biceps curl The biceps is an important muscle for carrying and lifting. You can use 3–5 lb (1–2 kg) weights for this sequence if you're a regular exerciser. Stand with feet hip-width apart, knees slightly bent, back straight, and arms at your sides. Breathe in, then exhale as you bend one elbow, raising your hand to shoulder level. Alternate arms until you've done 20 curls on each side (40 in total). If you find this easy, try doing a total of 60 curls.

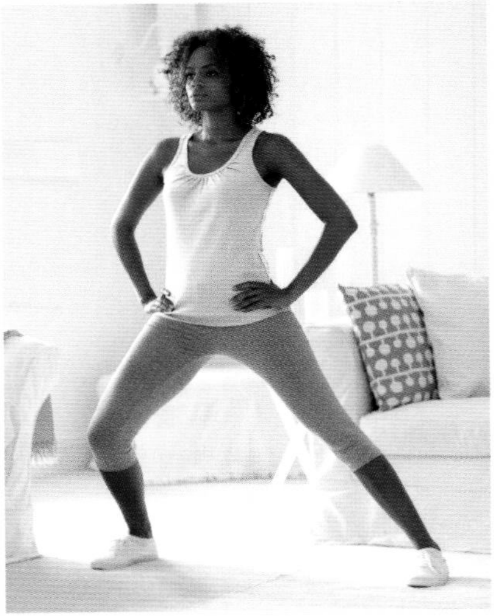

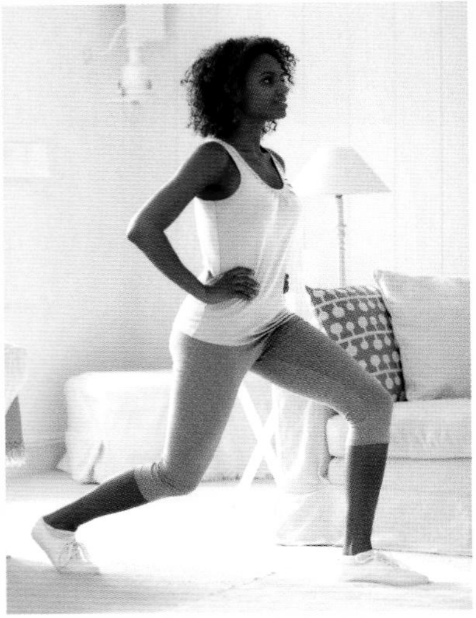

Side lunges (above left) These (and the forward lunges) strengthen the abdominal and thigh muscles. Start with hands on hips, legs hip-width apart. Step one leg out to the side, bending the knee. Keep the other leg straight. Step back to the starting position, keeping the tummy pulled in and torso straight. Do 10 lunges on each leg. **Forward lunges** (above right) Start with hands on hips, feet hip-width apart. Step one leg forward; bend the opposite knee toward the floor, allowing the heel to lift off the floor. Return to the starting position. Do 10 lunges on each leg.

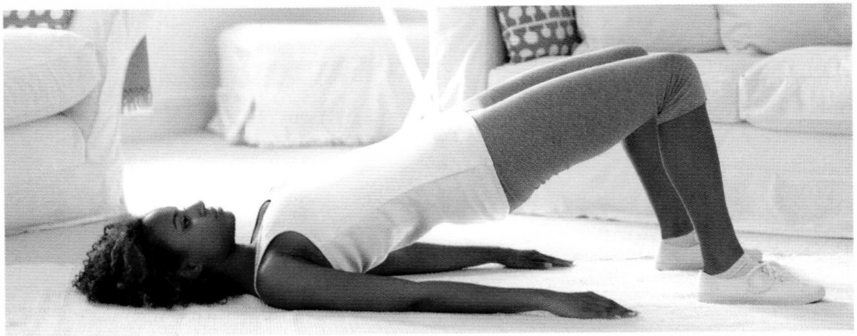

The bridge This exercise works your bottom, hamstrings, and inner thighs, and builds strength in your lower body to support your growing belly. Lie on your back with your feet flat on the floor and knees slightly apart. Raise your hips (this relieves pressure on your back and is safe in the second and third trimesters). Keep your hands on the floor next to you, arms straight. Slowly bring your knees together while clenching your bottom; open and close your knees 10 times. Slowly lower your hips and roll onto your left side to end.

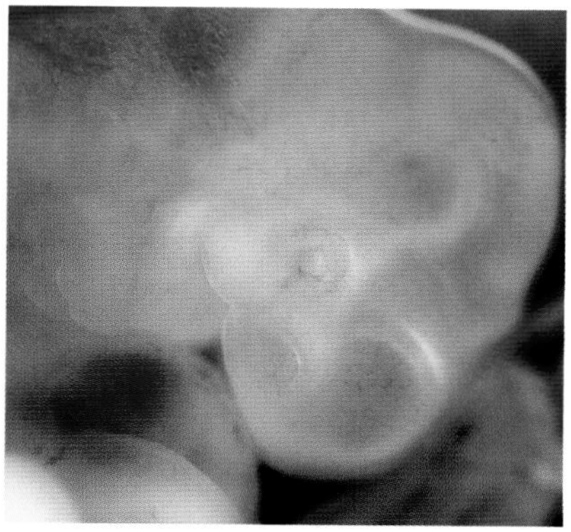

YOU ARE **6 WEEKS AND 2 DAYS**

236 days to go

YOUR BABY TODAY

The first recognizable facial feature to be formed is the eye, visible as a black dot in the center of this image. The gray areas are the fluid-filled chambers of the underlying brain.

> "Try not to dwell on your lifestyle before you realized you were pregnant, but start making changes now."

Have you only just discovered you're pregnant? Not all women realize they are pregnant immediately, especially if it wasn't planned. If you've only just found out, it's natural to be concerned about things that you did before you knew, such as drinking alcohol or taking drugs. You may be worried that you've harmed your unborn baby. Use your pregnancy as an opportunity to assess your lifestyle and improve your health.

Because of how pregnancy is dated (see p.35), your baby is still only a little over four weeks old. If you have not been taking folic acid (see p.35), start taking supplements starting today.

PRENATAL CARE

The options for prenatal care in the US are outlined on p.102, but they do vary from area to area. Whatever your type of prenatal care, any ultrasound scans, tests, and investigations may also take place at a hospital. Your options are likely to be:

- **Group medical practice** with your OB
- **Solo medical practice** midwifery-led
- **Combination practice** if you are high risk
- **Maternity Center–based practice**

GOING SOLO

The prospect of being pregnant and single, especially if it wasn't your choice, can be tough. Here are some useful things to consider:

Take care of yourself: plan a healthy diet, and an exercise routine. Get as much rest as you can. Ask a friend to spur you on or go online and seek support from other single pregnant women locally—you will have a ready-made support network after the birth.

- **Ask for help** from family and friends. You will probably find they are delighted to be involved in your pregnancy and are willing to come to prenatal appointments and classes with you: you may want to consider asking one of these people to be your birth partner.
- **Discuss support and access** with your baby's father (if appropriate), and if you can't agree, seek legal advice. You and your baby will benefit if an amicable arrangement is reached, and the sooner you start talking, the easier it will be.
- **Arrange support** for after the birth. A survey found that grandparents who are actively involved in their grandchildren's lives contribute positively to their well-being. If you don't have family close by, try to build a network of other support that will see you through the early weeks.
- **Start thinking early** about your career options for after the birth. You don't have to make any decisions, but it helps to know some of the choices you may have to make later.

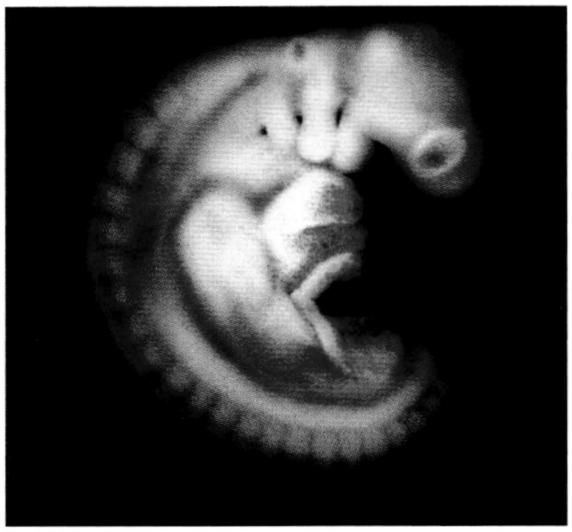

YOU ARE **6 WEEKS AND 3 DAYS**

235 days to go

YOUR BABY TODAY

The eyes begin life as shallow depressions, one on each side of the developing face. This image shows an early eye in the center right, together with the curve of the pale yellow somites of the developing musculoskeletal system.

> "Needing to urinate frequently is, unfortunately, one of the unwanted side effects of pregnancy."

Are you spending a lot of time in the bathroom? In addition to dealing with symptoms such as nausea and vomiting (see p.81), if you're like the majority of pregnant women, you'll need to urinate more frequently. It means you're unlikely to want to be too far away from the nearest bathroom.

It can feel as though your bladder cannot hold much urine so you may feel the need to go to the bathroom not long after you've just been, during the day and at night. This is because there is more blood being pumped through the kidneys so you produce more urine. As your uterus grows, it puts pressure on your bladder so it cannot expand as much as normal and will feel uncomfortably full earlier than usual. This can last throughout pregnancy, though you're most likely to experience it in the first and third trimesters.

If, however, you're concerned about the amount of urine you're passing, and/or develop pain or stinging while passing urine, you may have developed a urinary tract infection and should see your doctor immediately.

ASK A DOCTOR

Why do I have so much saliva in my mouth now that I'm pregnant? Called ptyalism, excess saliva is caused by increased hormone levels. Don't try to keep the saliva in your mouth; if you find yourself drooling, spit into a tissue or small cup. Place a towel on your pillow. Sucking lemon wedges or ice cubes may help. Pytalism usually subsides in later pregnancy.

KNOW YOUR CARBS

Make carbohydrates part of your balanced diet, but choose the right ones. Complex carbohydrates, such as whole grains, provide fiber that your body breaks down slowly, releasing glucose into the bloodstream gradually. These are low glycemic index (GI) foods. Other carbohydrates are metabolized quickly (high GI); examples are white bread and rice, mashed potatoes, and high-sugar products. These make the body release more insulin to control blood sugar. This is not good for you or your unborn baby. Fluctuating glucose and insulin levels may lead to gestational diabetes as well as influence the growth of the placenta and baby. Don't restrict your intake of carbohydrate-rich foods such as pasta, rice, grains, breakfast cereals, and bread because your baby is constantly drawing glucose from your bloodstream, so a steady release of glucose leaves you both with plenty of fuel. However, choose whole grains, such as quinoa, millet, and barley, opt for whole-wheat pasta and brown rice, and enjoy oatmeal or muesli for breakfast. The fiber will also help keep you feeling full and prevent constipation.

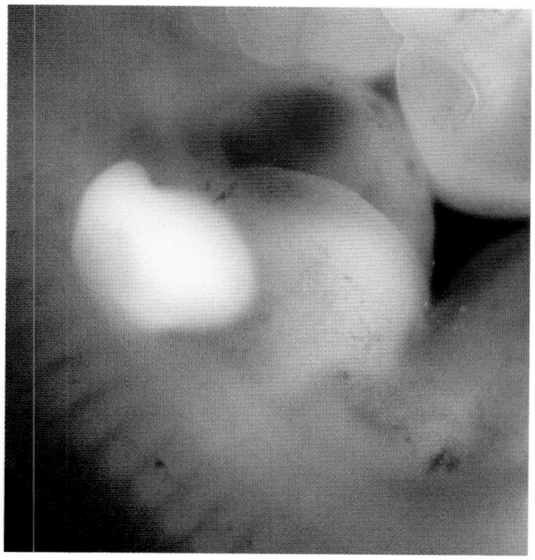

YOU ARE **6 WEEKS AND 4 DAYS**

234 days to go

YOUR BABY TODAY

The early limb bud that will form your baby's right arm can be seen here (white area). The upper limb buds appear before the lower limb buds. At this early stage, the hands and fingers are not yet developed.

In this seventh week of pregnancy, your baby's lungs are starting to develop. This begins with a small lung bud branching out from the upper part of the tube (esophagus) between your baby's mouth and stomach. This lung bud forms the main windpipe or "trachea," which then divides into two main branches (bronchi) that will eventually form your baby's right and left lungs. These bronchi continue to branch into smaller tubes, a process that will be repeated many times.

Your baby's gut is also starting to develop, from the mouth downward. At the beginning of this week, his future digestive system consisted of a simple tube, closed at each end, that lay along his entire length. The tube remains closed but the esophagus has now started to separate from the trachea and connect to the stomach. The swelling that will become your baby's stomach forms around the center of his body, but undergoes a 90-degree rotation to lie more on the left-hand side.

Buds arise from the duodenum (the first part of the bowel that leaves the stomach) that will form the pancreas and bile duct to the gall bladder.

In just a couple of weeks, your baby will have all its major organs and body systems.

> "Your baby's lungs won't be fully developed until late in pregnancy, but the foundations are being laid down right now."

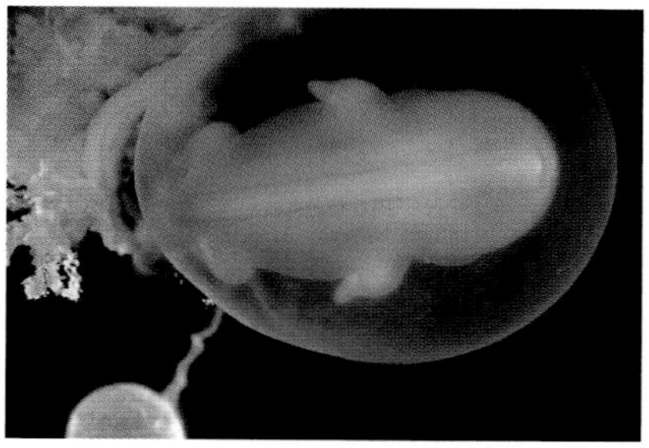

The embryo is safely cocooned in the fluid-filled amniotic sac. The yolk sac can be seen at the bottom of the image, attached by what is now a very fine thread; its function is gradually replaced by the placenta.

ECTOPIC PREGNANCY

An ectopic pregnancy can cause abdominal pain on one side and irregular vaginal bleeding. Some women get shoulder-tip pain caused by internal bleeding. An ectopic pregnancy can rupture the fallopian tube, causing severe pain and bleeding. Emergency medical attention is essential.

If an ectopic pregnancy is suspected, you will be given a scan. Sometimes the pregnancy will naturally regress; if not medication or surgery will be necessary.

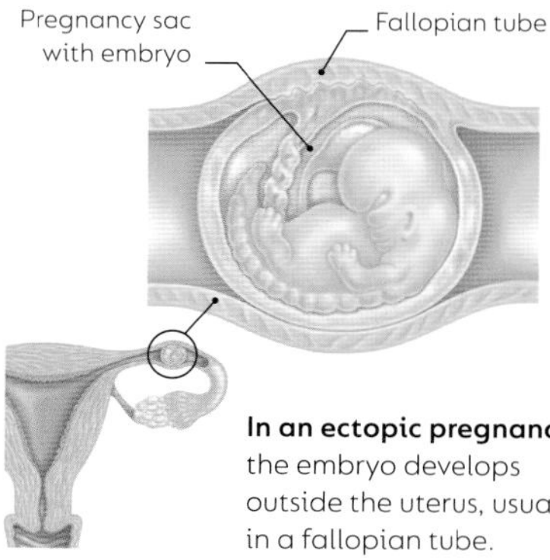
Pregnancy sac with embryo
Fallopian tube

In an ectopic pregnancy, the embryo develops outside the uterus, usually in a fallopian tube.

STRESS-REDUCING MUSIC

Listening to music can enhance well-being. A study found that pregnant women who listened to music that mimicked the human heartbeat had reduced stress levels compared to those who did not receive the treatment.

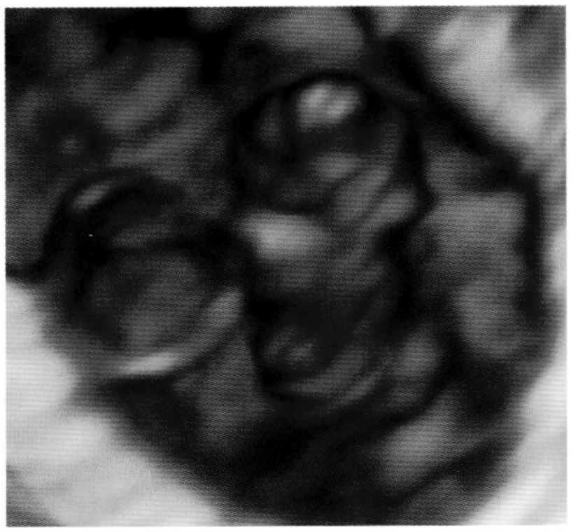

YOU ARE **6 WEEKS AND 5 DAYS**

233 days to go

YOUR BABY TODAY

This 3-D ultrasound scan shows the embryo and its yolk sac, attached to the wall of the uterus. The yolk sac provides nourishment for the embryo until the placenta is fully functional, and produces blood cells until the liver can take over this role.

If you feel lightheaded, especially when you get up from lying down, be extra careful. Dizzy spells are common, especially as your pregnancy progresses and you get bigger, since your heart has to work harder against the forces of gravity to get blood to the brain.

Try to stand up very gradually, in stages, from lying to sitting to standing. Dizziness can also occur if you have been standing for a long period of time, since blood may collect in your legs. Keep moving to encourage the blood to be pumped back to your heart.

Alternatively, you may feel dizzy due to low blood-sugar levels. Other symptoms of low blood sugar include feeling sweaty, shaky, and hungry. Even if you're feeling or being sick, try to eat little and often to ensure that your blood-sugar levels remain stable.

If you regularly feel dizzy, speak to your doctor, who will perform some basic health checks.

"By this stage, you may have experienced bouts of dizziness. It's all part of your body and brain adjusting to the pregnancy."

KEEP ON MOVING

The last thing you may feel like doing is exercising, but it can play a significant role in alleviating and preventing pregnancy symptoms. Although a run through the park or a walk downtown may not sound as inviting as a cozy nap on the sofa, exercise is invigorating and the effects will last. Try to think of it as being active, rather than "exercising."

If after completing a physical activity you feel even more fatigued, decrease how hard and long you exercise. Always listen to your body. As you become more fit and your pregnancy progresses, these feelings of fatigue should diminish, usually by weeks 12–14.

Exercising regularly can help you sleep more deeply. Insomnia is common in pregnancy, due to anxiety or difficulty in getting comfortable. Exercise is a destresser and will tire you out, increasing your chance of a good night's sleep.

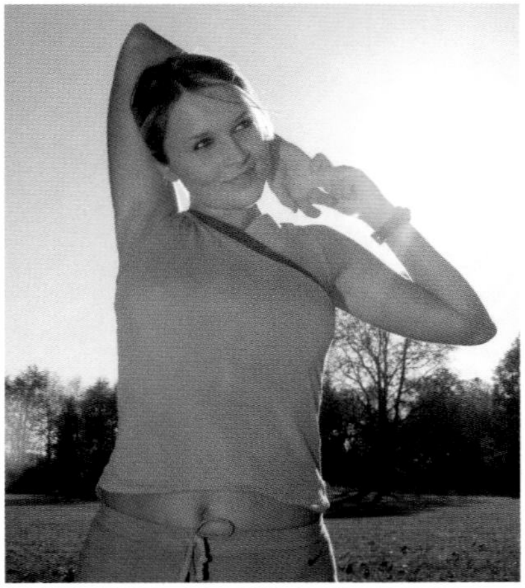

ASK A DOCTOR

Can exercising increase the risk of miscarriage? There is no evidence to suggest that, as long as you're healthy and have been given the all-clear from your doctor, exercise will put you at a greater risk of having a miscarriage. In fact, the benefits of getting regular moderate exercise while you're pregnant far outweigh the risks to you and your baby.

The most important factors at this stage of your pregnancy are to exercise at the same level you did prior to being pregnant. Do not attempt any new high-impact and strenuous activity or take up a new sport. Follow the guidelines that are set out on page 18.

Miscarriage

Miscarriage is the spontaneous loss of a pregnancy before the fetus is mature enough to survive outside the uterus. Miscarriage affects 15–20 percent of pregnancies—the majority occur in the first 12 weeks. Less than 5 percent of miscarriages occur in the second trimester.

Why miscarriage happens

An early miscarriage is usually due to a problem such as chromosomal or structural abnormality in the fetus; a fibroid (a noncancerous growth in the uterus); an infection; or an immune system disorder. Miscarriage occurs more commonly in older women, in smokers, and in multiple pregnancies.

If you miscarry, it's important to know that it wasn't linked to anything you did, such as exercise, sex, or travel. Also, no evidence suggests that rest reduces the risk of a threatened miscarriage going on to become inevitable (see box, below).

What will be done

If you have bleeding in early pregnancy, contact your doctor, who may recommend an ultrasound. If the ultrasound shows a normal fetal heart rate, the chance of miscarriage is reduced. If there is no heartbeat, you have a missed miscarriage, which means the pregnancy failed but your body has not passed the miscarriage. In a missed miscarriage, you may not have developed any bleeding or cramping yet. If you have not completed the miscarriage, you may be offered medication to induce the miscarriage or a procedure to remove the pregnancy. Medication means that you avoid general anesthesia and risks such as infection or, rarely, damage to the uterus. You may, however, bleed more heavily and for longer. Another option is to wait to see if miscarriage occurs naturally.

If you have three or more miscarriages in a row, your doctor may recommend tests to see if there is an underlying reason that may increase your risk of future miscarriages. Discovering a cause is unusual, but some rare abnormalities of the blood clotting system are associated with miscarriage.

After a miscarriage

You will bleed for a few days, like the end of a period. Use sanitary pads, not tampons, and avoid having intercourse until the bleeding settles. You could conceive again before your next period, which usually occurs 4–6 weeks after the miscarriage and may be heavier than usual.

There is no medical reason to avoid pregnancy, but it can be beneficial to wait to allow yourself time to grieve and to enable accurate dating.

SPOTLIGHT ON

TYPES OF MISCARRIAGES

Different terms are used to describe miscarriage, depending on what is found during an ultrasound scan or an internal examination.

- **Threatened miscarriage** is the term given to bleeding early in pregnancy, but in which the cervix remains closed. In this case, the bleeding stops after a few days, and the pregnancy is likely to continue.
- **Inevitable miscarriage** occurs when there is bleeding and the cervix is open, meaning that the fetus will be lost. If the pregnancy is less than eight weeks, the bleeding may be like a heavy, painful period. After eight weeks, the bleeding may be considerably heavier.
- **Incomplete miscarriage** occurs when there is bleeding and the cervix opens, but the uterus doesn't expel its entire contents and some pregnancy tissue is left behind.
- **Complete miscarriage** is when there is bleeding, the cervix opens, and the uterus expels all the pregnancy tissues.
- **Missed miscarriage** occurs when there may not be any bleeding or cramping but the pregnancy stops developing and the miscarriage isn't diagnosed until the routine scan at around 12 weeks.

LATE MISCARRIAGE

Losing a pregnancy after the first trimester is much more unusual than an early miscarriage. After 20 weeks, a pregnancy loss is referred to as a stillbirth. There are several reasons why late pregnancy loss may occur, including infection, uterine abnormalities or abnormalities in the baby, and a weak cervix. If you have a late miscarriage, your doctor will discuss the possible causes with you and, if a cause is identified, whether anything needs to be done in a future pregnancy.

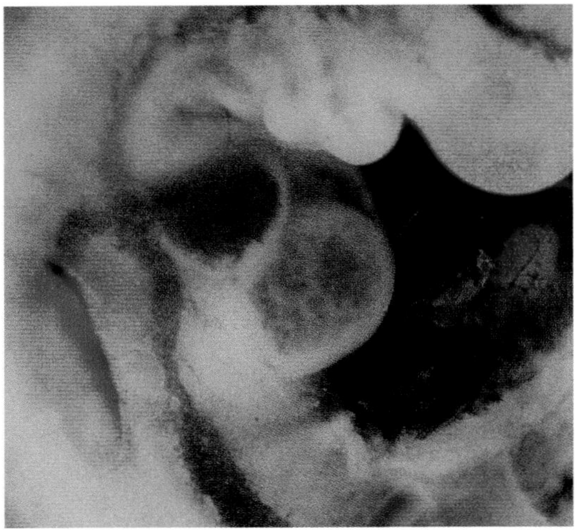

YOU ARE **6 WEEKS AND 6 DAYS**

232 days to go

YOUR BABY TODAY

At this stage of your baby's development, the heart is a tubular structure, visible in the center of this image. It is, however, already providing your baby with a very simple circulation.

> "What will become your baby's tiny arms and legs are beginning to develop during this seventh week of pregnancy."

It's still some weeks before your baby—still an embryo—will become recognizable as a human fetus. At the end of this seventh week, however, there are four simple limb buds, each slightly flattened at the end where, over the next two weeks, a hand or foot will form.

With the exception of muscle tone, which comes much later on, all stages of your baby's upper limb development precede any developments in his lower limbs.

The eyes are the first recognizable landmarks to form on the face. At this stage, the eyes consist of two simple surface indentations, which then develop a second indentation within the first; the inner one will become the lens and the outer the eyeball. Your baby's eyes are wide apart at this stage and his ears and nose have yet to form.

KNOW YOUR FISH

Fish is a great source of both protein and omega-3 fatty acids, which are essential for your baby's development (see p.169).

Eat at least two portions of fish a week, including one portion of oily fish. Include responsibly sourced white fish, such as haddock, cod, pollock, and flounder, since they are a good source of B vitamins and iodine.

There is concern that some fish may contain pollutants. Don't eat more than two portions a week of dogfish, sea bass or bream, halibut, turbot, or crab; or of oily fish, including salmon, mackerel, herring, sardines, and trout.

Large oily fish may contain high levels of mercury, so don't eat shark, marlin, or swordfish. For the same reason, limit yourself to four medium-sized cans of tuna (5 oz/140 g when drained) or two fresh tuna steaks (weighing about 5 oz/140 g cooked or 6 oz/170 g raw) a week.

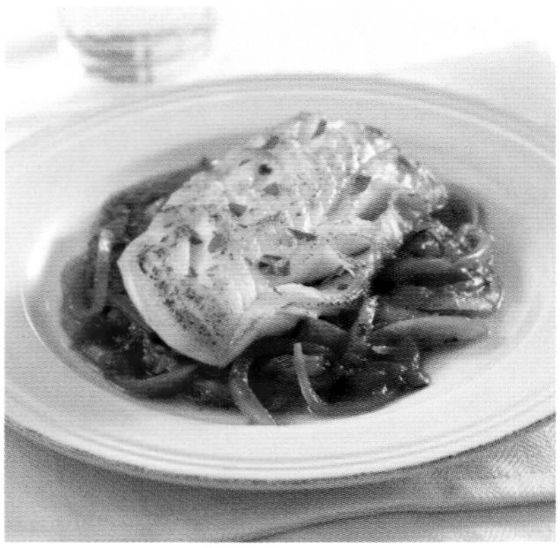

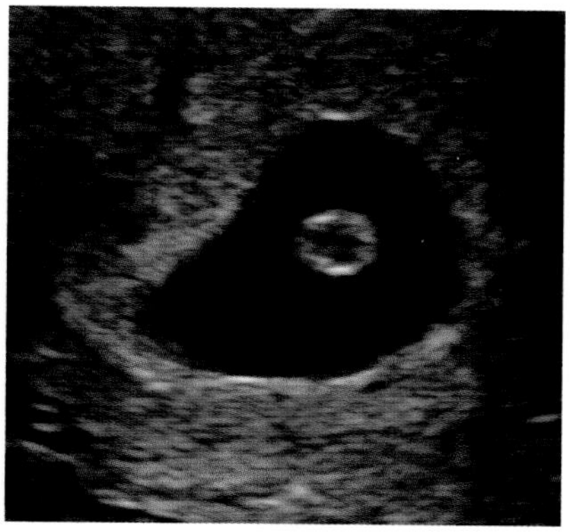

YOU ARE **7 WEEKS EXACTLY**

231 days to go

YOUR BABY TODAY

This early vaginal ultrasound scan shows the first signs of pregnancy: the black central area is the fluid-filled cavity in which your baby (not visible) is developing. Within this is a small circular area, which is the yolk sac.

> “As your baby’s body continues to develop, it won’t be long before some very general movements will be visible on a scan.”

ACTUAL SIZE OF YOUR BABY

At 7 weeks, your baby’s crown to rump length is 0.31 in (8 mm).

5 weeks

6 weeks

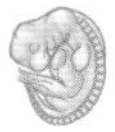

7 weeks

While you’re dealing with pregnancy symptoms, your tiny embryo is tightly curled in your uterus. In other species, a short portion at the lower end of the spine develops into a tail. This portion starts to disappear as more recognizably human features appear.

The ends of your baby’s limb buds flatten and begin to form short digits. At first these are fused together—then, like the rest of the skeleton, they grow around a soft framework of cartilage that gradually hardens into bone and become your baby’s tiny fingers and toes. As the upper limb buds lengthen, your baby’s elbows begin to form.

Your baby’s eyes continue to develop but won’t be fully formed until around week 20; his nostrils now appear as two shallow nasal pits.

FINDING A CONFIDANTE

Whether you want to tell people you’re pregnant is a matter of personal choice, but there’s a good reason to keep it quiet for the time being (see p.83).

You may, however, need to talk to someone (other than your partner), so confide in a friend. Choose someone who will indulge your need to discuss everything—from pregnancy symptoms to birth fears and baby names. The ideal candidate will find your food cravings and 4 am trips to the bathroom riveting... and provide bowls of ice cream and pickles, and advice around the clock.

ASK A DOCTOR

Help! I’m pregnant again and my little boy is only 18 months old. How will I cope? Pregnancy can be exhausting, particularly in the first trimester, when your body is adjusting to the new demands placed upon it. Having a toddler to contend with at this time makes it even harder. Most important of all, don’t feel guilty about putting your feet up—it’s important to take a step back and remember that your most important job right now is “growing” your baby. If there was ever a time to accept offers of help and call in favors from friends and relatives, it is in the coming months and after the new baby is born. Meanwhile, here are some simple things to try:

- Focus on quiet activities to enjoy with your toddler and leave the rough-and-tumble play to someone else.
- Take time to nurture yourself, sleeping when your toddler naps.
- In good weather, sit outside and let your toddler burn off energy.

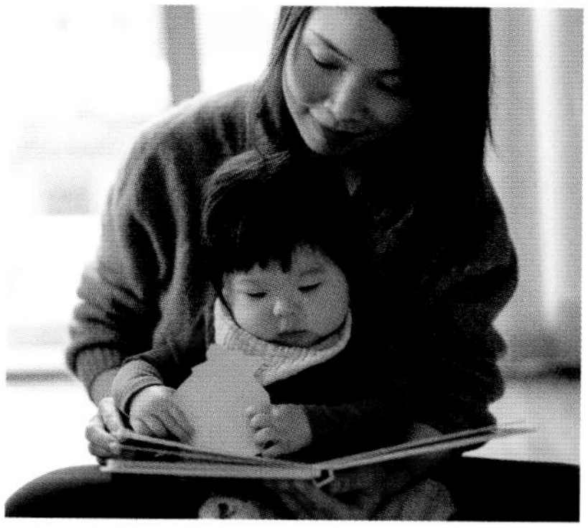

Your 8th week

YOUR MOOD MAY SWING FROM HIGH TO LOW AS HORMONES AND EMOTIONS TAKE HOLD. You're probably beginning to feel different, even though you don't look pregnant. You may feel a bit low and irritable at times; this is largely due to the changing levels of hormones in your body. You may sometimes have mixed feelings about being pregnant, however much you long for a baby. If the idea of going on vacation appeals to you, opt for short trips and a safe climate, and take extra care of yourself.

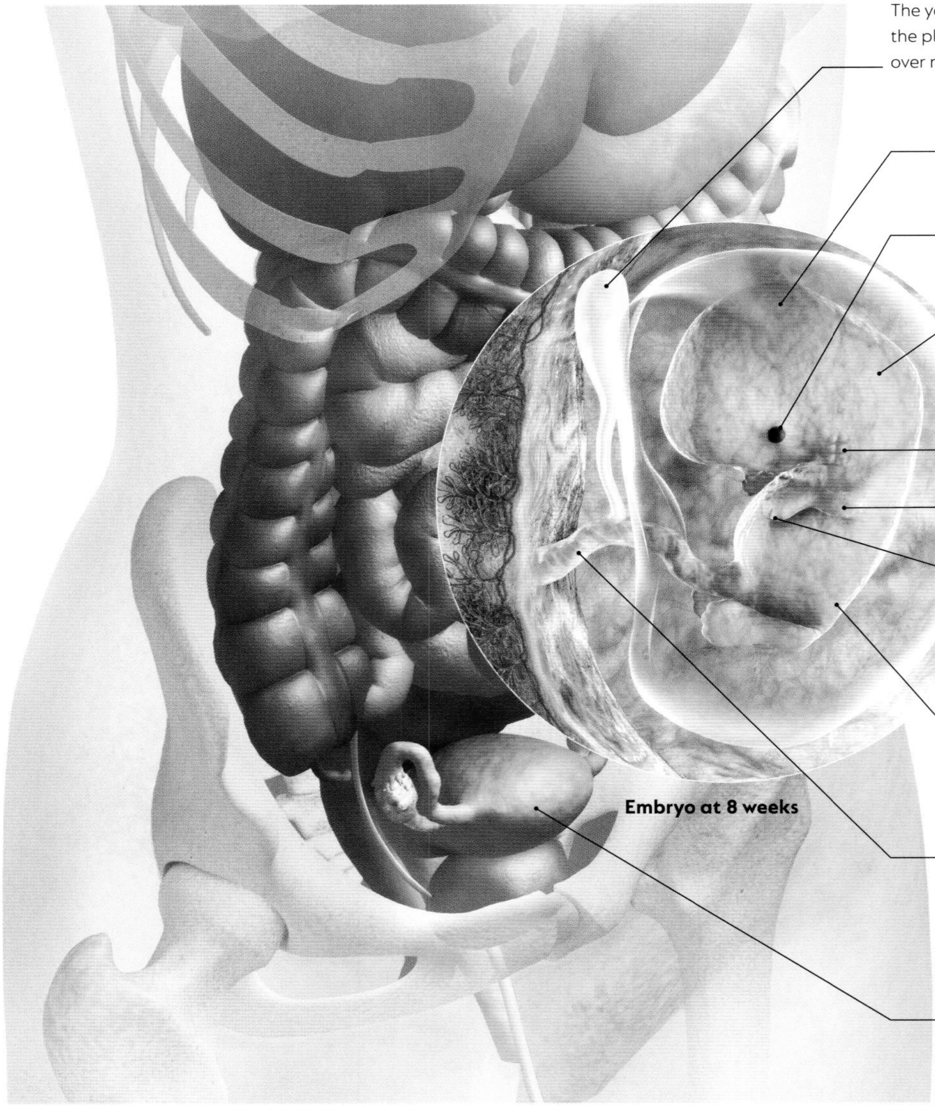
The yolk sac continues to shrink as the placenta now starts to take over nourishment of the embryo.
The baby's head is large relative to the trunk.
The eyes are getting larger and darkening with pigment.
The embryo measures 0.63 in (1.6 cm) from crown to rump.
The ears are just starting to develop; the small swellings will form part of the outer ear.
Elbows are now visible.
Digits begin to form on the hands and feet, although they are still fused together.
The baby's spine is straightening up, although the large head still topples forwards.
The umbilical cord contains blood vessels that are beginning to transport nutrients to the embryo and remove waste products.
Your uterus is starting to enlarge, but you won't notice any changes in your shape yet.

Embryo at 8 weeks

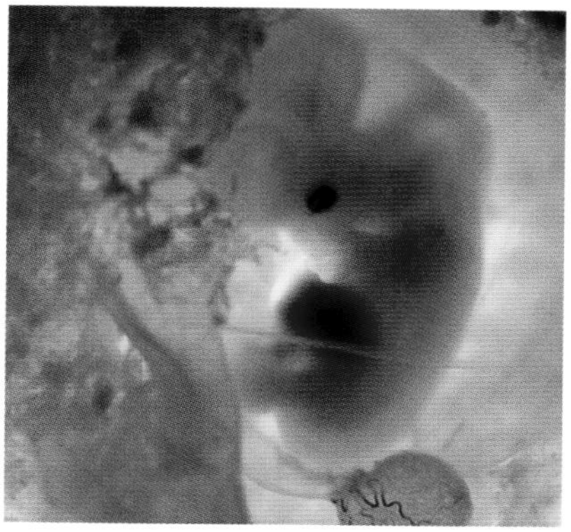

YOU ARE **7 WEEKS AND 1 DAY**

230 days to go

YOUR BABY TODAY

The fronds that will form the early placenta can be clearly seen on the right here. At the bottom and separate from the embryo is the yolk sac, which is becoming ever smaller as its role is taken over by the placenta.

> "As your body begins to change shape, you may begin to worry about gaining too much weight."

Pregnancy is not a time to overeat; neither is it a time for fad or restrictive diets. By eating sensibly and exercising moderately, you should gain a healthy amount of weight.

How much weight you should gain depends on your starting weight. If you were underweight when you became pregnant, you should put on more weight than someone who is a higher weight. The starting weight is calculated by figuring out your BMI (see p.16), which is a measure of weight in relation to height. It's a useful tool to figure out approximately how much weight you should gain during your pregnancy.

If you are underweight (a BMI of less than 18.5), your expected weight gain is 28–40 lb (12.5–18 kg). If you are a healthy weight (a BMI of 18.5–24.9), your expected weight gain is 25–35 lb (11.5–16 kg). If you are overweight (a BMI of 25–30), your expected weight gain is 15–25 lb (7–11.5 kg). If you are obese (a BMI of over 30), your expected weight gain is 11–20 lb (5–9 kg).Expected weight gain will be more for a multiple pregnancy.

It is unsafe for pregnant overweight and obese women to diet, but not unsafe to manage weight gain through exercise and healthy eating.

HOW MUCH WEIGHT WILL YOU GAIN?

Every woman will gain weight at a different rate depending on her starting weight.

Try not to be too focused on weight and expect to gain a little in the first trimester, then more, maybe 1.5–2 lb (750 g–1 kg) a week in the second and third trimesters.

In the final weeks of pregnancy, it's normal to gain a few more pounds. Remember that the amount you gain will depend on many individual factors; and where you gain weight can also differ from woman to woman. Consult your doctor if you are concerned about weight gain. Also exercise regularly.

COMPONENTS OF WEIGHT GAIN

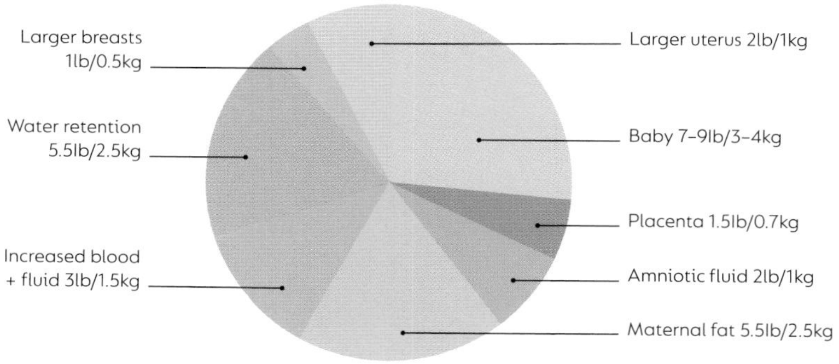
Larger breasts 1lb/0.5kg
Water retention 5.5lb/2.5kg
Increased blood + fluid 3lb/1.5kg
Larger uterus 2lb/1kg
Baby 7–9lb/3–4kg
Placenta 1.5lb/0.7kg
Amniotic fluid 2lb/1kg
Maternal fat 5.5lb/2.5kg

The weight you'll gain during pregnancy is a combination of your baby and their support system, the increased size of your breasts and uterus, essential fat reserves, and additional bodily fluids and blood.

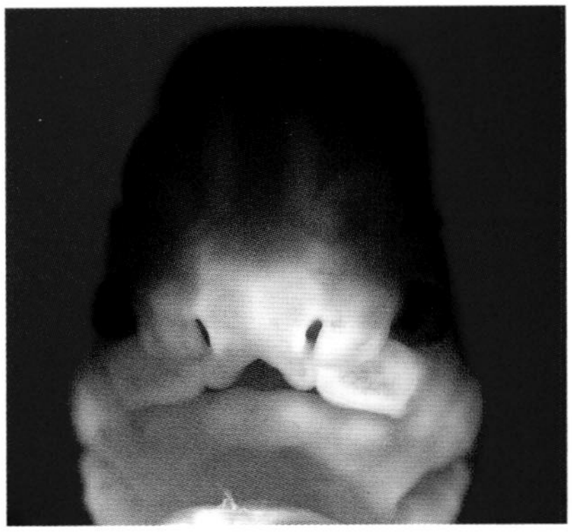

YOU ARE **7 WEEKS AND 2 DAYS**

229 days to go

YOUR BABY TODAY

Your baby won't look recognizably human yet, but the lower lip and jaw are formed; the upper lip is not yet complete, and the mouth appears very wide. The external ears are developing low down at the jaw line and the eyes are wide apart.

> “ Although your baby's brain is still very simply formed, it's undergoing some remarkable changes. ”

This is a really important stage of development. The baby's brain is a hollow structure, joined to the spinal cord, but it's now starting to fold and form five distinct areas.

The lowest part, or hindbrain, is the first part to grow rapidly and will become structures known as the pons, medulla, and cerebellum. These structures are the most primitive areas of the brain and determine many basic actions that we do without conscious effort, such as breathing and keeping our balance.

Above this is the midbrain that conveys signals from the hindbrain, peripheral nerves, and spinal cord to the forebrain. This part of the brain consists of the thalamus—involved with emotions and sensory perception—and the two cerebral hemispheres. Each hemisphere has a fluid-filled chamber and within that the cerebrospinal fluid is produced.

At the 11–14 week scan (see p.139), brain development checks will be carried out.

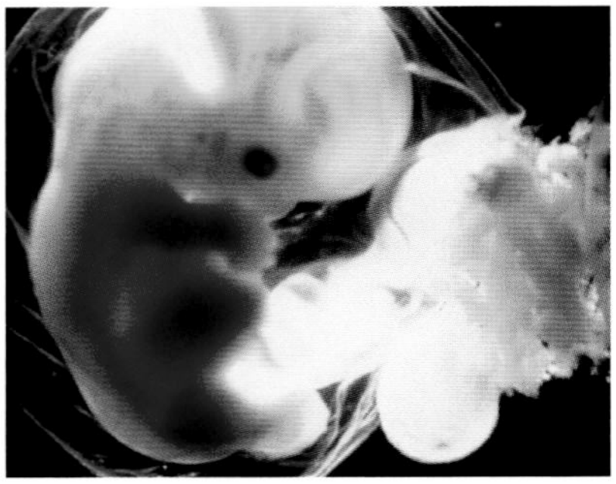

The dots that will form the eyes are clearly visible now. At the side of the head, the deep cleft can be seen between the front and back of the brain; this is normal at this stage.

EATING FISH

Fish really is brain food! Fish contains iodine (see p.80) as well as omega-3 fatty acids, which are essential for your baby's developing brain. Make sure you eat some fish every week, but be aware of the precautions you need to take with some varieties (see p.96).

ASK A DOCTOR

I'm eight weeks pregnant and have had some bleeding. Should I be concerned? If the bleeding is light, and there are no abdominal cramps or pain, then it's unlikely that there is anything wrong. However, consult your doctor if you have bleeding at any stage of pregnancy to rule out any complications.

Bleeding in early pregnancy can sometimes be due to a cervical ectropian, which is when the surface of the cervix becomes more delicate. This results from hormonal changes and is not harmful to the baby. A cervical ectropian can be aggravated by having sex.

Bleeding in late pregnancy may be more serious as it can mean there is placental abruption, when the placenta detaches from the wall of the uterus, or be due to a low-lying placenta (see p.212). A mucus discharge tinged with blood in late pregnancy may be a "show" (see p.391).

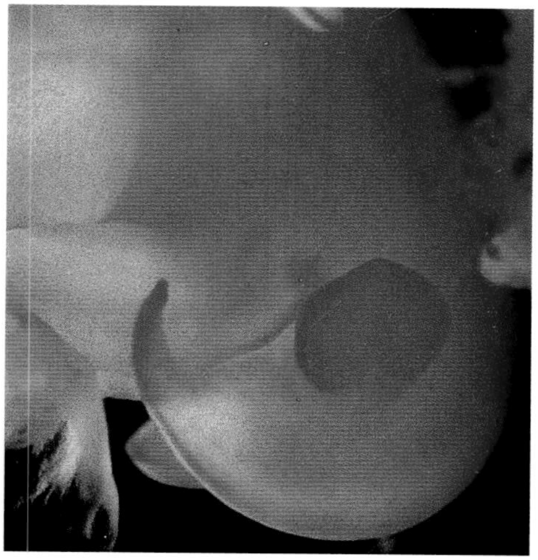

YOU ARE **7 WEEKS AND 3 DAYS**

228 days to go

YOUR BABY TODAY

At this stage, the embryo's "tail," shown curving up on the left, is starting to disappear. The somites of this area of the musculoskeletal system will eventually form the four fused bones of your baby's coccyx—the lowest part of the spine.

> "Even if you're happy about having a baby, it's natural to have mixed emotions at times."

At this early stage of pregnancy, changing hormone levels may cause mood swings and unexpected emotional responses. Your emotions may fluctuate—one minute you're laughing and the next you're irritable and yelling, or crying. Sometimes things that have never been a problem, such as hearing a particular piece of music or seeing an ad, might make you cry, or you may snap at your loved ones over something trivial. You might be confused that at a time when you should be happy, you often feel tense and tearful. Be reassured that this is a normal and temporary part of pregnancy and try not to be too hard on yourself.

These changing moods are caused mainly by pregnancy hormones, which is something out of your control. They are the same hormones that cause the symptoms of PMS—rapid mood swings, crying, and irritability—that you might have experienced before.

Be kind to yourself during these down times and do what works best for you, whether it's taking time out to be alone or sharing your feelings with others.

One in 10 pregnant women have symptoms of depression. If you are concerned that you might be depressed, seek the advice and help of your doctor. Having a supportive partner can make all the difference to managing mood swings during pregnancy. As a partner, all you can do is be as patient, and understanding as you can. Until the mood passes, which it will, just bide your time, bite your tongue, and give your partner a hug.

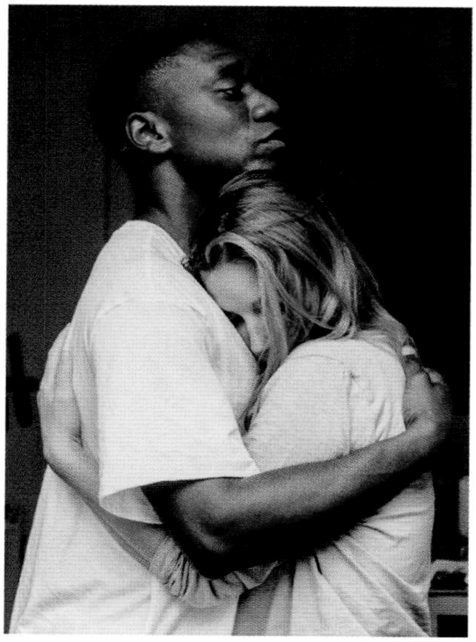

When you're a bit down, ask for a hug from your partner or a close friend or relative, and remember the negative feeing will pass.

TOXOPLASMOSIS

Toxoplasmosis is a rare disorder caused by a parasite living in some animals that can harm a developing fetus. The symptoms may resemble those of mononucleosis with a fever and/or swollen glands in the neck.

It can be spread through cat feces, so avoid changing cat litter boxes, and avoid handling newborn lambs. Be scrupulous about hygiene in the kitchen and make sure you cook meats fully. Home-cured meats, such as salami and chorizo, should be avoided or cooked, since the salting and curing alone may not destroy the parasite. Alternatively, freeze them first to destroy the parasites.

Prenatal care options

Throughout your pregnancy, you may be cared for by a family-practice doctor, obstetrician, or a combination of the two. The goal of your prenatal care is to monitor you and your baby so that problems can be identified and managed.

Your care during pregnancy

Early in pregnancy, you will need to think about who you would like to care for you during pregnancy, labor, and the postpartum period. You will also need to consider where you want to give birth since this will have an influence on your choice of care provider. The main options are outlined below, although these may vary depending on where you live. When you attend your first prenatal appointment at 8–12 weeks, you will be given information about the prenatal services you can access in your area. The medical checkups that are done during this appointment will also help establish the best choice for you prenatal care.

Types of prenatal care

The majority of your care will usually be provided by an ob/gyn. At your first appointment, they will outline the prenatal services you will receive.

Group medical practice With this type of care, you will see two or more doctors (typically ob/gyns and/or family practitioners throughout your pregnancy on a rotation basis. One of these doctors will be present at the hospital when you deliver.

Solo medical practice You'll have one doctor, and you will see them at every prenatal visit. They'll attend your birth at the hospital, unless they're unavailable and arrange for another doctor to be present for your delivery.

Combination practice With this type of care, you'll get to see both doctors and midwives. At least one ob/gyn and one nurse-midwife sees patients on a rotating basis. Depending on the practice, a midwife may be able to assist in delivery at the hospital. Expect a doctor to be present.

Maternity center-based practice If your pregnancy is low-risk, you can see certified nurse-midwives for most of your appointments throughout pregnancy. Ob/gyns are available for consultations as required. If you choose this option, you'll deliver your baby at the maternity or birthing center that is associated with the practice, unless complications arise, in which case your care would be transferred to the affiliated hospital.

Independent certified nurse-midwife practice Some states permit midwives to practice without a doctor in the office. If this type of care is available in your area and you have a low-risk pregnancy, you can see midwives for all of your appointments, and a midwife would be present at your delivery in a hospital, birthing center, or at home. The midwives generally have arrangements with doctors, who are available for consultations as needed.

Where you give birth

This important decision doesn't have to be made at your initial

INFORMED CHOICE

Being able to choose the type of care you receive is one of the most important aspects of pregnancy and childbirth. Make sure that you have the most up-to-date, evidence-based information available so that you can make informed decisions.

You will be able to discuss the options with your doctor and feel free to ask them whatever you want, change your mind, and know that your preferences, regardless of the recommendations made by the doctor, will be considered.

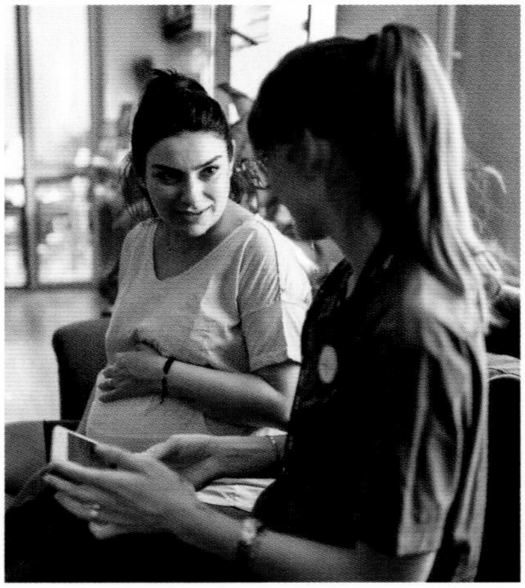

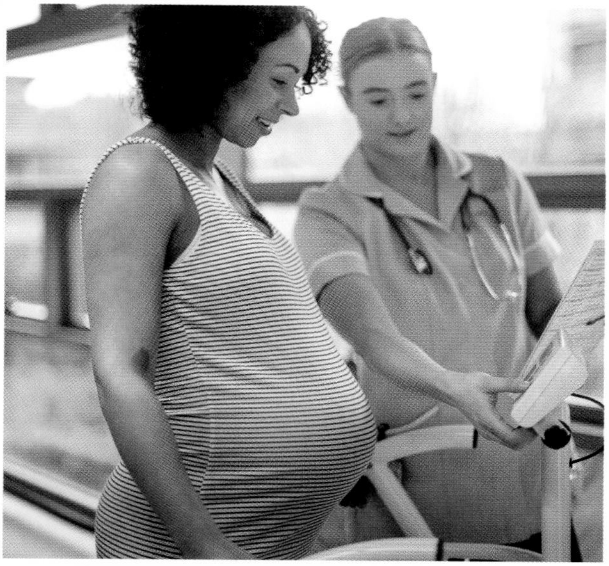

Midwives may provide care at doctors' offices, maternity centers, or their own practices.

appointment, but your midwife or doctor may discuss the options at this time. It's wise to be aware of the risks, benefits, and consequences of your choice. If you have a preexisting problem, or one that develops during pregnancy, this must be factored into your decision on where to give birth.

In the hospital Some women prefer to give birth in a hospital with doctors and medical equipment close by. Also, some women need specialized care and input from obstetricians because of existing conditions or problems that develop in labor. In this case, the obstetrician and the midwife will work closely together. Other specialists may also need to be involved during labor, for example, if a woman has diabetes or a heart condition.

In a birth center These units provide a homelike setting. They are led by midwives with no obstetric input and have facilities such as birthing tubs and pools. The goal at a birthing center is to make labor and birth more natural, with less monitoring and fewer routine medical procedures and interventions. Some pain medication may be available, but epidurals are not. Some birthing centers are next to or affiliated with hospitals so that, if necessary, you can be transferred quickly. Birthing centers are an option that is recommended for low-risk pregnancies.

At home A home birth is an option for women who want to give birth in familiar surroundings. However, a home birth is advised only for women who have low-risk pregnancies and for those with no preexisting medical problems. In the US, home births are considered controversial because complications can develop during the labor or the delivery, even in women with low-risk pregnancies. The American College of Obstetricians and Gynecologists and the American Medical Association oppose home births because of the potential for complications.

YOUR CARE PROVIDERS

Several different health-care professionals will care for you during pregnancy and labor, and in the postpartum period:

Ob/gyns provide the vast majority of care for women in pregnancy, labor, and the postpartum period. They're specially trained to handle all phases of pregnancy and postpartum recovery. If you have a preexisting condition that could complicate your pregnancy, like diabetes or high blood pressure, or if you're pregnant with twins, you should see an ob/gyn. Special doctors known as high-risk obstetricians, or maternal-fetal medicine specialists, may see you for some appointments if you have a very high-risk pregnancy, such as a baby diagnosed with a serious medical condition or a history of pregnancy complications or repeated loss.

General practitioners (GPs) may alternate appointments with ob/gyns.

Midwives can provide care for women with low-risk pregnancies throughout all phases of pregnancy and the postpartum period. Certified-nurse midwives often work in a practice with ob/gyns but sometimes can practice on their own. They are registered nurses with extra education and training who are certified by the American College of Nurse-Midwives.

Pediatricians are doctors with special training in the health of babies and children. All babies that are born in a hospital have a newborn checkup by a pediatrician before being discharged.

Neonatologists specialize in the care of newborns with problems.

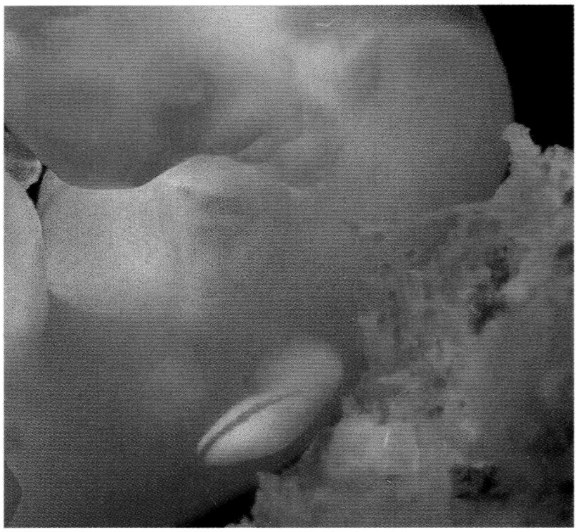

YOU ARE **7 WEEKS AND 4 DAYS**

227 days to go

YOUR BABY TODAY

The upper and lower limb buds that will form the legs and arms are clearly visible by now. The baby's head is still curled over the chest, but the beginnings of the ears can just be detected as raised areas at the base of the head.

> " Your baby's facial features are beginning to develop and over the next few weeks will become much more defined. "

Your baby has ears! Low down, near the jaw line, the ears form, each arising from six small mounds, fusing together to give your baby his unique and individual ear shape. As the face and jaw forms and your baby's neck extends moving away from the chest wall, the ears migrate upward; they will come to lie at the same level as his eyes by 11 weeks.

The baby's lips and nose are now beginning to take shape. To form the upper lip, two separate ridges of tissue grow from each side of your baby's face to fuse with the small piece of tissue in the midline extending downward beneath the nose (the grooved part of the upper lip).

At around this stage, your baby's small and large bowel lengthen. Because they have insufficient room to expand inside the still very curled-up embryo, the intestines appear as a bulge on the surface of the abdominal wall. This bulge is covered by a membrane, into which the umbilical cord becomes attached. The bowel will continue to grow in this embryonic sac until 11–12 weeks when it will be reabsorbed into the abdominal cavity, leaving just the surface attachment of the cord.

ALLERGIES

The risk of a baby developing allergies is not reduced by avoiding common allergens. In a recent study, pregnant and breastfeeding women avoided allergens such as peanuts and delayed introducing certain foods into their babies' diet. It did not decrease allergic disease in babies and toddlers.

CAREFUL COOKING

Your immune system is under extra pressure during pregnancy, making you more susceptible to food poisoning, and some food-borne illnesses can cross the placenta and affect your unborn baby. Always be careful to do the following:

• Wash your hands carefully and regularly, with hot water and soap. Dry them completely before preparing food, since bacteria spread more easily on damp skin. Also thoroughly wash utensils and work surfaces.

• Keep your fridge below 41º F (5º C). Keep food chilled until you prepare it.

• Cook food thoroughly and serve it hot. Red meat must reach 160º F (70º C) internally and the juices must run clear when you insert a sharp knife.

• Refrigerate leftovers immediately, and reheat until piping hot, only once.

• Cook prepared meals thoroughly, until they are piping hot, especially if they contain poultry.

• Use food before the use-by date.

• Wash fruit and vegetables fully.

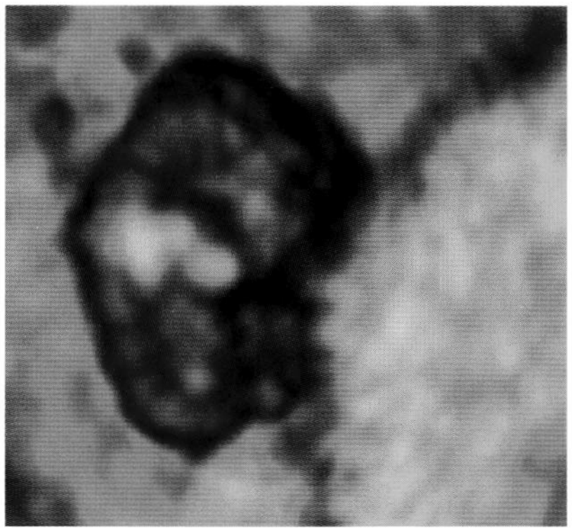

YOU ARE **7 WEEKS AND 5 DAYS**

226 days to go

YOUR BABY TODAY

This ultrasound scan is a side view of the baby. It shows that the head (at top) is relatively large compared to the rest of the body. The lighter, elongated area at the center of the baby's darker body is an upper arm bud.

> “ Life goes on even though you're pregnant, but make sure you seek the right help if you're becoming overly tired. ”

ASK A DOCTOR

I'm going on vacation to a tropical climate. Can I have vaccinations? It's advisable to avoid traveling to parts of the world where there is a high risk of disease unless you really need to. Local health care might not be adequate and food and water may be contaminated. If you can't postpone your vacation, be aware of the following:

- Oral vaccines to protect against yellow fever, typhoid, polio, and anthrax, for example, are contraindicated during pregnancy. Your doctor may decide that if you need to travel, the risk of having the vaccine is lower than the risks associated with contracting the disease.
- Some vaccines (polio and typhoid) are safe when given by injection. Mefloquine tablets, to prevent malaria, are considered safe after week 16.
- It's safe to have a tetanus vaccination if you're pregnant; check whether yours is up-to-date.

You may find work a strain at times. If you have symptoms, such as fatigue, and still haven't told your colleagues that you're pregnant, it can make for a stressful and difficult day. If you've told some colleagues, or your boss, you're expecting it may be easier but you might feel you have to prove you can still do your job as efficiently as before.

Traveling can be tiring so explore the possibility of doing more flexible hours, so that you can commute when it's less busy. Be reassured that even though you aren't feeling your best, your unborn baby is unlikely to be affected. Do, however, take care of yourself and be aware of your limitations when it comes to work and commuting.

If you find that you're struggling to deal with your workload, consider speaking to your boss (you can ask him or her to keep your pregnancy a secret until you are ready to tell), or someone in the human resources department, to give yourself a little breathing space. Lean on any colleagues who are close friends for support in these early weeks.

ARE YOU NESTING ALREADY?

There's nothing like a new arrival to inspire you to get all those do-it-yourself (DIY) jobs done around the home. For most women, the nesting bug occurs in the later weeks of pregnancy, but if you're itching to get your house in order before then, make sure you exercise a little caution.

First of all, avoid putting yourself and your baby at risk: don't stand on tall ladders, and don't bend and crouch for long periods since this may affect your circulation. Avoid contact with oil-based paints, polyurethane (used for flooring), spray paints, turpentine, and other paint removers, and avoid inhaling plaster dust.

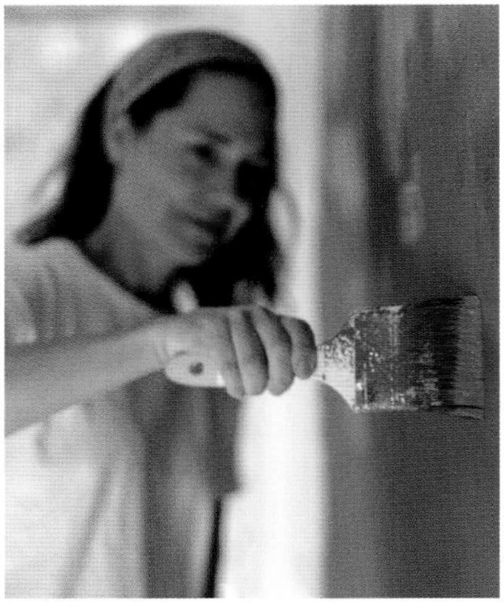

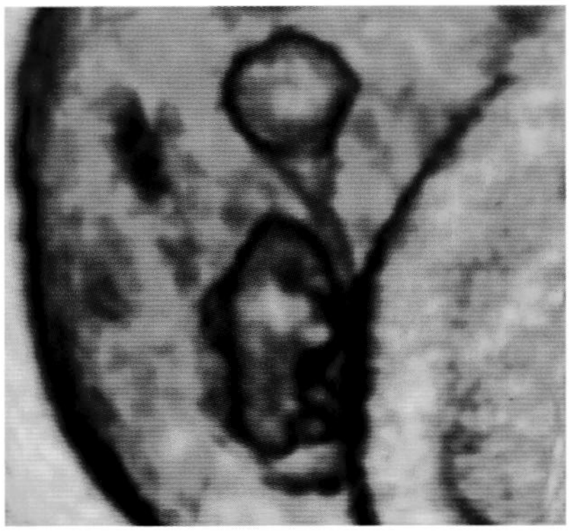

YOU ARE **7 WEEKS AND 6 DAYS**

225 days to go

YOUR BABY TODAY

The yolk sac can be seen floating like a balloon in the amniotic cavity on its fine stalk. As the embryo has drawn nutrition from the yolk sac it has gradually reduced in both size and importance. Meanwhile the placenta (on the right) is becoming established.

> "If you're planning a vacation, take into account that you may not feel up to a long trip."

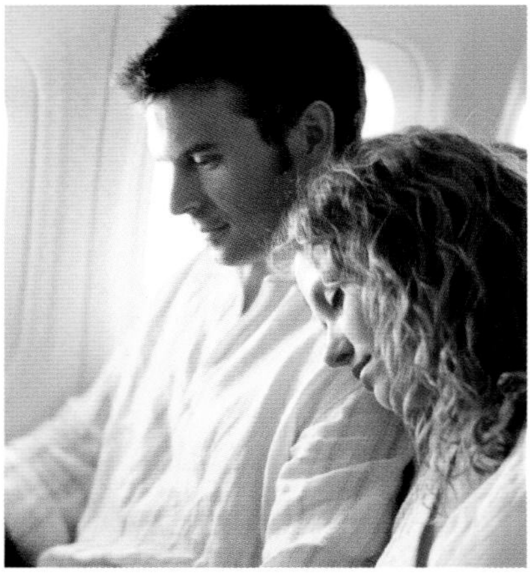

Be aware of your self-care on the flight. Rest but make sure you get up regularly to stretch your legs. It's even more important to keep the blood circulating when you're pregnant. Drink plenty of water to avoid dehydration.

You may have planned a vacation before you found out you were pregnant, or just feel like getting away. If you're feeling tired and have morning sickness, however, you may not feel up to traveling too far.

One advantage of going away is being able to spend quality time with your partner and fully embrace the fact that you're going to be parents.

When going on vacation, check with travel insurance companies to see if you can get coverage during pregnancy and check the medical facilities at your destination. If you have prenatal records, take them with you. Some airlines may not accept pregnant women on flights after 36 weeks without a doctor's letter written within 72 hours of the flight confirming your due date and your fitness to fly.

BREATHE EASY

Exercise can help keep breathlessness at bay, and increase the efficiency of your heart and lungs (cardiovascular system), helping you to deal with the physical demands of pregnancy now and in later months.

A cardiovascular workout involves increasing your heart rate for at least 20–30 minutes. However, pregnancy is not a time to start training for a marathon; stick to moderate-intensity workouts. A way to test if you are exercising at the right level is to talk while you are working out (see p.161)—if you can't, lower the intensity.

Try doing interval training, which involves alternating five minutes of cardiovascular workouts with five minutes of toning for the upper body (see p.196). Breathe in to begin and exhale as you lift the weights.

Breathing deeply allows oxygen to travel to your vital organs and helps the cardiovascular system to function effectively. During pregnancy, avoid taking short, shallow breaths. Focus on expanding your rib cage and filling your lungs with air by breathing deeply.

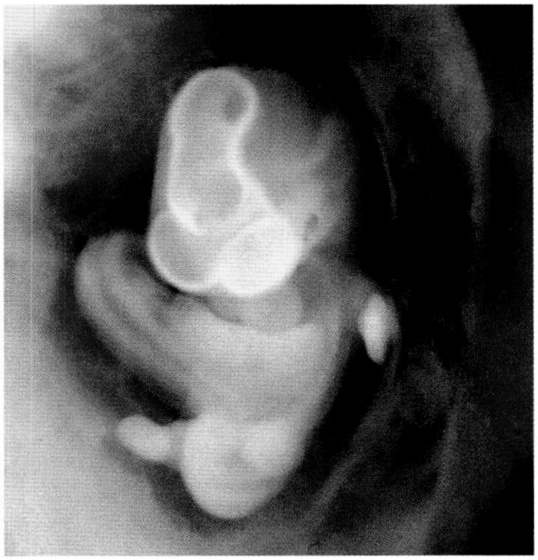

YOU ARE **8 WEEKS EXACTLY**

224 days to go

YOUR BABY TODAY

The head is disproportionately large at this stage. In the center of this image, the underlying structures of the brain can be seen: the forebrain has divided into two and these two halves will become the two cerebral hemispheres of your baby's brain.

> "You're probably wondering if you're having a boy or a girl, but the physical signs of gender aren't apparent yet."

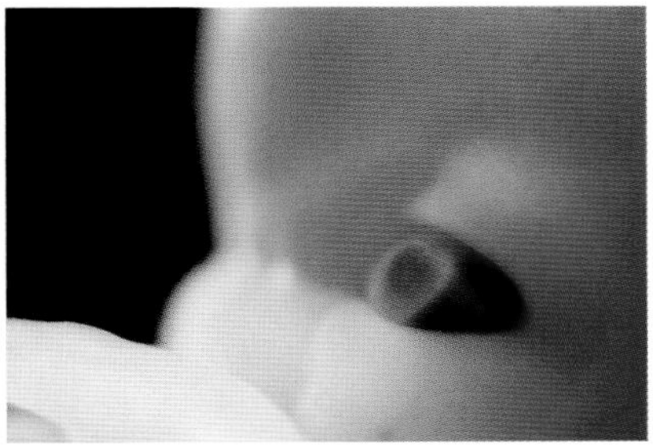

Your baby's head is large at this stage due to rapid underlying brain expansion that gives the impression of an overhanging forehead.

ACTUAL SIZE OF YOUR BABY

At 8 weeks, your baby's crown to rump length is 0.63 in (1.6 cm).

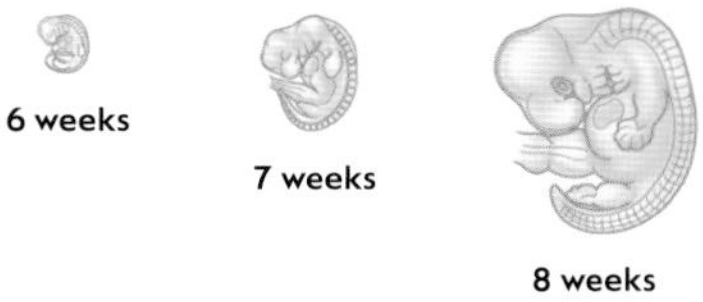
6 weeks
7 weeks
8 weeks

Although the sex of your baby was determined at the moment of fertilization, it will not yet be apparent whether the embryo is male or female.

At this stage of development, the external genitalia have exactly the same appearance (almost nonexistent). In a girl, no uterus or tubes have formed internally. The ovary in a female embryo and testes in a male embryo are currently just ridges of tissue, without any of the characteristics of either reproductive organ.

Incredibly, your baby's heart has already developed, with four chambers beating at about 160 beats per minute. The common tube leaving the heart has divided into the two main blood vessels: the aorta takes your baby's oxygen-carrying blood to his body and the pulmonary trunk takes his blood to the lungs. Valves within the heart ensure that the blood only travels one way and all of the major blood vessels are now established.

Your baby's eyes appear open because the eyelids have just started to appear and have yet to fuse. In reality, they won't properly open until week 26. Pigment is just starting to accumulate within the retina of the eye. The developing lens is supplied by a single blood vessel in the optic nerve, which will later disappear.

ASK A DOCTOR

I'm eight weeks pregnant and have an ear and throat infection. Will I be allowed to take antibiotics? You may be prescribed antibiotics by your doctor since there are some that can be taken during pregnancy. Penicillin-based antibiotics are usually prescribed, or if you are allergic to these your doctor will be able to offer other safe alternatives.

Never take antibiotics that have not been prescribed for you. The following should not be taken during pregnancy:

- **Tetracylines** taken during pregnancy can adversely affect the development of an unborn baby's bones, and may cause some discoloration of the enamel on the baby's teeth.
- **Streptomycin** can cause damage to the ears of the developing baby and result in hearing loss.
- **Sulfonamides** can cause jaundice in the baby.

Your 9th week

YOUR BABY HAS HANDS AND FEET, AND HIS BONES ARE GROWING. During this week, your baby starts to make tiny movements. You won't be aware of this, but it's exciting to think about. On the downside, you could be in the throes of nausea and sickness. However, many women find that the nausea starts to lessen from now on. There are various measures you can take to relieve the sickness, but if it's making life miserable, talk to your doctor.

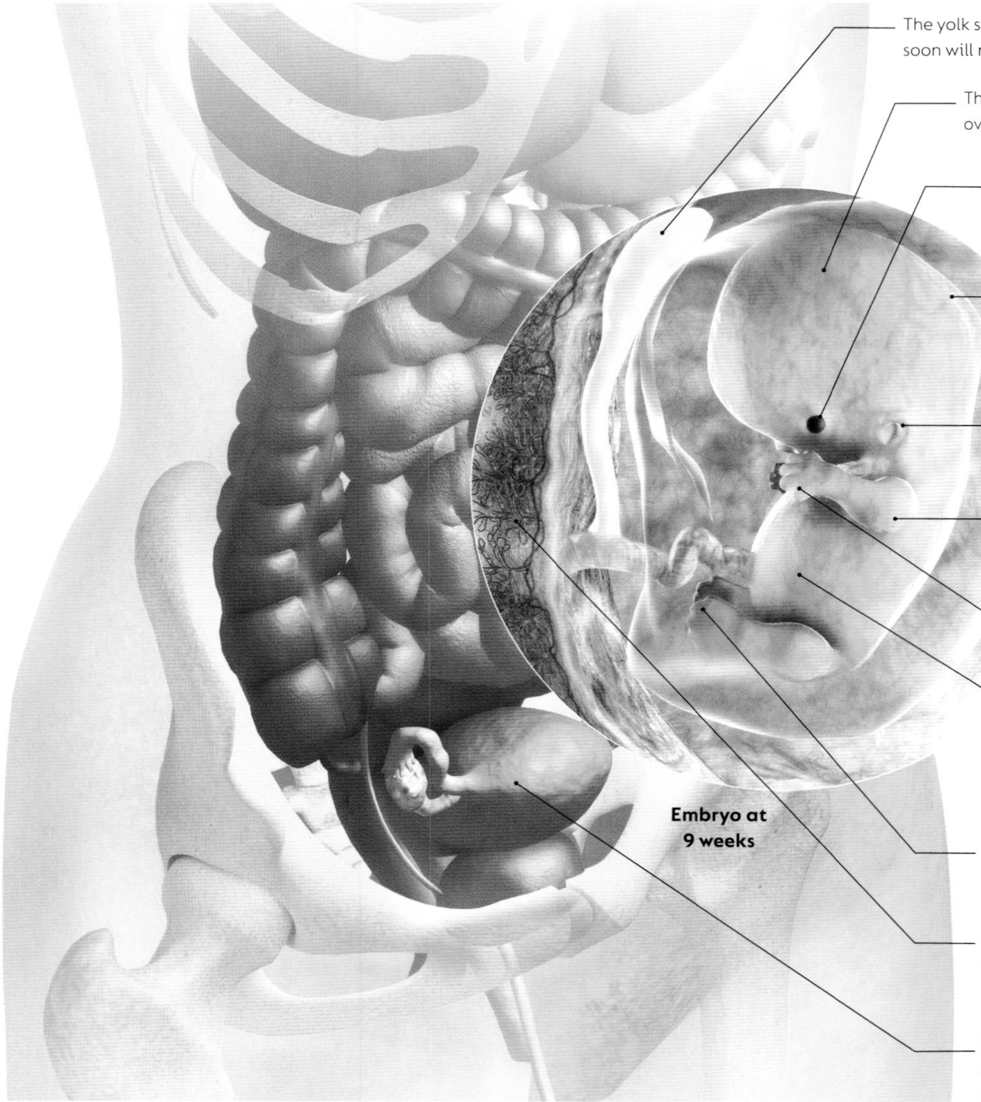
The yolk sac shrinks further and soon will not be needed.
The baby's head is still bowed over the bulge of his stomach.
The eyes, which until now have been on the side of the baby's head, have migrated around to the front.
The embryo now measures 0.9 in (2.3 cm) from crown to rump.
The outer ears are starting to take shape.
Elbows are now able to move.
Individual fingers are distinct, but are still not totally separate.
The major organs of the baby's digestive system have all started to develop but are not ready to carry out any digestive functions.
Embryo at 9 weeks
The toes are less advanced than the fingers and still appear budlike.
Chorionic villi continue to branch as the placenta matures and so that it can fulfill all your baby's needs.
Your uterus is growing to accommodate the baby and now starts to tilt upward.

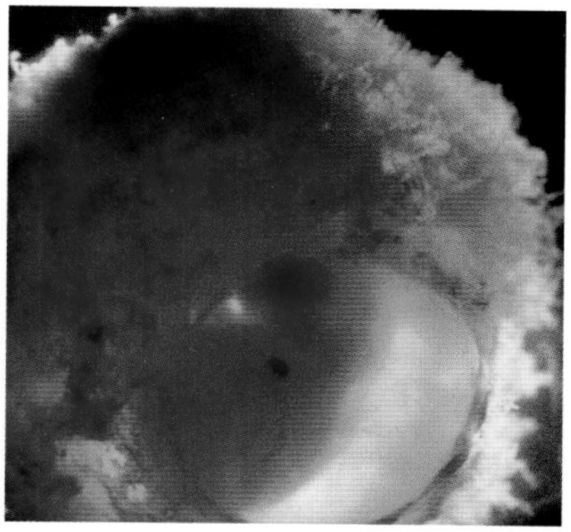

YOU ARE **8 WEEKS AND 1 DAY**

223 days to go

YOUR BABY TODAY

At this early stage in the pregnancy the placenta is much larger than the fetus. The fetus can just be seen within the amniotic sac. The fronds (white area) on the surface of the sac make up the placenta and at this stage surround nearly all of the amniotic sac.

> “Not all pregnant women have cravings, but many women do experience a change in their food preferences.”

When it comes to being pregnant, it seems your body instinctively knows what you like to eat. Experts are not sure how this can happen but it seems your body has natural protective mechanisms; certain foods are not good for the developing baby so your body turns you away from them; or your body is deficient in certain nutrients, so craves foods that will provide them.

Suddenly you can't stand the thought of food and drinks that you have always loved and find yourself craving things you never previously liked, or you long for bizarre combinations of foods. Aversions and cravings are often associated with nausea. It's common to be turned off by fatty foods since the smell alone can make you feel sick. You may start to dislike the taste or the smell of coffee or tea, cigarettes, and alcohol.

It is common to crave strong-tasting foods such as pickles, which may be due to the fact your taste buds change during pregnancy. What's termed “pica” is an unhealthy craving for bizzare items (see p.121).

You should try to eat healthily, but there are a few foods which should be avoided (see p.17). Otherwise eat whatever combinations you desire—and don't worry about the strange looks you might get in the sandwich shop!

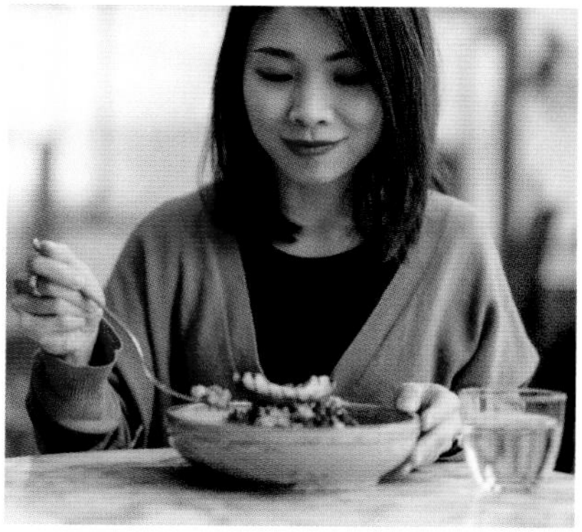

Your appetite is likely to change when you are pregnant and craving foods you don't usually eat is normal.

FOCUS ON PARTNERS

If it's your partner's responsibility to play host to the baby for nine months, it most definitely falls to you to see that your partner gets everything she needs. A word of warning: cravings usually occur the minute the local store has closed, or in the evening when you're relaxing. Forget the pickles and ice cream you've been told to expect. Instead, be prepared for a last-minute dash to the local pizza place, a trek to a 24-hour supermarket that carries organic sour-cream-and-onion-flavored potato chips, beets, or a chocolate doughnut.

Help by honing your cooking skills and preparing nutritious meals and snacks you can both enjoy. Your partner will appreciate your lovingly prepared meals and it may mean less temptation to eat unhealthy foods.

ASK A NUTRITIONIST

Should I stop adding salt to my food during pregnancy? No, but do stick to the recommended daily allowance of salt, which is 6g a day. To do this, avoid eating processed foods and sauces and, instead, get the salt you need from healthy snacks and homemade food. Most people consume too much salt and a lot of it comes from foods such as breads and chips, as well as prepared meals, sauces, pizza, and cured foods such as ham and bacon.

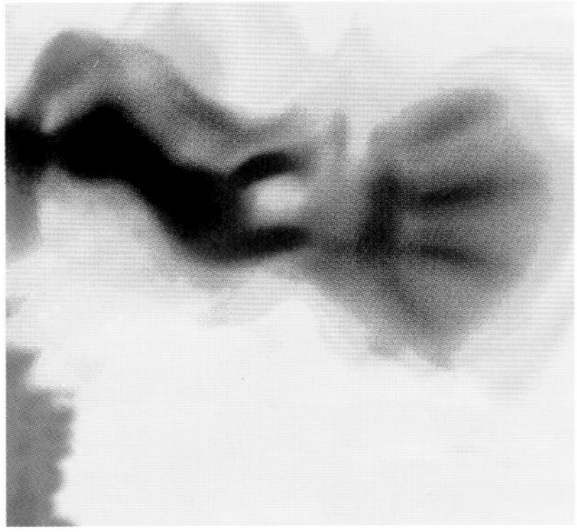

YOU ARE **8 WEEKS AND 2 DAYS**

222 days to go

YOUR BABY TODAY

The baby's hands (seen here) and feet are gradually developing and they are formed of cartilage, not bone, at this early stage. On the right, the fused rays of the hand plate that will become the fingers can be seen. The ribs are in the background.

“ Who will your baby look like? His unique facial features are beginning to take shape this week. ”

If you were to have an ultrasound scan this week, it would be possible to recognize several of your baby's facial features.

The eyelids fuse and will remain closed until around the 26th week. The lips have already formed and with the surrounding skin will have the greatest concentration of nerves. The muscular tongue arises from the base of your baby's mouth, but it will be two weeks before the first taste buds appear. The hard palate that forms the roof of the mouth arises from two "shelves" that start to grow, one each side, beneath the tongue; these shelves will lift upward to connect horizontally, allowing the tongue to drop down in to the mouth. Once they have joined together, the septum of the nose grows downward to meet them.

Your baby's tiny tooth buds are in place and this is critical to adequate jaw development. One branch of tooth buds will form the first milk teeth and a separate branch will eventually form the permanent teeth. The milk teeth develop slowly and it will not be until the six month of pregnancy that they acquire their hard enamel coating.

The embryo is still very curled up, with the head resting on the chest. Over the next two weeks as the jaw and neck grow, the head will gradually lift.

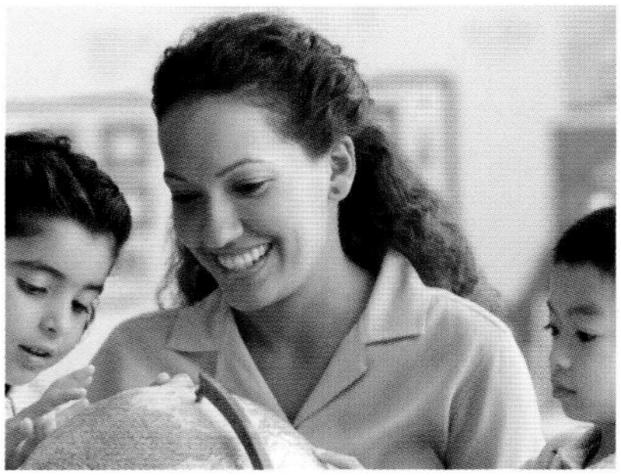

If you are in regular contact with young children, it's even more important that you check your immunity to childhood illnesses.

ASK A DOCTOR

I work for a dry cleaner. Could the chemicals harm my unborn baby? Concerns about dry-cleaning chemicals stem from research showing that women who operated dry-cleaning machines had a higher risk of miscarriage. If touched or inhaled, some organic (carbon-containing) solvents used in dry-cleaning machines can pass through the placenta and some are thought to increase the risk of miscarriage or birth defects.

Talk to your employer to find out how your duties can be changed for the duration of your pregnancy to limit your contact with organic solvents and industrial chemicals.

CHILDHOOD ILLNESSES

Having immunity against common infectious illnesses will protect your unborn baby. You may have natural immunity from having conditions such as chicken pox and fifth disease as a child. You will almost certainly have been vaccinated against mumps and measles, so your unborn baby will be protected from these.

If you are unsure about your immunity or medical history, or think you may have been in contact with any of these infections during pregnancy, contact your doctor immediately for further medical advice. They will be able to do a checkup and provide reassurance.

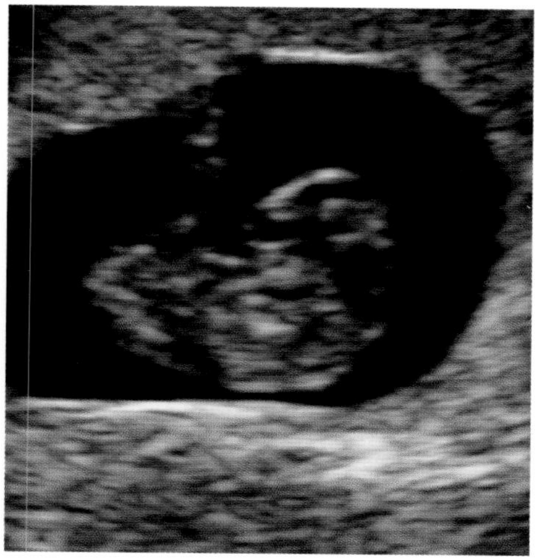

YOU ARE **8 WEEKS AND 3 DAYS**

221 days to go

YOUR BABY TODAY

In a matter of days, your baby's eyes have developed from slight ridges to clear depressions, on each side of the face. The face is developing rapidly at this stage, and your baby's heartbeat would be seen on an ultrasound scan.

" It's a few weeks before the hormone responsible for morning sickness subsides, but the nausea will pass soon. "

You may be wondering when you'll wake up and no longer feel sick. HCG (human chorionic gonadotropin) levels, which may be responsible for feelings of nausea, will begin to fall in about three weeks' time and most women begin to feel better then. For some women the sickness may continue beyond this time.

You may have just started to feel nauseous or your sickness may have begun weeks ago and now be worse, but by around week 12 you should be over the worst. Nausea that happens daily, especially if it is associated with fatigue, can be very wearing so try to remember that it's temporary.

It's normal to have some morning sickness and you should be able to keep some foods and fluids down. However, for a small minority of pregnant women—about 1 percent—the vomiting is severe, occurring regularly and lasting over a period of weeks. This more serious form of morning sickness is called hyperemesis gravidarum and can lead to dehydration. Hospital treatment with intravenous fluids and anti-nausea drugs may be required to rehydrate you.

Seek advice from your doctor if you're concerned about the amount of times you're vomiting or if you're struggling to keep fluids and food down.

About 70–80 percent of pregnant women suffer from nausea and vomiting. If you are one of the 20–30 percent who don't, be thankful. You may get anxious if you're not feeling sick because it is such a common symptom, but don't worry and just count yourself lucky.

EXERCISE AND NAUSEA

If you're feeling particularly nauseated, try going for a brisk walk while concentrating on your breathing and posture. Sometimes taking frequent sips of water helps these feelings and will allow you to exercise longer. Regular exercisers may find that nausea is absent during exercise, although it may resume after the session. Slow yoga moves can help with nausea. Be careful—extreme nausea and vomiting can be a sign of overexercising. Drink water before, during, and after physical activity.

ACUPRESSURE WRISTBANDS

One simple solution to help relieve feelings of nausea during pregnancy is to wear acupressure wristbands.

Available from pharmacists, acupressure bands have been clinically tested in the treatment of pregnancy-induced nausea. Unlike anti-nausea drugs, they don't have any side effects and are easy to use.

The elastic bands—one band is worn on each arm—work by applying pressure on the Nei Kuan acupressure point (known as P6). They can be washed and reused as necessary.

Your baby's life support system

The placenta links your baby's blood supply to your own and carries out all the functions that your baby can't perform for himself. The placenta is rooted to the lining of your uterus and linked to the baby by the umbilical cord.

How the placenta develops

The placenta forms from cells in the embryo shortly after the egg implants in the lining of the uterus. Early placental growth is rapid, and at the beginning of the first trimester, the placenta is larger than the baby. However, the baby's growth catches up by 16 weeks, and by the end of pregnancy the baby is almost six times heavier. The final weight of the placenta is between 12 oz (350 g) and 1 lb 5 oz (700 g). Once its structure is complete at the end of the first trimester, it takes on many important functions for the rest of the pregnancy (see opposite).

Growth after the first trimester The placenta grows throughout the second trimester of pregnancy. By the third trimester, growth slows, but placental efficiency continually improves as extra villi (through which substances are exchanged; see right) grow and increase the available surface area of the placenta by nearly fourfold. Cell layers also become thinner so that substances can be exchanged efficiently.

Placental blood flow is massive and many of the changes in your circulation are designed to meet its needs. By term, a tenfold increase in placental blood supply results in a fifth of your circulation supplying the placenta with up to half a liter of blood (almost a pint) each minute.

The aging placenta The placenta ages toward the end of pregnancy,

INSIDE THE PLACENTA

The placenta contains a huge network of tiny projections called chorionic villi that branch out from a thin membrane, the chorion, and contain fetal blood vessels. The chorionic villi are bathed in maternal blood within the intervillous space. Each villus is only one or two cells thick, which allows the transfer of gases and nutrients between the mother and the baby, while ensuring that the two circulations never come into direct contact. Through the process of diffusion, oxygen and nutrients such as glucose, your baby's primary source of energy, from the mother pass into the fetal circulation, and waste products from the baby are picked up and carried away in the mother's bloodstream. The chorionic membrane also acts as a protective barrier, preventing many harmful substances and infections from reaching the baby.

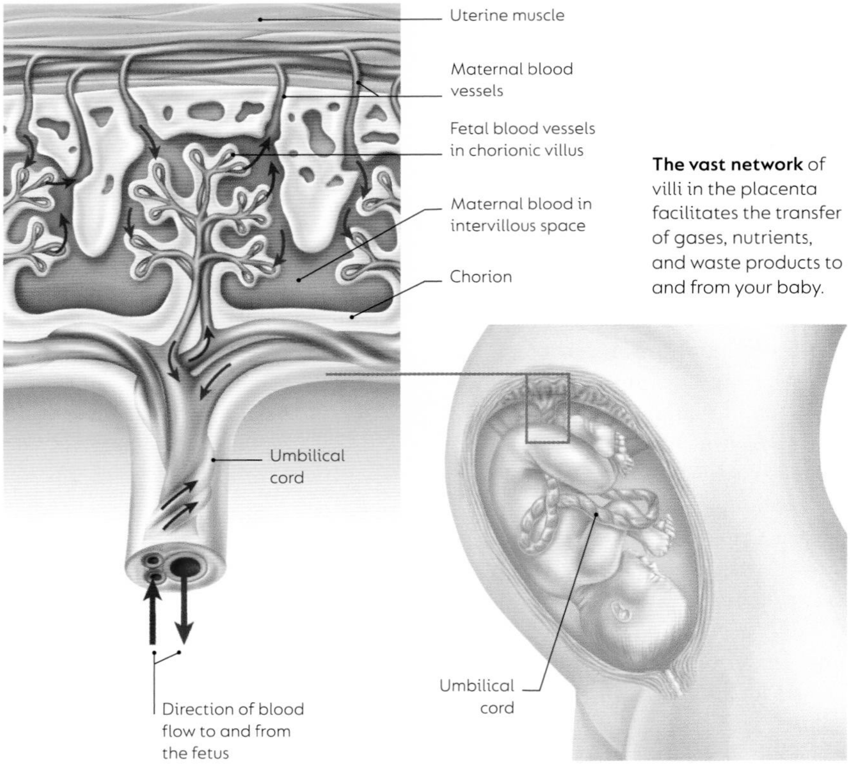

Uterine muscle
Maternal blood vessels
Fetal blood vessels in chorionic villus
Maternal blood in intervillous space
Chorion
Umbilical cord
Direction of blood flow to and from the fetus
Umbilical cord

The vast network of villi in the placenta facilitates the transfer of gases, nutrients, and waste products to and from your baby.

especially after 40 weeks. However, at least 60–80 percent of its function would need to be lost before there were any signs of problems with blood flow in the umbilical cord.

The role of the placenta

The placenta fulfills many essential roles that help sustain the pregnancy and enable the baby to develop.

The exchange of substances. The placenta transports substances to and from your baby, acting as your baby's lungs, kidneys, and digestive system.

To obtain oxygen, the baby's blood cells grab oxygen molecules from your own hemoglobin (the oxygen-carrying subtance in blood). Fetal hemoglobin has a modified structure that makes it bind readily to oxygen. Your baby requires twice as much oxygen weight for weight, as you, so the transfer of oxygen needs to be efficient. The placenta's enhanced blood supply, large surface area, and the characteristics of fetal hemoglobin all ensure the efficient transfer of oxygen from mother to baby. As your hemoglobin gives up oxygen, it accepts carbon dioxide molecules. Your lungs breathe out air rich with the baby's carbon dioxide as well as your own, and the cycle begins again.

To grow and develop, your baby also needs amino acids, the building blocks for proteins, and minerals like calcium and iron, and these all pass from your own circulation via the placenta to the baby.

Protecting your baby The placenta protects your baby from infections and harmful substances. Since your baby hasn't encountered any external threats, the baby doesn't yet make protective antibodies, immunoglobins, that can identify threats, such as viruses or bacteria. Instead, your baby is reliant on the transfer of these from your circulation via the placenta and into his circulation. This means that you are able to protect your baby in the uterus from illnesses such as chickenpox. After your baby is born, the immunoglobulins acquired from you will eventually be lost, which means that later your child becomes susceptible to chickenpox.

Hormone production The placenta produces hormones, such as estrogen and progesterone, that are vital to your baby's well-being and lead to many of the changes in your body during pregnancy.

Heat transfer A baby's high metabolic rate generates heat. The placenta's big surface area and high blood flow disperses heat, controlling the baby's temperature.

Medication Some harmful substances can cross the placenta, so always take medical advice before you use any type of medication.

THE UMBILICAL CORD

The umbilical cord, which connects your baby to the placenta, contains three vessels: two arteries, which carry blood from the baby to the placenta, and one vein, which carries blood back to the baby. The blood in the arteries contains waste products, such as carbon dioxide, from the baby's metabolism. Carbon dioxide is transferred across the placenta to your bloodstream and then to your lungs, where it's breathed out. Oxygen is transported from red blood cells in your circulation, across the placenta to the baby in the umbilical vein. In addition to oxygen, the umbilical vein transports nutrients from the placenta to your baby.

The vessels in the umbilical cord have a protective coating called Wharton's jelly, and the cord is coiled like a spring so that the baby is free to move around. The coiling pattern of the cord has usually established itself by week nine and is usually in a counterclockwise direction. However, the cord can coil later, and sometimes isn't established until 20 weeks. The baby's movements seem to encourage the cord to coil.

The cord is usually attached to the center of the placenta, although sometimes it's attached near the edge. Very occasionally, it divides into its separate vessels before finally entering the placenta. The cord is usually under 1 in (1–2 cm) in diameter and 23 in (60 cm) long, which is twice the length needed to ensure that there are no problems at delivery.

After delivery, the cord vessels close by themselves. The arteries close first, helped by their thicker muscular walls. This prevents blood loss to the placenta from your baby. The umbilical vein closes slightly later (starting at 15 seconds, but only completed by 3 or 4 minutes). This allows blood to continue to return to your baby. As a result, many feel that a slight delay before clamping the cord can be beneficial to the baby. There are no nerves within the cord, so cutting it after delivery is painless for your baby.

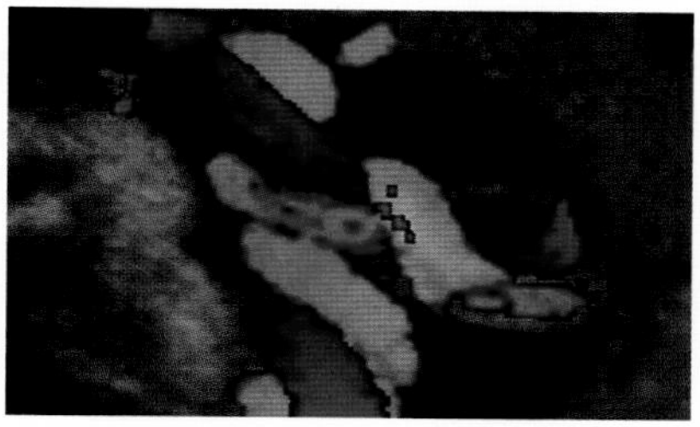

This Doppler scan shows the blood vessels in the umbilical cord. Blood flows through a single vein (blue) and two arteries (red).

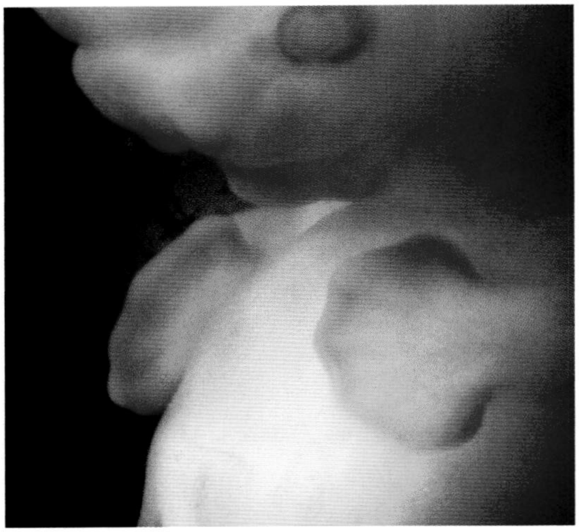

YOU ARE **8 WEEKS AND 4 DAYS**

220 days to go

YOUR BABY TODAY

In the upper limb bud, the flat expansion that will form the hand can be identified. The fingers are becoming more distinct and there will now be the first signs of movement at the elbows.

“ Your baby's bones are beginning to develop—and they will continue to lengthen from now until the teenage years. ”

You won't be aware of your developing baby's activities inside the uterus for some months yet, but the fact that their elbows are forming allows them to make some small movements; the wrists do not yet move.

Your baby is looking more human as each day passes. Their vertebrae and ribs are now in place, and their fingers are gradually lengthening. Their body is less curled up than it was a few weeks ago.

The skeleton will gradually calcify and harden. With the exception of the cranial skull bones, all your baby's bones have a soft cartilage core that will later be reabsorbed as it is converted into hard bone. This process of hardening, known as ossification, starts in so-called primary ossification centers during the next five weeks of your pregnancy. Within these primary centers, specialized cells form spongy then hard bone as calcium salts are laid down. Within the hard bone is red bone marrow, which in later weeks will become the main producer of the baby's red blood cells.

Secondary ossification centers develop in the second trimester at the ends of each of your baby's bones.

The portion of bone between the hardening primary and secondary centers is known as the growth plate. This plate is responsible for the continued lengthening of your unborn baby's bones.

MORE CHEESE PLEASE

There is a lot of confusion about which cheeses are safe to eat in pregnancy. The ones that should be avoided are those made from unpasteurized milk, and those that have a mold-ripened crust, such as Brie, Camembert, or chevre (a soft goat cheese). These could contain a food spoilage organism called Listeria. Soft blue cheese such as Roquefort, or Danish Blue, are susceptible to Listeria as well.

However, all other cheeses are safe to eat and provide essential protein, calcium, phosphorus, zinc, and vitamin B12. You can enjoy:

- Hard cheeses, such as Cheddar and Parmesan
- Emmental and Swiss
- Feta
- Ricotta and cottage cheese
- Mascarpone and cream cheese
- Mozzarella
- Processed cheese, such as spreads.

CALCIUM BOOST

The most easily absorbed source of calcium is in dairy products. If you can't or don't eat this make sure you get sufficient calcium from:

- Calcium-fortified dairy alternatives, such as soy or nut yogurts and milk.
- Canned fish with soft bones, such as sardines and salmon.
- Dried figs or apricots.
- Green vegetables, such as okra, watercress, spinach, or kale.
- Soy products, such as tofu.

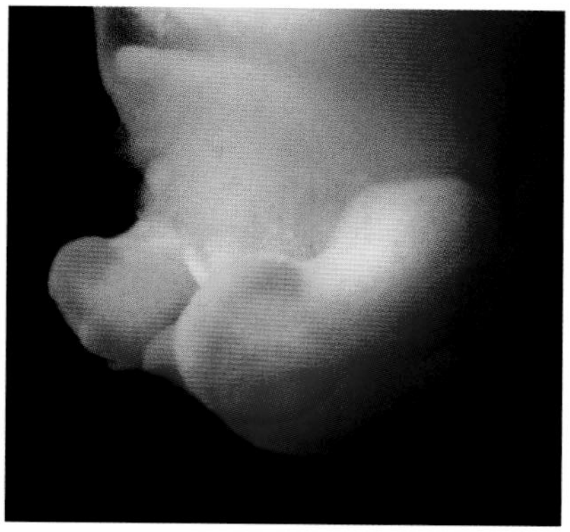

YOU ARE **8 WEEKS AND 5 DAYS**

219 days to go

YOUR BABY TODAY

The development of the baby's lower limbs always lags slightly behind that of the upper limbs. At this stage, the toes are not distinct and the legs are not yet bending at the knee.

Going through pregnancy together is momentous, and at a time when you want to feel close to your partner, you may find that your relationship is changing, and it may be quite fraught with issues. Your relationship will inevitably change—but as long as you keep communicating, you will be able to support each other. Being united now will stand you in good stead for the first year of parenting.

During the early stages of pregnancy, your partner may find it hard to relate to the fact that you're expecting a baby; the physical changes to your body won't be that visible at this stage and there won't be a scan photo yet. Conversely, you will be very aware of the pregnancy and undergoing many physical and emotional changes.

Your partner may need more time than you to adjust to the idea of being a parent and may be concerned about practical issues, such as the changes to your lifestyle and the financial implications of having a baby. Talking openly to each other can help ease anxieties for you both. Remember, that although many changes are happening to your body, your partner does have feelings and this is a big life change. If you've told your family and close friends about the pregnancy, all the attention may be on you. Your partner may be feeling left out and this is something that often gets worse as the pregnancy progresses and after the baby arrives.

Look for ways to involve your partner more in the pregnancy and encourage them to spend time with friends who have been through the expectant partner experience.

“ It's understandable that your pregnancy will be on your mind. Try to find ways to communicate this to your partner. ”

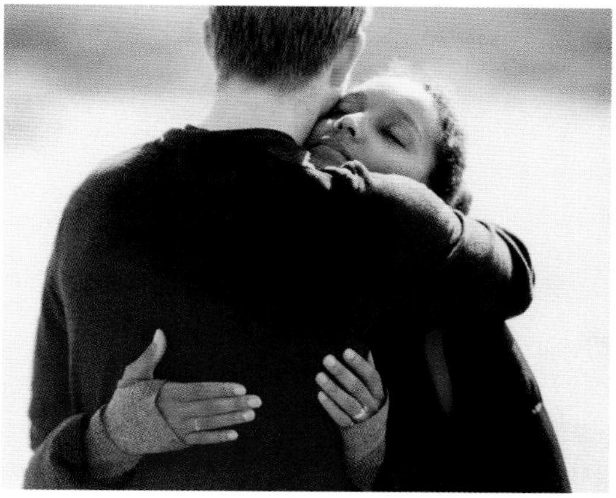

ASK A MOM

I'm worried we won't have space in our small apartment once the baby is born, but is a house move advisable while I'm pregnant? We started the process but thankfully it fell through since it was proving quite stressful, and it's not advisable to deal with those kinds of pressures while you're pregnant. We stayed in our apartment until our baby was one and it was fine. Remember that small babies have very few needs, other than being fed, loved, changed, and stimulated, and much of the paraphernalia that you think you need is unnecessary. If you have room for a crib, a stroller, a drawer for your baby's clothes, and a corner for toys, you'll be fine in a small space for the time being.

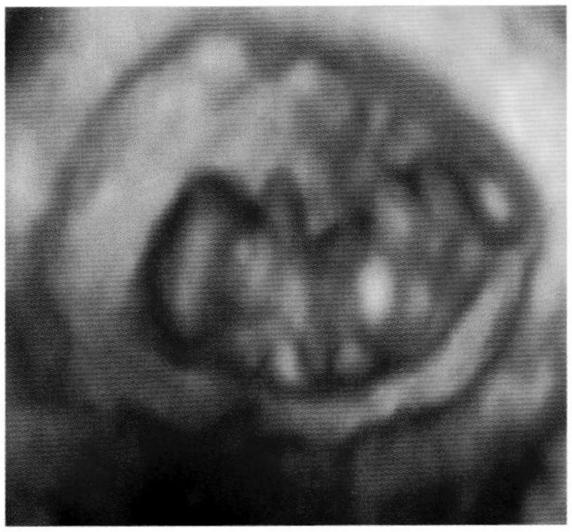

YOU ARE **8 WEEKS AND 6 DAYS**

218 days to go

YOUR BABY TODAY

This 3D ultrasound scan shows a baby lying on its back, in exactly the same orientation as the image opposite. It is just possible to pick out the limb buds on an ultrasound scan taken at this stage.

> " It's not long until you have your first prenatal appointment and will see your doctor. "

Soon you will have your initial appointment (see p.129) with the doctor. If you haven't made an appointment for this yet, contact your doctor or local maternity unit to arrange it. You may or may not have a choice of hospitals.

If you do have options, talk to women you know locally who have had their babies at those hospitals to find out about their experience. For example, some hospitals may have a birth center attached, and have a less medically managed approach to childbirth.

Start thinking now about the kind of questions you want to ask your doctor. It's a good idea to write these down before you attend the appointment. Also make a note, in advance, of the key details of your medical history, medication you're taking, and any pregnancy symptoms.

TACKLING COLDS

Cold medicines contain a variety of ingredients, including antihistamines, that are best avoided in pregnancy. Check the label and talk to your doctor or pharmacist before taking any medications.

Try natural remedies, such as steam inhalations or saline nasal sprays, before resorting to medication.

ASK A PANEL ABOUT HOME BIRTH

It's my first pregnancy. Can I have a home birth?

Midwife: if you're in good health with no complications, giving birth at home is an option. Many women enjoy the experience of giving birth at home, because they may feel more comfortable with familiar surroundings and people. Some women find labor easier when they get into water, either a familiar bathtub at home or a birthing pool that has been purchased or rented.

Obstetrician: there is no problem with this in general, but take advice from your doctor. You should avoid taking risks. If there is a history of long or complicated labors in your family, your baby is breech or very small, there are issues about the location of the cord or the placenta, you are very overweight or unhealthy, or you suffer from conditions such as diabetes, it might be worth erring on the side of caution. If you have your baby in a hospital, quick and early intervention can take place if needed. You may want to have a home birth; however, it is sensible to listen to the experts. Keep in mind that delivery of a healthy baby is the most important thing.

Mom: I had my first baby at home, and it was wonderful. I was nervous about what might go wrong, but my midwife reassured me that she would be monitoring me and would get me to the hospital if there was a problem. She also explained I could change my mind if I didn't think things were going well, and go to the hospital for the birth (and some pain relief!).

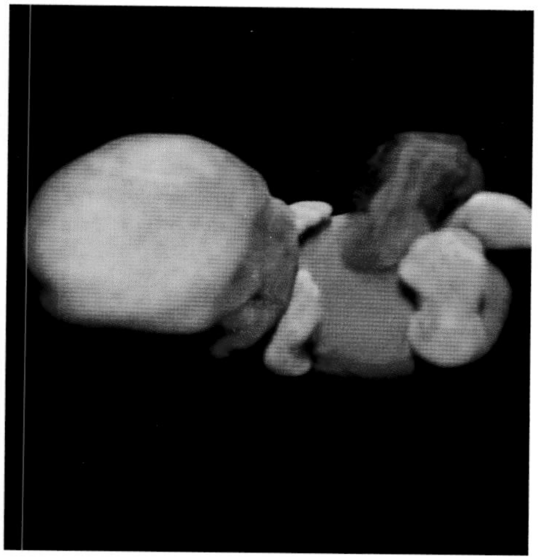

YOU ARE **9 WEEKS EXACTLY**

217 days to go

YOUR BABY TODAY

The baby's hands can be clearly seen here but the fingers are still fused at this stage. The fingers will be completely separate in just one week's time and wrist movement is just about to begin.

> "By the end of this ninth week, your baby's digestive system is rapidly developing but won't function properly for some time."

Your baby is developing quickly inside the uterus. The simple tube forming along his gut has undergone most changes at the upper end. Now the lower part dilates as the single tube then divides into what will become the rectum at the back and then the bladder and urethra at the front.

Although the mouth is open to the amniotic fluid, there is still a membrane in place, which will disappear in one to two weeks' time. The lower bowel is not yet mature and does not move material along its length.

The remainder of the large bowel and small bowel is still lengthening. The duodenum is the first part of the small bowel and it is still a solid tube. The pancreas, gall bladder, and liver have all formed buds leading off from the upper small bowel, but none are yet contributing any digestive function.

ACTUAL SIZE OF YOUR BABY

At 9 weeks your baby's crown to rump length is 0.9 in (2.3 cm).

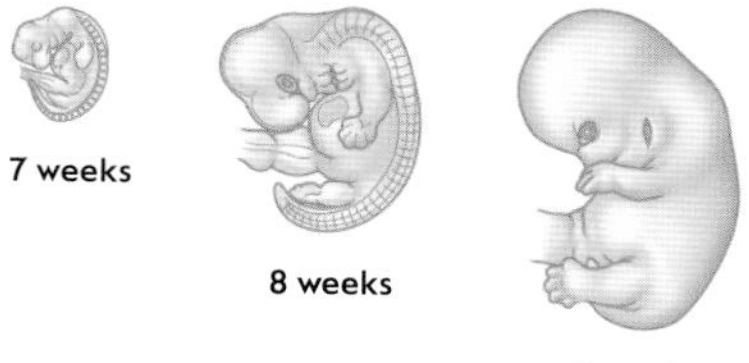
7 weeks
8 weeks
9 weeks

ASK A DOCTOR

Since I've been pregnant, I've had terrible headaches. Could staring at a computer screen for work be the cause?
Tension headaches and migraines are common in pregnancy, probably due to fluctuating hormones, and it is not uncommon to have severe headaches with prolonged computer use. Headaches are often worse in the first trimester. This could be due to eye strain and the fact that you are immobile, which can cause tension. Take even more breaks from your computer screen now that you're pregnant. You'll probably find you need more bathroom breaks anyway. If this doesn't help, ask if you can do tasks that don't require computer use for a short time. Drink plenty of water, too, as you work as dehydration can cause headaches.

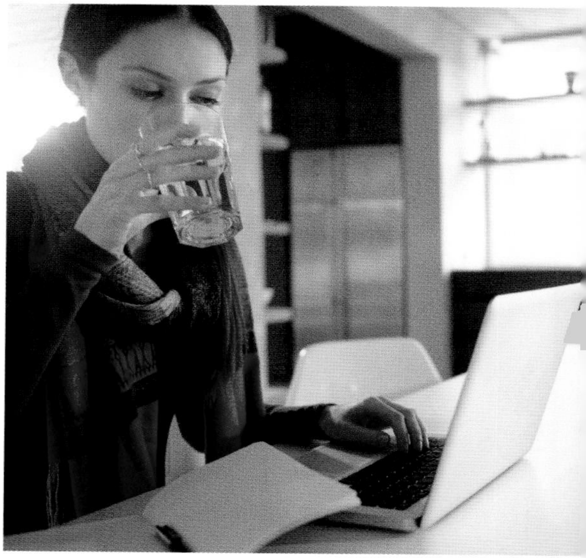

Your 10th week

YOUR BABY'S MAJOR ORGANS ARE IN PLACE, BUT NOT WORKING YET. This is your baby's last week as an embryo; next week they will be a fetus. The major organs are in place, although by no means in working order. The body systems will continue to mature for the rest of the pregnancy and beyond. The most noticeable difference to your body will be in your breasts. You may well have gone up a cup size—or more.

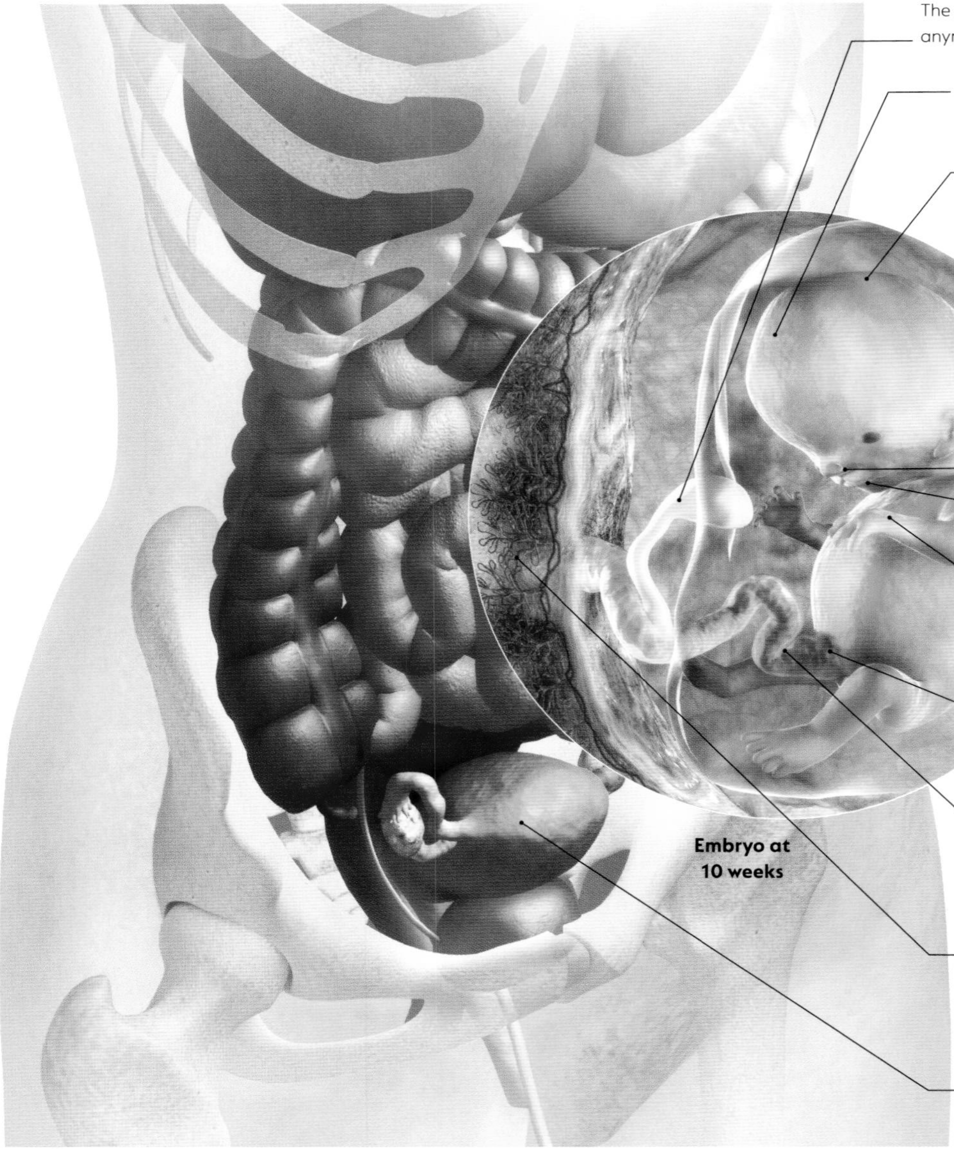

The yolk sac is not needed anymore and is shrinking away.
The baby's head has lifted slightly off the chest.
The embryo measures 1.2 in (3 cm) crown to rump.
The outer ear is fully formed but not yet in its final position, which will be higher up.
The nose protrudes from the face and now has a definite shape.
The mouth lips are nearly fully developed.
The wrist has formed and is able to bend.
The bulge at the base o f the umbilical cord contains the developing intestines.
The umbilical cord takes blood between the baby and the placenta.
The placenta is now fully functioning. It will be the baby's lifeline until the end of your pregnancy.
The uterus continues to enlarge and lift upward.
Embryo at 10 weeks

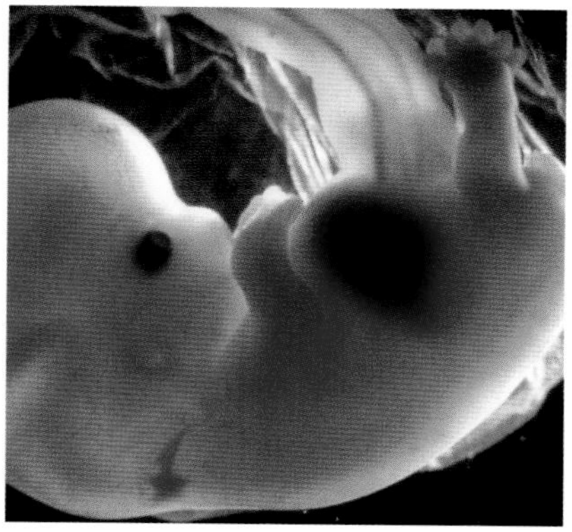

YOU ARE **9 WEEKS AND 1 DAY**

216 days to go

YOUR BABY TODAY

At about nine weeks, the human embryo measures about 1.2 in (3 cm). Most of the primitive organ systems are formed: the arms and legs have budded; the retina of the eye, and the nose, can be seen. The large dark mass is the enlarged liver.

> "Your baby's welfare will be your main concern, but rest assured that, however you're feeling, she'll be getting sustenance."

You may be conscious of your health and well-being, but even if you've felt unwell, your baby has been taking what she needs from you: you have internal reserves of various minerals and substances, such as iron, and will still be absorbing some nutrients from what you eat. If you are eating a balanced diet, you will be getting most of the minerals and vitamins you and your baby need. You should also be taking 400 mcg of folic acid and 600–800 IU of vitamin D daily. You can take these as separate supplements or as a multivitamin. The latter should be one designed for pregnancy to ensure it does not contain harmful substances such as animal-derived vitamin A.

There is no cause for concern if you do not put on any weight in the first trimester, or even if you lose a bit of weight. The majority of weight gain takes place in the second and third trimesters (see p.99).

If you're vomiting a lot and struggling to keep food down (see p.111), don't hesitate to see your ob/gyn.

COUVADE SYNDROME

Can your partner ever really understand what you're going through? According to a recent study, some dads don't need a fake pregnancy belly to empathize. Known as Couvade syndrome, symptoms experienced by expectant fathers ranged from morning sickness to backaches, mood swings, and food cravings. Although, interestingly, often it was the woman claiming her partner had these symptoms.

Couvade is thought to happen because men are so deeply involved in the pregnancy. While others believe it could be jealousy (you're getting all the attention) or guilt that he's responsible for your condition and therefore your symptoms.

YOUR CHANGING BREASTS

Breast changes are caused by both an increased blood supply and a rise in pregnancy hormones, particularly in the first 12 weeks.

Before your pregnancy was confirmed, you may have felt tingling sensations (especially in the nipple area) as the blood supply increased.

- As early as 6–8 weeks, your breasts will have become larger and more tender and may have begun to look different, with threadlike veins starting to appear.
- At around 8–12 weeks, the nipples darken and can become more erect.
- As early as the 16th week of pregnancy, colostrum, the first milk, may leak from your breasts.

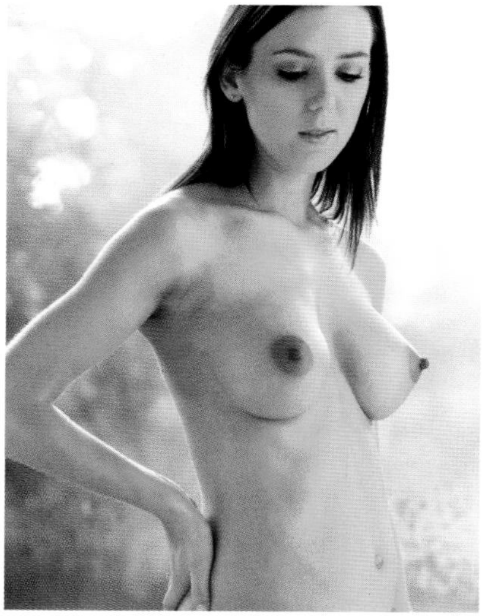

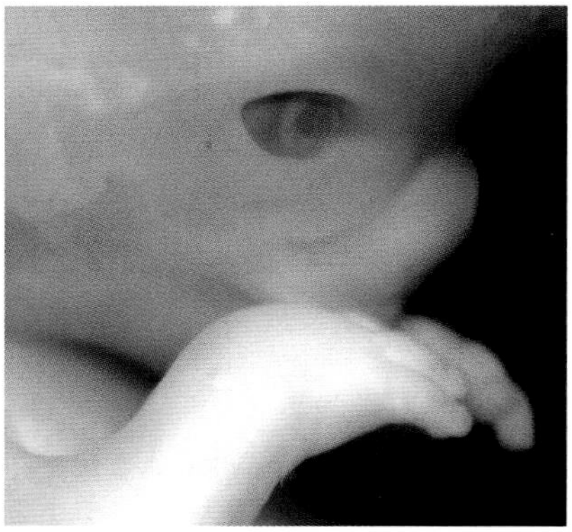

YOU ARE **9 WEEKS AND 2 DAYS**

215 days to go

YOUR BABY TODAY

The baby now begins to bend their wrists. The natural position is for the limbs to be slightly bent at all joints, especially in the early stages. There is a more distinct neck area as the baby's head is now slightly lifted off the chest.

"The muscular diaphragm that will eventually enable your baby to breathe—and hiccup—is developing now."

HAVING SCREENING AND DIAGNOSTIC TESTS

It's useful to be aware of the screening tests (see pp.142–143) and diagnostic tests (see pp.152–153) that will be available in the weeks to come.

- **Screening tests:** these tests identify the "risk factor" for a particular condition, but do not confirm that your baby definitely has a condition. For example, a screening test for Down syndrome may give a risk factor of 1:200. This means that your baby has a 1 in 200 chance of being affected by Down syndrome, but it does not mean that the baby actually has the condition.
- **Diagnostic tests:** if screening tests reveal your baby has a high risk factor for a chromosomal abnormality, you will be offered a diagnostic test, such as amniocentesis or chorionic villus sampling, which gives a definite result as to whether or not a condition is present.

As your baby's lungs develop in the chest, there is nothing to separate them from the stomach, liver, and bowel in what will later become their abdominal cavity.

In adults, the chest is separated from the abdomen by the muscular diaphragm. When we breathe, the diaphragm moves downward and the ribs expand outward. This process allows air to enter the lungs.

Your baby's diaphragm forms from four in-folds of tissue. First seen at around this week of pregnancy, these folds gradually expand inward, fusing together and closing the space by the end of this week.

In the center of the diaphragm there are openings for the esophagus to the stomach, main artery to the body—the aorta, and main vein returning blood from the lower body, the inferior vena cava. As your pregnancy progresses, muscle fibers gradually strengthen your baby's diaphragm, and later in the pregnancy your baby will make breathing movements.

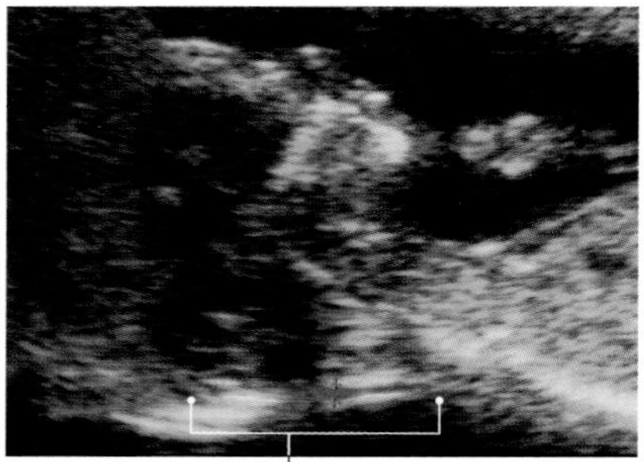

Red area shows the fluid under the skin at the back of the baby's neck

The nuchal translucency scan (see p.143) measures the depth of fluid under the skin in the nuchal fold at the back of the baby's neck. Excess fluid increases the chance of the baby having a chromosomal abnormality, such as Down syndrome, or a heart problem. More tests are always needed for a final diagnosis.

TWIN TESTS

If you're expecting twins or more, blood-based screening tests for Down syndrome can mislead, since they rely on measuring the amounts of circulating AFP (alfa-fetoprotein) and other markers, which are present in much higher levels when there's more than one baby. That's why your best bet for screening is the nuchal translucency test at 11–14 weeks (see right and p.143).

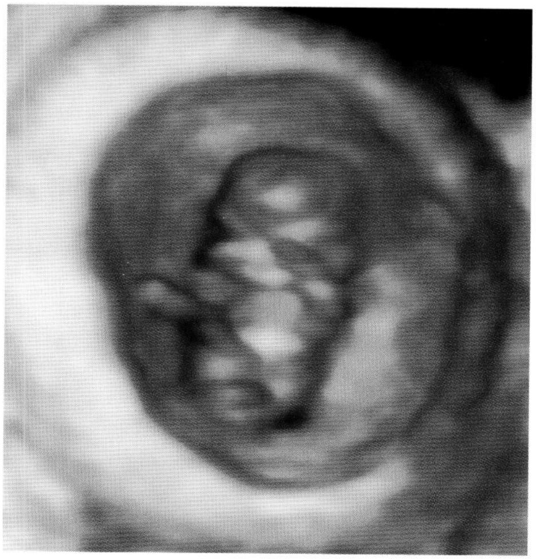

YOU ARE **9 WEEKS AND 3 DAYS**

214 days to go

YOUR BABY TODAY

The shoulders, elbows, and wrists are flexed leaving the hands in front of the face. It's far too early to be aware of them but several fetal movements will start to become apparent on an ultrasound scan at this stage.

> "You don't need to shop for a maternity wardrobe just yet, but it might be time to purchase some bigger bras."

If your normal bras are starting to feel a little uncomfortable, it's time to go for a professional fitting if you have not done so already, get yourself measured professionally. Wearing a good and supportive bra during pregnancy is essential to prevent backaches and will help ease any breast discomfort you may be feeling. Whenever you feel you need a new bra, get measured properly to ensure that you're wearing the right size. Although your breasts may be growing very quickly at this time, you should find that by the end of the first trimester the growth has stabilized. There is then unlikely to be much more breast growth until you're in your third trimester and after the baby is born.

Wearing underwire bras during pregnancy is not recommended because they can dig into developing breast tissue and damage it, and may even cause problems with milk production. Wireless bras with wide supportive straps, such as sports bras, are good in pregnancy.

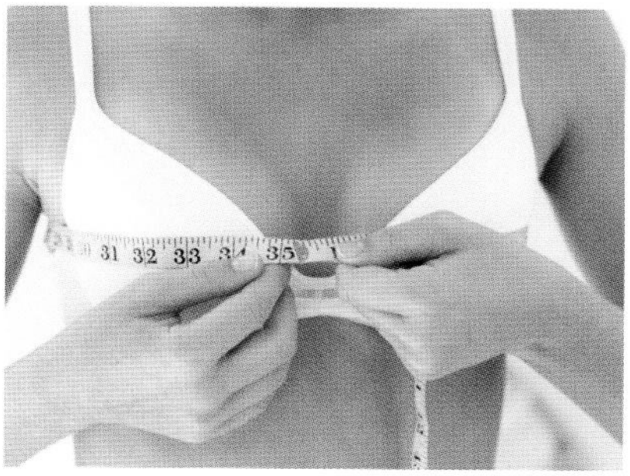

Measure your breasts so you can buy the correct bra size and ease any discomfort.

INEDIBLE CRAVINGS

Pica means craving inedible substances and comes from the Latin for magpie, a bird that scavenges indiscriminately. If you like crunching coal, eating snow, or licking the toothpaste, you probably have pica—a fairly common condition. There are several theories about the cause of pica, one being that it is due to a diet deficient in iron or zinc. Avoid eating toxic items such as chalk, glue, soil, and soap and seek advice from your doctor.

VEGAN DIETS

If you are a vegan and pregnant, make sure your diet covers the key nutrients you and your baby need. A well-planned vegan diet provides plenty of fiber folate, vitamins C and E, and complex carbohydrates. The nutrients you need to be aware of including are:

- Protein (see p.14)
- Iron (see p.84)
- Zinc (see p.17)
- Calcium (see p.114)
- Vitamin A (see p.17)
- Vitamin B12 (see p.17)
- Iodine (see p.80)
- Omega-3 fatty acids (see p.169)

Hardly any plant foods contain vitamin B12, so take a supplement and eat B12 fortified foods, such as yeast extract. Zinc, which is vital for many metabolic functions, including helping your body use folic acid, is supplied by seeds, especially sesame, nuts, and wheat germ.

Your first prenatal visit

Your first prenatal appointment usually takes place between 8 and 12 weeks. At this visit, your prenatal records will be started and you will have a chance to discuss any concerns or issues with your doctor.

At your initial visit, you will meet the doctor who will be providing your care. She will ask you questions about your past and present health and about medical conditions in your family. You will also have a physical examination and blood and urine tests. Your due date will be estimated based on the date of your last menstrual period (see p.35).

Medical history

The doctor will take a full medical history to check for health problems, and identify your pregnancy as high or low risk. If there is a problem, she will explain how this could affect your pregnancy. If you have an existing condition, she'll discuss how your pregnancy may affect your health and if your treatment needs to change. Inform the doctor of any medications you're taking; certain ones, such as some of those for high blood pressure, may need to be changed (see pp.20–1).

You will be asked about drug use and sexually transmitted diseases. It's important to be honest so that your doctor can identify and prevent potential problems. You may also be asked about your previous obstetric history, including any previous miscarriages or terminations of pregnancy. If your partner is unaware of a past event and you feel sensitive about this, tell your doctor privately and ask for it to remain confidential.

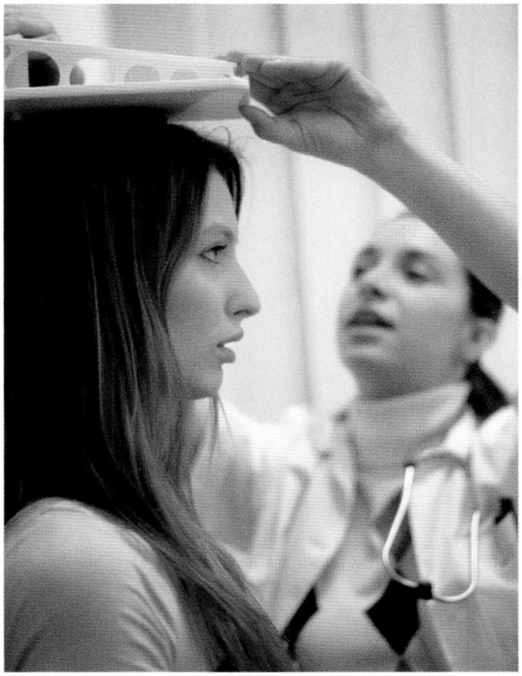

A baseline height and weight measurement is taken at your first prental appointment.

Family history

The doctor will ask about any health problems in your own and your partner's family. This is important because some conditions can be passed on, and testing may be available to identify whether your baby is affected.

Height and weight

A baseline height and weight measurement will be taken to calculate your body mass index (BMI; see p.16). A BMI of more than 30 puts you in a higher risk group for complications. Losing weight in pregnancy is not recommended, but your doctor will give you advice about healthy eating and exercise to avoid excessive weight gain.

Blood pressure

A baseline blood pressure measurement will be taken at your first visit. Blood pressure usually goes down at the start of pregnancy, rises around week 26, and by the 32nd week, returns to its original prepregnancy value. So if your initial blood pressure is in the normal-to-high range, it's likely to rise to above normal during the third trimester and need treatment.

Routine blood tests

Bloodwork will be collected to determine your blood type and tested for anemia and various infections, such as HIV, syphilis, and hepatitis B. Detecting and treating infections early can prevent or greatly reduce the risk of transmission to your baby.

Complete blood count This is a screening for anemia, which occurs most commonly from low levels of iron in the blood. If you're anemic, you'll be advised to eat iron-rich foods (see p.84) and may need an iron supplement.

Blood type A blood test will determine your blood type (A, B, O, or AB) and if you're rhesus positive (Rh+) or rhesus negative (Rh–) (see p.127). During pregnancy and at the birth, a small number of fetal red blood cells may cross the placenta into maternal circulation. This happens most commonly during the birthing process or if you have any bleeding in pregnancy.. If you are Rh– and your baby is Rh+, your body will develop antibodies to destroy the fetal cells in your circulation. This is known as sensitization. These antibodies in turn can cross to the placenta, destroying the baby's cells and causing anemia. This is unlikely to be problematic in a first pregnancy, but may get more severe with each subsequent pregnancy.

To prevent this from happening, you will be given an anti-D injection during pregnancy at about 28 weeks. After delivery your baby's blood type will be checked and, if confirmed to be Rh+, you will be given another dose of anti-D. If you have any bleeding in pregnancy or after an amniocentesis, you may also need an anti-D injection.

There is a new test becoming available to check the baby's Rh status. Tiny fragments of the baby's blood in your circulation can be tested to determine whether your baby is Rh+ or Rh-. If your baby is negative, you won't need anti-D.

Rubella This blood test checks your immunity to rubella. Infection with rubella in early pregnancy may cause serious problems for the baby. If you aren't immune, you can't be vaccinated in pregnancy, but will usually be vaccinated after delivery so you're protected in future pregnancies.

Hepatitis B This test identifies women who are infected with hepatitis B, a viral liver disease that can be transmitted to the baby.

Syphilis The blood test checks if you have ever had syphilis. Active syphilis can cross the placenta and cause serious complications in your baby.

HIV You will be offered a test for human immunodeficiency virus (HIV). If you have HIV, you can reduce the chances of passing this on to your baby by taking antiviral agents and not breast-feeding.

Sickle-cell disease or thalassemia You are tested to see if you are a carrier of sickle-cell disease or thalassemia, genetic disorders that affect the oxygen-carrying ability of red blood cells. These are most common in people of African, Hispanic, or Mediterranean origins. If you're found to be a carrier, the baby's father will need to be tested; if he is a carrier, there is a chance that your baby could develop the disease.

Routine urine tests

Routine urine tests are no longer needed; however, there may be times when your doctor recommends checking your urine for protein. If present, this may indicate an infection or, less commonly, kidney disease. Around 15 percent of women have bacteria,but no signs of infection. If bacteria are found, you may need antibiotics to stop kidney infection, which is more common in pregnancy and can cause complications. If no infection is found, more tests will check your kidney function. Later in pregnancy, protein in the urine can be a sign of preeclampsia (see p.476).

Getting your results

If all is well, you will be given the blood test results at your next visit. If there are any concerns, you will be contacted to discuss the results.

EXTRA SCREENING

Some additional tests may be offered.

- **Cervical cultures** Chlamydia and gonorrhea can be symptomless, so get tested if you think you're at risk.
- **Hepatitis C** You may be offered screening if you are high risk.
- **Varicella** A test can confirm whether you have chickenpox (varicella) immunity. If you're not immune and are exposed to the infection, treatment can help prevent severe chickenpox in pregnancy.
- **Toxoplasmosis** Being infected in the past will protect you from infection in pregnancy.

PRENATAL APPOINTMENTS

If your pregnancy is low risk, you will have about 10 prenatal appointments for a first pregnancy and about seven for second and subsequent pregnancies. After the first appointment with your doctor, your next visit will be at about 16 weeks.

At each appointment, your doctor will perform routine checkups, including taking your blood pressure and checking your urine for protein, the presence of which could indicate an infection or, later in pregnancy, preeclampsia (see p.476). You will be weighed regularly even if there are no particular concerns.

Before 16 weeks, your doctor will start to listen to your baby's heartbeat. Before 25 weeks, she will measure your abdomen to monitor growth (see p.284).

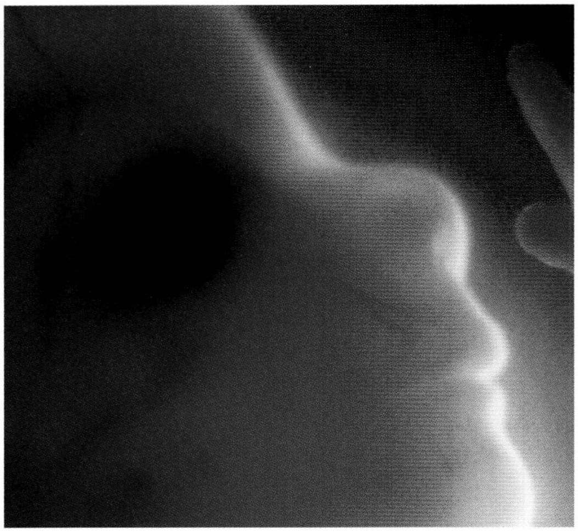

YOU ARE **9 WEEKS AND 4 DAYS**

213 days to go

YOUR BABY TODAY

The baby's facial features are becoming more distinctive by this stage. The very fine eyelids have now completely fused over the developing eye and will remain closed until approximately the 26th week of pregnancy.

> "Just as you've become used to the idea you're pregnant, you may discover that you're carrying more than one baby."

Do you have an instinct that you're having twins? Some women, even very early in pregnancy, suspect they're carrying more than one baby simply because they feel "more pregnant." Signs of a multiple pregnancy include highly sensitive breasts, and extreme morning sickness and fatigue. In a multiple pregnancy, your uterus might also be larger than expected. Your doctor may be able to feel it rising into your lower belly from this week, instead of from 12 weeks.

Whether or not you suspect anything, the first ultrasound scan (see p.137) will show definitely if you are carrying more than one baby.

ASK A MOM

I'm delighted we're having twins but how will I manage? I felt the same when I was expecting and had so many worries—"Will I be able to breast-feed two babies? How many cribs will I need?" At first, your head is likely to be spinning with these thoughts, as you get used to the idea of your twin pregnancy.

To give yourself time to come to terms with the news, you may prefer to keep it to yourselves for a few weeks. What you'll find is that family and friends react differently. Responses can range from pure joy (usually from thrilled grandparents) to envy or a bit of scaremongering (from friends and strangers).

We found it helpful to talk to others who were expecting twins or who were already parents to twins. Visit the website of the National Organization of Mothers of Twins Clubs to find a local group.

THE SHOCKING NEWS

The news that you're having two or more babies may not always be delivered with the greatest tact. For instance, the sonographer may look at the scan and say that "something needs checking." This sounds worrying, of course, but remember, they are only being cautious before giving you the life-changing news. The sonographer may also be checking your twins for size, to rule out any major problems. Once this is done, however, there are likely to be hearty congratulations.

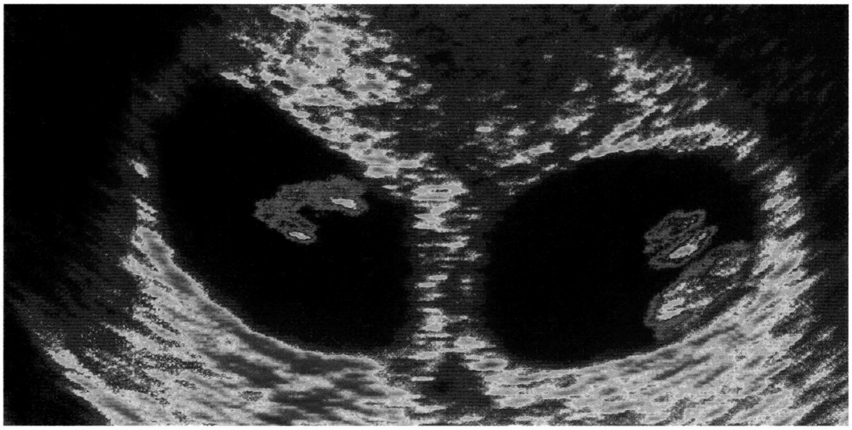

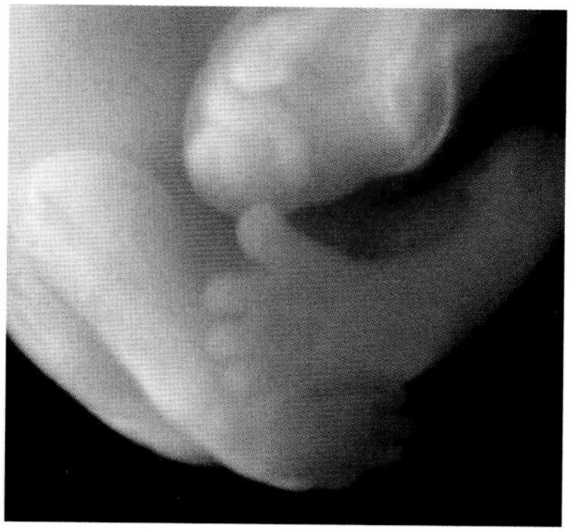

YOU ARE **9 WEEKS AND 5 DAYS**

212 days to go

YOUR BABY TODAY

The lower limbs are now held flexed at the hip and knee joints, leading to a slightly crossed-legs position. The separate toes can be distinguished. Further growth of the thigh and shin bones will bring the foot length into proportion with the rest of the leg.

> " One of the downsides of pregnancy is being at greater risk of urinary tract infections, so you need to be aware of the signs. "

Be on the lookout for any signs of a urinary tract infection. Although not very serious and easily treated, it's a complication you can do without.

An infection may cause you to urinate more frequently, but this is also a symptom of early pregnancy so it can be hard to spot. If, however, you also have stinging or discomfort when you actually urinate, lower abdominal pain, or even blood in the urine you may have developed a urinary tract infection. These infections are very common in women in general, because the urethra (tube which carries urine from the bladder to the outside) is very close to the anus and so bacteria do not have far to travel to create an infection.

In pregnancy, there are high levels of the hormone progesterone; this relaxes the tubes of the urinary system making it even easier for bacteria to enter and infect the bladder or even the kidneys. It is important to have your urine tested if you have the symptoms of a urinary-tract infection. They are usually easily treatable in pregnancy. If there is an infection, you will be prescribed antibiotics that are safe to take. The infection must be treated because, if not, it may cause a kidney infection and increase the risk of preterm labor.

STAYING IN SHAPE

If you were a regular exerciser prior to becoming pregnant, it is important to continue with some form of exercise. Stopping entirely, just because you're pregnant, would be a shock to your fit body and you may lose the benefits of the fitness you have achieved up to now.

There are some contraindications to exercising during pregnancy (see p.18), but if you have clearance from your doctor, take the following steps to make sure you are exercising safely and effectively:

- **Continue with activities,** such as fast walking and swimming, as long as you feel comfortable.
- **Listen to your body**—look for signs that you should take a break, such as pain, extreme fatigue, and dizziness.
- **Get adequate rest** between workouts, and drink water before, during, and after all forms of exercise.
- **Exercise at a moderate level**—you should be able to do the talk test (see page 161).
- **Keep to low-impact** and low-risk activities (avoid sports that involve contact and the risk of falling).
- **Wear the right clothing:** cotton will enable your body to dissipate heat, and a supportive sports bra is vital for your growing breasts, especially if you're jogging.

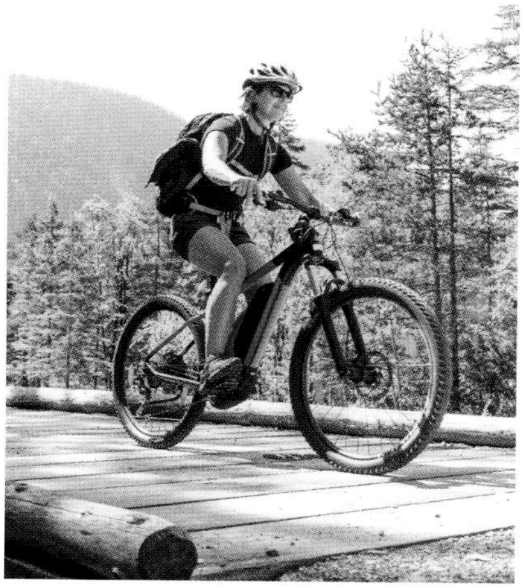

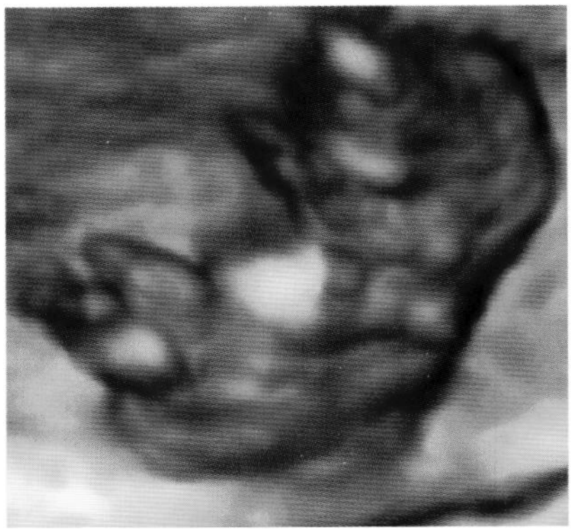

YOU ARE **9 WEEKS AND 6 DAYS**

211 days to go

YOUR BABY TODAY

The umbilical cord widens where it enters the baby's abdomen. This bulge is necessary to accommodate the bowel that is forming underneath at this stage of development. The bones of the head are not yet fully formed.

" Your baby's organ systems are now present, in a basic form, so at this point she changes from being an embryo to a fetus. "

NONINVASIVE PRENATAL TEST

A noninvasive prenatal test (NIPT) to screen for Down syndrome is available (see p.142). This blood test, which also tests for Edwards syndrome and Patau syndrome, detects 99 percent of chromosomal abnormalities.

The early embryonic period of the baby's development of the embryo was characterized by the three cell lines each developing into their own types of tissues and organs, as it grew from a flat disk of cells into a human shape. Many of the changes took place concurrently, but it was the heart, circulation, and nervous systems that developed initially with the gut, limbs, and face development following.

During next week (your 11th week), your baby's kidneys and genital system will undergo their most rapid development. All your baby's organs need to mature fully, and many of them, such as the brain, lungs, and kidneys, will continue to mature throughout pregnancy and after birth.

During the eleventh week, your baby's facial features will begin to become more recognizable. The ears will take on their final shape, although they will still be positioned low.

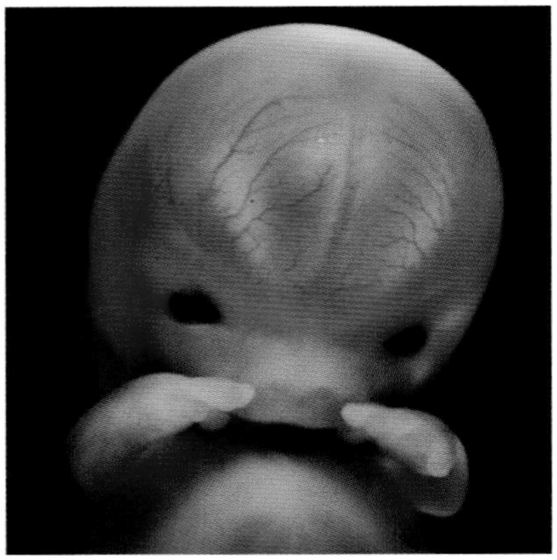

The eyes, which started on the side of the face start to move more centrally, the nose is visible, and the head achieves a more rounded contour.

VEGETARIAN MOM-TO-BE

Most vegetarians get sufficient protein for their pregnancy needs, if they eat eggs and dairy products.

Few vegetarians lack dietary fiber if they are eating vegetables and whole grains but should be aware that iron can be bound by other plant compounds, and drinking tea or coffee with meals hinders absorption. An iron supplement may be needed.

Biotin, a B vitamin, is vital for the early development of a baby's genetic structure. The best sources are meat, fish, and poultry, but vegetarians can obtain biotin from eggs, peanuts, and almonds.

Although the body can convert the omega-3 fatty acid called alpha linoleic acid (ALA) into the EPA and DHA your baby needs (see p.169), it makes sense for vegetarians to take a supplement providing these marine- based omega-3 fatty acids. Algae provide fish with the DHA and EPA, so look for vegetarian-friendly EPA/DHA supplements.

If you are vegetarian, also eat plenty of foods rich in ALA, including canola oil, flaxseed, pumpkin seeds, and walnuts, as regularly as you can.

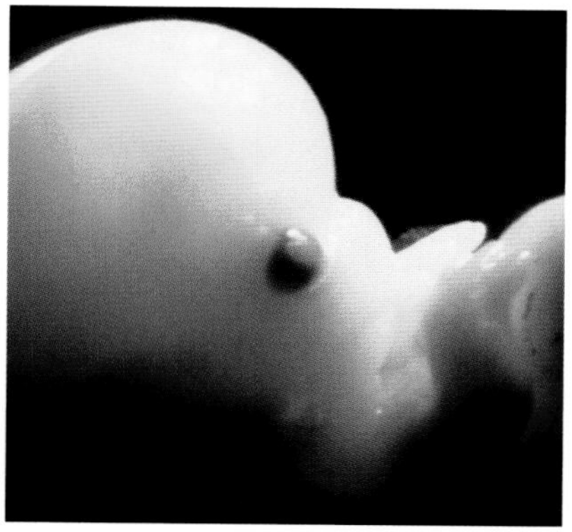

YOU ARE **10 WEEKS EXACTLY**

210 days to go

YOUR BABY TODAY

The bones of the front of the skull are starting to grow over the baby's forehead and harden from cartilage to bone. The forehead is still very prominent and the top of the head still very flexible to accommodate the baby's rapidly developing brain.

> "The placenta is rapidly developing and once it's fully formed, will supply all your baby's needs."

A milestone in your baby's development—the placenta takes over from the yolk sac to provide the baby with nutrients. Just like your baby, the placenta has needed to grow and develop a circulation to support the ever-increasing demands that are being placed on it.

One week into the pregnancy, the placenta formed a distinct inner and outer layer of cells that gradually penetrated the lining of the uterus, with fingerlike fronds. You may have noticed a very slight bleed at this implantation stage (see pp.67). More and more fronds spread out into the lining of the uterus, which itself undergoes a transformation process that enables each frond or villus to be bathed by small pools of maternal blood, enabling oxygen and nutrient transfer to take place.

Up until now, this blood flow has been limited by plugs of tissue, but at this stage of pregnancy these plugs begin to disappear. This means the placenta is sufficiently developed to withstand the pressure of maternal blood on each delicate villus. Villi will continue to branch out until around 30 weeks of pregnancy.

ACTUAL SIZE OF YOUR BABY

After 10 weeks your baby's crown to rump length is 1.2 in (3 cm).

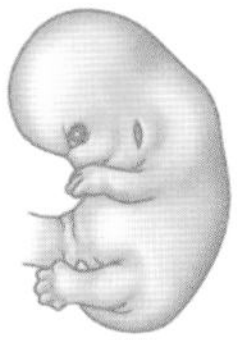

9 weeks

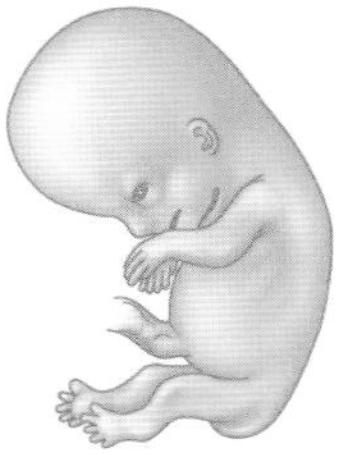

10 weeks

ASK A DOCTOR

I've been told I might be rhesus negative. What does this mean? Red blood carries a positive or negative rhesus factor (Rh-factor). Problems arise if an Rh-negative woman carries an Rh-positive baby who has inherited the Rh-positive status from the father. If the mother's blood comes into contact with the baby's during delivery, she may produce antibodies against it. Although this may not be a problem in the first pregnancy, the antibodies can affect a baby in subsequent pregnancies, leading to anemia. To prevent this from happening, anti-D injections are given at week 28 and possibly again after the birth.

In some units, it is also possible to have your blood tested for fragments of your baby's blood to determine whether the baby is rhesus negative or positive.

Your 11th week

YOU'LL NOW BE SETTING UP THE HEALTH CARE THAT WILL SUPPORT YOU OVER THE COMING MONTHS. Your baby is now unmistakably human and is undergoing many sophisticated changes, such as development of the sense organs. To mark his new status, he's now called a fetus. If pregnancy hasn't seemed quite real to you so far, it soon will. It's time to get down to such practicalities as your first prenatal checkup. Procedures such as ultrasound scans and blood tests are about to become part of your normal pregnancy routine.

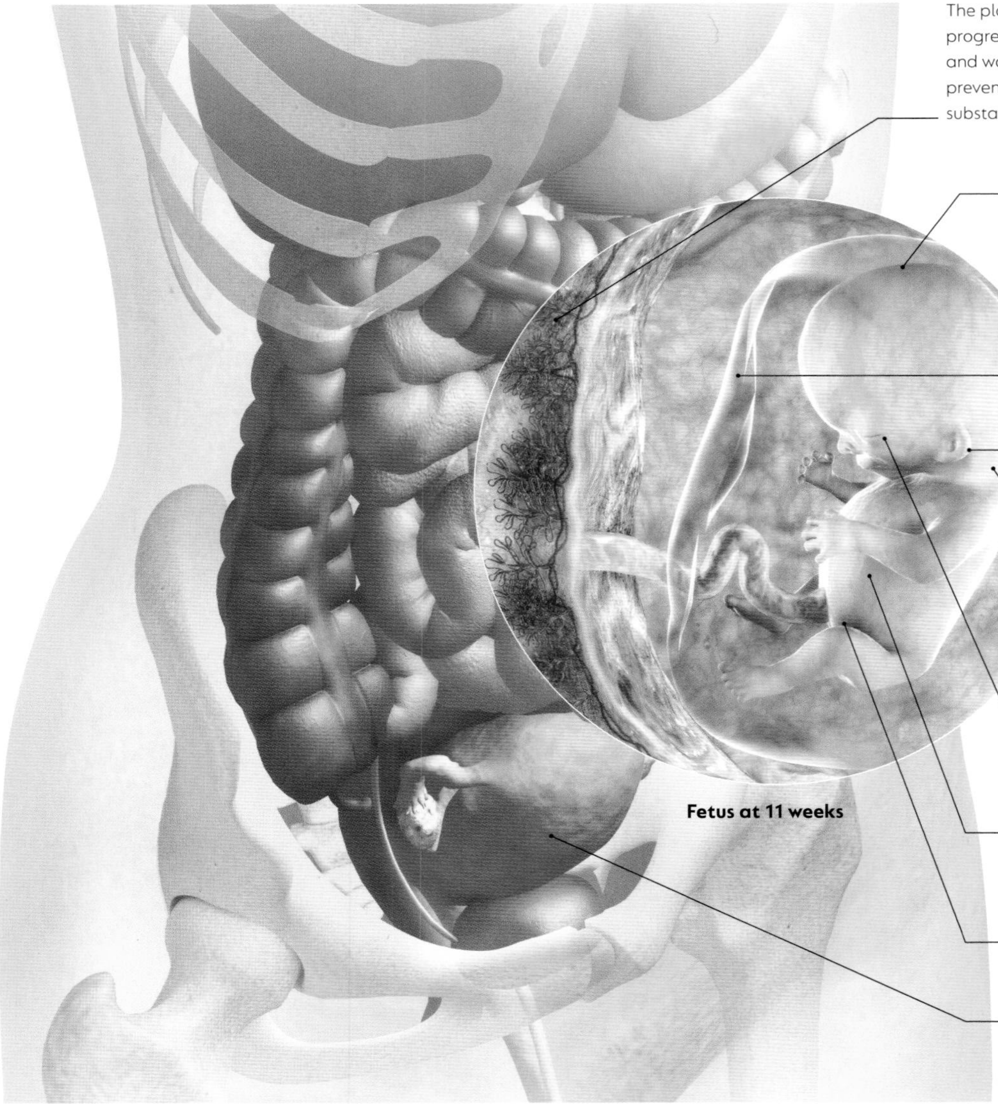

The placenta will get larger as pregnancy progresses. In addition to allowing food and wastes to circulate, the placenta helps prevent harmful microorganisms and substances from reaching the baby.
The fetus measures 1.6 in (4.1 cm) from crown to rump.
Within the amniotic sac, the baby is becoming very active, kicking and squirming. You cannot feel any movements yet.
The ear has started to move into its final position.
The neck has lengthened, allowing the baby to nod and shake his head from side to side.
The eyelids are sealed shut and will remain this way until the 26th week.
The diaphragm is complete, and your baby can make breathing movements.
The ovaries or testes are beginning to develop.
Your growing uterus may begin to cause discomfort as ligaments and muscles stretch to make room.

Fetus at 11 weeks

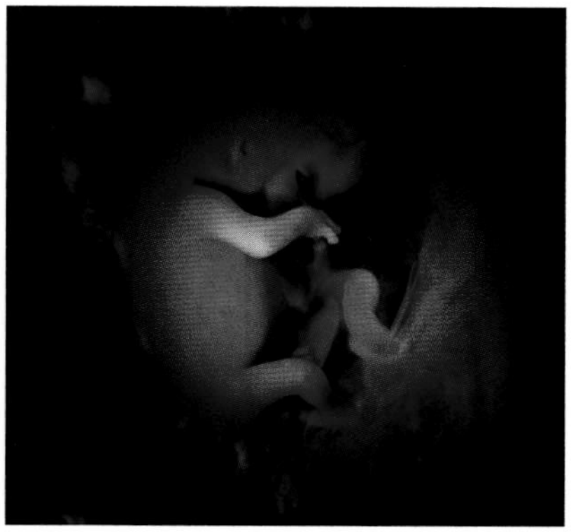

YOU ARE **10 WEEKS AND 1 DAY**

209 days to go...

YOUR BABY TODAY

In this side view of a fetus, the right ear and eye are just visible and the right hand and leg can be seen in characteristically bent positions. The reddish, tubelike structure, to the right of the image, is the umbilical cord.

> " Your prenatal care begins with your first appointment, where you will get to talk with your ob/gyn about your pregnancy care. "

You should have your first prenatal appointment around now. The exact timing of it will vary depending on when your doctor sees pregnant patients for the first time. This is the first time you will see your ob/gyn during pregnancy. Unless your doctor has a solo practice (see p.102), your prenatal team is likely to consist of several doctors who will take care of you throughout your pregnancy.

The purpose of this appointment is for a doctor to obtain your medical history, provide information, and plan your care for pregnancy and the birth. It's also an opportunity for you to ask any questions you may have and discuss the schedule for appointments, blood tests, scans, and prenatal classes. You will be given booklets, information leaflets, and important contact telephone numbers.

The doctor will ask you about your medical history; your family's medical history; your partner and your partner's family's medical history; about any previous pregnancies you have had; and how this pregnancy has been so far.

Your answers will help the doctor identify factors that may affect your pregnancy, for example, if there is a family history of preeclampsia. The doctor will also do some health tests, such as urine tests, at this and other prenatal appointments.

THE ROLE OF A MIDWIFE

Midwife comes from the anglo-saxon word "mit wif," meaning "with woman." A midwife's role is to respect the ability of a woman to give birth independently, and to only intervene when it is essential to do so.

ASK A DOCTOR

How should I decide which tests I want? Your doctor will give you a lot of information regarding tests, and you have to decide whether you want them. There are two different types: screening tests (see pp.142–143) and diagnostic tests (see pp.152–153). The goal of screening tests is to figure out the risk of there being a problem—based on the result, you may be advised to have a diagnostic test.

Most women opt to have the screening tests, but it's worth considering how far you would continue with the process. For example, if you had a high-risk result from the screening test, would you opt to have a diagnostic test? If you did, and the results of that were positive, would you want to continue with the pregnancy?

Such considerations are difficult but important. For example, if you know that, no matter what, you and your partner would want to continue with the pregnancy, then you may decide not to have a test or decide to have the test so you can prepare yourself for a baby with potential problems.

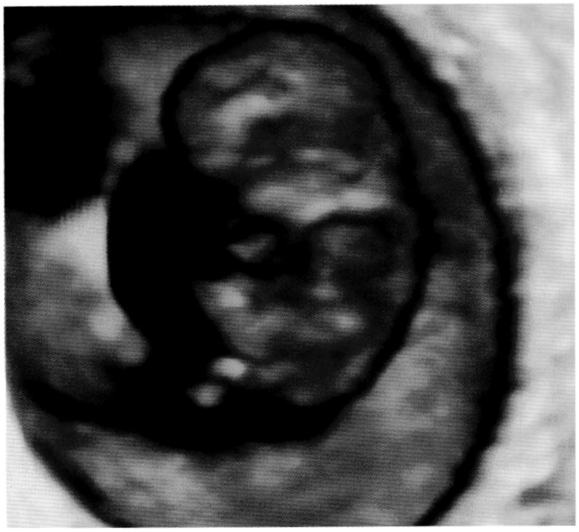

YOU ARE **10 WEEKS AND 2 DAYS**

208 days to go

YOUR BABY TODAY

The baby's head is just under half the length of his body. His limbs are still relatively short but the hands and feet can look quite big. Early basic trunk and limb movements are taking place but it's too early to feel them at this stage.

" Will it be a boy or a girl? Significant changes are taking place that enable your baby's sexual organs to develop. "

The unborn baby's ovaries or testes now begin to form. The testes will gradually descend but their structural development won't be complete until your child hits puberty. The ovary will produce eggs (see p.226), but these will remain in the early stages of development.

A minute genital tube forms the external genitalia but each sex appears the same at this stage. This is not entirely surprising since the phallus is only 0.09 in (2.5 mm) long.

Your baby's bladder and rectum have now separated. The kidneys will take some time to fully develop: two buds grow up from the bladder to the tissue that will become the kidneys. These form the ureters—the tubes that transport urine from the kidney to the bladder. The buds must successfully fuse with the kidney tissue in the pelvis. As the buds expand upward, the early kidneys developing in the pelvis will move upward to lie in the abdomen.

ASK A DOCTOR

I have hay fever. Can I take antihistamines? The potential effects of taking antihistamines in pregnancy aren't known, so it's best to err on the side of caution and not take them. However, if your symptoms are severe, there are oral antihistamines that can be taken during pregnancy. Nasal sprays and eye drops are also available. Speak to your doctor.

FOCUS ON TWINS

Nonidentical twins are always in separate amniotic sacs with a placenta each. If your babies are identical (from one fertilized egg) they may share the same placenta and/or amniotic sac, with a single membrane called the chorion surrounding them. These are known as monochorionic twins and will require greater monitoring. The arrangement of the placenta and amniotic sacs can be analyzed on an ultrasound scan.

When twins share a placenta, a blood vessel directly connects them. This can cause one twin to receive too much blood, which can cause heart problems; the other twin will get too little blood and not grow at the correct rate. This is called twin-to-twin transfusion and happens in about 10–15 percent of monochorionic pregnancies. The imbalance can sometimes be corrected by draining amniotic fluid from around the twin with the greater blood supply, or by using laser treatment to seal off some blood vessels in the placenta. An early delivery may be necessary.

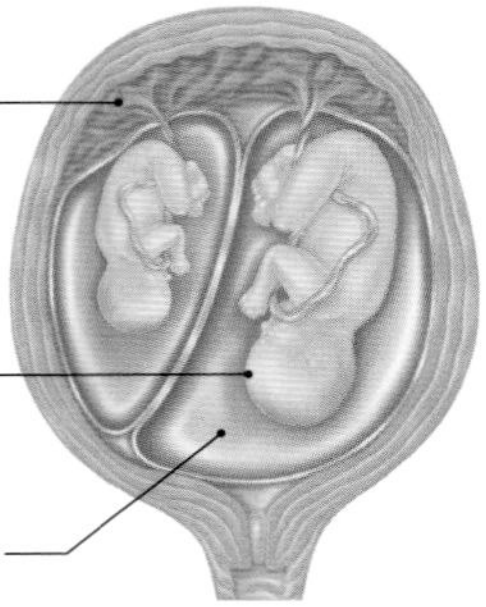
Shared placenta
One baby is bigger than the other
Amniotic sac

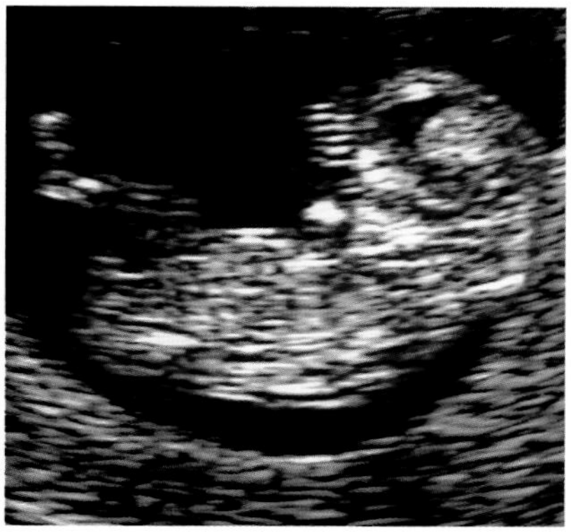

YOU ARE **10 WEEKS AND 3 DAYS**

207 days to go

YOUR BABY TODAY

This color 2-D ultrasound scan shows a baby lying on its back with its head to the right. This is the ideal position when measuring the crown (head) to rump (bottom) length to accurately date the pregnancy: it simply measures in a straight line.

> "You may begin to notice some discomfort around your pelvis as your body begins to accommodate your growing uterus."

Having a few minor aches and pains during pregnancy is nothing to be concerned about. They occur because the ligaments and muscles of your pelvis are stretching to fit your ever-growing uterus. This can cause some discomfort but should not be painful.

If you're experiencing cramplike period pain, and there is any bleeding, or if the pain becomes very severe and constant, then you should go to the doctor or the hospital to be checked. You will be examined to rule out a miscarriage (see p.94) or ectopic pregnancy (see p.93).

SAFETY WHILE TRAVELING

When traveling, it's important to be prepared (see also pp.28–9):

- **Check that you're healthy enough to travel—**speak to your doctor.
- **Find out whether you need any vaccinations** and discuss these with your doctor (see p.105). It's advisable to avoid traveling to areas where there is a high risk of disease.
- **Get travel insurance** and make sure it covers you during pregnancy.
- **Carry your prenatal records** with you at all times and stay within reach of medical help.
- **Don't stay seated** for long periods in transit and stay hydrated. Wear support socks to reduce the risk of DVT (see p.186).
- **Wear adequate sun protection** if you're going to a hot climate.
- **Be careful** about what you eat and drink bottled water.
- **Avoid eating street food** since it may put you at risk of food poisoning.

ASK A NUTRITIONIST

I'm intolerant to dairy products. What can I eat to make sure my baby gets the nutrients these provide? Dairy products are an excellent source of protein, calcium, and phosphorus—these are all essential nutrients that are required for the development of your baby's teeth and bones—riboflavin (vitamin B2), which helps with the production of energy; and iodine (see p.80), which helps the baby's brain development. Vitamin A is also found in dairy fat, so cheese and whole and low-fat milk all provide some.

- **For calcium:** Have fortified alternatives such as soy or nut milks, tofu, and dried figs. Eat canned fish with small bones, such as sardines.
- **For riboflavin (vitamin B2):** Choose fortified breakfast cereals, lean beef, chicken, and turkey.
- **For vitamin A:** As retinol (see p.46), eat egg yolk, mackerel, salmon, or other oily fish. As carotenes (from plants), eat carrots, sweet potatoes, red peppers, spinach, kale, cantaloupe, mango, and papaya.

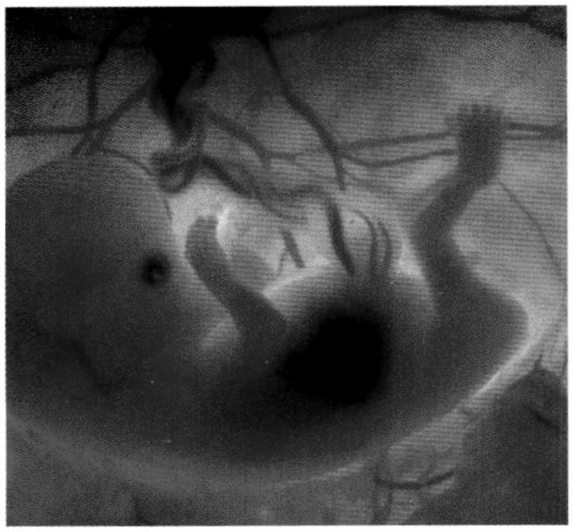

YOU ARE **10 WEEKS AND 4 DAYS**

206 days to go

YOUR BABY TODAY

The umbilical cord gradually becomes more coiled as the pregnancy progresses—as seen here on the left of the image. This coiling is thought to occur because of the many movements the embryo makes.

> "Your baby's limbs are more developed now, enabling him to move, and his hands and fingers can be clearly seen on a scan."

Your baby takes on a more human form as his neck lengthens and his head is seen as separate from his body. The head is still about half the total length of your baby. The length of your baby can be measured on an ultrasound by measuring the distance between your baby's head (crown) and his bottom (rump). This is noted as the CRL (crown-rump length) measurement. The head is also measured: this is the biparietal diameter (BPD), which is the distance between the two parietal bones on each side of the baby's head.

Now that the neck is more developed and all the limb joints have formed, your baby can begin to make several movements. The completed diaphragm allows for breathing movements. In the gut, the duodenum opens up along its length, the small bowel starts to rotate and prepares to re-enter the abdominal cavity.

Within your baby's mouth, the hard palate has formed; the relatively large tongue makes it easier for your baby to move amniotic fluid through the nostrils rather than through his mouth with each breath.

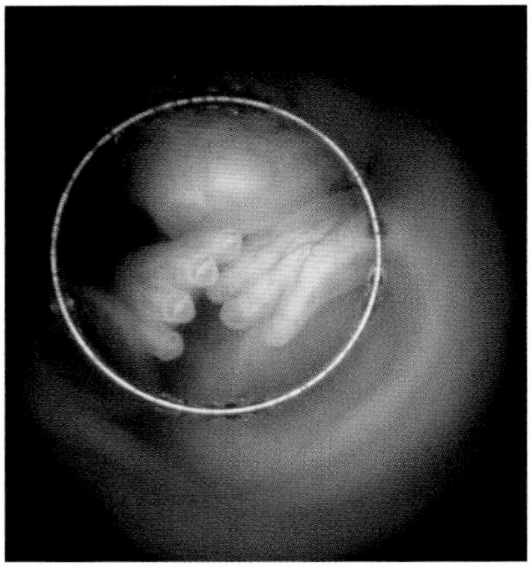

This endoscopic image, obtained by passing a fine light-emitting tube into the uterus, shows the hands obscuring the fetus's face.

FOCUS ON TWINS

Since your body is growing two or more babies, there will be physical effects. But there is a positive side: Since your growing size and hormones are the cause, these symptoms are often worse if the babies are doing well.

- **In the first three months,** your heart has to work harder to pump more fluid around your body, which can lead to a greater feeling of fatigue.
- **Morning sickness** can be more severe because you have higher amounts of pregnancy hormones.

Mention severe symptoms if you're suffering, but remember these symptoms are not serious. You may be seen earlier if you suspect you're having twins, and will go on to have more prenatal appointments and ultrasound scans. You may be asked to limit activities like travel and exercise as your pregnancy progresses.

TESTS FOR DOWN SYNDROME

After 10 weeks of pregnancy, it is possible to have a test to assess the risk of your baby having a chromosomal abnormality, such as Down syndrome.

- **This can either be with a blood test and scan** between 10–14 weeks, or a blood test after 14 weeks.
- **A blood test,** known as the noninvasive prenatal test (NIPT) is available after 10 weeks (see p.142).
- **If the results of any of these tests** show a high risk, a diagnostic test is offered (see pp.152–153).

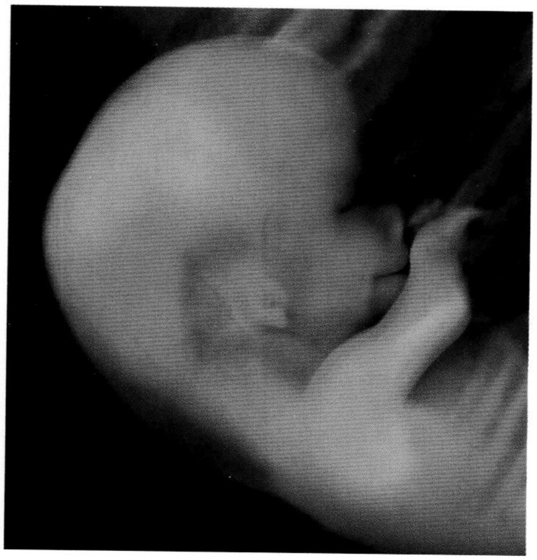

YOU ARE **10 WEEKS AND 5 DAYS**

205 days to go

YOUR BABY TODAY

The external ear is now more clearly seen as it makes its way to its final position. The eyes are also much closer to their final position and the neck continues to lengthen. The baby will often bring his hands up to his mouth, providing important sensory feedback.

> “Healthy teeth and gums are essential in pregnancy, so brush thoroughly and make regular dental appointments.”

Make sure you're taking care of your teeth and gums. The hormone progesterone causes gum tissue to soften and it's therefore more likely to bleed when brushed and to become infected.

It's even more important than usual to brush your teeth regularly and use dental floss at least once a day. Think about your diet, too. Avoid having sugary drinks and foods, and if you are suffering from morning sickness rinse out your mouth with water after vomiting to remove the acid from your stomach.

To keep your mouth healthy during your pregnancy, brush your teeth twice a day with a fluoride toothpaste and floss your teeth every day. Be sure to see your dentist regularly for cleanings as recommended. If you need antibiotics to treat an infection, make sure to remind your dentist you are pregnant so that medications that are safe in pregnancy are prescribed.

If your dentist needs to take X-rays of your mouth, he or she will protect your baby by covering your abdomen with a lead apron.

A TOOTH FOR EVERY CHILD

A US study found that, on average, those with one child were missing two or three teeth, and those with four or more children were missing between four and eight teeth.

So the old wives' tale that “You will lose a tooth for every child” could have some basis in truth. It might be because of the hormonal changes occurring during pregnancy that can cause gum disease (see above).

ASK A DOCTOR

Why am I getting more vaginal discharge since being pregnant? In pregnancy, the layer of muscle in the vagina thickens, and cells lining the vagina multiply in response to an increase in the pregnancy hormone estrogen. These changes prepare the vagina for childbirth. As a side effect, the extra cells mean that there is an increase in vaginal discharge, known as leukorrhea.

If you feel sore or itchy in the vaginal area and the discharge is anything other than cream or white, or smells, your doctor will need to take a swab to rule out infection.

Some infections, such as yeast, cause an abnormal discharge. They are common in pregnancy and are easily treated. Even if you've self-treated yeast infections before, call your doctor for advice this time. She'll likely recommend medication that's applied vaginally, but if she determines that you have bacterial vaginosis, oral medication may be required.

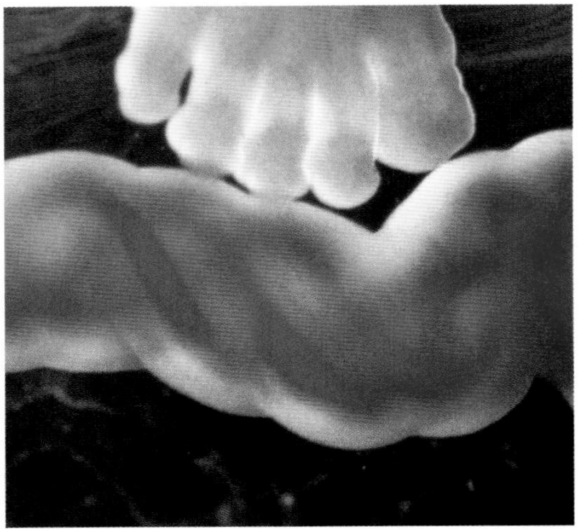

YOU ARE **10 WEEKS AND 6 DAYS**

204 days to go

YOUR BABY TODAY

This is the umbilical cord of an 11-week-old fetus. The cord is a strand of tissue that contains the two spiraling arteries that carry blood to the placenta and a vein that returns blood to the developing baby.

“Has sex been the last thing on your mind, or have you noticed an increase in your libido? It seems all women are different.”

Being expectant parents can bring you emotionally closer as a couple, but not necessarily physically. While some women find that their libido increases during pregnancy, often much to their partner's surprise, the majority find that their sex drive diminishes in the early weeks. In the first trimester many women are affected by fatigue and nausea, and so the last thing they want to do is have sex. If this is the case then make sure you explain how you feel to your partner, so that they don't feel rejected. Try to find other ways to stay physically connected with each other: perhaps you can still enjoy some aspects of foreplay, if not penetrative sex. If not, at least try to be affectionate to each other.

It may be your partner who's anxious about having sex due to worries about harming the baby through penetrative sex, although there is no chance of this happening.

Remember, if you do want to have sex, unless a doctor tells you otherwise, it's safe to do so while you are pregnant.

ASK A NUTRITIONIST

Is it safe to drink herbal teas? Herbal teas don't contain caffeine, but herbs and dietary supplements are not regulated by the Food and Drug Administration, and there's not much research about the effects of many herbs on pregnancy. Stick to decaffeinated black teas. If you want to drink fruit or ginger teas, make sure no herbs are present. Also, limit green tea, because it may interfere with fetal growth.

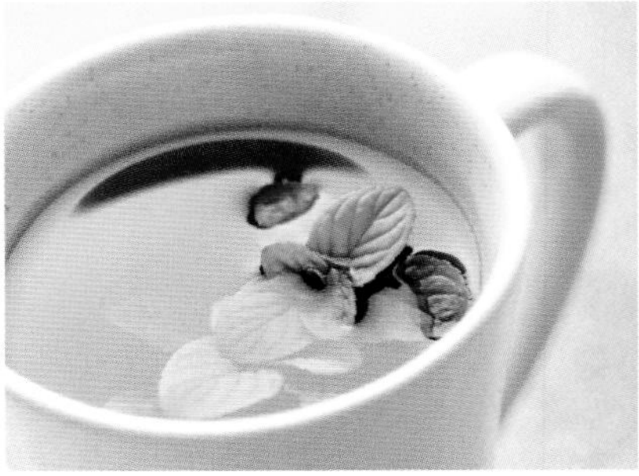

TACKLING SPIDER VEINS

Spider veins (or spider nevi) are tiny red blood vessels that branch outward, just under the skin. They are caused by an increase in the level of estrogen during pregnancy. They usually appear on the face, upper chest, neck, arms, and legs. Often disappearing soon after birth, spider veins are not a cause for concern and can usually be covered with makeup. You can discourage spider veins by:

- **Upping your intake of vitamin C,** which helps to strengthen your veins and capillaries.
- **Avoiding crossing your legs,** which can exacerbate the problem.
- **Getting regular exercise** because it keeps your blood circulating around your body.
- **Avoiding standing or sitting** for long periods, and elevating your feet when you do sit down.
- **Avoiding eating spicy food,** since some women have found that this helps reduce spider veins.

If you suddenly notice lots of broken veins appearing on your skin, see your doctor.

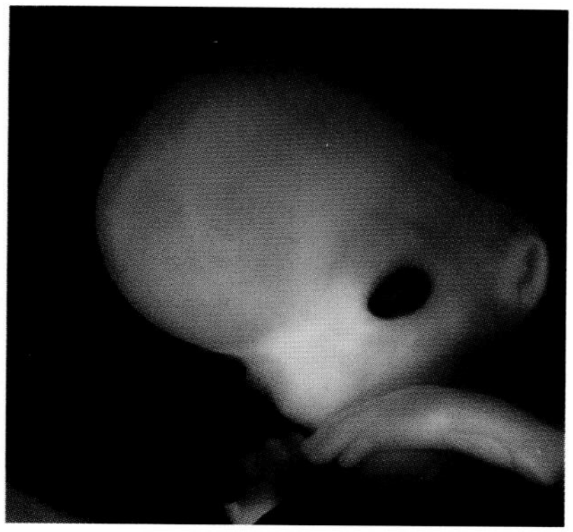

YOU ARE **11 WEEKS EXACTLY**

203 days to go

YOUR BABY TODAY

The hands can now be easily brought up to the face and the baby's neck has lengthened, which will enable him to flex it and make side-to-side movements. The baby's ear and eye are clearly visible.

" The key organs that enable your baby to see, hear, and taste are developing rapidly now, and he's starting to move around. "

The baby is developing hearing. The ears continue to move up toward their final destination, but your baby can't hear at this stage. Hearing requires the middle and inner ear to structurally mature and the inner ear to complete nerve connections to the brain. Hearing will, however, be one of the first senses to develop and can be tested by seeing if the baby responds to the sound waves that reach him in the uterus. Judging when taste is established is harder, but taste buds have started to appear on the tongue.

Your baby's eyes have a lens and early retina but even if the eyelids were open the eyes would not yet be able to see light signals. The lens is solid and the optic nerve is not yet responding to signals from the retina.

More signs of bodily movement appear but although your baby is quite active he is too light for you to feel the kicks. But you'll be fully aware of him in about two months (see p.213).

ACTUAL SIZE OF YOUR BABY

At 11 weeks your baby's crown to rump length is 1.6 in (4.1 cm).

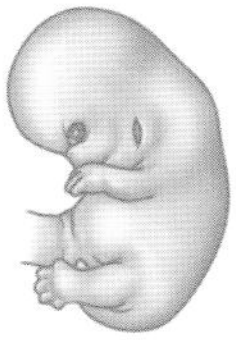

9 weeks

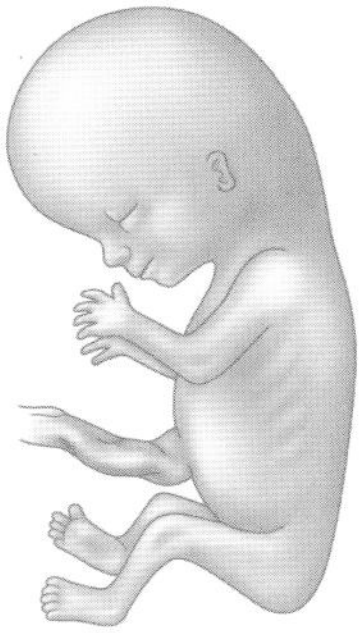

11 weeks

ASK A DOCTOR

I had some bleeding after I exercised. Should I be worried? If you have vaginal bleeding during exercise with or without cramping, stop immediately and seek medical advice. It's unlikely that exercise is the cause, but you should be checked as soon as possible and before you exercise again.

Bleeding in the first trimester may be due to a number of issues completely unrelated to exercise, but it's important to rule out any problems at the outset. Once you have the all-clear from your doctor, you can begin exercising again.

SUPERNUTRITIOUS SMOOTHIES

Smoothies and juices are a great vitamin C boost, but they are high in natural sugars. If you're suffering from gestational diabetes and need to maintain even blood-sugar levels even, keep your intake of smoothies and juices to mealtimes.

The recommended portion size for fruit juice and smoothies is 5oz. Here are a couple to try:

- **Strawberry/banana:** fresh or frozen strawberries, banana, plain yogurt, and orange juice.
- **Raspberry/orange:** fresh or frozen raspberries, orange sorbet, and orange juice.

Your 12th week

AN IMPORTANT MILESTONE IS PASSED AS THE FIRST TRIMESTER ENDS. Yawning, arms and legs waving—your baby is on the go and you can actually see it happening. Most women have their first scan this week, and it's the big thrill of the first trimester. Up until now, you may have preferred to keep your pregnancy a precious secret. After the scan, you'll probably feel more confident about making an announcement, especially when you have the photos to prove there's really something happening!

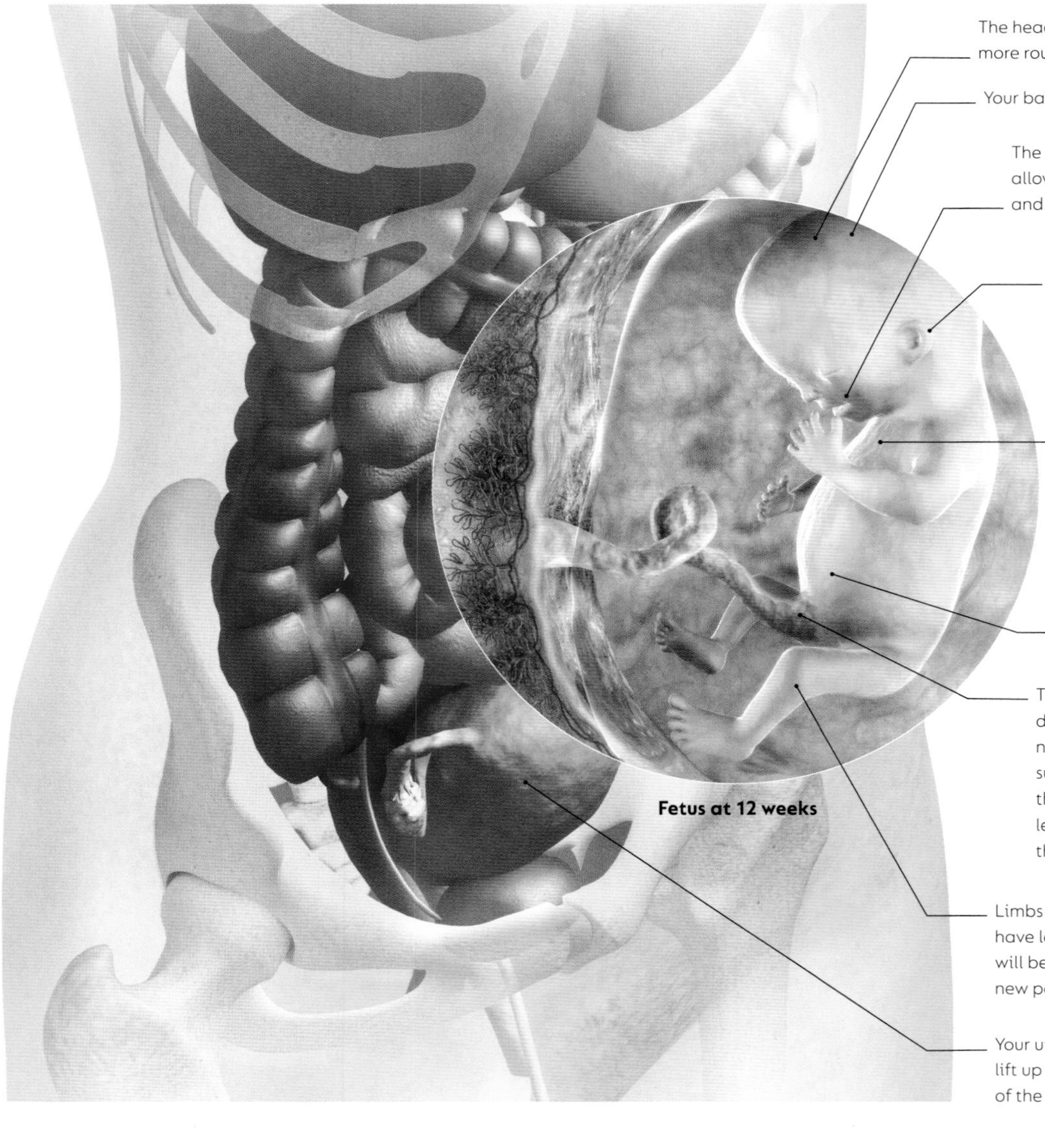

The head now has a more rounded shape.
Your baby measures 2.1 in (5.4 cm).
The mouth can open and close, allowing your baby to swallow and yawn.
Ears are nearly in their final position on the head.
Your baby's heart is beating rapidly, about 160 beats per minute, which is twice as fast as your own heart rate.
The intestines, previously contained in the base of the umbilical cord, move into the abdominal cavity where there is now room.
The umbilical cord is fully developed, ensuring that vital nutrients from your bloodstream, such as glucose, are carried to the baby from the placenta. It lengthens during the course of the pregnancy.
Limbs are fully formed and have lengthened; your baby will be trying out all sorts of new positions.
Your uterus is beginning to lift up out of the bony cavity of the pelvis.
Fetus at 12 weeks

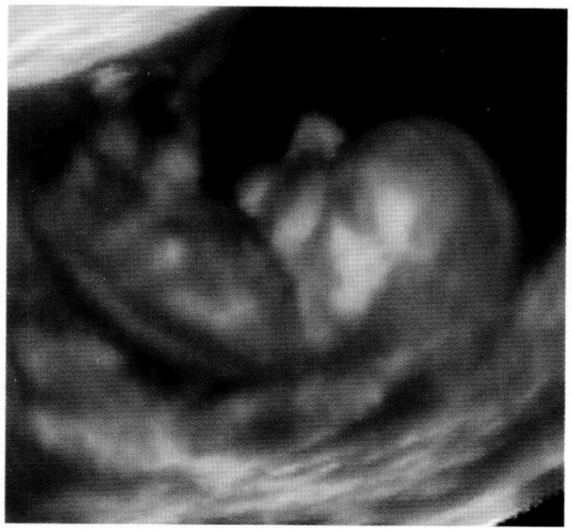

YOU ARE **11 WEEKS AND 1 DAY**

202 days to go

YOUR BABY TODAY

Although on a scan it might look as though the baby is resting on her back, the fluid in the amniotic sac means that she is floating in a near weightless environment and can easily move into any position within the uterus.

You and your partner have reached an exciting milestone. You'll have your first ultrasound around now and see your baby; this may help you feel closer to her. For many partners, seeing the baby on the scan may be the first time the pregnancy becomes a reality.

At this scan, your baby's length will be measured (see p.139) and this will be used to figure out her age. Up until about 14 weeks of pregnancy, all babies grow at around the same rate so irrespective of whether you and your partner are tall or short, until this time your baby will be the same size as others at this stage of fetal development.

Figuring out your due date (see p.74) using the first day of your period isn't always accurate, especially if your menstrual cycle is long or irregular. The dating scan can give a more accurate expected date of delivery, but it by no means tells you for certain—very few babies arrive on their actual due date.

> “In this final week of your first trimester, you'll probably have your first ultrasound scan and see your baby for the first time.”

FOCUS ON PARTNERS

You and your pregnant partner will be looking forward to the first scan, but it is normal to worry that there may be a problem with your baby.

The first scan may seem quite technical since it is used to detect your baby's heartbeat and take some measurements, but it's also very emotional. In reality, the first scan gives you the first look at this new life. It lets you see your baby moving around, with legs kicking and arms flailing, even though those movements can't be felt yet.

Perhaps, as the nonpregnant partner, the biggest shock of the scan is the fact that it confronts you for the first time with the physical evidence that your baby really exists. Your partner is likely to be more used to the idea of pregnancy, because she's carrying the baby, but the scan will make the pregnancy much more real to you, and you may be surprised at how emotional you feel.

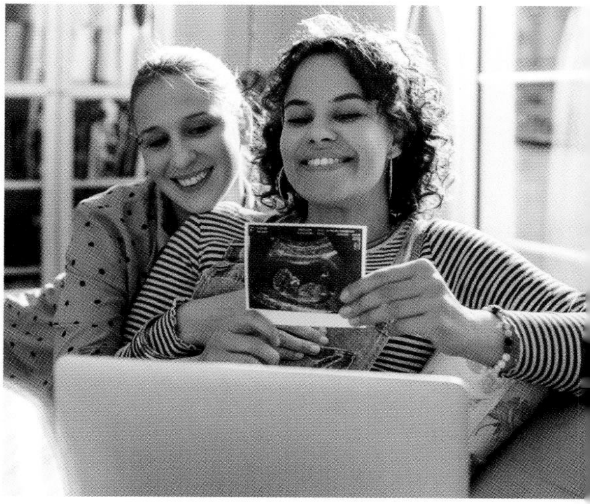

You will be given a scan picture of your baby. Don't be surprised to find yourself looking at it again, and again, and again! It's also a great way to share the news with others.

First ultrasound scan

Your first scan at 10–14 weeks can pinpoint the length of your pregnancy to within a five- to seven-day window. Such accurate dating helps estimate your due date and determine the right time to perform tests later in pregnancy.

Your first scan

This ultrasound helps to accurately establish your baby's gestational age. This is particularly useful if you are not sure of the date of your last menstrual period, if you have irregular periods, or you became pregnant immediately after you stopped using contraception such as the pill. At this stage of pregnancy, your baby can be measured from crown to rump (from the top of the baby's head to its bottom).

Accurate dating of your pregnancy is important not only for establishing your due date and the timing of screening and diagnostic tests, but also because it helps to avoid misdiagnosis of problems such as poor fetal growth (see p.284). Your due date will usually be changed at this scan if there is more than a five- to seven-day difference between your menstrual dates and the dates based on the crown–rump length.

A scan may be given before 10 weeks if you have bleeding or pain to rule out the possibility of a miscarriage or ectopic pregnancy (see p.93).

How the scan is done During an ultrasound scan, high-frequency sound waves are emitted through the abdomen via a handheld device called a transducer. As the sound waves hit solid tissue, they translate into an image that is viewed on a computer screen and interpreted by the sonographer.

At this scan, you will need to drink plenty of water to raise the uterus and provide a clearer image. The sonographer will put some cold gel on your abdomen to maximize contact with the skin and will then move the transducer gently over the area.

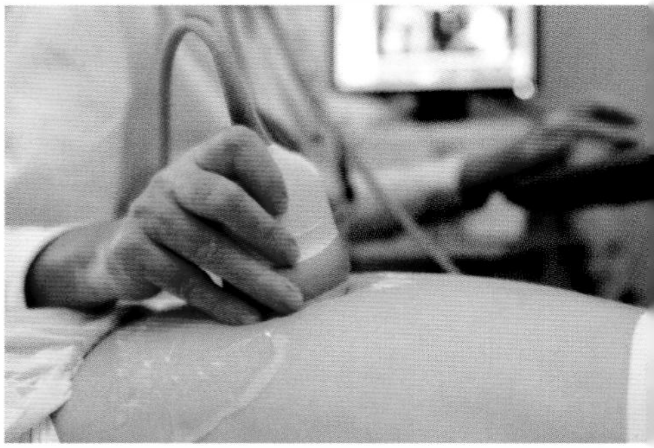

As the transducer is passed over your abdomen during the ultrasound scan, you will see your baby on the screen.

WHAT THE SCAN SHOWS

In addition to confirming your dates, your first scan may reveal some other useful information.

- **This scan usually confirms whether** you have a single or multiple pregnancy (twins, triplets, or more).
- **Uterine anomalies** can be seen, such as a double uterus, although this is rare. Uterine fibroids (benign tumors) will also be identified.
- **The scan may reveal an ovarian cyst** (corpus luteum) on the ovary that produced the egg. These are common and can persist in the first trimester.
- **Major anomalies** may be seen, but most are diagnosed at the 20-week scan when the organs are seen (see p.214).

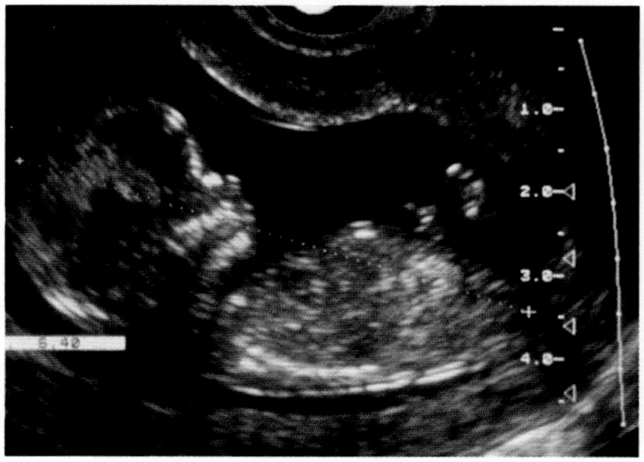

By 12 weeks the fetus has taken on a human appearance. The forehead, eye sockets, and small button nose are all visible in profile.

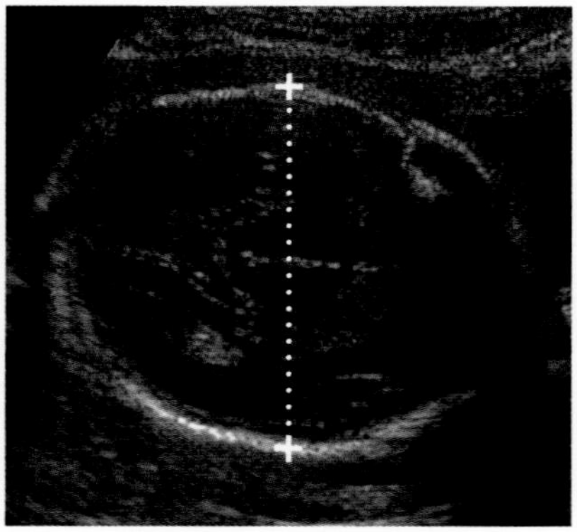

Measuring the diameter of your baby's head (the biparietal diameter) helps assess your baby's growth and date your pregnancy.

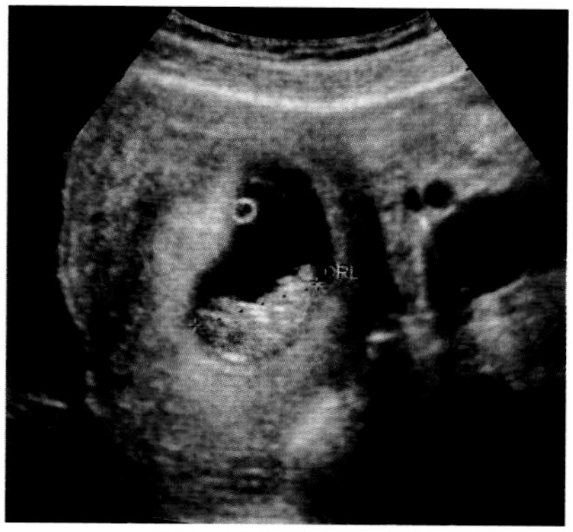

YOU ARE **11 WEEKS AND 2 DAYS**

201 days to go

YOUR BABY TODAY

This image shows the yolk sac at the 12 o'clock position with the placenta seen as a thickening to the lining of the uterus on the left. The baby is in the lower part of the uterus and is positioned lying on her back.

" The dating scan is reassuring because it's an opportunity for your baby's progress and development to be thoroughly checked. "

At your ultrasound scan, the pregnancy is dated according to your baby's length from crown (head) to rump (bottom) because he is—and will remain—quite curled up. This is known as the CRL (crown–rump length).

Since your baby can flex their spine and stretch their neck, this measurement needs to be taken with the baby in a specific position so it can take some time to achieve. The measurement is used to estimate your baby's date of delivery and this may be different than the EDD you calculated (see p.74)

On this first ultrasound scan it should be possible to recognize all four limbs, your baby's hands and feet, the spine, some aspects of brain development, the fluid-filled stomach, and the bladder. From now on your baby's kidneys will be producing small amounts of very dilute urine and the bladder will start to fill.

ASK A DOCTOR

I've had quite a few pregnancy symptoms and don't feel as though my body is my own. How can I relax and enjoy being pregnant? Not all women adapt well to pregnancy and for some dealing with the symptoms and worrying about issues such as weight gain makes them feel out of control. The best way to cope with these feelings is to embrace the changes and remain in touch with your body by exercising and taking time to focus on what is happening inside you. We spend most of our lives listening to all the things that happen on the outside, but very little time focusing on the inside.

Try to practice deep breathing and relaxation and consider learning pregnancy yoga and meditation techniques.

The dramatic changes happening to your body may be mirrored in the wide swings of emotions and feelings you experience throughout your pregnancy. Some days you may feel excited and elated at the prospect of being a parent, and on other days you may feel quite overwhelmed and anxious.

Perhaps the nine months' gestation period is nature's way of giving us time to get used to the idea of becoming a parent and allowing us time to deal with our emotions and prepare for the birth. So try to relax, but if you're feeling really anxious, speak to your doctor.

THE DUE DATE

Dating scans are only an estimate. The chance of delivering on your due date is only around 5 percent. So keep the estimated due date in mind but don't expect your baby to abide by it!

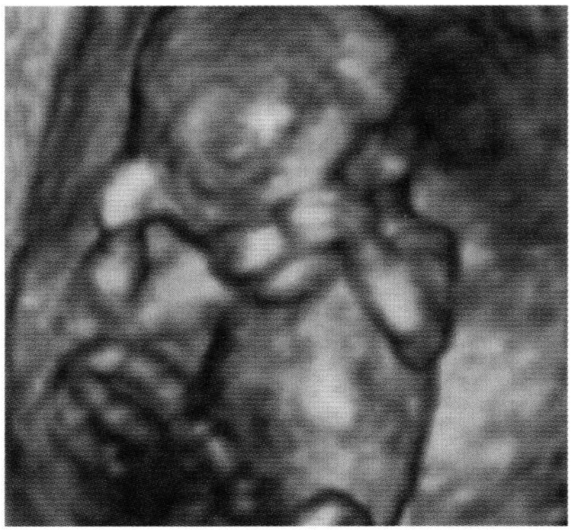

YOU ARE **11 WEEKS AND 3 DAYS**

200 days to go...

YOUR BABY TODAY

As the baby floats in the amniotic fluid, their limbs are now more fully developed, allowing them to make many movements. The lips and fingers—which are now completely separated—stimulate sensory feelings.

“ Does your face resemble the pimply complexion of your teenage years? Don’t worry, it’s those hormones again and it will pass. ”

Your skin is likely to change during pregnancy. Some women find that they develop pimples or acne due to the high levels of progesterone. Conversely, you may get dry skin, also due to pregnancy hormones. The dryness may become worse over your abdomen as your belly grows and the skin is stretched.

Freckles and moles may get darker. You may also notice tiny red lines on your chest or legs: these are called spider nevi (see p.134) and are due to the increased blood supply to the skin which makes the vessels dilate and become more visible.

Other women find that the high levels of estrogen mean that their skin is in a better condition than before they were pregnant. The “glow” of pregnancy is due to the increased blood supply that occurs in pregnancy, which gives you a rosy, healthy-looking complexion.

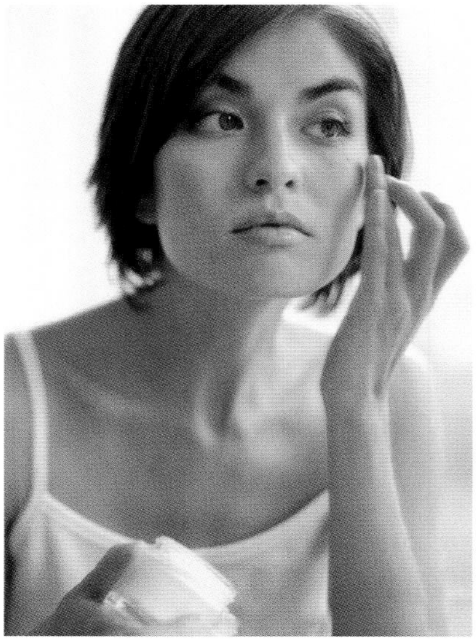

As hormonal changes can affect your skin, you may want to change the skincare products that you use during pregnancy.

TELLING YOUR EMPLOYER

As soon as your employer knows you’re pregnant, you should be protected by the Pregnancy Discrimination Act, which says that pregnant employees must be treated the same as other employees with disabilities or limitations. Most parents-to-be wait until 12 weeks when the risk of miscarriage is lower. Some wait longer.

- **Each company has its own policy** on maternity leave. Some offer paid or unpaid leave for a set period. Others let employees use sick leave or vacation days. Meet with a human resources representative to learn your options.
- **You can discuss** when your maternity leave will start. If your baby is born early or your maternity leave starts earlier than planned due to illness, the arrangements can be altered at short notice.
- **Your employer** should respect your right to confidentiality. If you want the news of your pregnancy to remain under wraps until a certain date, make this known.

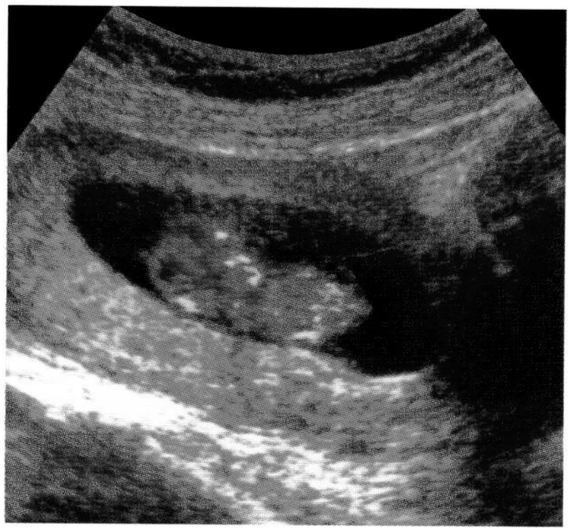

YOU ARE **11 WEEKS AND 4 DAYS**

199 days to go...

YOUR BABY TODAY

The fetus can be seen inside the uterus on this color ultrasound scan. At this stage of development, the fetus measures approximately 2.1 in (5.4 cm) crown to rump and weighs around 0.5 oz (14 g).

> " At around 12 weeks, the doctor might be able to hear your baby's heartbeat with a handheld monitor. "

At this stage, your baby's heart beats at approximately 140 beats per minute; at least twice as fast as your own. The heart and its internal electrical conducting system are structurally complete but its external nerve supply is still quite immature. The nerves to the heart influence its rhythm, gradually slowing the rate as the pregnancy advances.

The heart is tiny, and to maintain an adequate output the heart is unable to increase the amount of blood it pumps with each beat (as we can), but instead increases the number of times it beats each minute.

The abdominal cavity is large enough to hold the intestines. Whereas before they were bulging outside of your baby's body, they now fit into her abdominal cavity. Having started to rotate while outside the body, the bowel completes its final rotation in the abdominal cavity. Once inside, the bowel position remains fixed, and its diameter increases as the loops of bowel become hollow.

FOCUS ON TWINS

If you're carrying twins, you're likely to have put on some weight by now, perhaps around 11 lb (5 kg). Early weight gain is usually a good thing, especially in your case, since this is a vital time for the formation and development for your babies organs. As a rough guide, a good recommended weight gain is:

- **For twins,** total weight gain of 35–45 lb (16–20 kg), preferably 24 lb (11 kg) by week 24, then a gradual increase until the birth.
- **For triplets,** a total weight gain of 50–60 lb (23–27 kg), preferably 35 lb (16 kg) by week 24, then a gradual increase until the birth.
- **For quads,** total weight gain of 65–80 lb (31–36 kg), ideally 50 pounds of it by week 24.

SMOKING: THE FACTS

At your first prenatal appointment, the doctor will discuss with you whether you, your partner, and anyone else you live with smokes.

Here's how smoking affects your baby:

- **The carbon monoxide,** nicotine, and other substances that you inhale pass from your lungs into your bloodstream and cross the placenta.
- **Nicotine** makes your baby's heart beat faster as they struggle for oxygen, which can affect their growth rate.
- **Smoking increases the risk** of miscarriage, premature birth, and low birth weight, and exposure to tobacco chemicals makes your baby more likely to suffer from conditions such as asthma and chest infections after the birth.
- **There is also a higher risk** of crib death (see p.64) if you or your partner smoke. Your partner should stop, too.
- **If you live with a smoker,** you will be inhaling thousands of toxic carcinogenic chemicals that are released into the hair around you from the burning end of the cigarette and the exhaled smoke.
- **Several studies** have shown that even passive smoking can be dangerous in pregnancy.

Tests for chromosomal abnormalities

Optional routine screening tests in the first trimester assess the risk of your baby having a chromosomal disorder such as Down syndrome. If your risk is high, you will be offered a diagnostic test (see pp.152–3) for a definite result.

What is screened for

In addition to Down syndrome, screening tests also assess the risk of other chromosomal abnormalities such as Patau syndrome (trisomy 13) and Edwards syndrome (trisomy 18). Babies with these conditions have more severe mental and physical abnormalities than babies with Down syndrome and rarely survive beyond a year. These conditions are rare, with each year about 1 in 10,000 babies born with trisomy 13 and 1 in 6,000 born with trisomy 18, compared to 1 in 800 babies born with Down syndrome.

ACCURACY OF SCREENING TESTS

As more screening tests have become available, the detection rate for Down syndrome, which used to be assessed on maternal age alone, has significantly increased. The aim of screening tests is to provide a high detection rate for Down syndrome and a low "false positive" rate. A false positive means the screening test indicated a high risk of Down syndrome, but subsequent diagnostic tests gave the all clear, which means the mother would exposed to unnecessary testing.

TESTS	TIMING (WEEKS)	DETECTION RATE	FALSE POSITIVE RATE
Combined test	11–14	85%	5%
Integrated test	11–13/15–22	85%	1%
Quadruple test	15–22	76%	5%

The "combined" test

The recommended screening test for Down, and the one most commonly offered, is the "nuchal translucency screening," performed between 11 and 14 weeks. This test has a high accuracy rate and the results are produced quickly.

The test uses a combination of a maternal blood test and an ultrasound of your baby. The ultrasound measures the thickness of the skin at the back of your baby's neck, called the nuchal fold (see box, opposite). The blood test looks at the levels of two chemicals: pregnancy associated plasma protein A (PAPP-A) and one of the pregnancy hormones, human chorionic gonadotropin (hCG). The results of the blood test are combined with your age and the measurement of the nuchal fold. A mathematical formula is then used to calculate your baby's risk of Down syndrome.

If you have your blood test before your ultrasound, you will usually receive your results immediately following your ultrasound. If you have your blood drawn at the time of the ultrasound, you will receive your results a few days later. Your baby's risk of Down, Edwards, and Patau syndrome from the combined test may be higher, lower, or the same as her risk based on your age alone.

Noninvasive testing

DNA is the genetic material we get from our parents that determines characteristics such as eye color and any genetic diseases. During pregnancy free DNA from the baby is present in the maternal circulation. When blood from the mother is analyzed for the presence of chromosome 21, 18, and 13, higher than average amounts predicts that the baby may have one of these syndromes. This test is the most accurate screening test available for the detection of Down, Edwards, and Patau syndrome, with detection rates of 99 percent for Down and Edwards syndrome and 92–99 percent for Patau syndrome. Blood is taken after 10 completed weeks from the mother and the results are available within 10 days.

The test can predict the sex and blood type of the baby, and it can also be used to screen twin pregnancies, although not to determine the sex of the babies. The result of this test is either positive, negative, or inconclusive. If the result is inconclusive, it just means there was not enough free fetal DNA, so you will be offered a repeat test.

Quadruple tests

These screening tests are done in the second trimester, and assess your baby's risk of Down syndrome from blood tests alone. If after 14 weeks you'd like to have a screening test for Down syndrome, you will be offered the quadruple test, which measures levels of hCG, AFP, estriol, and inhibin A, levels of which are altered in pregnancies with a baby who has Down syndrome. Screening for Edwards and Patau syndrome is done by ultrasound at 20 weeks.

A positive screen

A positive result does not mean your baby has Down syndrome. If your risk is higher than 1 in 150, this is a higher risk result. However, a risk of 1 in 150 means that there is a 149 out of 150 chance that your baby does not have a chromosomal syndrome. Talking to your doctor or a genetic counselor can help to understand your risk and decide whether you want to have a diagnostic test (see pp.152–153) for a definite result. Factors that might affect your decision could be your anxiety levels, your fears about pregnancy loss, and what you would do if you found out your baby had a chromosomal syndrome. Research suggests that women are more likely to enjoy their pregnancy and come to terms with the diagnosis if they know in advance that their baby has Down syndrome. So diagnostic tests aren't only about deciding whether or not to continue your pregnancy.

If you have a positive screening test for another more severe chromosomal disorder, such as trisomy 13 or 18, your doctor will talk to you about the outcomes for the baby as most will die at a young age, sometimes within the first week—to help you decide what to do. In some cases these disorders are associated with abnormalities detected during the dating scan (see p.138), and the presence of these abnormalities combined with a positive test may confirm the diagnosis. Nevertheless, many women opt to have a diagnostic test before deciding whether or not to terminate their pregnancy.

More screening

Another option is to have a special ultrasound scan to look for Down syndrome markers between 17 and 22 weeks. However, a second-trimester ultrasound is not such an accurate test for Down syndrome as other tests, so only consider this path only if you are strongly against having a diagnostic test such as amniocentesis and feel that you don't need a definite diagnosis.

NUCHAL TRANSLUCENCY SCREENING

An ultrasound scan, known as the nuchal translucency screening, is done between 11 and 14 weeks of pregnancy and is used to help assess your baby's risk of Down syndrome. During this test, the sonographer measures the depth of fluid under the skin at the back of the baby's neck, known as the nuchal fold. If this measurement is high, it indicates that excess fluid is present, which means that the baby has a higher risk of Down syndrome. The measurement is then combined with the results of blood tests and the average risk based on your age to give your baby's individual risk for Down syndrome. If your risk is higher than 1 in 250, you will be counseled and offered a diagnostic test, such as amniocentesis or chorionic villus sampling, to give a definitive result (see p.152).

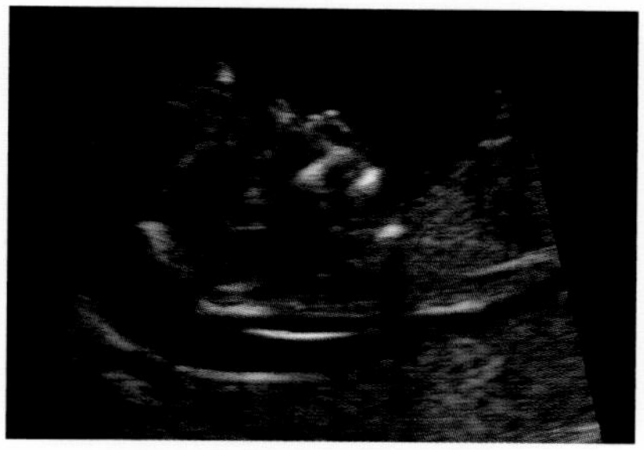

The small depth of fluid seen in the neck's nuchal fold in this scan means that the fetus has a low risk of developing Down syndrome.

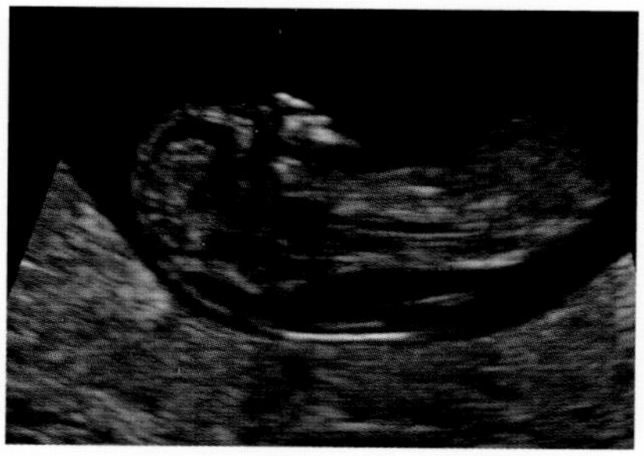

The thicker nuchal fold seen here indicates an increased risk of Down syndrome in this fetus, and a diagnostic test will be recommended.

PAPP-A

PAPP-A (Pregnancy Associated Plasma Protein-A) is produced by the placenta and can be used to screen for growth problems and preeclampsia (see p.476). If a blood test shows the PAPP-A level is low (this occurs in about 5 percent of pregnancies), there is an increased risk of preeclampsia or of having a low birthweight baby.

You will be offered a specialized scan at 20 weeks to look at the blood flow to the placenta and extra growth scans later on in pregnancy. Low-dose aspirin, which can reduce the risk of preeclampsia, will also be suggested as long as you do not have an allergy to aspirin. If you smoke, this is definitely the time to quit.

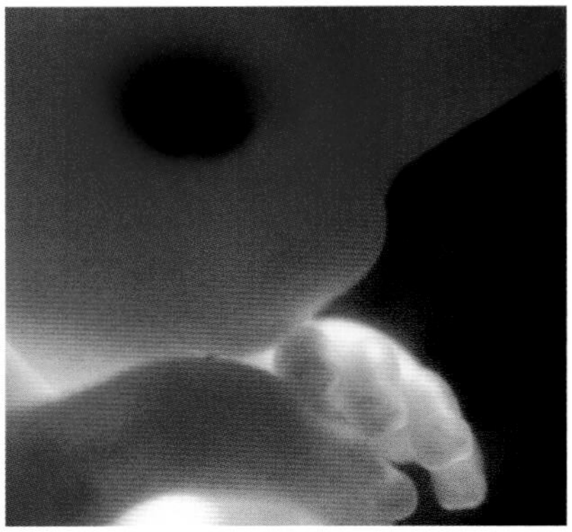

YOU ARE **11 WEEKS AND 5 DAYS**

198 days to go

YOUR BABY TODAY

At this stage the eye—not yet in its final position—still dominates the appearance of the face. The eye is not yet responsive to light and remains well protected behind the covering eyelid.

> "Having your first scan this week, and knowing your risk of miscarriage is reduced now, should mean you can start to relax."

This can be a very positive time for you, especially if you've been anxious from day one of your pregnancy. The risk of miscarriage falls as your pregnancy progresses and by the end of this 12th week, it's no more than 1 percent.

As you enter the second trimester, you should begin to feel better (see opposite), and this, combined with the knowledge that you have passed the most risky time, may help you relax. If you've been keeping your pregnancy a secret, you can also enjoy telling others.

SAFE SCANS

Medical ultrasound has been used since the early 1960s. However, the first discovery of high-frequency echo-sounding techniques, was as long ago as 1880 in Paris. It was not until the 1940s that research began into its use as a diagnostic tool.

Children who've been exposed to prenatal ultrasound do not have differences in speech, hearing, vision, or school performance, or an increased risk of cancer.

Although it is safe, ultrasound should only be carried out when it is necessary to do so.

ASK A NUTRITIONIST

I have a really sweet tooth. Is it okay to indulge this while I'm pregnant? You don't want to deny yourself sweet foods for the whole pregnancy, but too many candies and cookies may fill you up without providing other vital nutrients your baby needs. So occasional treats are fine, but don't let them take the place of more nutritious foods. A small treat after you've eaten a meal is preferable to replacing your lunch with cake.

It's a good idea to carry nutritious snacks with you or keep them at work. That way when you feel like a nibble you have something on hand rather than being tempted by a sweet treat from a deli or vending machine. Small bags of dried apricots, prunes, and raisins are sweet and also provide fiber and essential iron.

To help curb your sweet tooth, eat regular meals. This helps to steady your blood-sugar level and may reduce cravings. Try to drink plenty of water each day, since sometimes you may be dehydrated, not hungry. Have a glass of water before you are tempted with something sweet, and if you're still hungry, have a healthy snack such as a sandwich, yogurt, dip with vegetables, or a piece of fruit.

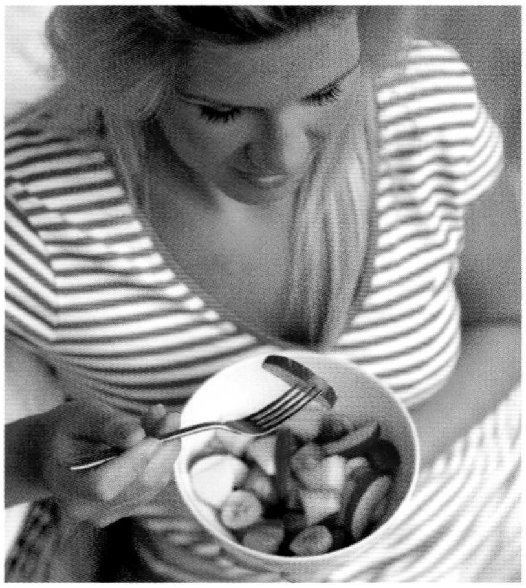

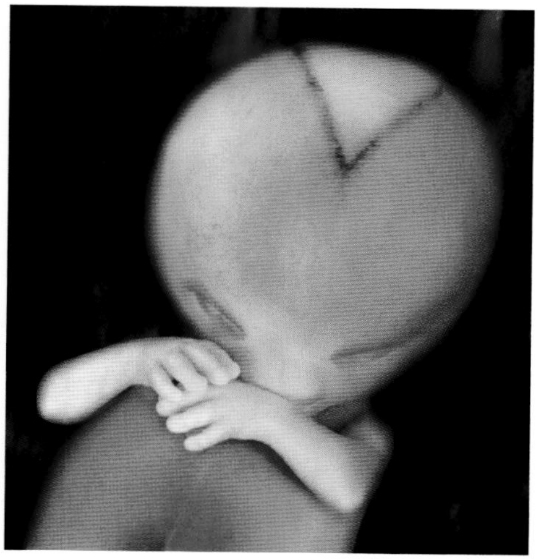

YOU ARE **11 WEEKS AND 6 DAYS**

197 days to go

YOUR BABY TODAY

The bones of the front of the skull have continued to expand and cover the head, protecting the delicate brain structures beneath. The soft spot in between the skull bones (center) remains through pregnancy and into babyhood.

“If you’re finding you’re out of breath when you get to the top of the stairs, accept this as a normal side effect of pregnancy.”

ASK A DOCTOR

My bra size has gone from an A cup to C cup. Will this increase last forever? The majority of women who have had babies do report a permanent increase in breast size. The effects of estrogen cause fat to be deposited in the breasts and when your milk comes in after the birth your breasts will get bigger, but reduce again once you have stopped breastfeeding.

By the end of the first trimester it’s normal to begin feeling a little breathless. This is because your heart and lungs are having to work much harder to supply your body with oxygen due to all the changes that are taking place.

The amount of oxygen you need in pregnancy is about 20 percent more than normal; some of this goes to the placenta (see p.127) and baby and the rest to your other organs. To get this increased amount of oxygen you breathe faster and deeper, almost hyperventilating so you feel short of breath, especially when you exercise.

This shortness of breath, or feeling that you are not breathing deeply may continue or worsen as the baby grows. Your uterus will expand upward and your other abdominal organs will rearrange themselves to create more room. Your organs and uterus push up against your diaphragm so it becomes more difficult to take a deep breath, so in order to get all the oxygen you need, you then have to breathe much faster. The hormone progesterone may also affect the rate at which you breathe.

If you have any concerns about breathlessness, don’t hesitate to speak to your doctor.

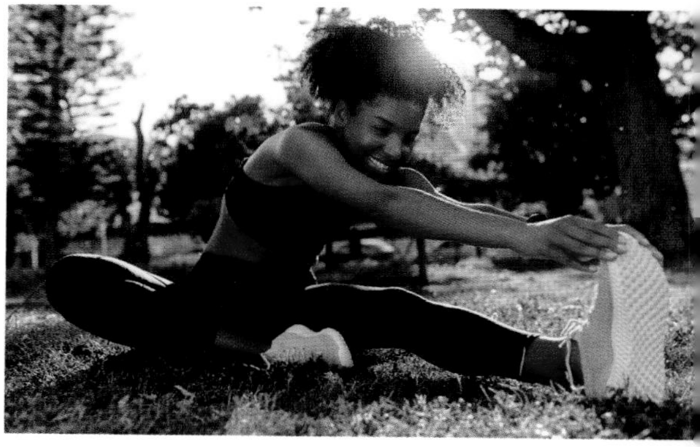

Some of your usual vitality should begin to return toward the end of the first trimester.

FEELING BETTER?

By the end of this trimester, many of the early pregnancy symptoms are likely to have passed.

- **Nausea** may have begun to lessen and it can be a complete relief to wake up in the morning without feeling sick. Your lost appetite will return, and you can stop worrying about whether your baby is being properly nourished, which is often a common concern for women who suffer from morning sickness.
- **You won’t need to urinate** quite so often. This is because your uterus is now moving up the abdominal cavity and therefore is placing less pressure on your bladder.
- **The fatigue** that you may have felt in these early months is likely to have lifted by now, and you may be sleeping more deeply now that you’re relaxing into your pregnancy.

If your sickness hasn’t passed yet, don’t worry—for some women, it does last longer (see p.159).

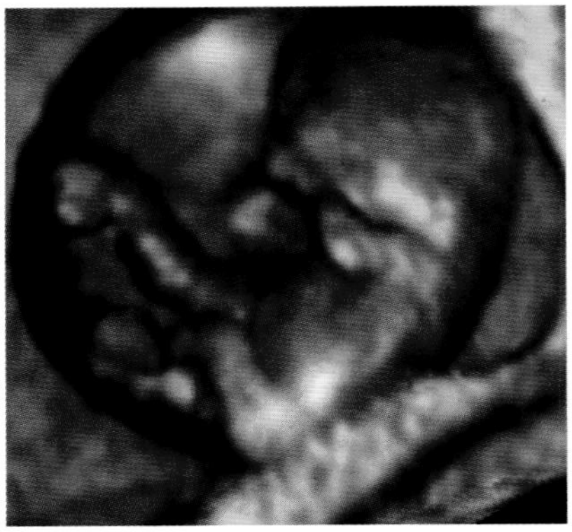

YOU ARE **12 WEEKS EXACTLY**

196 days to go

YOUR BABY TODAY

Here the legs are crossed and the arms outstretched. The umbilical cord is short and thick at this stage, but will lengthen as the baby grows, and become much thinner with many coils.

> "You've reached the end of the first trimester and in this time your baby has developed from a ball of cells to an active fetus."

Your amazing baby can do so many things already, including being able to open her mouth and yawn, and swallow. Swallowing develops earlier than sucking. Your baby will be swallowing the amniotic fluid regularly but the more complex sucking movements cannot be identified until 18–20 weeks. Swallowing will encourage gut development. The amniotic fluid enters into the stomach not the lungs, which are protected now by the vocal cords and the higher pressure of the lung's own fluid. The amniotic fluid will later be excreted as urine when the fetal kidneys start to function.

After the stomach, the amniotic fluid will enter the small bowel. The intestinal walls are developing muscular layers but these do not yet contract in a coordinated way to move the fluid along the digestive tract. It will be 20 weeks before the structural organization of the gut is finally complete. Many digestive enzymes are starting to be released into the gut but these currently act as a stimulus to development rather than for the absorption of nutrients.

Your baby is reliant on a steady stream of glucose, which is stored as glycogen in the liver. This continues throughout pregnancy and at birth your baby will, for her size, have significantly larger glycogen reserves than adults do. The correct level of glucose is controlled by insulin secreted by the pancreas. The placenta, however, has little control over the amount it takes from your blood-stream and passes on. For this reason if your glucose level is very high, for example in poorly controlled diabetes, the baby will be presented with high levels of glucose. To maintain a normal glucose level she will secrete insulin but this will lead to increased fat deposition and weight gain.

ACTUAL SIZE OF YOUR BABY

At 12 weeks your baby's crown to rump length is 2.1 in (5.4 cm).

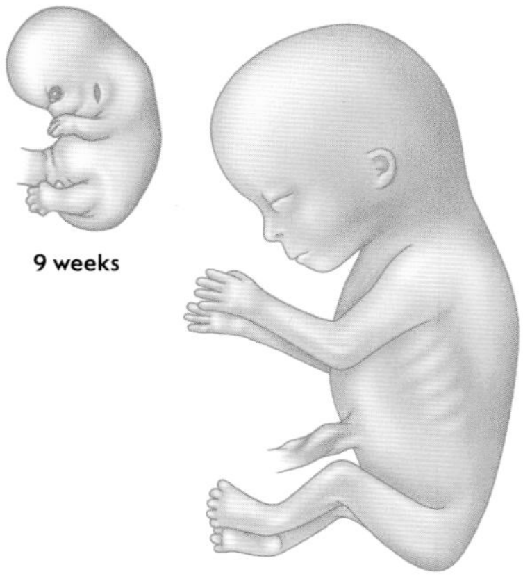

YOUR DOCTOR

Most pregnant women develop a good relationship with their doctor, who can be a fountain of fantastic information, and a wonderful source of comfort and reassurance.

It's important that you are as honest as you can be with your doctor. Like many women, you may be reluctant to reveal concerns, or to admit to unhealthy habits for fear of being embarrassed or scolded. It's very likely that your doctor will have heard it all before, and will be able to help and advise—with a few tried-and-tested tricks up her sleeve.

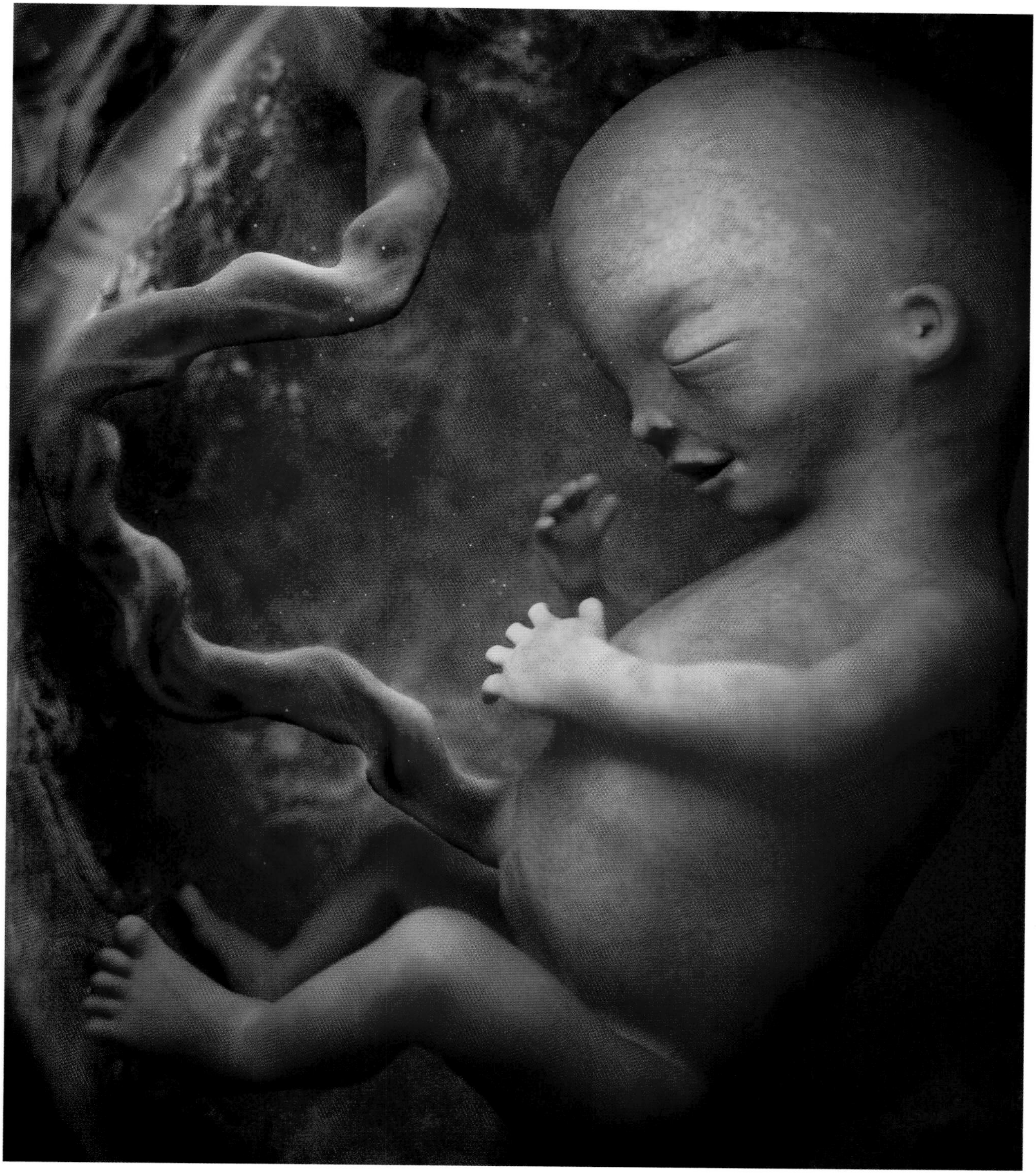

All your baby's organs, limbs, and facial features are in place, but their head is still disproportionately large. They can open and close their mouth; their eyes are developing behind closed lids.

Welcome to your second trimester

WEEK 13 | WEEK 14 | WEEK 15 | WEEK 16 | WEEK 17 | WEEK 18 | WEEK 19

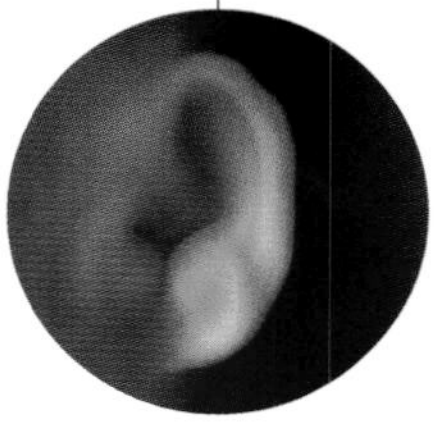

Although your baby can't **hear** anything yet, the **ears** are nearly fully **developed** and visible by this stage of pregnancy.

Your baby's **hands** and **feet** look quite large by now. The **limbs** will soon catch up.

WEEK 13: SHARING YOUR NEWS WITH OTHERS

Now that you have safely completed the first trimester and the risk of miscarriage significantly decreases, many people decide to share news of their pregnancy with friends, family, and colleagues.

WEEKS 18–22: FEELING YOUR BABY MOVE

Some women feel their baby's movements for the first time as early as 18 weeks, but for many it happens closer to 22 weeks. Keep in mind that you're more likely to feel your baby move when you're resting than when you're active.

“Now your pregnancy starts to feel “real” as your body changes rapidly and you feel your baby move.”

WEEK 20

WEEK 21

WEEK 22

WEEK 23

WEEK 24

WEEK 25

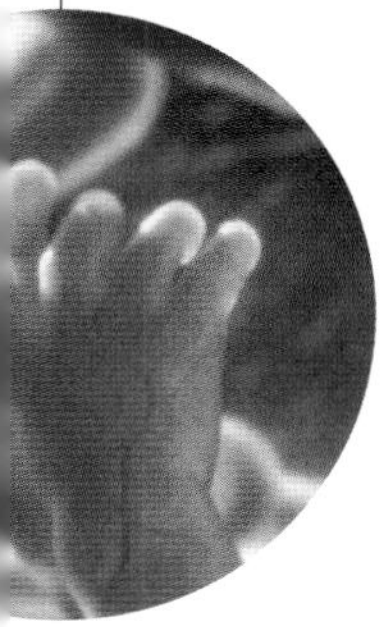

The **mouth** and **nose** are well developed and the baby will **suck** in amniotic fluid.

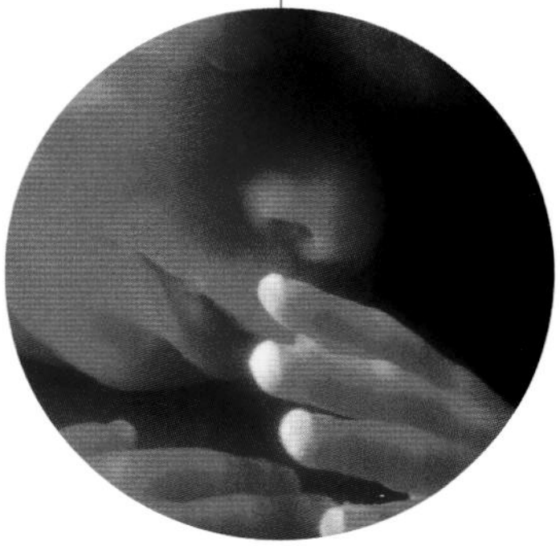

YOU AND YOUR BABY **AT 25 WEEKS**

Your baby is beginning to look more proportional, even though the head is still much larger than the body. Hearing is well developed and your baby may react to outside sounds by moving around. By the end of the second trimester, you may find yourself slowing down as you adjust to your growing bump.

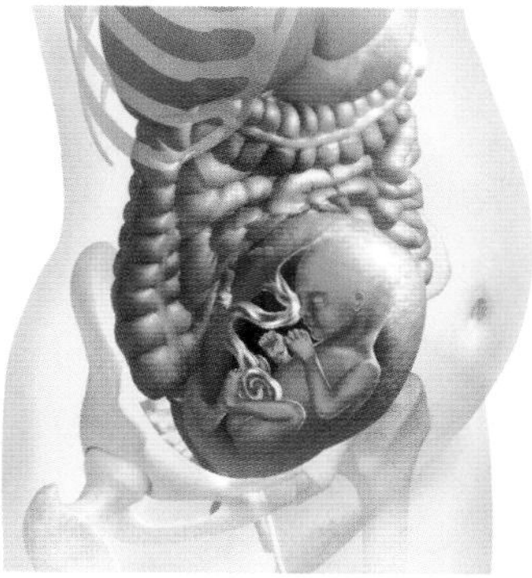

WEEK 20: FINDING OUT THE SEX OF YOUR BABY

Your anatomy ultrasound typically occurs around 20 weeks. The purpose of this scan is to take a detailed look at all of your baby’s developing parts and measure how your baby is growing. At this scan, you can also find out the sex of your baby, if you wish—that is, as long as they cooperate!

Your 13th week

AS YOU ENTER THIS SECOND TRIMESTER, YOUR BODY WILL SETTLE INTO PREGNANCY. For most women, any discomforts of early pregnancy start to disappear this trimester. The high levels of pregnancy hormones, which are thought to contribute to sickness, are subsiding, and fatigue should begin to diminish. Meanwhile, your baby floats peacefully in the amniotic sac. As he goes on growing, the sac will expand to give him plenty of room to kick and stretch. His brain is developing at a rapid rate.

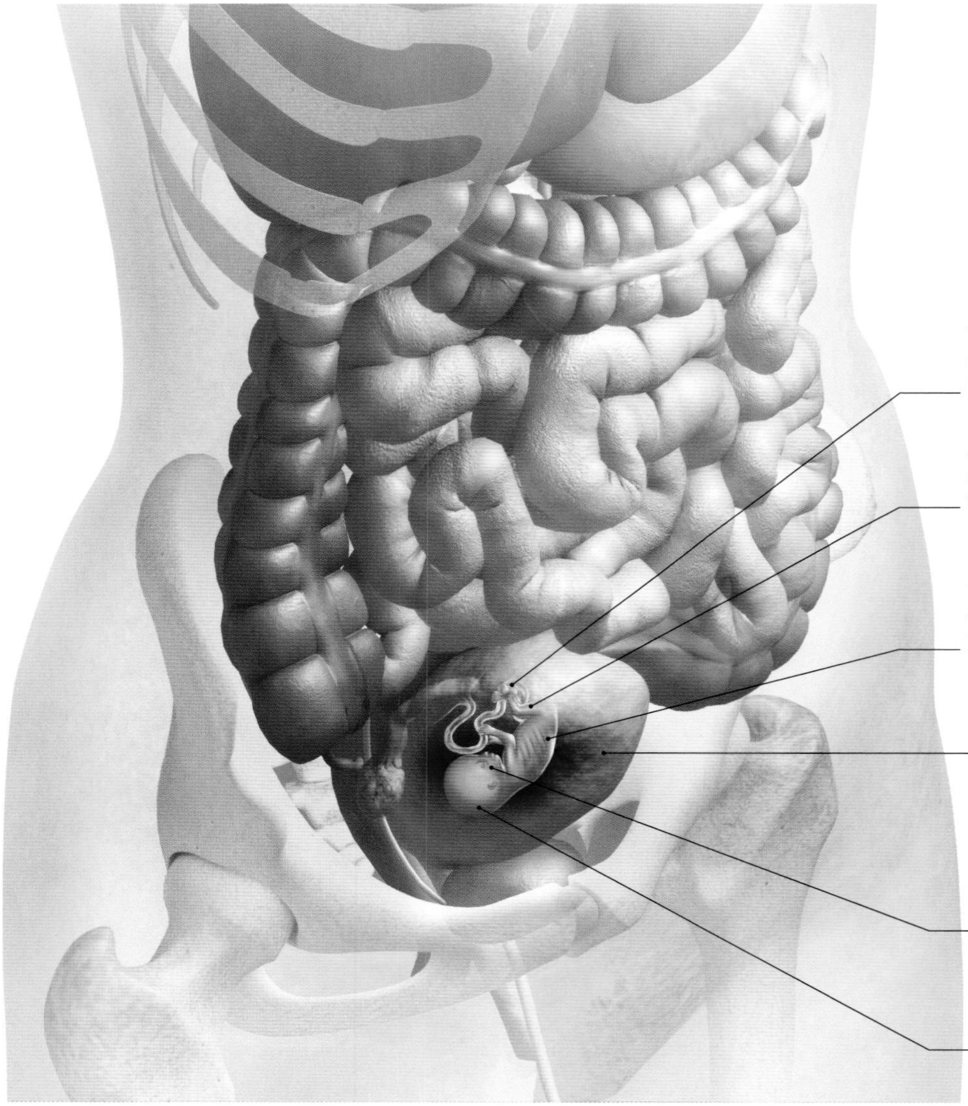
The ankle joints have matured and the toes have separated.
Arms and legs are lengthening rapidly and muscle control is developing.
The baby's body has no underlying fat, and the bones look prominent beneath the delicate skin.
In the amniotic sac, there is room to move freely and your baby is very active. Amniotic fluid cushions the kicks and wiggles, so you won't feel any movements.
The eyes have moved more toward the front of the face but they are still tightly closed.
At 13 weeks the average crown to rump length is 2.9 in (7.4 cm) and the average weight is 0.8 oz (23 g).

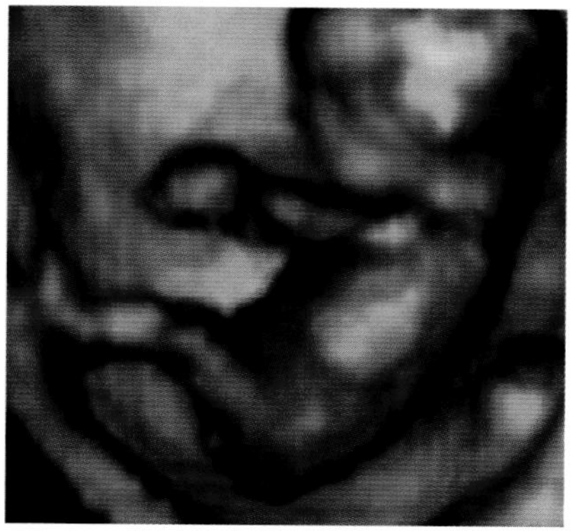

YOU ARE **12 WEEKS AND 1 DAY**

195 days to go

YOUR BABY TODAY

This 3-D ultrasound scan clearly demonstrates that the baby's arms and legs are now fully formed and much more in proportion with the trunk. All of the baby's joints are now formed, enabling a full range of movement.

Now that you're in your second trimester and have had your dating scan (see p.138), you may want to start telling a wider circle of people that you're pregnant. You can feel confident doing this, knowing that the risk of miscarriage is reduced to no more than 1 percent after the 12th week of pregnancy. Besides this, your belly will begin to show in a few weeks, if it hasn't already, so hiding the pregnancy will become difficult.

If you and your partner have been keeping the pregnancy a secret for the past three months, announcing it will be a huge relief and it can be a positive experience to share your good news with others. However, be prepared for an onslaught of advice and people's tales of their pregnancy and birth experiences!

Sometimes letting others know that you're pregnant can be difficult. Be sensitive to other people's feelings: friends who also want to have a baby, but are having difficulty conceiving, may find it difficult to share your happiness right away. It's preferable to tell these people face to face rather than them hearing it through the grapevine. Even if they don't react positively, and don't want to talk about your pregnancy all the time, give them time to come to terms with it at their own pace. Remember they can be sad for themselves while being happy for you.

" This is a good time to start telling the important people in your life your exciting news—before they guess for themselves. "

CLOTHING ADJUSTMENTS

Although your clothes may be feeling a little tight by this stage, you probably aren't ready to wear voluminous maternity clothing just yet, so it's time to get creative! Simply bridge the gap between your button and button-hole with an elastic band or by sewing in an elastic panel. Assuming your partner is bigger than you, try raiding their wardrobe—their T-shirts, shirts, and sweaters can be gathered in with a low-slung belt.

Check what's in your wardrobe already: empire-cut dresses will see you through most of your pregnancy; looser smock tops can be layered over tight-fitting T-shirts; low-slung pants can sit neatly under your belly, topped with an oversize shirt. You might want to buy a pair of maternity pants—something stretchy with an adjustable waist.

SECOND TRIMESTER TESTS

If you have not yet had a screening test for Down syndrome, you will be offered either the combined test or the quadruple test depending on your gestation.

- The combined test can be carried out at between 10 weeks and 14 weeks, and from 14 to 20 weeks the quadruple test is offered (see p.143).
- You may also want to have the NIPT blood test (see p.142).
- Screening for other abnormalities is done by ultrasound.

Diagnostic tests

If you've had a positive screening test for Down syndrome or another genetic abnormality, you will be offered a diagnostic test, which gives a definitive answer as to whether or not your baby has an abnormality.

What are diagnostic tests?

Diagnostic tests are tests that involve taking a sample of the placenta, the amniotic fluid, or fetal blood. The samples are then sent away and examined in a laboratory for chromosomal or genetic abnormalities. The two main diagnostic tests are amniocentesis and chorionic villus sampling, or CVS. Since both of these tests carry a small risk of miscarriage (see right), you will need to carefully consider the advantages and disadvantages of the tests before going ahead with either of them.

Chorionic villus sampling (CVS) Chorionic villi are fragments of placental tissue. Because the placenta originates from the fertilized egg, the chromosomes in the cells that make up the placenta are representative of your baby's chromosomes. During CVS, a small amount of tissue from your placenta is removed and tested in a laboratory to reveal if your baby has a chromosomal disorder such as Down syndrome or another trisomy disorder, such as Edwards or Patau syndrome. CVS is done between 11 and 14 weeks' gestation and the results are usually available within 7 to 10 days. The procedure can also definitely identify your baby's sex, if you want to know. If you don't want to have this information, make your wishes clear before the test. In rare cases, the doctor will be unable to perform CVS due to the placenta's position. In this case, you may be asked to return for an amniocentesis at 15 weeks.

Amniocentesis This is the most common diagnostic test, done at around 15 to 20 weeks of pregnancy. The amniotic fluid around your baby mainly consists of your baby's urine and contains cells from your baby's skin and urinary tract. During amniocentesis, a number of cells are collected from the amniotic fluid. They are then sent to a laboratory and grown in a cell culture, until there is a sufficient number of cells to examine your baby's chromosomes and identify whether your baby has a chromosomal abnormality such as Down syndrome.

Sometimes, for very specific reasons, the amniotic fluid is tested for the presence of toxoplasmosis or cytomegalovirus.

CHORIONIC VILLUS SAMPLING

There are two ways of doing chorionic villus sampling. In the transabdominal method, a fine needle is placed through the abdomen to collect placental fragments. In the transcervical procedure, a thin tube (catheter) is inserted into the cervix. It is most usually performed using the transabdominal method. During the procedure, ultrasound guidance is used so that the doctor can see the placenta's position.

CVS can also be done in a multiple pregnancy; in this case both the transabdominal and transcervical methods of collection may be used.

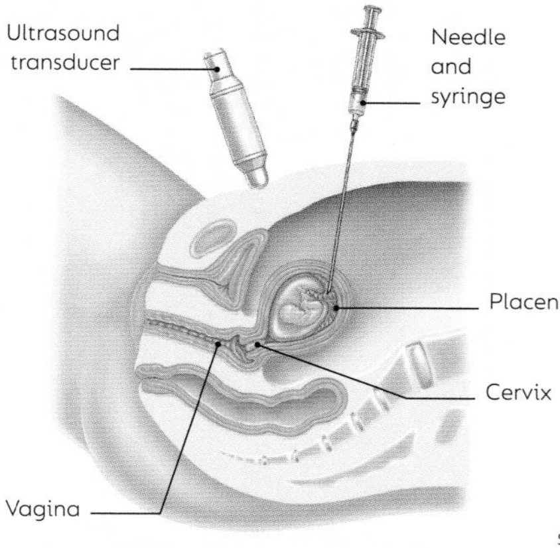
Ultrasound transducer
Needle and syringe
Placenta
Cervix
Vagina
Transabdominal procedure

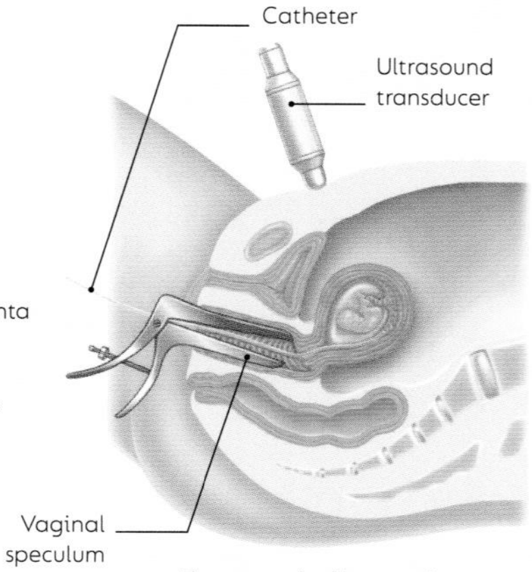
Catheter
Ultrasound transducer
Vaginal speculum
Transcervical procedure

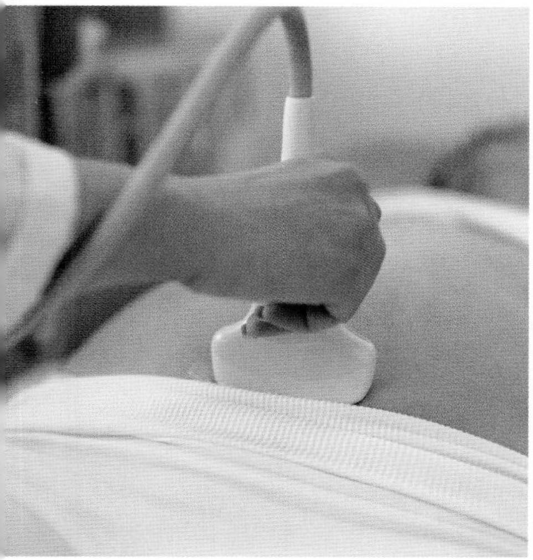

In a diagnostic test, the doctor uses ultrasound to guide a fine needle into the abdomen to take a sample of amniotic fluid (amniocentesis) or tissue from the placenta (chorionic villus sampling).

A COMPARISON BETWEEN CVS AND AMNIOCENTESIS

Before deciding which test to have, you should consider the advantages and disadvantages. Both tests carry a 0.5–1 in 100 risk of miscarriage, but there are other things to consider before making a decision.

CVS: the pros

- CVS can be done up to five weeks earlier than amniocentesis, so if an abnormality is found and you decide to terminate, it can be done in a safer, less traumatic way.
- Because more genetic material is collected, the results may arrive sooner, decreasing the anxious wait.

CVS: the cons

- The risk of miscarriage after CVS is higher than amniocentesis, because it is done at an earlier stage of gestation. The risk is the same for a transabdominal and transvaginal procedure (see opposite).
- In the past, some women who had a CVS had babies with limb abnormalities. These cases occurred when CVS was done before 10 weeks when the limbs were starting to form. The risk of limb defects without CVS is 1 in 1,700 and 1 in 1,000 with CVS.

Amniocentesis: the pros

- Amniocentesis is highly accurate.

Amniocentesis: the cons

- Since this is done later than CVS and the results may take longer, if you terminate you'll be induced and have a vaginal delivery.

How you might feel

You may be concerned about having a procedure during pregnancy, but the majority of women find it is not particularly painful. In a transabdominal procedure, the needle usually doesn't hurt any more than a blood test. Sometimes the doctor will give a small amount of local anesthetic before the transabdominal procedure to numb the area—the anesthetic itself may sting. Although afterward it's common to experience uterine cramps, similar to menstruation cramps, rest assured that these alone do not mean that you have an increased risk of miscarriage.

If your blood type is Rh negative (Rh−; see p.127), you should receive an injection of anti-Rh after the procedure to prevent complications from occurring during this and future pregnancies.

After the procedure

It's thought that being active after a CVS or amniocentesis does not increase your risk of miscarriage. However you may feel better if you don't exercise heavily right away; it's not necessary to remain in bed. In most cases, you should be physically able to return to work within a day or so after a diagnostic procedure, although emotionally you may want to return to work right away.

Getting the results

The initial results from both procedures are available within 48 hours and the result confirmed about two weeks later.

AMNIOCENTESIS

During amniocentesis, the doctor uses ultrasound to locate an open pocket of amniotic fluid. Under continued ultrasound guidance, a thin needle is placed through the skin of the abdomen and then through the uterus and into the amniotic fluid. A small amount of the fluid is drawn up into the needle and an attached syringe. A local anesthetic may be applied to your abdomen before the procedure to ease any discomfort.

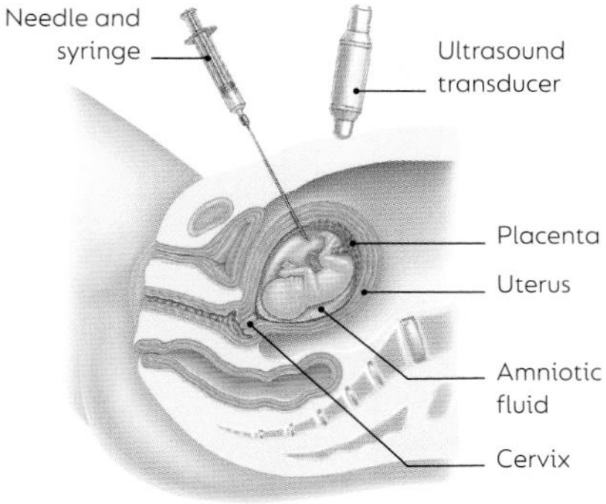

Needle and syringe
Ultrasound transducer
Placenta
Uterus
Amniotic fluid
Cervix

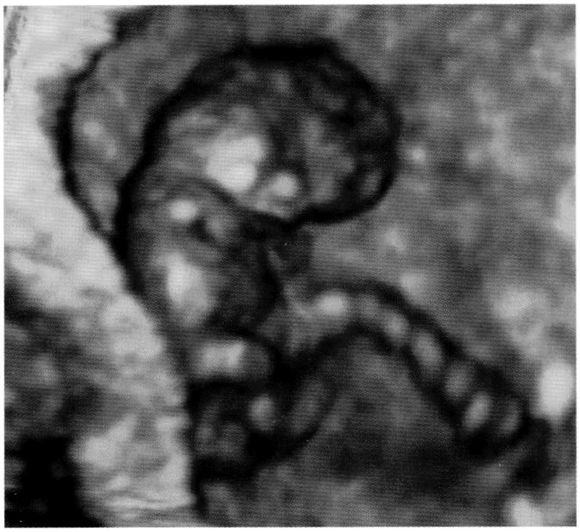

YOU ARE **12 WEEKS AND 2 DAYS**

194 days to go

YOUR BABY TODAY

In this ultrasound scan, the baby is seen floating in amniotic fluid, which provides plenty of space for him to move around. Later in pregnancy, your baby will excrete waste products into the fluid, but his bladder is still tiny and kidney function not yet established.

“ The bag of amniotic fluid is your baby’s home—it will keep him safe and free from infection until he is ready to be born. ”

Your baby is safely cushioned in the amniotic fluid, which gives space for them to move and grow and helps them maintain a constant temperature.

The volume of amniotic fluid is only 1 ml at seven weeks but is 25 ml by this stage of your pregnancy. In about six weeks’ time, there will be around 60 ml of fluid, with plenty of room for your baby to move around and to do lots of somersaults.

The amniotic fluid increases steadily until around 32 weeks of pregnancy, then stays constant until 37 weeks. It begins to reduce slightly thereafter by about 8 percent per week.

Further on in the pregnancy, waste products excreted in your baby’s urine will be absorbed from the fluid back into your bloodstream. At 37 weeks, a baby urinates an astonishing one-quarter to one-third of his body weight every day. Compare this with your own production of 2–3 percent body weight as urine.

Your temperature directly influences your baby’s temperature. Temperature control is not an important requirement until later in pregnancy when your baby’s high metabolic rate means that heat needs to be transferred to you in order to cool down.

ASK A NUTRITIONIST

My appetite has come back, but how many calories should I be eating at this stage of my pregnancy? Like many women, you’re finding that the second trimester has brought relief from the discomforts of early pregnancy. As a result, you may have noticed you’re less nauseated and have more of an appetite.

Technically your caloric needs don’t increase at this stage of pregnancy, although if you’ve been very nauseated in the first trimester and not gained weight you may feel hungrier now. Be guided by your doctor and don’t restrict your eating, but continue to eat meals and snacks that are nutritious. Snack on a glass of milk and a banana, a handful of dried fruit and nuts, or a slice of toast with peanut butter or cheese.

If you’re exercising regularly, you need to allow yourself to have additional energy. After exercising, avoid the sports drinks and opt for a glass of milk—it’s hydrating and provides protein, too.

IRON-RICH FOODS

Anemia is fairly common in pregnancy and is more likely to occur when you start pregnancy with low iron reserves. This can be because you became pregnant unexpectedly, had a baby in the last 18 months, have had very heavy periods, or don’t eat any red meat or fish. While you can’t undo these, you can start to increase your intake of iron-rich foods. Anemia in pregnancy can influence not only the size of your placenta, but could increase your risk of giving birth prematurely or to a smaller baby.

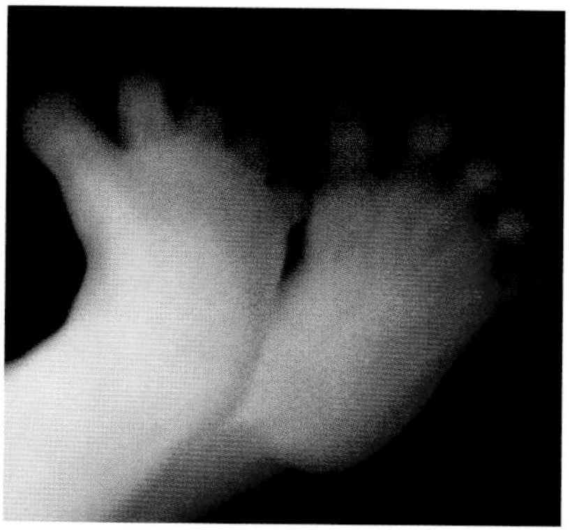

YOU ARE **12 WEEKS AND 3 DAYS**

193 days to go

YOUR BABY TODAY

The toes are now separate and are all the same length. The ankle joints are now mature enough to be working, although it will still be many weeks before you are likely to be conscious of any kicks.

There's a strong band of connective tissue in your pelvis, supporting your uterus. Known as the round ligament, this band has to stretch as your uterus expands, which can cause some discomfort. The pain is generally felt in the groin or lower abdomen and can be on either side. Although the pain starts in the pelvis, it may travel up to your hips. You may feel a short, sharp, stabbing pain or a more prolonged, dull ache.

You will soon adapt and find sitting and lying positions that cause you the least discomfort and which may relieve discomfort. Also, try other common methods of pain relief, too, such as taking a warm bath or resting comfortably with your feet up.

Round ligament pain is common in pregnancy and isn't a cause for concern. See your doctor, however, if you have sharp abdominal or pelvic pains that don't resolve quickly or if your pain becomes crampy; if there is any bleeding; if there is a burning sensation when you urinate; or if you're feverish. If you're in any doubt, always seek medical advice.

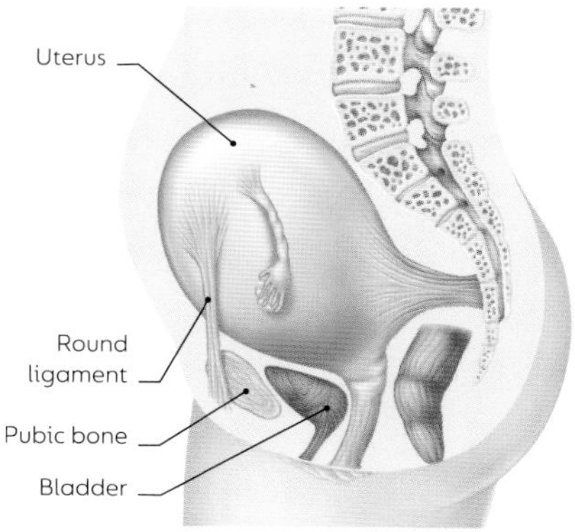

The round ligaments, which help support the uterus, stretch as the uterus enlarges and pull on nearby nerve fibers and sensitive structures, causing discomfort.

> " As your uterus grows to accommodate your baby, you may begin to notice a few twinges around your pelvis. "

FERTILITY TREATMENT AND MULTIPLE BIRTHS

Fertility treatment has had a huge impact on the number of multiple pregnancies. In 1977, the year before the world's first "test tube baby" was born, the natural occurrence of multiples in live births in the US was: twins 1 in 53; triplets and other multiple births, 1 in 3,092.

Today, with the increased use of fertility treatments, those numbers are 1 in 618 for triplets and other multiple births.

FOCUS ON TWINS

If you're expecting twins or more, it's good to know that most multiple pregnancies are straightforward and without complications. However, being pregnant with multiple babies is going to be more challenging for your body to handle than if you were carrying just one baby.

It's wise to know about the slightly higher risk of certain conditions that can occur. These include:

- Placenta previa (see p.212)
- Polyhydramnios (see p.475)
- Poor growth of one or more babies, which may be caused by twin-to-twin transfusion syndrome (see p.130)
- Premature labor (see p.431).

The fact that any of these conditions can develop is the reason why you'll have more prenatal checkups to preempt problems and minimize their effects.

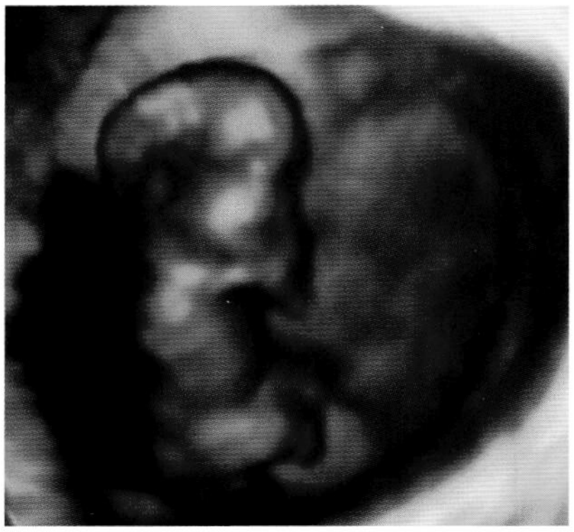

YOU ARE **12 WEEKS AND 4 DAYS**

192 days to go

YOUR BABY TODAY

By now the fetus's forehead is high and bulging, with visible joins in the plates of bone that comprise the skull. The eyes have migrated from the sides of the head at this stage of development.

"Complex brain development is gradually enabling your unborn baby to become more responsive and mobile."

Your baby's brain is under-going rapid development. The right and left cerebral hemispheres begin to connect. Each hemisphere controls the opposite side of the body, so the right side of the brain controls muscles on the left side of the body and vice versa.

Motor fibers (those that control movement) mature first, so your baby can make increasingly complex limb movements. Sensory nerves (those that control feeding) mature later and are first present on your baby's hands and in his mouth. The brain matures quickly over the next three weeks and will be complete in around 10 weeks' time, as the rest of the upper and lower limbs and trunk achieve adult levels of sensitivity to stimuli. All your baby's nerves are very immature at this stage and he doesn't have any perception of position, pain, temperature, or touch.

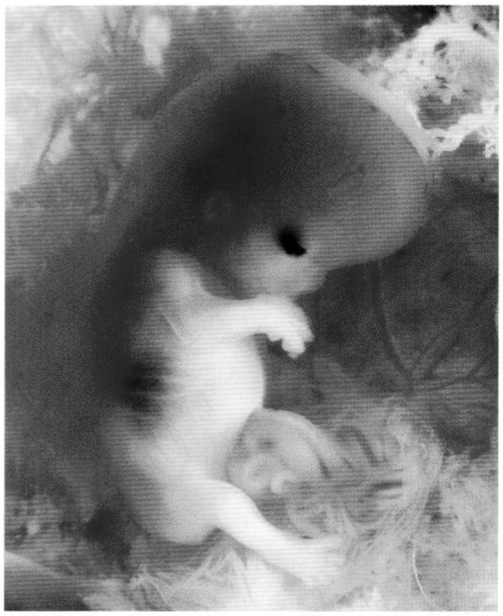

As your baby's brain develops, he is able to make larger movements with his arms and legs, but this activity won't be well coordinated at this stage.

YUMMY YOGURT

For a calcium-packed snack, stock up on yogurt. Those that contain so-called friendly bacteria are okay to eat during pregnancy and may help your digestion. Choose plain varieties or those with the least amount of sugar. If you eat dairy-free yogurt, make sure it's fortified with calcium.

ASK A DOCTOR

I have diabetes. How will this affect my pregnancy? Whether you develop diabetes in pregnancy (known as gestational diabetes), or have preexisting diabetes, you will require special care from a diabetic health-care team and an obstetrician. This is because diabetes poses risks in pregnancy, particularly if there is poor control of blood-sugar levels.

Insulin requirements increase during pregnancy. You will be taught how to measure your blood sugar at home and the results will determine whether you require additional treatment for diabetes with oral medication or insulin injections.

Pregnant women who are diabetic are at a greater risk of high blood pressure, blood clots, and preeclampsia (see p.476). If you have diabetic kidney disease or diabetic retinopathy, a condition that affects the retina in the eye, there's a chance it will worsen during pregnancy. For your baby, there is an increased risk of congenital abnormalities and growth may be too fast or too slow.

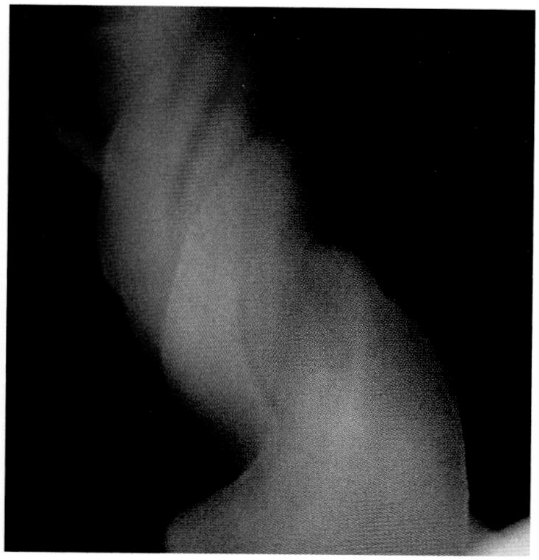

YOU ARE **12 WEEKS AND 5 DAYS**

191 days to go

YOUR BABY TODAY

This image is a close-up of your baby's umbilical cord. The umbilical arteries can be seen as they carry blood from the baby to the placenta. Since there are no nerve fibers in the cord, your baby is unaware that this is happening—or even that the cord is there.

At this point in your pregnancy, you won't be able to feel your baby move. It will also be a little while before your baby will be able to hear (see p.238) and recognize your voice and that of your partner, or hear other sounds, such as music. Nevertheless, some pregnant women still enjoy talking to their babies, feeling that it brings them closer to the baby; and it certainly does no harm! Do whatever feels natural to you, whether that is talking out loud or in your head.

You might want to think of an interim name for your baby. This might be "the bump" or "the bun" or an inside joke between you and your partner. It can be helpful to give your baby an identity because it's difficult to talk about them at this relatively early stage, especially given that in most cases you won't know the sex.

If you are still keeping the pregnancy a secret from people in some quarters, using a code phrase to refer to the pregnancy may be useful in some circumstances.

> **"You and your partner will be developing your own special relationship with your baby."**

ACTIVITIES TO AVOID IN THE SECOND TRIMESTER

The second trimester is generally when fatigue lifts, and you begin to feel more energetic. This is a great time to continue your exercise program, making good use of your increased energy levels before you are too big and too uncomfortable to move and enjoy being fully active.

While you're encouraged to continue to exercise during the second trimester, there are some high-risk exercises that should be avoided. You should avoid any activity that potentially could cause you to fall, activities that involve a high degree of balance and agility, and specifically exercises that require lying on your back for extended periods, or twisting of the upper body. Changes to your center of gravity due to the increased size of your belly can increase the chances of stumbling, risking injury to you and your baby.

The following activities are best avoided during your second (and third) trimesters of pregnancy:

- Vigorous exercise at a high altitude (unless you are used to it)
- Diving and scuba diving
- Road or mountain bicycling
- Rock climbing
- Skiing, snowboarding, and waterskiing
- Ice skating/ice hockey
- Horse riding
- Bungee-jumping!

YOUR ACTIVE BABY

Your baby's many different movements are vital for his development. As your baby twists and stretches their body, flails their arms and legs, and moves their head, they're helping their skin grow and their bones, muscles, and joints to mature.

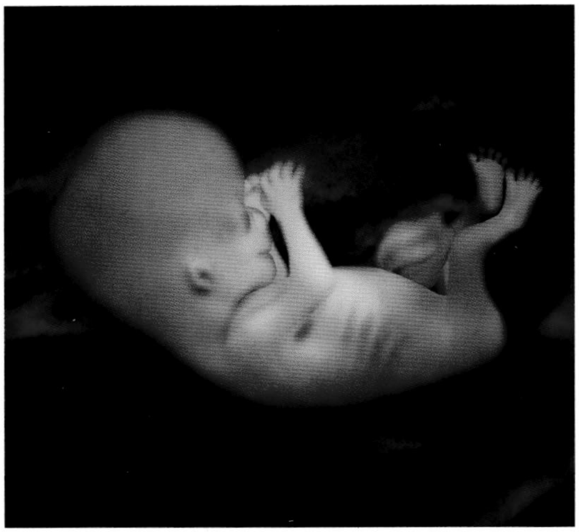

YOU ARE **12 WEEKS AND 6 DAYS**

190 days to go

YOUR BABY TODAY

The developing eyes are now facing forward. The right eye, along with the baby's right ear, can be seen here. Your baby spends most of the time in a curled position, often with legs crossed, and hands close to the face.

"It's never too early to start planning what you'll need to buy for your baby, even if you don't want to start shopping just yet."

Now that you're in your safer second trimester, you may be tempted to start buying a few baby items, unless you're superstitious and would prefer to wait. A good reason to start shopping in this trimester is that your energy levels should be at their pregnancy peak. In later months, you will find it too tiring to carry your belly, as well as your bags, around the stores and a shopping trip may not be your favorite pastime. Even if you're not shopping yet, start planning. Ask friends to recommend their favorite strollers, cribs, slings, and car seats, then check prices so you can plan your budget. You might also find that family and friends offer used goods you can buy or borrow.

If you purchase new baby clothes, leave the tags on and check the store's return policy in case you have a baby who's too big for the newborn clothes or you decide against the items you've bought.

MANAGING HAIR GROWTH

Changing hormones can play havoc with hair growth. To deal with any new unwanted hair:

- **Shave larger areas** and pluck out the odd stray hair.
- **Depilatory creams and hair-lightening bleaches** may be absorbed through the skin so shaving and tweezing are safer. If you feel you must use depilatory creams and bleaches, do a patch test first and keep the room well ventilated to avoid fumes.
- **If you're waxing**, be aware that your skin may be more sensitive during pregnancy.

ASK A DOCTOR

I've just told my parents I'm pregnant but they reacted very negatively because they don't approve of my partner. What can I do? First, give them time to come to terms with the news. Creating a baby with someone is the ultimate commitment, and marks an important life-changing event. For your parents, it is a signal that your partner isn't going anywhere, however much they might disapprove of him.

Once things have calmed down, suggest that your parents take the pregnancy as an opportunity to reestablish their relationship with your partner and wipe the slate clean. Reassure them that you and your partner very much want them to be a part of their grandchild's life, and that you'd rather clear the air now, so there aren't any negative feelings and tension once your baby is born.

Remember that all is likely to be forgotten when your parents hold a much-loved grandchild in their arms, and since part of that baby will be your partner's that should help them to feel warmer toward him.

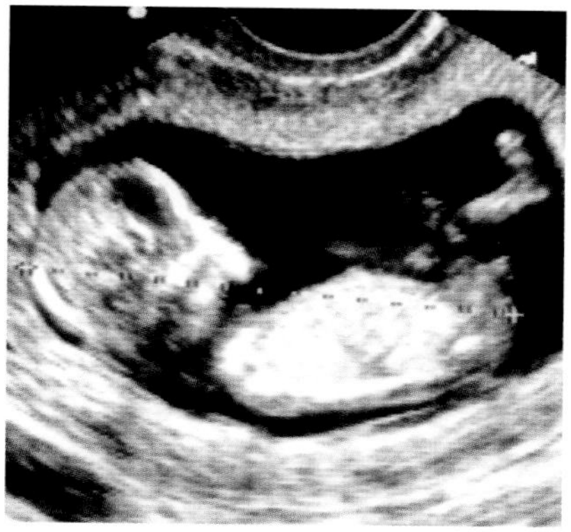

YOU ARE **13 WEEKS EXACTLY**

189 days to go

YOUR BABY TODAY

This 2-D black-and-white ultrasound scan is similar to the scan you may see and may be given. The baby is the white area, and the amniotic fluid is black. This type of scan is the best way to measure your baby's length at this stage.

"Your hormones have done all the hard work to establish your pregnancy and as they settle down, so should your nausea."

YOUR IMMUNE SYSTEM

Your immune system weakens during pregnancy to stop your body from rejecting your developing baby. This, unfortunately, makes you more prone to colds and bugs. As an added burden, pregnancy hormones can worsen a stuffed nose and nausea.

Morning sickness usually subsides around the start of the second trimester. It's believed that the rapid hormonal changes required to establish and maintain the pregnancy in the early stages may cause the sickness. By this stage your pregnancy is well established and your baby's major internal organs and support system are fully formed, so these hormone levels start to stabilize. This may be why the nausea passes.

Furthermore, there is a theory that nausea is the body's way of protecting the baby from harmful substances in the early crucial stages of development, so a pregnant woman becomes naturally adverse to alcohol and junk food, for example.

If your nausea and sickness hasn't begun to subside, don't worry; for some women, it does continue into the second trimester. See your doctor if you are concerned about your level of sickness.

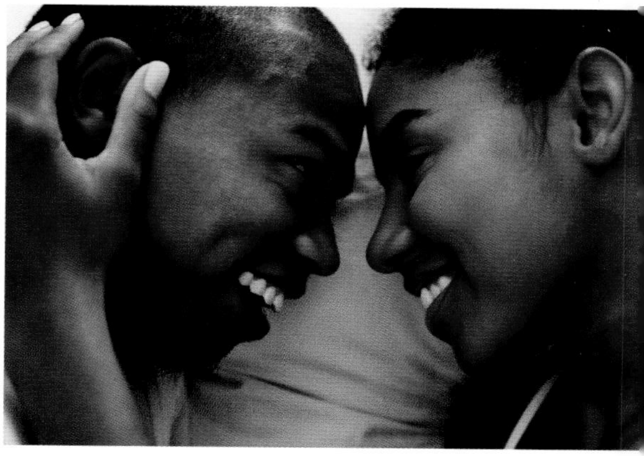

Even if you are having less sex, take the time to be affectionate and show your partner you want to be physically close.

ASK A MOM

My partner hasn't wanted sex at all since I've become pregnant. Will they ever desire me again? Yes! Although it's difficult, try not to take their reluctance to have sex personally. When I was pregnant, my husband didn't want to have penetrative sex, and most of his fears centered around harming the baby or me. This was made worse by the fact that I'd taken a long time to get pregnant and was also having a difficult pregnancy, with lots of nausea and sickness.

We spoke to our doctor and she was able to reassure my partner that he couldn't harm the baby in any way by having penetrative sex. She also told us that it wasn't uncommon for either partner to experience a reduced sexual desire in pregnancy for a variety of reasons. Although many women experience an increased libido at this stage of pregnancy, the same may not be true for their partner. It's important that you talk to your partner to find out their fears and explain your own thoughts and feelings.

Don't let this issue cause an argument between you. Each couple is different and you will need to talk to each other to find your way through this problem. You may also find it helpful to talk to someone who isn't so closely involved, such as your doctor or a trusted friend.

Your 14th week

THERE ARE SUBTLE CHANGES HAPPENING TO YOUR SHAPE THAT ONLY YOU WILL NOTICE . Your baby isn't big enough to give you an obvious pregnancy belly, but you'll definitely notice your waistline become thicker. At this stage of pregnancy, many women feel re-energized and have a strong sense of well-being. Healthy eating is very important, so be clued in about the best food choices. In particular, your body needs plenty of protein; and your baby needs it, too, to sustain her rapid growth.

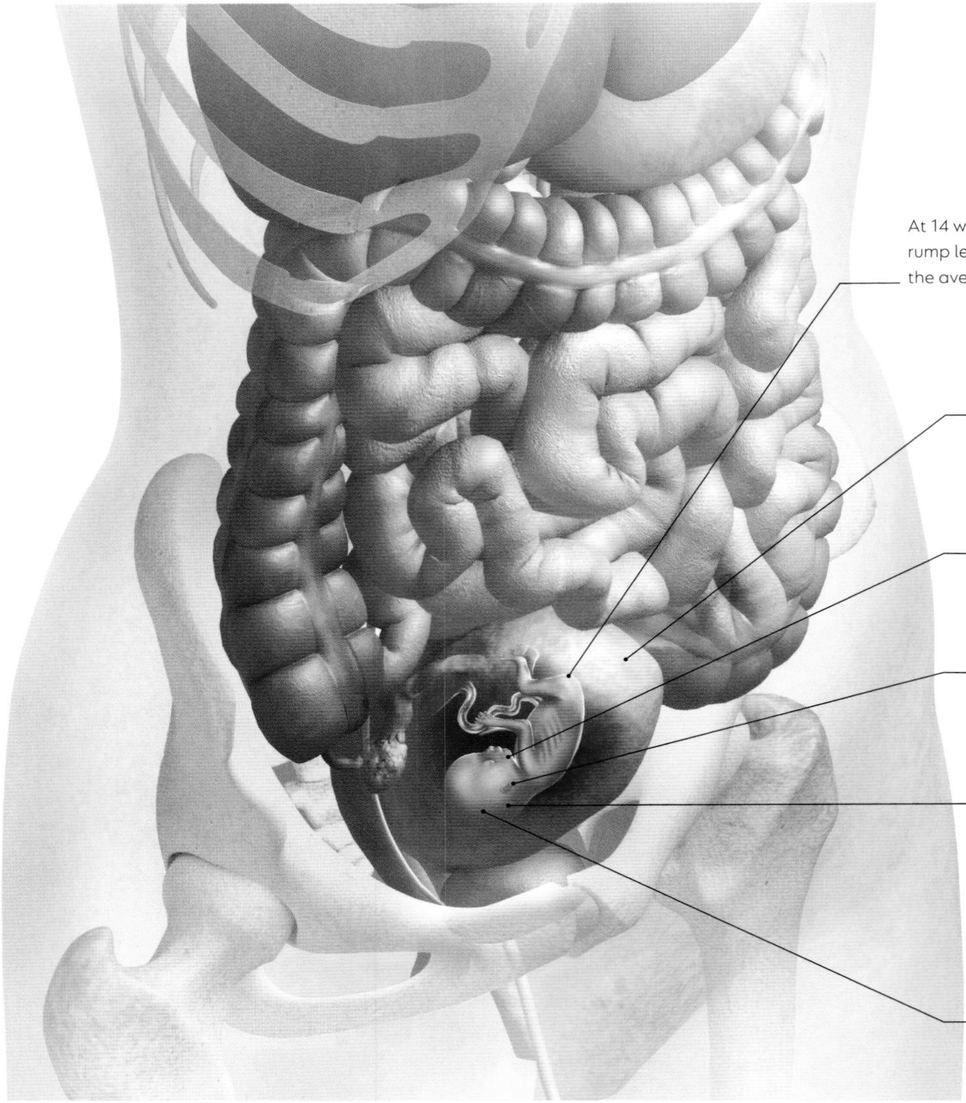
At 14 weeks the average crown to rump length is 3.4 in (8.7 cm) and the average weight is 1.5 oz (43 g).
The fundus, the top of the uterus, can now be felt in your abdomen.
Facial features are becoming more clearly defined. The eyes and ears have reached their final positions.
The ears have already developed their helical pattern, although your baby cannot hear yet.
The first hairs of the baby's scalp and eyebrows often appear at this stage.
The brain is developing rapidly, and your baby's head accounts for about half her total length.

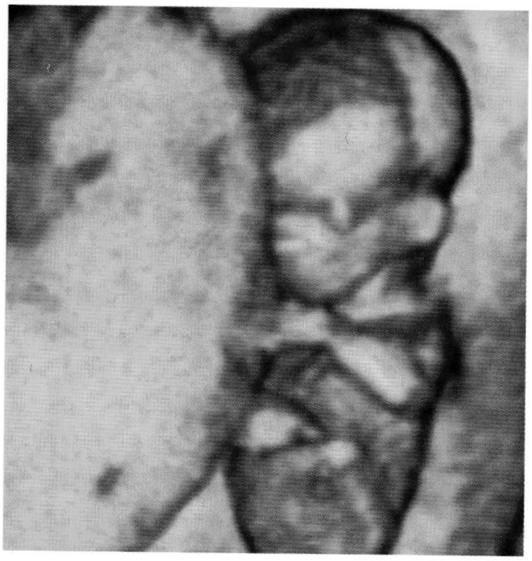

YOU ARE **13 WEEKS AND 1 DAY**

188 days to go

YOUR BABY TODAY

It's easy to see where your baby's bones are on an ultrasound because they show up as brighter areas. Other features may be harder to see. If you have a scan and are unsure what you are looking at, ask your doctor to interpret it for you.

While you're undoubtedly feeling better physically, and probably have lots more energy, you may still be up and down emotionally. This is completely normal.

This stage of pregnancy can be a very emotional time: reaching the second trimester is a pregnancy milestone and coincides with seeing your baby on the scan (see p.138). You know that, with the chances of miscarrying now being so minimal, you're really going to have a baby. However, like many pregnant women, you may find that the feeling of relief at reaching this stage is followed by occasional anxieties.

One good outlet for all this emotional energy is exercising, which you may find easier now that you're over the first trimester fatigue. Exercise releases endorphins, the feel-good hormones, and can improve your emotional as well as physical well-being; but always exercise safely (see box, below).

“Relief, excitement, apprehension... it's normal to feel all this and more at this stage of your pregnancy.”

LISTENING TO YOUR BODY

Check with your doctor whether there's any reason why you shouldn't be exercising; there are certain pregnancy conditions, such as placenta previa (see p.212) and the risk of premature labor, that may preclude you from exercising.

When exercising, always use your common sense—listen to your body and watch for symptoms that may indicate you are exercising too hard. Aerobic exercise is often tracked by measuring the heart rate, but this is difficult during pregnancy since there is a natural increase in your heart rate, even at rest. So the most effective way to keep your exercise at a safe level is the talk test: you should be able to carry on a conversation while exercising. This will indicate that you are not exercising to exhaustion and potentially restricting the oxygen flow to your baby.

There are other symptoms that indicate you're exercising too hard or should not be exercising at all:

- Vaginal bleeding
- Dizziness and headaches
- Chest or sharp abdominal pain
- Extreme and sudden muscle weakness
- Calf pain and leg swelling
- Leakage of amniotic fluid.

If you suffer from any of the above symptoms, even momentarily, stop exercising and seek medical advice.

THE IMPACT OF EXERCISE ON LABOR

Exercising may reduce the time you are in labor. Research has shown that women who exercise at a moderate to high intensity can cut their time in labor by up to three hours, and they tend to have less complicated deliveries than those who don't exercise.

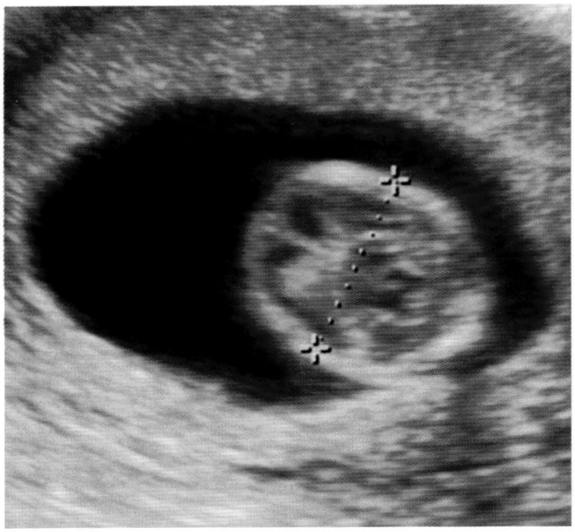

YOU ARE **13 WEEKS AND 2 DAYS**

187 days to go

YOUR BABY TODAY

This scan shows a cross section of your baby's brain, with the two hemispheres clearly seen. From this point on, your baby's brain measurement from one side to the other, taken just above the ear, is used as a reliable indicator of her growth and development.

“Even at this early stage of development, your baby has started to urinate, although in very small quantities.”

Your baby's bladder now fills and empties every 30 minutes. The amniotic fluid is swallowed, filters through your baby's kidneys, and then passes into the amniotic sac as urine. The bladder volume is tiny at this stage, and even by 32 weeks it will only be 10 ml, reaching 40 ml by 40 weeks. Your baby produces very dilute urine, having only a limited capacity to reabsorb water in the kidney to concentrate the urine. However, the placenta performs most of the kidney functions until birth.

Your baby's blood system can now make and break down blood clots. The placenta has been able to form clots for some time, reducing the risk of bleeding. A small number of white blood cells are now being produced by your baby but she is still relying on yours to fight infection. Her red blood cells contain hemoglobin that transfers oxygen to all the cells of the body. Before birth she has several forms of hemoglobin that differ from yours. These are more stable at a lower acidity and bind more easily to oxygen. This allows your baby's body to extract the oxygen in your hemoglobin for her own use.

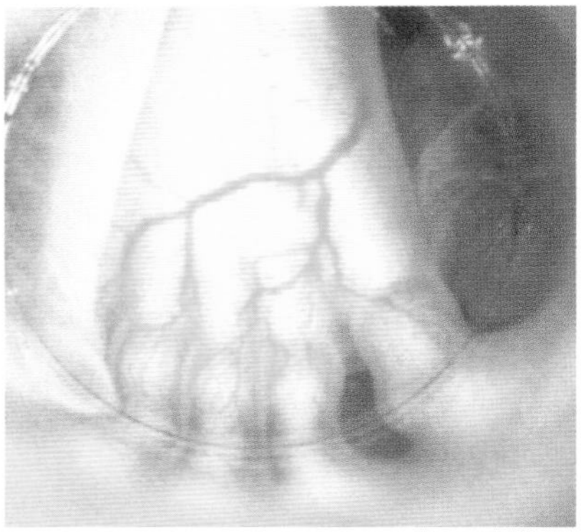

The toes are now fully formed and separated, and their individual bones can be clearly discerned on an ultrasound.

AMNIOCENTESIS

This involves testing the amniotic fluid that surrounds the baby and is normally done at 15–20 weeks (see pp.152–3). It may be offered in the following circumstances:

- When there's a family or pregnancy history of a genetic problem.
- When a screening test (see pp. 142–3) has shown that there is a high risk of the baby being born with a chromosomal abnormality.

ASK A DOCTOR

I'm expecting triplets. How will my prenatal care differ? All the usual risks are increased for a multiple pregnancy, partly because hormone levels are higher when there is more than one baby, and because it will be hard work for your body to carry and nourish three fetuses. You will be referred to an obstetrician and have more frequent checkups and scans.

The average pregnancy length for triplets is 34 weeks. You will probably need to have a Cesarean. For more information about multiple pregnancy and details of local support groups, check out Multiples of America (see p.483).

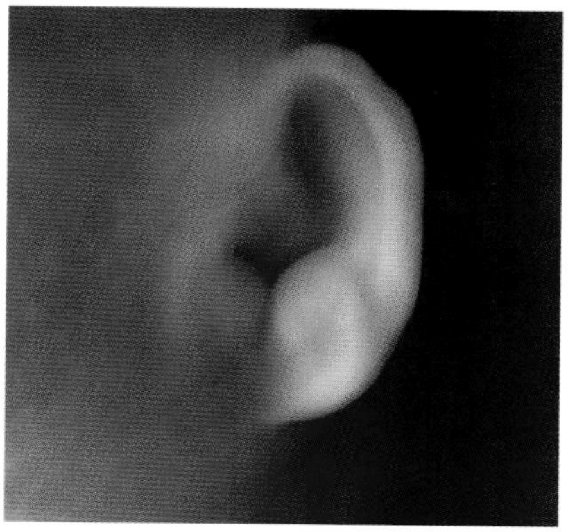

YOU ARE **13 WEEKS AND 3 DAYS**

186 days to go

YOUR BABY TODAY

It is surprising how much detail is already present in your baby's body. This close-up of an ear shows that its helical pattern of folds is nearly fully developed, although it is still too soon for your baby to hear anything.

" Your waistline will be increasing and your body shape changing but your belly is unlikely to be very prominent for several weeks. "

By week 14, if you stand in your underwear in front of the mirror, you will see a change in your body shape, but to the outside world you may not look very different. Women who have previously been pregnant tend to show earlier than those who are pregnant for the first time, because their stomach muscles have already been stretched once so they stretch much more quickly.

Women often say that this is the time when they look as though they have put on weight and feel fat, not pregnant! But it won't be long before your belly will be visible for the world to see.

If you're feeling uncomfortable and heavy, make sure you choose the right clothes. See page 151 for some tips on how to adapt your wardrobe without having to spend any money yet.

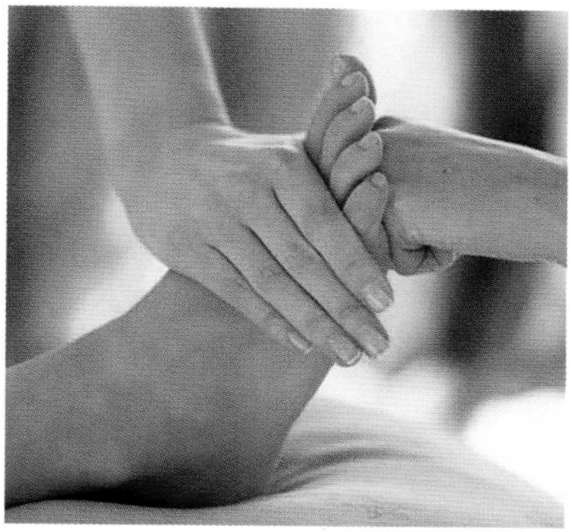

Reflexology involves applying pressure to reflexes on the feet. It can help with nausea, backache, fluid retention, and swelling.

SLEEP PROBLEMS

Now that you're in the second trimester, you may be sleeping better. Or maybe not, since sleep-related problems can affect women during the entire pregnancy. Here are some common problems and solutions:

- **Heartburn** Lying down soon after a big meal can cause acid reflux, known as heartburn. To lessen the possibility of disrupted sleep due to heartburn, avoid eating big meals 2–3 hours before bed. If your heartburn is severe, discuss options with your doctor.
- **Restless leg syndrome** This condition makes you feel the need to move your legs around to relieve a creepy-crawly feeling while you're lying in bed. It's a good idea to mention it to your doctor, since it can sometimes be caused by a deficiency that can be treated by taking supplements.
- **Napping** If pregnancy makes you tired, you may want to nap in the afternoon. But for some pregnant women, this extra shut-eye makes it more difficult to fall asleep at night. If this happens to you, skip the nap and go to bed a little earlier.

ASK A DOCTOR

Is it safe to use complementary therapies? Check with your doctor before opting for complementary and alternative medicine. This umbrella term covers medical practices and products that are not considered part of conventional medicine, and studies of their effects on pregnancy may not have been done. "Natural" doesn't mean "safe."

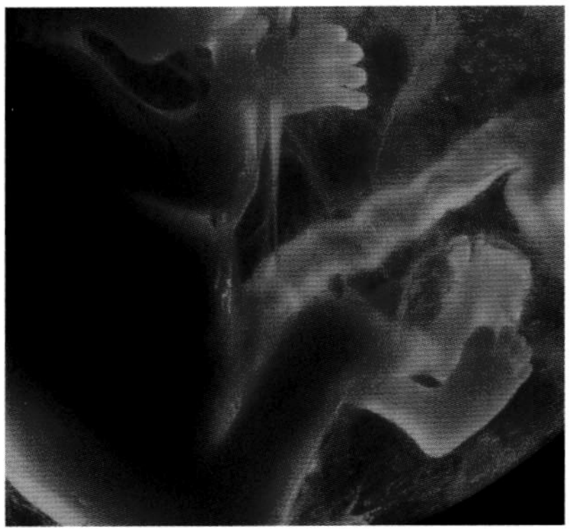

YOU ARE **13 WEEKS AND 4 DAYS**

185 days to go

YOUR BABY TODAY

Whether your baby's legs are crossed or uncrossed, it is very difficult to tell from an ultrasound at this stage whether your baby is a boy or girl: male and female look too similar to reliably tell them apart.

" Your baby's central nervous system, including the brain and the spine, now has all its basic components. "

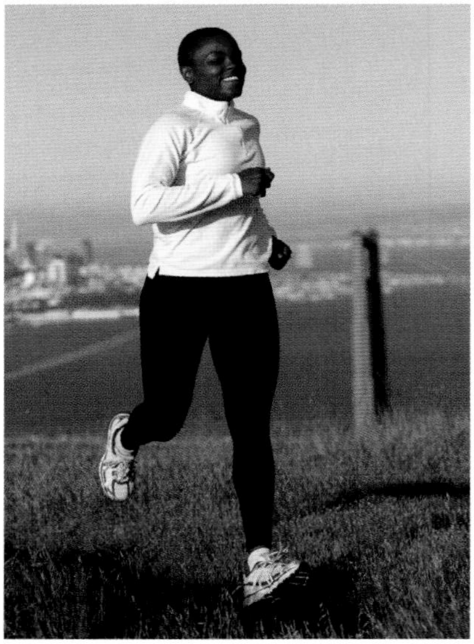

Relaxed jogging is a good aerobic activity, but only if you're used to running. Don't take it up as a new activity in pregnancy. Switch to brisk walking in later pregnancy.

The core development of your baby's central nervous system has taken place, and it will now progress further using four overlapping processes. The number of nerve cells increases and their positions alter during migration—a process by which cells move to their final locations and develop specific functions. The connections between individual nerve cells become more organized, and the fibers become insulated.

The growth of the nervous system now enters its most active phase. Reflecting this, the head accounts for half of the entire length of the baby. Both the nerves and their supporting cells increase in number. Although most of the nerve cells are produced during pregnancy, the supporting cells continue to increase in number during your baby's first year. The supporting cells assist in the migration process, which is largely completed by 22 weeks.

VITAMIN C

This important vitamin can't be stored in the body Vitamin C so it is needed in the diet. It has a huge number of roles, one being its protective antioxidant function. In pregnancy vitamin C, along with vitamins A and E, supports the immune system, so regularly eating vegetables and fruit rich in vitamin C will help boost your immunity.

You can't have too much of a good thing with vitamin C since excess is passed in urine. However, vitamins don't behave in the same way when taken as a supplement, so don't exceed 2 g a day of vitamin C in supplement form.

Vitamin C helps your body absorb iron from food, so have a glass of citrus juice or tomatoes with meals. It is easily destroyed, however, so to minimize losses cut vegetables into large pieces before cooking them, use minimal water, and serve as soon as possible. Steaming or microwaving will preserve vitamin C. Leftover vegetables retain little vitamin C, so just cook the amount you need.

ASK A DOCTOR

Can I continue jogging? There's no reason why not if you were a regular runner before you became pregnant, but take it easy—now is not the time to run a marathon!

You need to avoid becoming overheated so don't run on hot days and drink plenty of water, regardless of the temperature. Wear sports gear that supports your growing breasts and belly. Try to run on soft surfaces, such as grass, to reduce the stress on your joints, especially your knees.

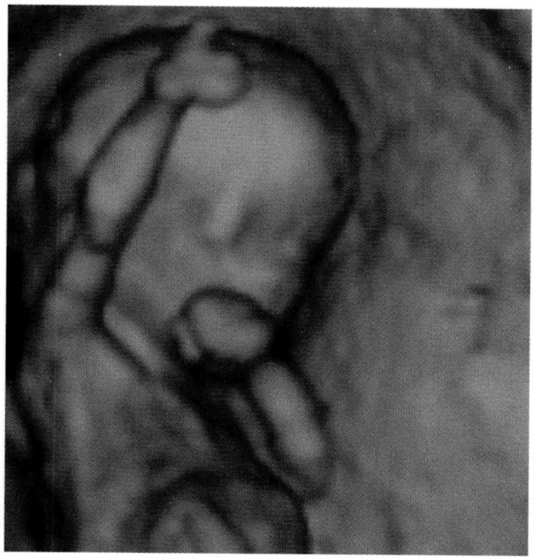

YOU ARE **13 WEEKS AND 5 DAYS**

184 days to go

YOUR BABY TODAY

At this stage the head, although still large, has a much more rounded shape than before and, as the jaw and neck lengthen, the chin moves away from the neck. An ultrasound now will show the thumb as distinct from the fingers.

Is your partner nudging you in the night because you're keeping them awake? It's common for pregnant women to snore. This is largely due to increased swelling of the nasal passages, but it can also be caused by increased weight and the fact that you may roll over onto your back during the night.

Your stuffy nose is due to the increased volume of blood in your body while you're pregnant. This can cause congestion and make your ears feel blocked, too. Nosebleeds are also very common in pregnancy; some women find that every time they blow their nose they have a small amount of bleeding. This is because the blood vessels in the nose are very fragile, and with the increased volume of blood flowing through them, they tend to bleed more easily. However, the bleeding should be very light.

To treat a nosebleed, tip your head forward and pinch the middle of your nose (in the soft part) hard. It should stop quickly. If it doesn't, try an icepack on the nose to help the blood vessels constrict. In the rare situation of heavy bleeding, go to the hospital. Seek medical advice if you are getting heavy bleeding regularly.

> "It's only a minor pregnancy symptom, but nasal congestion can happen most days—and make you a snorer at night!"

ASK A NUTRITIONIST

Is it safe for me to eat peanuts or nuts while I'm pregnant? All women, unless they have an allergy to peanuts or nuts, can safely eat them during pregnancy. This advice updates the previous position of avoiding having peanuts during pregnancy. When eating nuts, always opt for the unsalted varieties if possible.

Here are some good reasons to keep eating nuts:

- Peanuts are a good source of protein, healthy fat, and vitamin E.
- Peanuts provide valuable copper, which helps your body to make red blood cells.
- Other nuts, such as almonds, Brazil nuts, and cashews are also great snacks. They are an especially good snack for vegetarians because they provide some of the minerals that vegetarians find hard to obtain from their diet.
- Brazil nuts are very high in vitamin E and the antioxidant selenium, and almonds and hazelnuts are both rich in biotin.

FOCUS ON PARTNERS

During the first trimester, you probably anxiously awaited developments in the pregnancy and supported your partner when the going got tough. Now that her early pregnancy symptoms such as nausea, sickness, and fatigue are likely to have passed, and the risk of miscarriage is reduced, you may begin to feel differently about the pregnancy and your future.

As your partner starts to show increasing strength and vigor, and as you begin to notice her changing body shape and belly, you may find that the reality of the pregnancy hits you and your sense of trepidation is replaced by optimism as you both look forward.

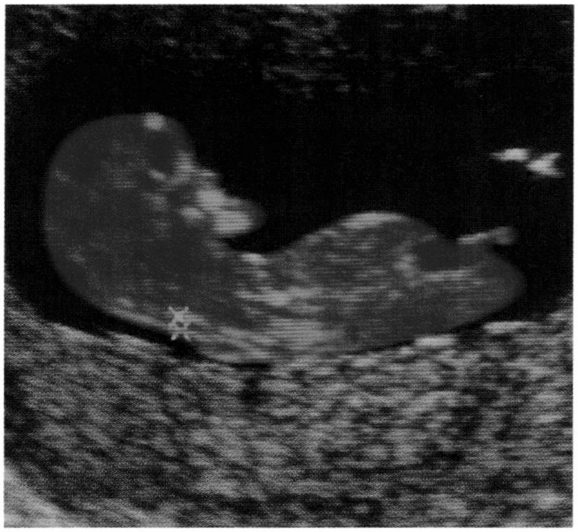

YOU ARE **13 WEEKS AND 6 DAYS**

183 days to go

YOUR BABY TODAY

In this color ultrasound image the baby is red and the placenta green. It is just possible to see the two crosses that measure the depth of fluid in the nuchal fold at the back of the neck (see p.143). Now is the last opportunity to measure this reliably.

“Your baby is growing and getting stronger every day, and it’s all thanks to her life support system—the placenta.”

Your baby’s rapid growth continues and her weight will increase during the next three weeks from 1.5 oz (43 g) to 5 oz (140 g). Muscle and bone growth advances, but, although all joints are present, it will be three weeks before the skeleton begins to harden.

Your baby is now totally dependent on the placenta for her nourishment. Environmental factors have almost no influence on your baby’s size at this stage; all babies up until around 20 weeks’ gestation are the same size.

The placenta is larger than your baby and supplies all the nutrients she needs. To aid her growth, the placenta extracts amino acids from your circulation, giving her high levels. Amino acids are the building blocks of protein, from which muscles and organs develop.

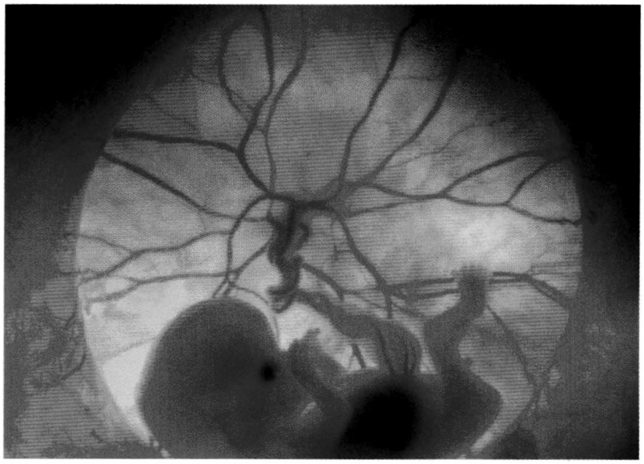

The umbilical cord can be seen connecting this 13-week-old fetus with the placenta, which nourishes your baby. The incredible blood vessels of the placenta are clearly visible in the background.

PROTEIN PLUS

Both you and your baby need a regular supply of protein throughout pregnancy for the physical development of cells for your baby and the placenta, and for the expansion of tissues you’re starting to see in your own body.

Most pregnant women easily achieve the right amount of protein (around 51 g) in their diet because it is widely distributed in foods. Those most at risk of inadequate protein are vegans or women who restrict their diet. By eating a range of different foods at each meal including beans, peas, and lentil products as well as grains, nuts, and seeds, vegans will get all the essential amino acids.

Lean meat, fish, poultry, and eggs are high in protein, so try to eat a portion at two meals a day. These protein-rich foods also supply vital vitamins and minerals (see p.17).

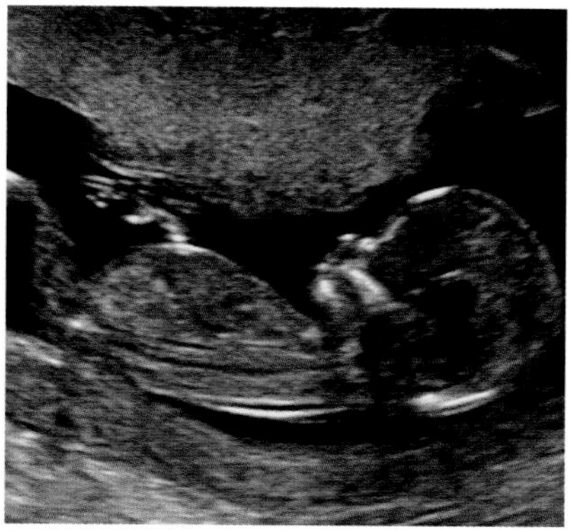

YOU ARE **14 WEEKS EXACTLY**

182 days to go

YOUR BABY TODAY

This 2D ultrasound shows the profile of the baby particularly well. The nasal bone can just be seen at the bridge of the nose, as can bright echoes from the lower and upper jaws; the umbilical cord is rising from the center of the abdomen.

One side effect of pregnancy all women have to deal with is conflicting information and advice. One article says to do something, while a friend says the exact opposite. It can be confusing and irritating. While you can choose to stop reading a newspaper or turn to a different television channel, it's more difficult to avoid the unwanted advice of other women. Even more difficult is the advice from close relatives, such as your mother and mother-in-law. You'll need the support of your family and friends, so you won't want to alienate them, but don't feel pressured to act in a certain way. Also don't reject everything immediately as some of the advice may in fact be useful and accurate.

If someone is persistently advising you, explain that you're overwhelmed by information and would rather not talk about the pregnancy at this time. Or listen to the person's advice, smile politely, and then do what you want. You could subtly hint that you will ask for advice as and when you need it.

> **"It can be difficult to avoid information overload—everyone, it seems, will have advice to share with you."**

USING HAIR DYES

There is no evidence that the chemicals in hair dyes are dangerous in pregnancy. Most permanent and non-permanent dyes contain chemicals that are unlikely to be toxic when used in the small amounts taken to dye hair, and only every few months.

If you're worried use natural dyes or stick to highlights, which don't expose the whole scalp to dye. When colouring your own hair, always do so in a well-ventilated space and always wear the gloves provided.

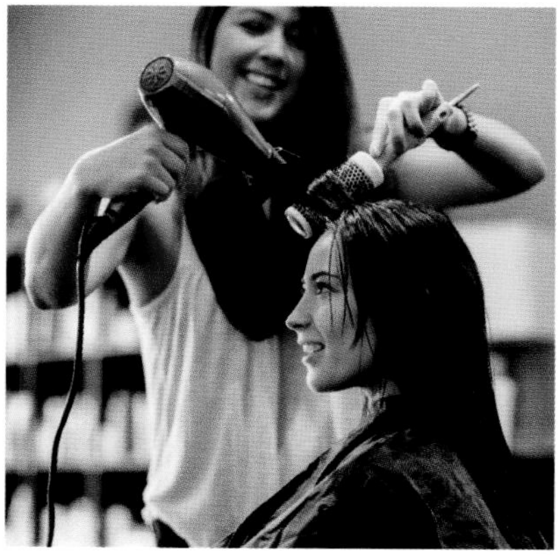

ASK A DOCTOR

Why are varicose veins common in pregnancy and what can I do to avoid getting them? Your blood volume increases up to 30 percent, due to the added needs of your baby and your expanding body. The hormone relaxin also softens the walls of your blood vessels. The blood vessels relax and the increased blood and extra weight of the baby make you susceptible to varicose veins.

To reduce the likelihood of getting varicose veins:

- **Avoid sitting or standing in one position** for prolonged periods: walk around, move your arms as you do so to increase the blood flow in your body.
- **Exercise daily:** most forms of cardiovascular exercise will help increase blood flow. Water aerobics is a good choice since the pressure of the water helps increase blood circulation.
- **Sleep with your legs slightly elevated** by placing a pillow under the fitted sheet at the end of your bed.

Your 15th week

START TALKING TO YOUR BABY—THEY CAN HEAR YOUR VOICE. Amazingly, your baby's ears have formed enough for them to hear you speaking. They'll recognize your voice—and your partner's—when they come out into the world. Like many pregnant women in the second trimester, you may now be reaping the benefits of the pregnancy "glow" as hormones improve the appearance of your skin and hair. Enjoy this time and the attention that often comes with it.

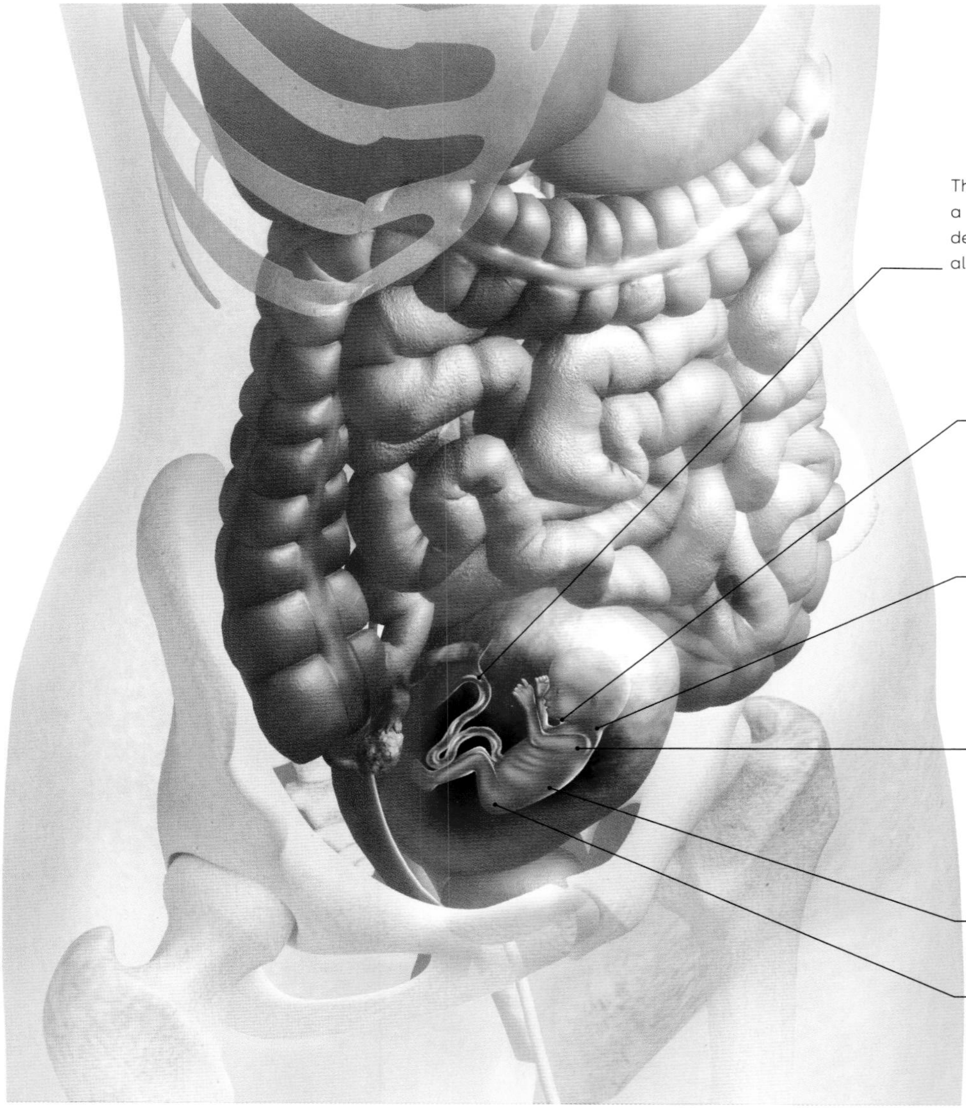
The placenta undergoes a new wave of development to meet all your baby's needs.
The thyroid gland is working, using iodine transported from your body via the placenta.
The neck is lengthening and the baby can raise his head further, lifting up his chin from his chest.
The arms have grown long enough to allow the baby to place his hands together in front of his face.
The fully formed spinal cord now extends the entire length of the vertebral canal, with nerves leaving between every vertebra.
At 15 weeks the average crown to rump length is 4 in (10.1 cm) and the average weight is 2.5 oz (70 g).

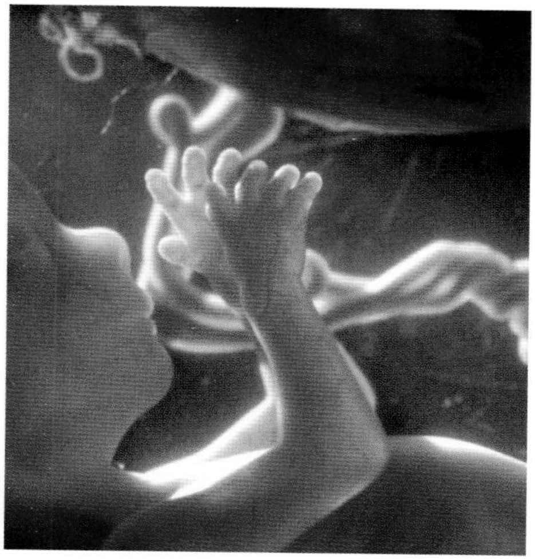

YOU ARE **14 WEEKS AND 1 DAY**

181 days to go

YOUR BABY TODAY

At this stage, the fetus's forearms, wrists, hands, and fingers are all well differentiated. The eyes, which are visible as dark areas behind the sealed eyelids, have migrated inward from the sides of the head.

You may not feel as though you are pregnant at the moment. The beginning of the second trimester is an interesting transition period: you know you're expecting a baby—you've seen the ultrasound scan—but you may not look or feel that pregnant, and you won't feel the baby move for several weeks yet (see p.213).

The physical reminders that were common in the first trimester—such as nausea and fatigue—may have greatly lessened or passed entirely. Many women say they feel completely normal, as they did before they were pregnant, and find this strange because they think that they "should" be feeling something. Try to enjoy this time and keep looking at that scan picture if you need a reminder that your baby is there. You may long to feel normal again once you hit the third trimester and some of that fatigue returns.

> "Now that some pregnancy discomforts have passed and while you await your baby you may feel strangely "normal.""

THE POWER OF OMEGA-3

Omega-3 fatty acids are essential and only obtained through what we eat—the main source is seafood, but they are also found in algae. DHA and EPA are needed to help the development of the baby's eyes, brain, and nervous system. In the last trimester your baby's brain is growing rapidly, so you need a diet rich in DHA. Your body can also store some DHA, so that when you are breast-feeding your baby will continue to receive DHA through your milk—this will help with brain development.

Guidelines vary, but 200 mg of DHA daily is often recommended. This is easily achieved by eating 140 g of baked salmon (around 2 g of DHA) or 140 g grilled mackerel (2.5 g DHA). White fish, such as sea bass and cod, contains much less. If you don't eat fish, consider taking a pregnancy omega-3 supplement. It is possible to buy vegetarian supplements based on algae.

Some studies have demonstrated improved language development, IQ, and cognitive development in babies whose mothers took omega-3 supplements in pregnancy, but more research is needed before routine supplementation in pregnancy can be recommended. Always make sure a supplement is safe in pregnancy and avoid those containing cod liver oil since this is not safe due to high levels of vitamin A.

FOCUS ON PARTNERS

Make the effort to set aside time The two of you for you and your partner to be alone together. Whether it's an evening out once a week, or that weekend away you've been promising yourselves—do it now! Remember, the second trimester is also a good time to go on vacation (see p.185).

It's common for there to be fundamental changes to a relationship when a baby arrives as you adapt to being parents. By spending time together now, you will build a greater bond for when the baby is born and feel satisfied that you enjoyed lots of pleasant time together during the pregnancy.

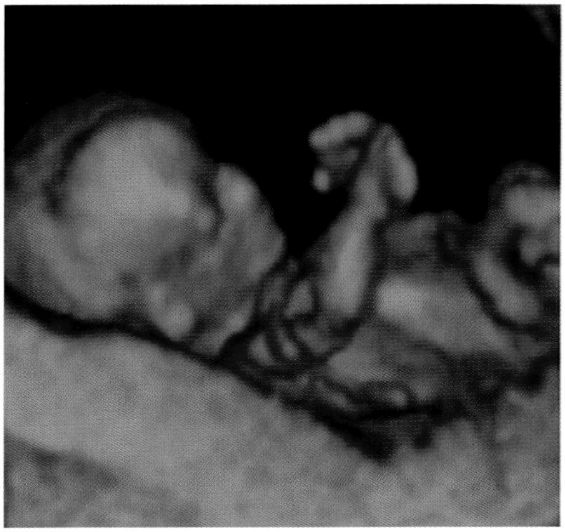

YOU ARE **14 WEEKS AND 2 DAYS**

180 days to go

YOUR BABY TODAY

In this 3D ultrasound scan, the baby is lying on his back. The arms and legs have lengthened and the baby is able to move them freely. His head is still relatively large compared to the trunk and the forehead bulges out.

> "He's well-developed on the outside, but complex changes are taking place as your baby's internal organs continue to mature."

Your baby's neck is growing and now looking more like a human. Internally, the thyroid gland first develops at the base of the tongue but moves to lie in the neck, overlying the trachea (windpipe). The thyroid gland is producing the hormone thyroxine, using iodine transported from your body across the placenta.

The baby's kidneys are starting to function. The nephrons in the kidneys are lengthening and maturing: these essential units enable the kidney to function by filtering the blood and eliminating waste from the body.

New nephrons will be produced up until the 37th week and the kidneys continue to lengthen by around 1 mm a week during the entire pregnancy.

WORKING DURING PREGNANCY

Most employers are supportive, but should a problem arise, employment law is in place to protect pregnant women:

- **You can't be fired,** unless you breach the terms of your agreement.
- **You can't be laid off** because you're pregnant or on maternity leave. However, if the reason for the lay off is a legitimate one, unconnected with your pregnancy, it is allowed.
- **Your employer** has extra responsibilities when you're pregnant, and these include ensuring that your workplace is safe. For example, you should be protected from handling or lifting heavy loads, standing for long periods of time, or handling toxic substances.
- **If you need time off** for a pregnancy-related absence, your employer must hold your job for you the same length of time that jobs are held for employees on sick or disability leave.

ASK A DOCTOR

I've developed a dark vertical line down the middle of my belly. What is this? This line is called the linea nigra, which occurs due to changes in skin pigmentation. It's extremely common, affecting 90 percent of all pregnant women in some way or another, and is often more noticeable if you are darker skinned.

You may also notice a darkening of the skin around your nipples and a darkening of freckles, moles, or birthmarks. A few women may also experience brown patches on their face called chloasma or the "mask of pregnancy" (see pp.190 and 469). These changes are caused by the extra amounts of the hormone estrogen during pregnancy, which affects the melanin-producing cells of the skin—these cells produce the pigment that darkens the skin. These color changes are normal and will usually fade once the baby is born.

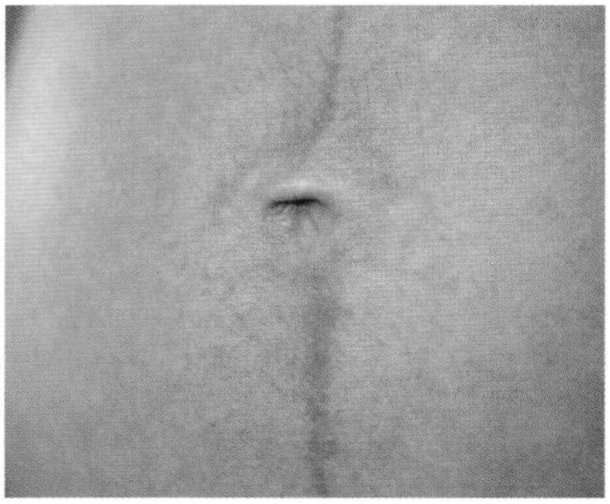

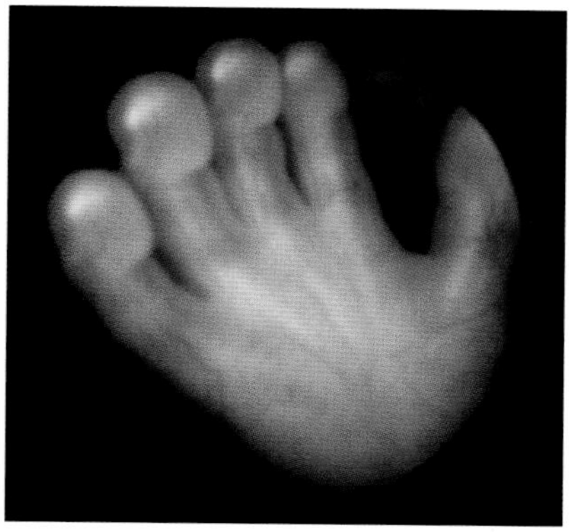

YOU ARE **14 WEEKS AND 3 DAYS**

179 days to go

YOUR BABY TODAY

The hands are well developed at this stage, but, as can be seen here, the skin is very thin and transparent, which means the developing bones of the fingers and the blood vessels can be seen.

> "Your baby's external sex organs are now visible and it may be possible to identify gender from an ultrasound scan."

Around this point in the second trimester, the sex of the baby's external genitals has become apparent. When the genitals first began to form at around four weeks, they were the same in males and females. They consisted of a rounded bump called the genital tubercle and two ridges called labioscrotal swellings separated by a membrane. From around six weeks, differences started to occur driven by the presence or absence of a male (Y) chromosome (see p.200). By the 14th week, in boys the genital tubercle has elongated to become the penis and the labioscrotal swellings have fused to form the scrotum. In girls the labioscrotal swellings remain separate, forming the labia (lips), while the genital tubercle forms the clitoris.

ANIMAL MAGIC

Living with a cat or dog in early childhood may reduce the risk of developing asthma. Children residing with cats were more likely to have allergy-related antibodies to felines. Do not leave a baby alone with a dog or cat.

ASK A DOCTOR

How can I relieve my constipation?
Constipation is a common symptom of pregnancy, mainly because progesterone slows down your bowel function, making everything more sluggish. Many women exercise less than usual during pregnancy, which can also cause things to become blocked. Finally, iron pills, which may be prescribed for anemia, can cause constipation. There are, thankfully, many ways to relieve it:

- **Eat more fiber:** Ensure that you are getting plenty of fiber in your diet, in the form of fresh fruit and vegetables and whole grains, and drink plenty of water.
- **Go natural:** Psyllium (or ispaghula), a common ingredient in some laxatives, appears to be safe during pregnancy, although studies in pregnant women have not been done.
- **Exercise regularly:** Exercise helps to reduce constipation.
- **Try reflexology:** Visit a registered therapist or do a little yourself at home. Massage the base the base of the heel and the arch, pushing your thumb evenly and deeply into the tissue of your foot.
- **Constipation during pregnancy can lead to itchy or painful hemorrhoids:** If this happens to you, ask your doctor what medicines you can use for soothing relief.
- **Don't ignore the urge to go:** Ignoring the urge too often can lead to constipation. Take care of your needs, even if you think you're too busy to stop what you're doing or you'll have to use a public toilet.

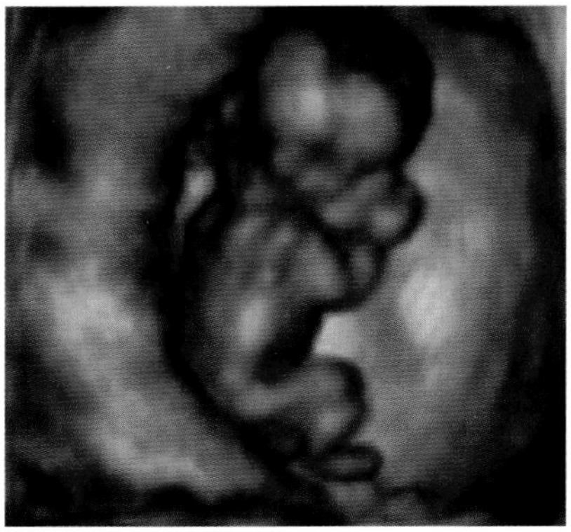

YOU ARE **14 WEEKS AND 4 DAYS**

178 days to go

YOUR BABY TODAY

In this image the placenta can be seen to the left of the baby. The placenta is still very much larger than your baby and is growing at a faster rate, preparing to meet the demands of your baby, who will later overtake it in size and weight.

“ To function successfully, the placenta needs a good maternal blood supply to the arteries in the wall of the uterus. ”

The placenta now starts a second wave of growth that will take almost six weeks. The outer layer of cells in the placenta move into the coiled, or spiral, arteries in the uterus, destroying their muscular wall. This causes the arteries to dilate, resulting in a low resistance to blood flow. Only those arteries beneath the placenta (80–100 vessels) are invaded by the placental cells in this way. If these cells move too deeply, they can fuse too tightly with the muscle of the uterus and have difficulty separating after delivery. If the wave of invading cells is inadequate, however, the low resistance to blood flow doesn't develop. This can increase the risk of the mother developing preeclampsia (see p.476), and cause the baby growth problems.

ASK A DOCTOR

I'm trying to stay out of the sun but is it okay to use fake tanning lotions? Sunless tanning lotions are safer than sunbathing or tanning beds but they have not been tested on pregnant women so their effects aren't known. It may be better to err on the side of caution and go without a tan while you're pregnant. Bear in mind that a fake tan does not protect your skin so, if you do wear it, you'll need to wear additional protection when you are in the sun.

No tanning pills of any kind have been approved by the Food and Drug Administration. They may contain canthaxanthin and can be toxic to your unborn baby, and also have been known to cause hepatitis and eye damage.

SLEEP REMEDIES

Even though you may not need to use the bathroom as much at night as you did in the first trimester, and may not yet be suffering from too many aches and pains, sleep may still escape you in the second trimester. You may find that during this life-changing time you are having especially vivid dreams, which can disrupt your sleep. Even if you're feeling well, it's essential to get adequate sleep: after all, your body is working hard to create another life.

To get more sleep:

- **Have a mug of warm milk** with honey or a yogurt before you go to bed.
- **Don't watch TV in bed** for an easier time falling asleep.
- **Avoid having caffeinated drinks** starting in the afternoon (see p.16) and make chamomile tea your bedtime drink instead.
- **Take a bath before bedtime,** and add a few drops of relaxing lavender oil to the bath water. Make sure the water isn't too hot as this can stimulate rather than relax.

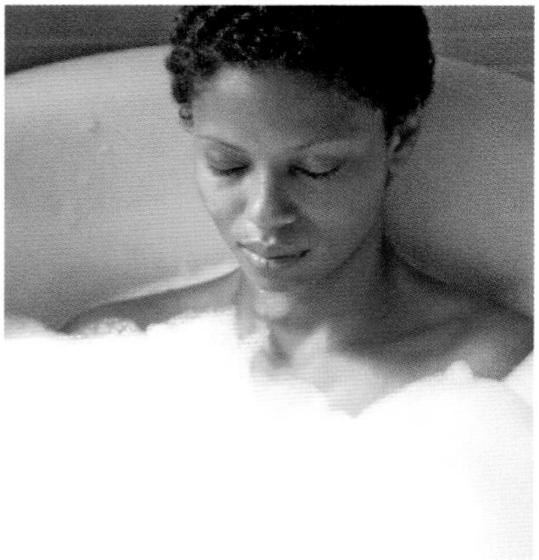

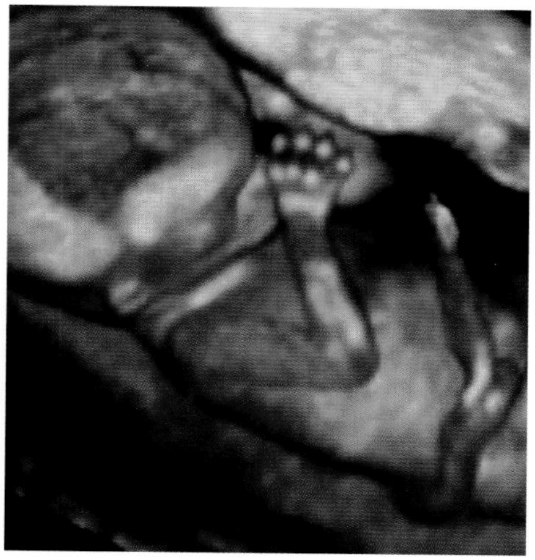

YOU ARE **14 WEEKS AND 5 DAYS**

177 days to go

YOUR BABY TODAY

This 3D ultrasound shows the hands held up in front of the face. The knees seem "knobby" with every bone clearly seen on the scan. The soft spot on the baby's head can also be seen: this protects the brain while still allowing for its rapid growth.

The terms "blooming" or "glowing" are often used to describe pregnant women, especially during the second trimester. The ideal image is a woman with thick shiny hair and perfect skin that has a healthy blush.

The improved condition of your skin is thanks to estrogen (pregnancy hormones can have positive effects, too!) and the increased blood supply to the skin; the many blood vessels just below the skin's surface give you a healthy glow, or at least stop you from looking pale and tired. The glands also secrete more oil, giving your skin a healthy-looking sheen.

Again due to hormonal changes, your hair may look thicker. Less hair than normal falls out during pregnancy and hair grows more quickly. After the birth you may find that your hair appears to be falling out more than normal as you lose the hair that's built up during the nine months. Normal hair loss is about 100–125 hairs a day; after the birth you might lose 500 hairs a day.

If you don't feel you match this picture of good health, it may just be that you can't see it yourself, especially if you're still adapting to your pregnancy. If you're looking pale and feeling tired, speak to your doctor because you may be anemic and need to boost your iron intake (see p.154).

> "You might receive some compliments, because at this stage of pregnancy you're likely to look glowing with good health."

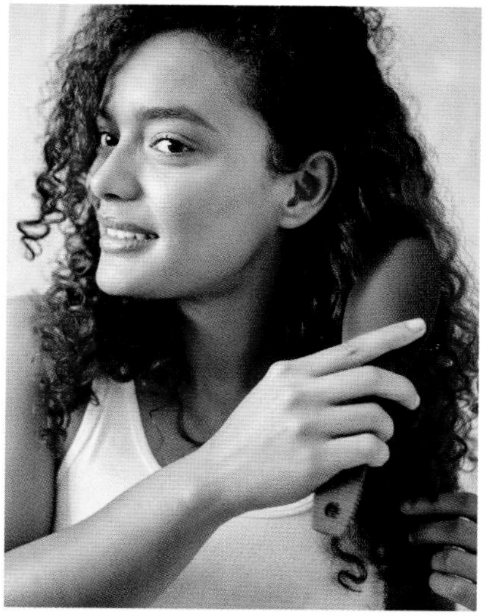

In the second trimester, the combination of thick, lustrous hair; rosy cheeks; and fewer pregnancy discomforts may make you look as though you're glowing.

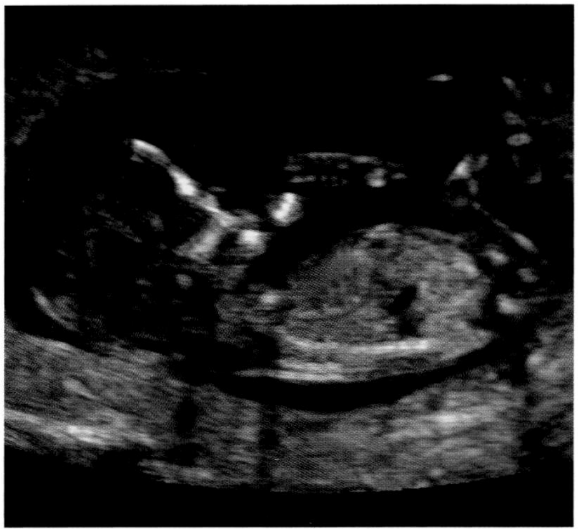

YOU ARE **14 WEEKS AND 6 DAYS**

176 days to go

YOUR BABY TODAY

Your baby is starting to swallow amniotic fluid more regularly: this enters the stomach (seen here as a dark circle in the center of the abdomen). The tiny bladder is also visible as a black fluid-filled structure within the lower pelvis.

> "The neural tube, the basis of your baby's spinal cord, developed in the very early weeks; now the spinal cord is fully formed."

Nerves from your baby's spinal cord are linked to each set of his vertebrae, but as your baby grows in length the spinal cord does not grow at the same rate.

Given this difference in growth rate, the lower tip of the spinal cord ends up lying at the mid-lumbar level,which is halfway between the hips and the lowest rib.

Below the mid-lumbar level of the spine, the nerves leaving the spinal cord have lengthened so that they still exit between the lowest vertebrae. In adult life, the cord will end slightly higher than it is at birth.

Because the spinal cord does not extend the entire length of the vertebral canal, a fluid-filled space fills the lower portion.

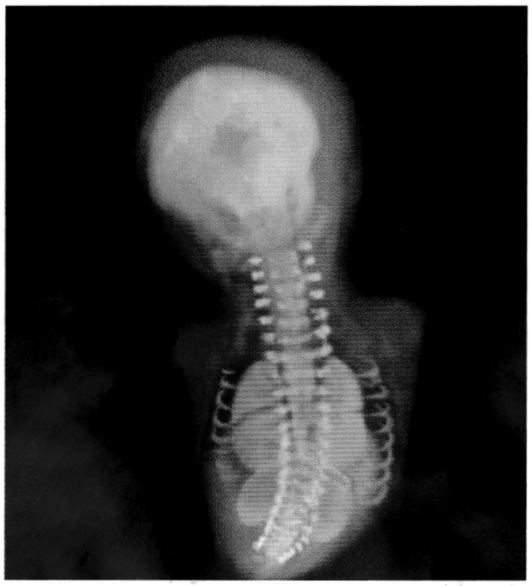

In this computer-generated image, the internal organs of the fetus can be seen. The skull, spine, and rib cage are also clearly visible. The lungs (pink) are protected by the rib cage; the kidneys (red) are below.

GIVING YOUR BABY ENERGY

You are constantly giving to your baby throughout pregnancy, and he gets all the energy he needs from you. Glucose from your bloodstream is transported from your blood to the baby's bloodstream through the placenta. Your blood sugar level is higher than your baby's to help this process. Protein in the form of amino acids (the building blocks of protein) are actively transported across the placenta, so levels in your baby's blood are always higher than those in your blood.

ASK A DOCTOR

When can my baby first suck their thumb? Ultrasound scans have shown unborn babies sucking their thumbs from as early as 12–14 weeks of pregnancy. However, this is likely to be a reflex at this stage as the brain does not have any conscious control over movement until the fetus is much more developed later on in pregnancy.

Some research has suggested that if an unborn baby shows a preference for sucking, for example, their right thumb, then they will prefer to lie with their head turned to the right after the birth. The same research suggested that this preference could be used to predict right- or left-handedness in the baby as they grow older.

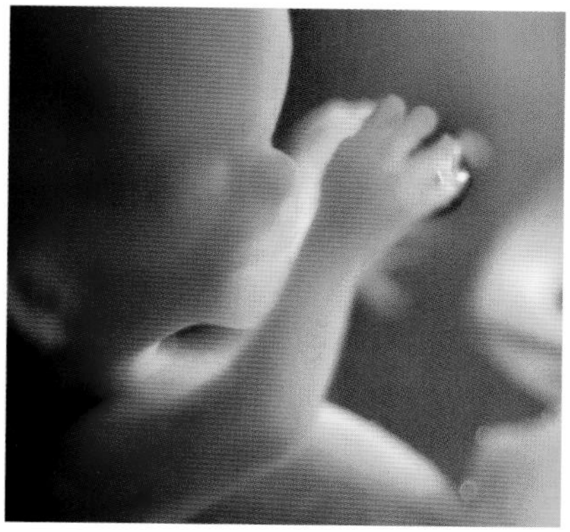

YOU ARE **15 WEEKS EXACTLY**

175 days to go

YOUR BABY TODAY

This profile view shows that the bridge of the nose is shallow and the eyes are still dominating the face. The jaw is lengthening and the chin held away from the chest. The hands (with outstretched fingers) are in a common position—close to the face.

Your belly will be getting bigger by the day and, as a result, you may find it increasingly difficult to get comfortable when you're lying down, especially during the night.

You should avoid sleeping on your back in the second half of your pregnancy, so start practicing some new positions now. This is because the weight of your uterus will press on the major veins that return blood to your heart, which may result in dizziness, low blood pressure, and possibly a reduction in blood flow to the uterus.

Ideally, lie on your left side as this is actually good for you and the baby, although it won't harm you or your baby to lie on your right side. It improves blood flow to the placenta and helps your kidneys eliminate fluids and waste products. Don't worry if you wake to find you're lying on your back: just roll onto your side and support yourself with pillows if necessary.

It's fine to lie on your front if you prefer (your baby is safely cushioned in the amniotic fluid), but the bigger you get, the more difficult this will become.

> "It's worthwhile finding comfortable sleeping positions now; these will stand you in good stead throughout pregnancy."

ASK A DOCTOR

My doctor is great but she's always in a hurry. How can I get her to answer my questions? This is a common problem. Doctors' practices are often very busy, with lots of women for the doctor to see. As a result, many doctors allow only a certain amount of time for each appointment—sometimes barely enough time to go through the basic physical checkup. However, it is important that your questions are addressed and it may be helpful to write them down so that you remember what you want to ask. If your doctor doesn't have time to discuss the issues during your appointment, ask her to arrange to talk to you at a mutually convenient time. This could be in the form of a phone call, or another appointment at her office. Or she may be able to direct you to other sources of information such as books, websites, or other health-care professionals.

It's a crucial part of your prenatal care that you feel comfortable with your caregivers and are given the opportunity to discuss any questions you have or issues that arise since they will be involved with your labor and delivery, which is a very important time for you.

QUIET TIMES

Times when you can focus quietly on your baby are precious bonding opportunities and a great way to relax. You may want to visualize your baby floating in the amniotic fluid.

Try this "butterfly" pose with the soles of your feet together. Place your hands on your abdomen and massage your baby using different strokes. Think of your baby and shed your preoccupations with each out-breath.

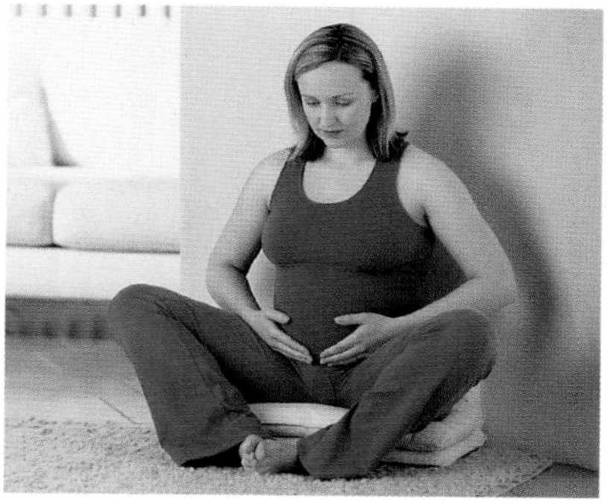

Your 16th week

THE BELLY STARTS HERE, ANNOUNCING YOUR PREGNANCY TO THE WORLD. Some days, you'll take huge pride in your emerging belly; on other days you may sigh for the loss of your figure. Enjoy your changing shape—you'll probably find that your partner loves it, too. For many couples, this can be a time of increased interest in sex. If you have any emotional or physical worries, there'll be an opportunity to discuss them with your doctor. Another prenatal checkup is likely to take place this week.

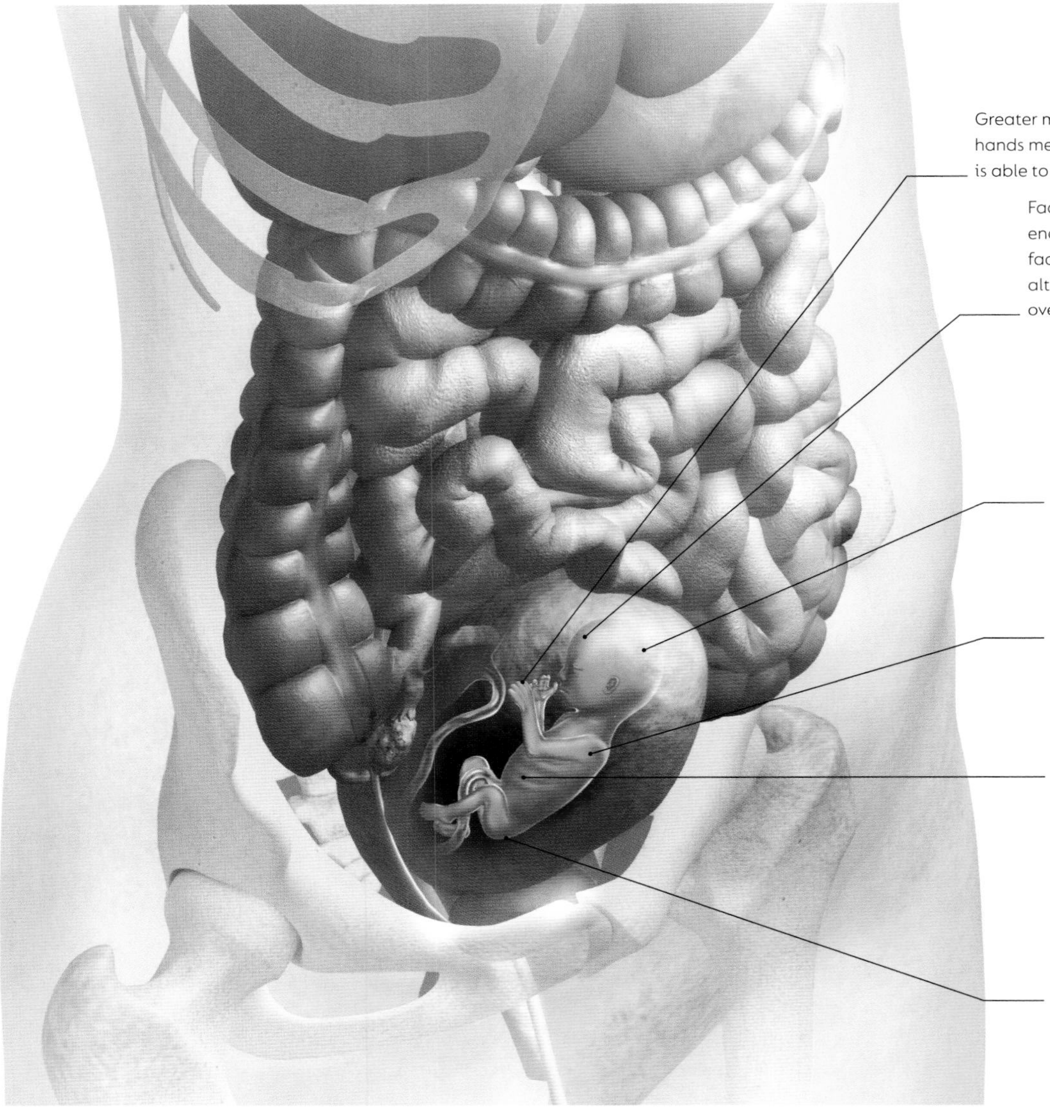

Greater mobility in the hands means that the baby is able to suck her thumb.

Facial muscles have developed enough for the baby to make faces, such as frowning, although she has no control over her expressions.

In the brain, nerve cells are forming and moving from the central to the outer areas. As yet, any neural activity is still very immature.

The skin is quite smooth and has a reddish tinge, since there is very little underlying fat.

The gut is too immature to function properly but it can take in the tiny amounts of amniotic fluid that the baby swallows at infrequent intervals.

At 16 weeks the average crown to rump length is 4.6 in (11.6 cm) and the average weight is 3.5 oz (100 g).

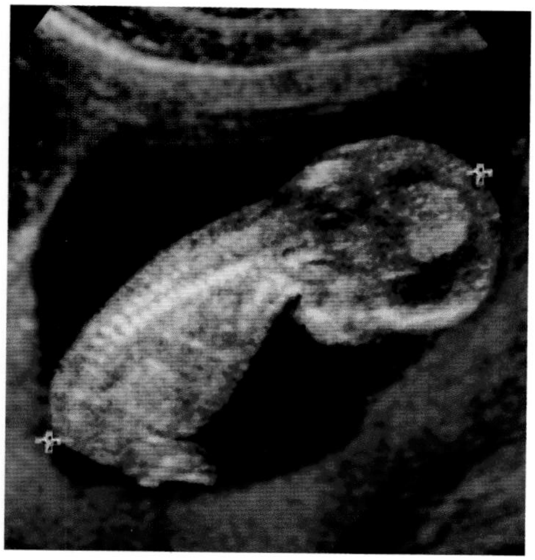

YOU ARE **15 WEEKS 1 DAYS**

174 days to go

YOUR BABY TODAY

In this artificially colored ultrasound scan of the baby within the uterus, the spine shows up especially clearly. The two blue crosses, at the top of the baby's head and at his bottom, indicate where the rump to crown measurement is taken.

" Your belly "bump" may be clearly visible by this 16th week of pregnancy, and you'll be amazed at how quickly it grows. "

At around this stage you may begin to "show," that is, instead of having a slightly bigger waist you develop a definite "bump" and start to look pregnant. You may begin to notice people's eyes are drawn toward your abdomen. If you'd rather keep the pregnancy quiet in some circles—for example, at work—wear baggy clothes.

While some women have neat little bellies positioned more to the front, others have bellies that are more spread out. The size and shape of yours will be individual to you, so try not to compare. There are old wives' tales that if you're carrying in front you're having a boy, and if you're carrying spread out over your hips you're carrying a girl, though this hasn't been proved.

If you haven't bought any maternity clothes, you may want to shop for some or adapt your clothes (see p.179).

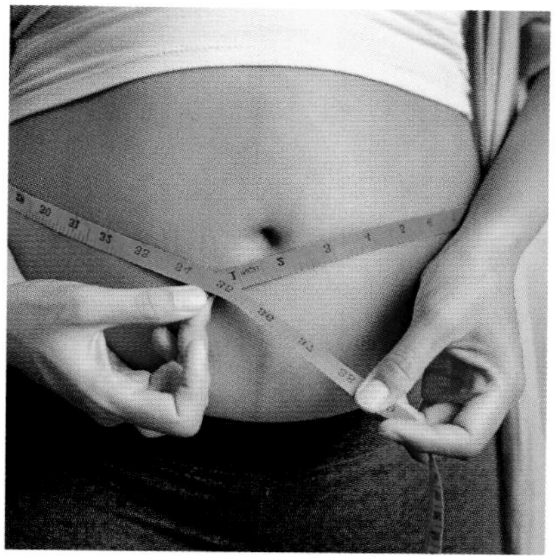

Although your shape changes gradually, some women find that their bump grows at a faster rate during some weeks than others.

FOCUS ON TWINS

Twin bonding occurs well before the babies are born. Advanced video technology has captured the special relationship between twins in the uterus. They have been seen to interact and even grasp each other's hands.

ASK A NUTRITIONIST

I keep waking up hungry at night—what should I do? It is normal to get the nighttime munchies during pregnancy, but annoying, especially if you're already having difficulties sleeping. Try eating a small snack before going to bed, and make sure that you have plenty of complex carbohydrates (see p.14) to help with a slow release of glucose.

- **Have a bowl of oatmeal** or a whole-grain breakfast cereal as a bedtime snack. Or try having whole grains, such as quinoa, or brown rice with your evening meal instead of pasta or potatoes.
- **Tryptophan,** an amino acid that is found in eggs, dairy, tuna, and turkey, may help with sleep because it produces the brain chemical serotonin.
- **Put a snack next to your bed** to keep those tummy rumbles at bay. Good options are nuts, a yogurt, or half a sandwich protected with plastic wrap. If you don't end up eating a perishable snack overnight, you can have it for your breakfast the next morning instead.

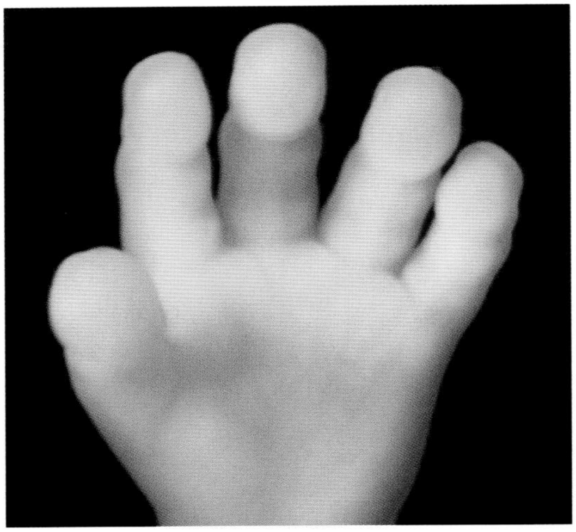

YOU ARE **15 WEEKS 2 DAYS**

173 days to go

YOUR BABY TODAY

The fingertips are prominent and the fingers still quite short. Each finger is separate and moves independently of the rest. This is the most comfortable position for the hand, with the thumb and fingers outstretched rather than curled into a fist.

" You're unlikely to feel any movements yet, but your baby is becoming increasingly active inside your uterus. "

ASK A DOCTOR

Can using tanning beds and hot tubs harm my unborn baby? Tanning beds expose you to ultraviolet light which can prevent you from absorbing folic acid, which the baby needs for development. Also, it's been reported that a rise in the mother's temperature, which can happen on a tanning bed, in a hot tub, or in a sauna, may increase the fetus's temperature. A temperature above 102° F (39° C) has been associated with spinal malformations in developing babies, and if a rise in temperature is maintained long enough, it may cause brain damage. The temperature of the amniotic fluid can also increase and it's thought that an extreme rise in your temperature can cause problems with the flow of blood to the baby.

So avoid tanning beds, hot tubs, and saunas while you're pregnant.

By now, your baby may be active for up to five minutes at a time. In the next few weeks, you may begin to feel some slight fluttering movements, particularly if this is not your first pregnancy (see p.193). You'll only be aware of those movements that cause your baby to make contact with the inner muscular wall of your uterus.

The placenta can act like a cushion absorbing the impact of all but the strongest of the baby's movements. This is why women with an anterior placenta (one lying on the front wall of the uterus, closest to the skin) often feel movements at a later stage than those with a posteriorly sited one (that lies closer to the back).

Your baby's brain is continuing to develop. The nerve cells that will form the outer gray matter start centrally within the brain, and need to move outward to their final position. This process takes place in waves that occur from 8 to 16 weeks. The migration process is not complete until 25 weeks and electrical activity cannot be detected until 29 weeks. Even after this point, gray matter continues to mature and organize neural connections in the brain throughout the pregnancy. Your baby's body is now longer than her head for the first time.

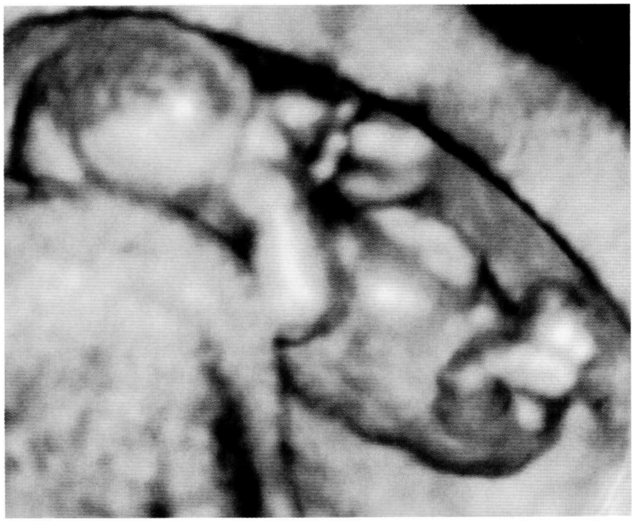

3-D ultrasound scanning uses computer technology to produce more detailed images than conventional 2D scans. This scan shows a 15-week-old fetus in the uterus. At this stage all of the organs are formed, as are the vocal cords.

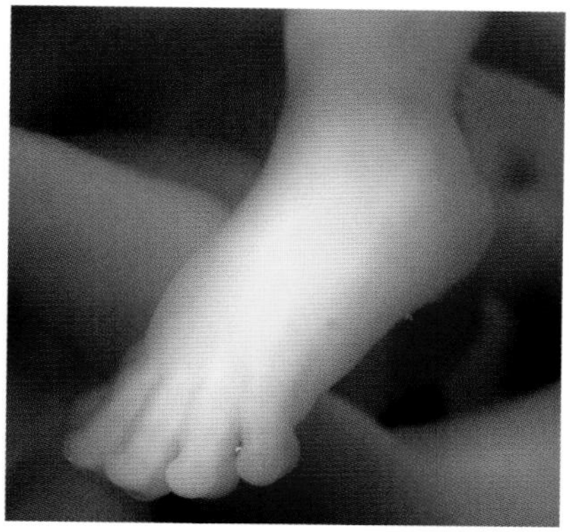

YOU ARE **15 WEEKS 3 DAYS**

172 days to go

YOUR BABY TODAY

Now the toes are lengthening and a gentle arch to the foot is beginning to take shape. Your baby can grasp her feet at will but has difficulty bringing them up to her mouth: this is not a problem a little later in pregnancy.

> "It's time for another routine prenatal appointment to ensure everything is progressing well with you and your baby."

You may have a prenatal appointment around 16 weeks, if you had your last appointment at around 12 weeks. You'll be weighed, your urine tested, and your blood pressure measured, and the baby's heart rate monitored. Furthermore, the doctor should be able to hear your baby's heartbeat (see p.188), which can be very reassuring.

Women who do not have the nuchal translucency scan (see p.143) at around 11–14 weeks of pregnancy, may be offered the quadruple test (see p.143), in the second trimester, which is a screening test for Down syndrome and other chromosomal abnormalities.

This appointment also offers you an opportunity to discuss any concerns you may have, and your doctor will report the results of the routine tests (see pp.122–3) you had at your first prenatal appointment, or shortly thereafter.

If your blood test results show that your hemoglobin levels were low, your doctor may offer you a prescription for iron.

MATERNITY WEAR

Maternity wear first appeared around the middle of the 19th century. At this time a prudish society felt that pregnancy should be hidden. For this same reason, and for the well-being of mother and child, women were encouraged to stay in bed in the weeks leading up to the birth.

YOUR GROWING BUMP

You'll need to choose clothes that accommodate your growing belly, but that doesn't have to mean investing in a whole new maternity wardrobe just yet.

The following innovations will help keep you comfortable and extend the life of your normal clothes for a few weeks at least:

- **Pregnancy support pants:** these stretch with you and ease the strain on your lower back, while giving you a smoother outline.
- **Pants expander:** an elastic belt that enables you to wear your jeans with a burgeoning belly. Alternatively, loop a rubber band—or, for extra girth, a slice cut from a pair of tights—around the button, through the buttonhole and back.
- **Belly band:** a wide band of stretchy fabric that you wear on your belly, to conceal the gap between your top and your waistband.
- **Bra extenders:** hook on to the fastening at the back of your bra to add up to 3 in (8 cm).
- **Borrowing:** you can borrow clothes from your partner or friends who are slightly larger than you.

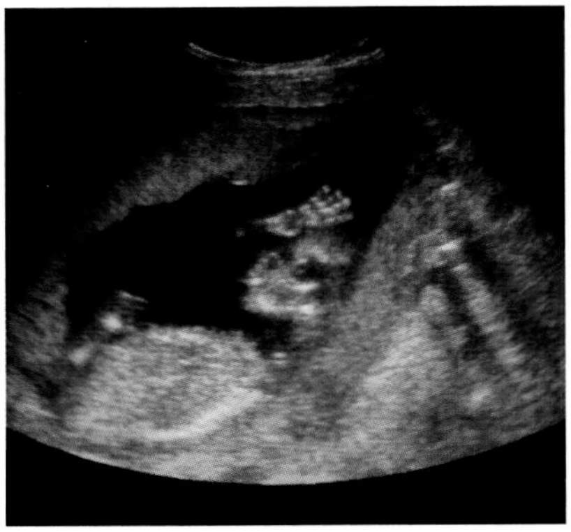

YOU ARE **15 WEEKS AND 4 DAYS**

171 days to go

YOUR BABY TODAY

In this 2-D ultrasound, the top of the baby's head is in shadow, although the hand can be seen in front of the face. All the bones are growing and maturing at this stage of pregnancy.

“ Your baby's skin is still transparent and there is little fat lying beneath it at this stage of the pregnancy. ”

Your baby's skin is made from three layers. The outer layer is the epidermis, and beneath this lie the dermis layer and the subcutaneous layer. The epidermis started as a single layer of cells but is now three or four cells thick. The most superficial layer of epidermal cells flatten but do not harden until much later.

The dermis is made from connective tissue comprising collagen (90 percent) and elastin fibers that allow for stretch and resistance. Within the dermis are blood vessels and nerves that support the epidermis and provide sensory feedback. At first, the junction between the dermis and epidermis is smooth, but dermal ridges form and it becomes increasingly irregular.

At the same time your baby starts to develop hair follicles. There is no significant subcutaneous fat present at this stage and the skin is almost transparent. Fat plays a part in temperature control and acts as a barrier to the passage of water. These barriers are not yet in place so the skin is still very permeable.

PREECLAMPSIA

Low-dose aspirin may reduce the risk of preeclampsia in women at the highest risk. Some research has shown that mothers who previously had severe early preeclampsia who take low-dose aspirin (81 mg daily) can lower their risk of getting it again. But don't use aspirin unless directed by your doctor, since it can cause serious side effects.

FOCUS ON PARTNERS

Your partner may have mixed feelings about her changing shape. She may at times appear to be a "pregnant goddess" who enjoys the fact that she's carrying a child. When she feels this way, she may seem strong and content.

However, at other times, rather than loving her belly she may feel down about gaining weight and losing her body shape. When some fashion magazines show extremely thin women as a symbol of "beauty," it is little wonder that the arrival of the belly can trigger a number of conflicting feelings in a pregnant woman, making her sometimes doubt her looks and knocking her self-esteem.

You can help by steering her toward her more positive "goddess" side and reassuring her about her looks. Remind her that what she's doing is amazing.

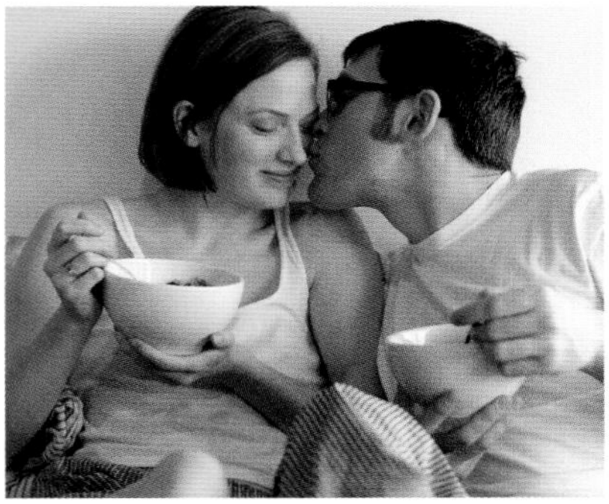

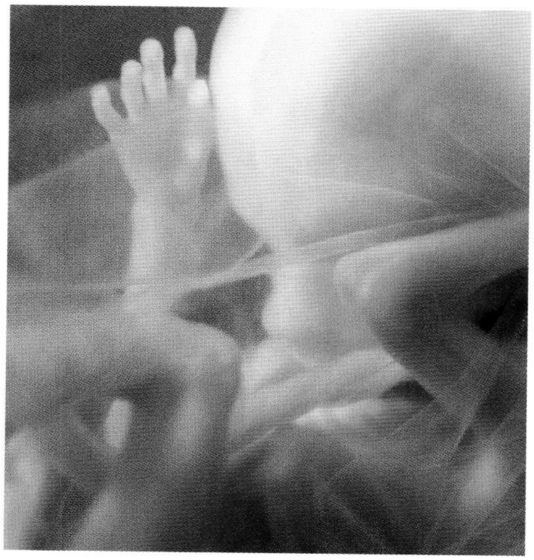

YOU ARE **15 WEEKS AND 5 DAYS**

170 days to go

YOUR BABY TODAY

Here the baby is seen within the amniotic sac. For the first time, her head is smaller than her body, marking another developmental milestone. Having a large, heavy head is not a problem in the nearly weightless environment of the uterus.

> "Your doctor may speak to you about writing a birth plan so she can get an idea of the type of labor and birth you want."

The purpose of a birth plan is to communicate your wishes for labor and birth to those who are caring for you. Writing a plan will help you to address different aspects of the labor, such as methods of pain relief and who you'd like to attend the birth. It also gives you a chance to ask questions about procedures such as induction and other types of medical intervention. Filling in a plan is also a useful way for your birth partner to be made aware of your wishes so that he or she can communicate these to the doctor while you're in labor.

Bear in mind that circumstances may dictate that not all of your preferences are met, but there's more chance of you getting the labor and birth you want if you've thought it through and written down your views. Being as informed as possible about labor and your choices (see pp.302–3) will help you to prepare in advance.

YOUR BIRTH PLAN

Scented candles, womb music, and beanbags... or serious pain relief from the first contraction? Writing a birth plan is an opportunity for you to think about how you'd like your labor and delivery to go. Give it some thought now and if there are parts of the plan you are unsure about, begin discussing this with your midwife

- **Start to think about:** your birth partner(s), pain-relief preferences, whether you'd like an active labor, and the environment you'd prefer to give birth in. You might know you want to give birth in the hospital or at home, or in a birth center, which offers a home-style setting with the backup of medical technology.
- **Consider your options**—for example, you might want to use a birthing pool or give birth in an upright position. You might want minimal medical intervention.
- **Be flexible** because labor doesn't always go according to plan and your baby's safe delivery is the most important thing.

ASK A DOCTOR

I have dry eyes and am finding it hard to wear my contact lenses. What can I do? During pregnancy, hormonal changes may cause your eyes to feel dry, and you may experience burning, itching, and a feeling that there is a foreign object under your eyelid. This is common in pregnancy. Dry eyes can also occur during menopause, when there are similar hormonal fluctuations. The condition appears to be caused by a change in the composition and quantity of tears, leaving the eye dry and inadequately lubricated. The discomfort can be remedied with "artificial tears," available from an optician or pharmacist, and it usually disappears once the baby is born. In the meantime, limit the time you wear your lenses and wear your glasses more often, especially if you are looking at a computer screen for long periods of time.

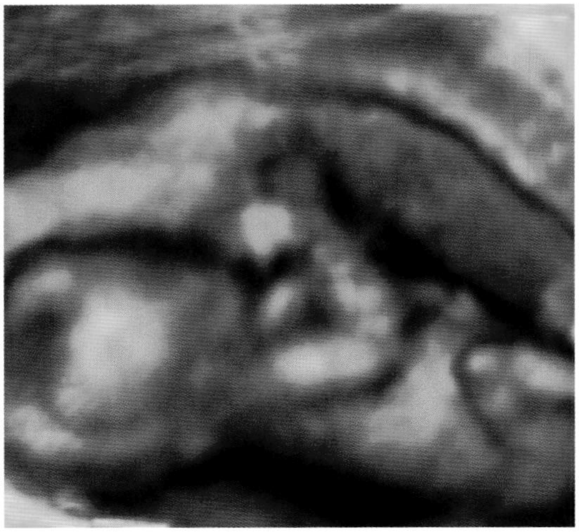

YOU ARE **15 WEEKS AND 6 DAYS**

169 days to go

YOUR BABY TODAY

The upper limbs are well differentiated into forearms, wrists, hands, and fingers; these develop at a faster rate than the lower limbs, a feature that continues even after the birth.

> "To help your baby's lungs expand and develop in preparation for breathing, the chest wall must be fully bathed in amniotic fluid."

Your baby's lungs continue to branch and divide. The cells lining the airways constantly produce fluid that leaves the lungs when your baby makes breathing movements. The release of this fluid is regulated by the vocal cords within the larynx.

In addition to fluid, the lungs have glands that produce mucus. Cells with tiny hairlike structures, known as cilia, have appeared that help move the mucus. This production of mucus is important once the baby is born to prevent the constant flow of air from drying the lining of the lungs, to trap dust particles, and to act as a barrier to infection.

Because the gut is still very immature, the gradual increase in amniotic fluid is due to the relatively low frequency of fetal swallowing. By 37 weeks your baby will be swallowing 1.75 pints (almost a liter), half of the total amniotic fluid volume, each day.

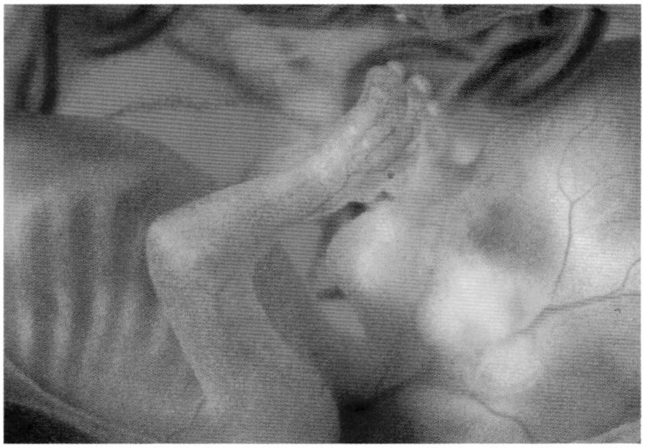

In this close-up the baby's left arm and chest wall can be seen. Because the skin is almost transparent the ribs are easy to see. They are very soft at this stage and still predominantly made of cartilage.

AN INCREASED LIBIDO

You may be taken aback by a sudden increase in your libido. Often, in the second trimester, women find that they feel far more energetic and sexy. The increased blood flow to the pelvic area combined with an increased lubrication of the vagina means that, in theory, having sex can be better than ever.

High levels of progesterone and estrogen make your breasts and vagina super sensitive so expect to become more easily aroused during foreplay. You may also find that you orgasm more quickly than usual. The uterus tightens when you orgasm, so be prepared for this.

Your partner may be delighted by this upturn in events, as well as approving of a beautiful rounded body to explore, but if they aren't responding positively, talk to them about how they are feeling.

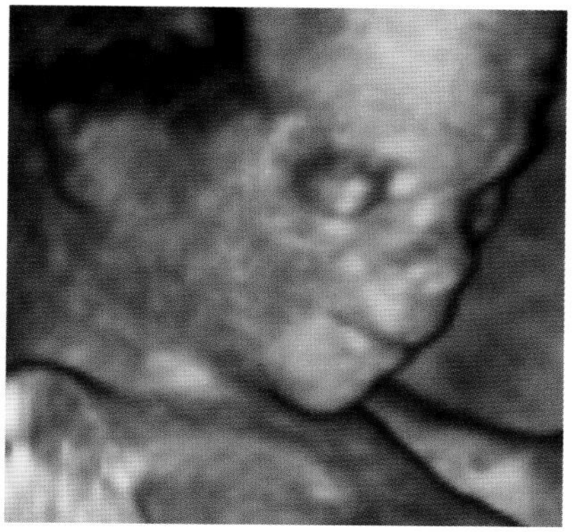

YOU ARE **16 WEEKS EXACTLY**

168 days to go

YOUR BABY TODAY

As your baby's skin starts to become more waterproof, the amniotic fluid is increasingly made from urine produced by your baby's kidneys and bladder. This urine does not contain waste products, since these are transported across the placenta.

Is your partner worried about you having a sip of wine or eating a tad too much chocolate, or are they constantly checking that you're getting enough rest? You may find that your partner becomes very protective of you and the baby and while some women enjoy the attention, others find it irritating.

If it bothers you, ask your partner why they feel the need to be so protective. If you can understand their feelings and concerns, it can help. Take the time tell them how you feel. Explain that pregnancy is not an illness and is a natural process, and reassure them that you're being well looked after by the doctor. For further reassurance, you could get them some reading material and involve them by inviting them along to a prenatal appointment. Encourage your partner to be involved, talk about your concerns, and include them in your prenatal visits.

“ It's natural that your partner will want to protect you and the baby, but you may need to help them get the balance right. ”

STRENGTHENING YOUR LEGS

A strong and toned lower body can be achieved by doing the exercises shown below. Strengthening these muscles will make day-to-day tasks, such as walking and climbing the stairs, a lot easier as your baby grows. Strengthening your leg muscles can also help prepare you for labor positions, such as squatting.

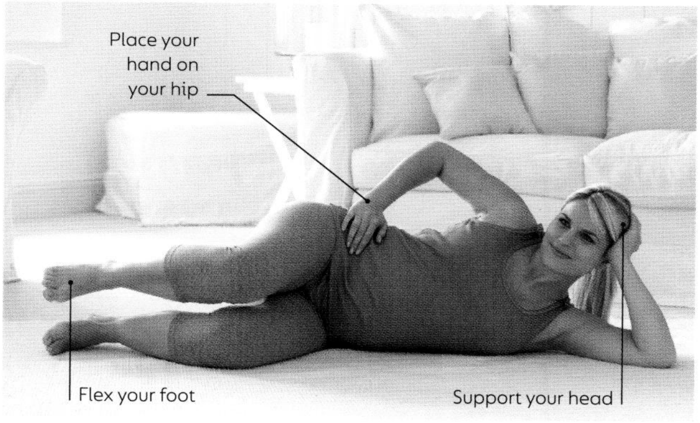
Place your hand on your hip
Flex your foot
Support your head

Lie on your side. Place both legs in front of your body, bent at the knee at a 90-degree angle. Slowly lift your top leg up and lower it to the starting position. Repeat 30 times, if comfortable. If you need to, you can place a pillow under your belly for support.

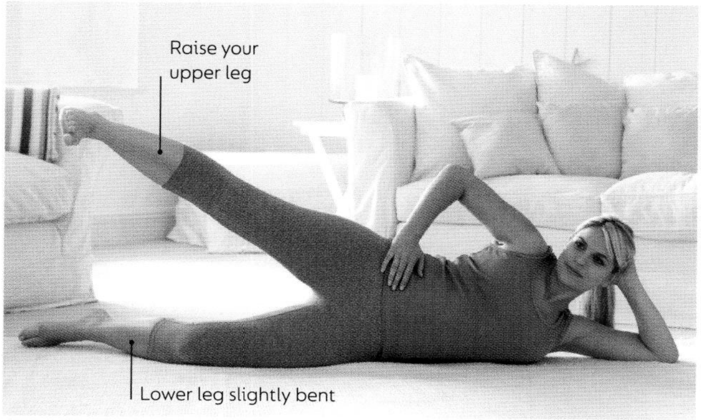
Raise your upper leg
Lower leg slightly bent

Lie on your side, with your lower leg slightly bent at the knee and top leg positioned at a 45-degree angle. Lift your leg slightly (about 4 in/10 cm), hold for 10 seconds, and then lower back to 45 degrees. Repeat 30 times, if comfortable.

Your 17th week

YOUR BABY IS INCREASING HIS MOVEMENTS AND EVEN DOING SOMERSAULTS. Things are becoming lively in your uterus. Your baby has plenty of room to move around and he's making the most of it, stretching and turning. All the activity is good for his future physical and mental development. You might feel like some relaxation, so think about taking a break. The second trimester is usually regarded as the best time in pregnancy for traveling and getting out and about.

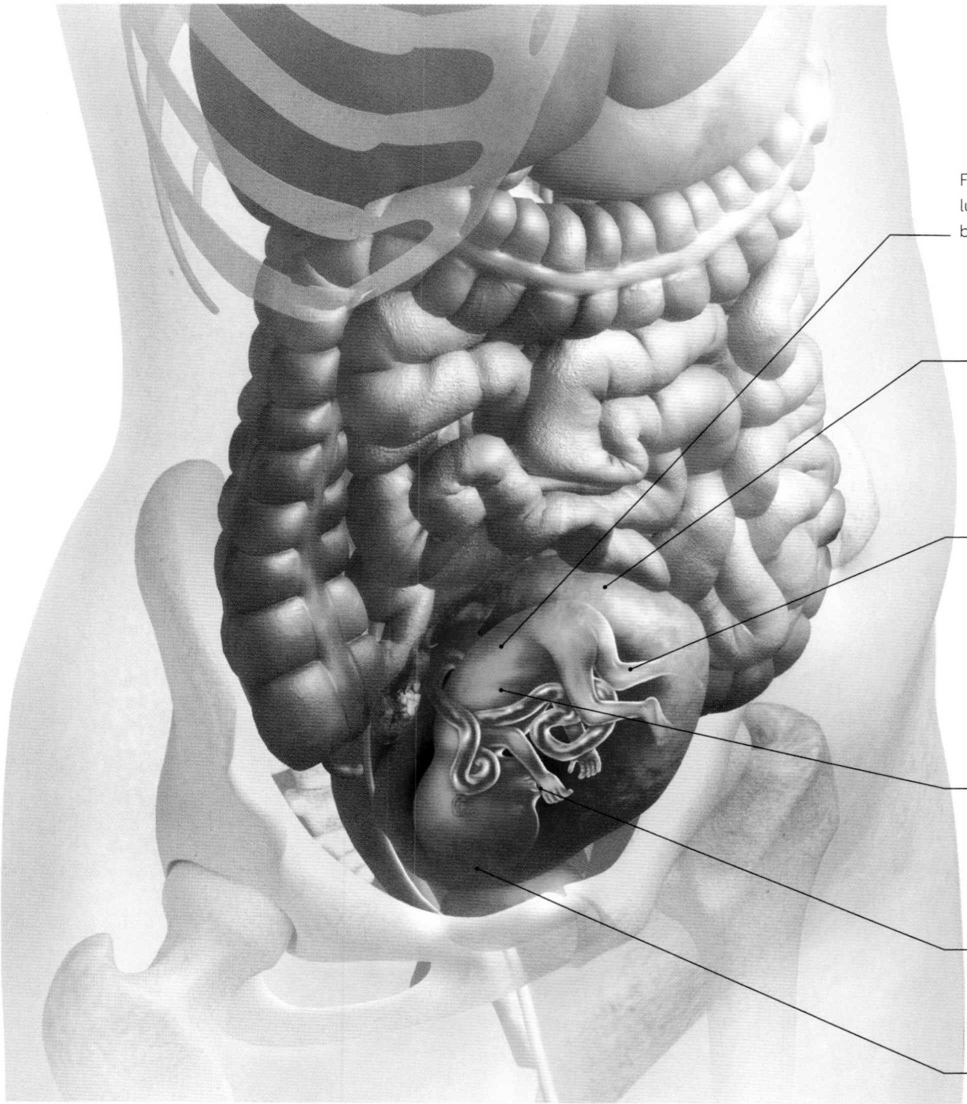
Fluid is pushed out of the lungs as the baby practices breathing movements.
The expanding uterus is now pushing up against your other abdominal organs.
Curling and stretching, arms and legs flailing, the baby is constantly changing position, lying first head-up and then head-down.
The baby's rapid heartbeat, easily distinguished from your own, may be strong enough for a doctor to detect with a handheld probe.
The mouth opens and shuts regularly, and your baby can swallow, may yawn, and occasionally hiccups.
At 17 weeks the average crown to rump length is 5.1 in (13 cm) and the average weight is 5 oz (140 g).

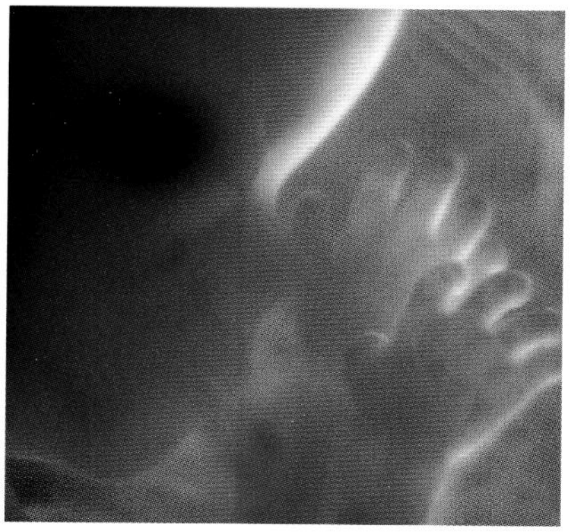

YOU ARE **16 WEEKS AND 1 DAY**

167 days to go

YOUR BABY TODAY

Your baby's lips and mouth are well formed. The mouth opens and closes and the baby can swallow. Inside the mouth, the taste buds are now mature, but the baby cannot taste anything yet because nerve connections are immature.

At this time, you're likely to be over the sickness and fatigue of the first trimester and not overburdened by, or uncomfortable from, a large belly yet. You can also rest easy knowing that your baby is developing well, with very little chance of a miscarriage occurring. Going on vacation is a great opportunity to spend quality time with your partner and pamper yourselves.

Relax and enjoy yourself, but be aware of the extra health precautions you need to take during pregnancy (see below and pp.28–9). If you've had any complications, check with your doctor that it is safe to go on vacation.

"Since this is considered to be a safe stage of pregnancy, with no, or few, symptoms to contend with, it's a great time to go on vacation."

ENJOY A HEALTHY VACATION

If you go on vacation while you're pregnant, there are a few additional factors to consider:

- **Give yourself plenty of time** when you're trying to finish all those prevacation preparations; getting ready for a vacation can be stressful. Pack hand luggage sensibly so you won't have to carry heavy bags.
- **Plan a road trip carefully,** keeping in mind that you may need snacks and more bathroom breaks than usual.
- **Be aware that sightseeing** will be more tiring than usual, so pace yourself and allow yourself to spend time in a cafe, just watching the world go by.
- **If you're abroad,** drink lots of bottled water, especially if you're in a hot climate. Avoid having ice in your drinks since it may be made using tap water.
- **Peel fruit** or wash fruit and vegetables with bottled water.
- **Carry snacks** with you in case you can't find somewhere to eat quickly. Mini bags of crackers and rice cakes are a great option.
- **If you get diarrhea,** it's even more important than usual to drink plenty of water to replace the fluid you've lost. Don't take diarrhea medication and check with your doctor before taking any type of treatment for diarrhea. If your urine is very concentrated and you can't keep fluid down, see a doctor.

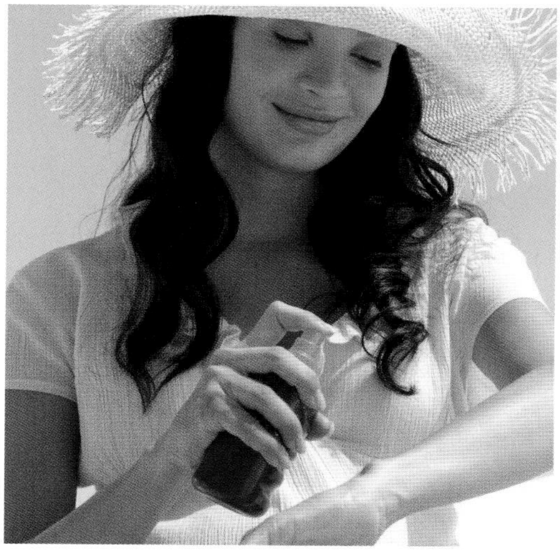

You can enjoy hot climates but if you're exposed to the sun, wear a high-SPF sunscreen because your skin is likely to be more sensitive to the sun while you're pregnant.

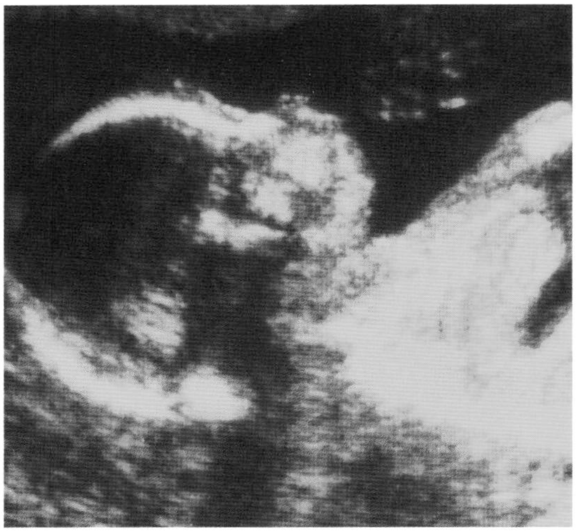

YOU ARE **16 WEEKS AND 2 DAYS**

166 days to go

YOUR BABY TODAY

In this color 2-D ultrasound scan the baby is facing upward. The skull bones reflect the ultrasound beam most effectively and show as bright areas. The curved frontal bone of the forehead is seen just above the short nasal bone forming the bridge of the nose.

> “ Your baby is at his most mobile about now, and he may even be doing somersaults in your uterus. ”

There are several ways in which your baby can now move: they can curl and stretch their trunk, move their head up and down and from side to side, and move their arms and legs independently. Regular chest wall breathing movements occur, along with occasional hiccups. The mouth can open and shut, and your baby can yawn and swallow amniotic fluid. The hands can be brought up to the face and the baby may prefer lying on their side rather than back. They have plenty of space in which to move.

Your baby's taste buds first appeared at 10 weeks and by now have an appearance very close to that of a mature taste bud. They also have their own nerve supply, connected to a branch of the facial nerve. Because these neural connections have not yet matured, it is too early for your baby to be able to taste anything.

ASK A DOCTOR

Am I at increased risk of DVT when I fly? Deep vein thrombosis (DVT) is a condition in which a blood clot forms in a deep leg vein. It blocks the blood flow in the vein, causing pain and discomfort. The most serious complication of DVT is a pulmonary embolism, when part of the clot travels to the lungs, blocking a pulmonary artery. This can cause chest pain, shortness of breath, and blood-tinged phlegm to be coughed up. A pulmonary embolism can be fatal.

Pregnancy is considered to be a pro-thrombotic condition, meaning that clots are more likely to form in blood vessels. Pregnant women who have previously had DVT, who are aged 35 or over, or who are obese are more at risk.

Wearing support hose (see p.225), drinking plenty, and moving around while flying can help. If you must fly and are at increased risk of DVT, talk to your doctor about medication that can reduce the risk of developing a clot.

FOCUS ON TWINS

By now, you may be starting to feel your twin babies move. Contact between them probably began a few weeks ago, long before you knew about it, and it becomes more complex as their brains develop. By this stage, babies have the elementary brain circuits that help them feel the parts of their body and appreciate their position, so it's no wonder that your babies can now interact at a basic level.

Your babies will move around 50 times an hour and can touch each other, even though in all but a tiny percentage of cases they're in separate amniotic sacs so there's a membrane between them. Ultrasound studies show that twin babies make physical contact and sometimes react to each other's touch and pressure.

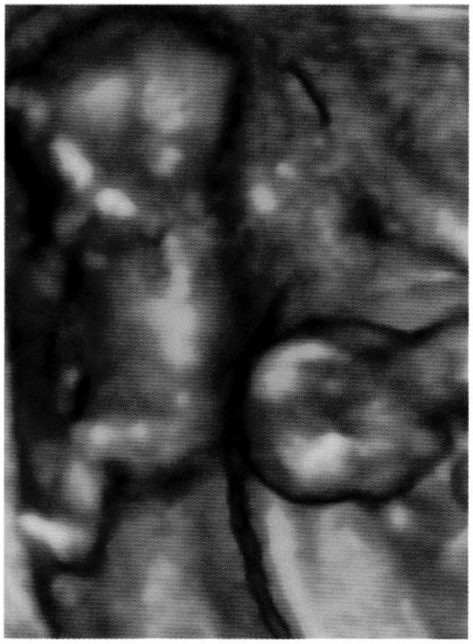

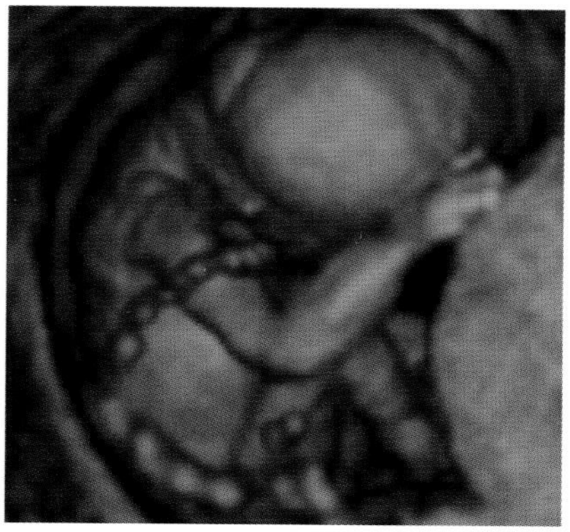

YOU ARE **16 WEEKS 3 DAYS**

165 days to go

YOUR BABY TODAY

This 3D scan is taken from a viewpoint above the baby's head and looking over the shoulder, but since the baby is curled up the face cannot be seen. The placenta is to the right of the image, with the umbilical cord over the baby's arm.

You may be pregnant and happy, but life goes on: this means you might still be working full time, in addition to running a home, and you're bound to have stressful days and times when you feel you can't manage. And, of course, even though you are in the second trimester now, you're still contending with those challenging pregnancy hormones that can cause some emotional ups and downs.

Like many women, you may become stressed about the big changes that are going to happen—there's no greater life change than becoming a parent—and worry about factors such as finances, whether you'll be a good mother, and how your relationship will change. It's important to keep worries in perspective and try to maintain an emotional balance since being stressed isn't good for your health or the health of your baby.

Find simple ways to handle and reduce your stress—see below for some suggestions. Activities such as going swimming may take some planning, but try to find a slot in your schedule to make time for this every week.

Sometimes relieving stress can be as simple as sharing it, so talk to others to put your concerns in perspective. Or if you don't want to share your worries, write them down instead.

> " While you're pregnant, it's even more important to find ways to relieve stress and keep any worries in perspective. "

RELIEVING STRESS

Learn to recognize the signs that you're stressed: you may feel your heart racing or a rise in your body temperature. When you know you're stressed, take action.

- **Identify the cause** and try to keep it in perspective. Let go of the stress by breathing deeply and relaxing your muscles. Imagine blowing the stress away as you exhale.
- **Stay busy**—sometimes having too much time to think can make you more stressed.
- **Going swimming** is a great stress reliever and a great way to stay in shape.
- **Take time to relax,** especially if you have a lot on your mind or are juggling lots of things. Put your feet up, watch TV, read a book, or just spend quiet time thinking about your growing baby.
- **Talk through your problems** with your partner or a close friend. If you're worrying about any aspect of your health or how your baby is developing, seek reassurance from your doctor.
- **If work is an issue,** be honest with your boss or the HR department and they may be able to help. Your most important job right now is to nurture your baby.

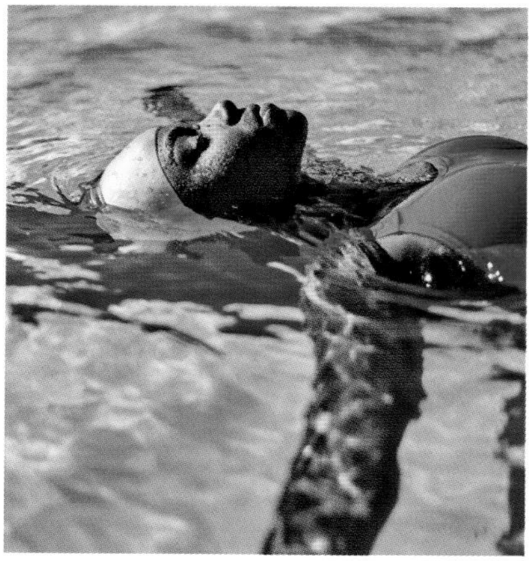

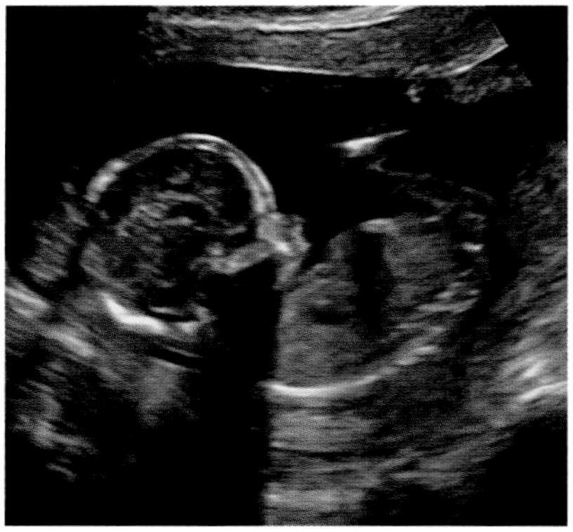

YOU ARE **16 WEEKS AND 4 DAYS**

164 days to go

YOUR BABY TODAY

In this 2-D ultrasound, the baby's head is to the left, with the arms not visible, although the knee and lower leg can be seen. At this stage, details of the brain developing under the skull are becoming much more apparent.

"Until you feel your baby move, hearing his heartbeat is the next best way for you to bond with him."

At this stage of pregnancy, your doctor may be able to hear your baby's heartbeat using a handheld Doppler ultrasound machine. Because ultrasound waves do not travel well in air, gel is applied to the end of the probe or "transducer" as it is placed on your abdomen. This then detects the heartbeat and converts it into a sound that we can hear.

It's quite easy to distinguish your baby's heartbeat from your own since it beats almost twice as fast. However, your baby's heart rate peaked around five weeks ago and, since then, has slowed down as the nerves controlling the heart's rhythm have matured.

During the second half of pregnancy, the range of the heartbeat is between 110 and 160 beats per minute and will be responsive to many stimuli, as well as to your baby's activity.

HEART RATE AND GENDER

The baby's heart rate is not an indication of gender. A study in the mid-1990s, using over 10,000 measurements, dispelled the theory that the speed of a baby's heartbeat predicted whether it would be a boy or a girl.

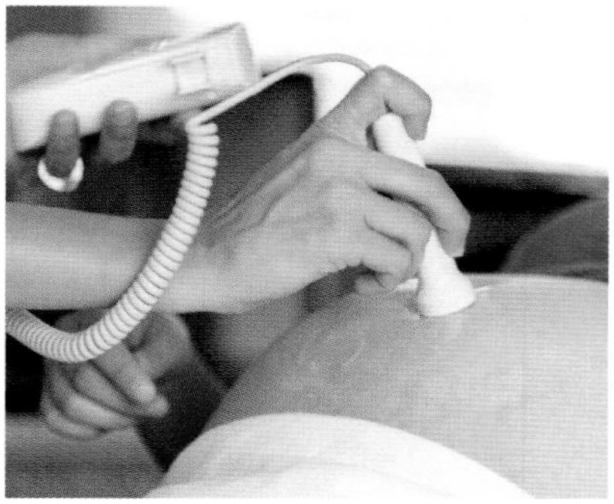

ASK A PANEL

My partner is eager to rent a handheld Doppler so we can listen to our baby's heartbeat. Is this is a good idea?

Doctor: Handheld ultrasound Doppler devices, which allow parents-to-be to listen to the fetal heartbeat at home, are currently sold over the counter in the US. Parents are told they can listen to their baby "in complete safety as early as 10 weeks of pregnancy" and "any time they want," implying there is no limit on frequency of exposure.

However, there has been no research into the effects of frequent scanning, which would be more than the baby receives during prenatal care. A Doppler is not a toy and using it in this way is an unnecessary risk.

Midwife: Using your own Doppler may help reassure you if you are very anxious about your baby's well-being, but it is just as likely to have the opposite effect if you can't pick up the heartbeat. Identifying different sounds takes practice and if you have difficulty finding the heartbeat (this happens to midwives, too!), it could be distressing. If you're worried about your baby for any reason, help and advice is only a phone call away.

Mom: I used a Doppler because I am a worrier and it really gave me peace of mind. I didn't use it very often and only when there was a good reason to. For example, at one stage of my pregnancy, I had an episode of bleeding and clots. After this, I was very worried about my baby's health and hearing his heartbeat really helped to calm me down, so it had benefits for the baby, too. I don't think a Doppler is a substitute for medical advice but it's a useful addition.

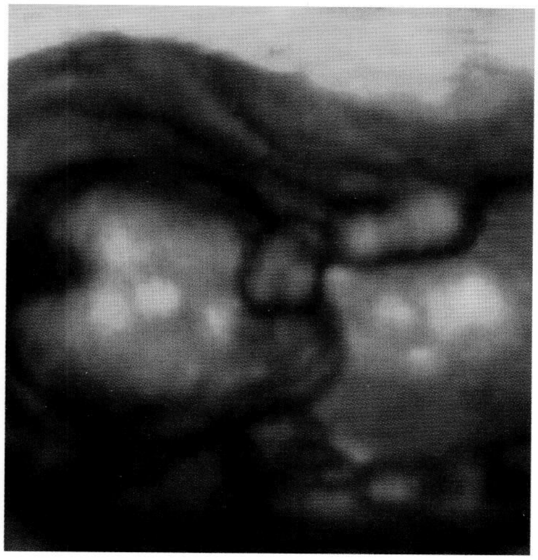

YOU ARE **16 WEEKS AND 5 DAYS**

163 days to go

YOUR BABY TODAY

The baby's face is partially obscured by the hand in this 3-D image. Babies at this stage are small enough to fit onto the ultrasound screen, but beyond 20 weeks it is increasingly only possible to see a smaller part of the baby at any one time.

Staying hydrated in pregnancy can be a challenge. Because of the hormonal changes taking place, some of the fluid you take in leaks into your body tissues, rather than staying within the bloodstream.

It's difficult to recommend an exact amount of fluid that should be drunk to keep you hydrated, since this depends on many factors, such as the foods you eat (some naturally contain water), your size, the amount you exercise, and the heat and humidity in the environment. Therefore, you need to listen to your own body to determine if you're adequately hydrated. One of the best ways to do this is to look at your urine. If it's clear to light yellow, you're adequately hydrated. If it's bright yellow or orange, you're likely to be dehydrated.

Drinking plenty of water is important. Sometimes, though, if you are nauseous, or just plain tired of drinking water, you may want to try other options for hydration, such as drinking a glass of milk; enjoying a light soup, miso, or broth; or having an unsweetened fruit juice. Remember that caffeinated beverages, such as coffee, tea, and cola are not hydrating; caffeine has a diuretic effect, which means that you will need to urinate more often.

A great way to stay hydrated is to eat fruit. Many fruits are very high in water, especially melons, grapes, and strawberries. This water is absorbed very well in your body because it is partnered with sugar, which helps the water stay in your bloodstream. And, of course, fruit is highly nutritious.

> “ Ensuring you drink enough is essential to good pregnancy health, so always carry a bottle of water with you when you go out. ”

NUTRITIOUS SEEDS

Seeds are a powerhouse of the essential fatty acid ALA (see p.169) as well as a source of vitamins and minerals. Pumpkin seeds and flaxseeds contain iron, magnesium, and zinc, and sesame seeds provide calcium. Snack on them, sprinkle them on your cereal, and enjoy tahini (sesame paste) in dips and sauces. All seeds contain vitamin E, which boosts immunity and may protect you against preeclampsia (see p.476).

ASK A DOCTOR

Should I stop picking up my toddler while I'm pregnant? You may be experiencing some back pain and discomfort as your hormones begin to soften your ligaments. This means that your joints are less stable than usual, and injury is more likely.

Lifting your toddler will not harm your baby, but it may cause you discomfort, and you may be more likely to lose your balance. Ask your toddler to climb onto a chair so that you don't need to lift from a bending position. To lift from floor level, squat down and use your legs to bear the weight. Avoid bending, which strains your back. Encourage your toddler to get onto your lap for a hug.

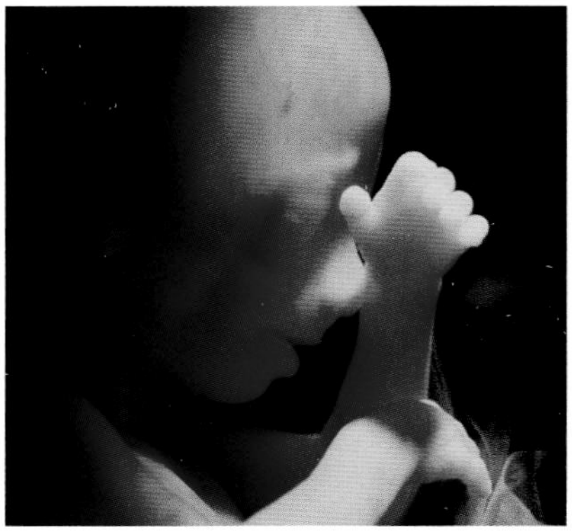

YOU ARE **16 WEEKS AND 6 DAYS**

162 days to go

YOUR BABY TODAY

The baby often brings their hands to their face and sometimes sucks their thumb; but the sucking action is not well coordinated and the thumb is likely to enter the mouth more by luck than design. The arms are now in proportion with the rest of the body.

> "Your baby is practicing his breathing movements, which are vital to develop his chest muscles and enable his lungs to grow."

While they're in the uterus, your baby is practicing their breathing movements, which aids their lung development. When they breathe in, the diaphragm moves downward and the chest wall moves inward.

Each "breath" the baby takes lasts less than a second. Breathing might only happen occasionally at this stage and when it does it can be either regular or irregular.

Your baby might also open their jaw and swallow at the same time as making a breathing movement. A single breathing movement with a large movement of the diaphragm may resemble a sigh.

For the chest wall movements to be effective, there must be an adequate amount of amniotic fluid (see p.182). This is especially true for the time of lung development (16–26 weeks).

By the 24th week of pregnancy, your baby will spend approximately three hours in a 24-hour period practicing breathing movements, and around eight hours in a 24-hour period in the last eight weeks.

When a pregnant woman smokes, it reduces the number of times her baby practices breathing movements. In a *British Medical Journal* study, the proportion of time the baby practiced breathing movements was found to fall within five minutes of the mother beginning to smoke her cigarette.

FOCUS ON TWINS

While most unborn twins grow at much the same pace, from now on some don't. Your babies are almost certainly developing all the right organs at the right time, even when there's a size discrepancy. If, however, a scan detects a growth difference between your twins, you'll have additional scans to monitor growth. Doctors aren't usually concerned unless there's a growth difference of more than 15 percent.

ASK A DOCTOR

Why am I beginning to get brown patches on my face? As many as 70 percent of pregnant women find the color of their skin changes. You may notice brown patches appearing on your forehead, cheeks, and neck, known as chloasma or the "mask of pregnancy." Darker-skinned women may develop lighter-colored patches.

Chloasma is caused by an increase in the production of melanin, the pigment that gives the skin and hair its natural color. It will gradually fade after the birth. To minimize the patches, stay out of the sun as much as possible, use a high protection sunscreen, and wear a hat outdoors. Try covering larger patches with a tinted moisturizer or foundation and use concealer on smaller patches.

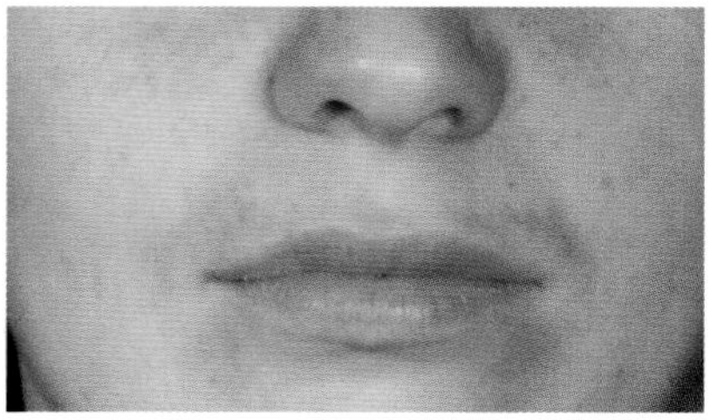

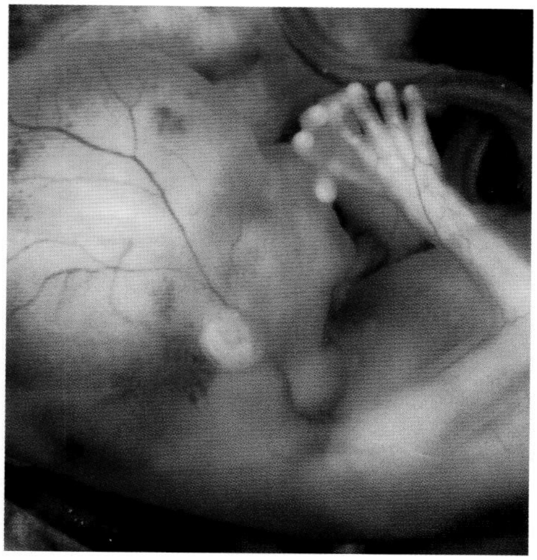

YOU ARE **17 WEEKS EXACTLY**

161 days to go

YOUR BABY TODAY

Every part of your baby has an enhanced blood supply bringing nutrients for growth. Blood vessels are easy to see on scans because the skin is still quite transparent, with little fat yet deposited beneath the skin.

It's possible to eat out safely. However, you may have to ask what's in particular dishes to avoid eating foods that aren't recommended during pregnancy (see p.16).

Request that your meat and poultry are cooked to well done. You can check this by inserting a sharp knife—if the juices are still pink, ask for it to be recooked. Ask if the dairy products, particularly cheeses you aren't familiar with, are made with pasteurized milk.

If fried or fatty foods upset your stomach and cause heartburn, stick with foods that have been oven baked or steamed, and avoid fatty cuts of meat.

A lot of sushi contains shellfish, but you should only eat cooked shellfish during pregnancy. Raw shellfish contains harmful viruses and bacteria. If you're served sushi, ask whether the shellfish has been cooked and whether any other fish used has been frozen first. If it has, it should be safe to eat.

> "While your energy levels are at a peak, make the most of eating out but choose your meals wisely."

ASK A NUTRITIONIST

I'm a vegetarian but keep craving meat. Is this normal? Yes, when you're pregnant, it is common for your body to crave certain foods. One theory is that, even as a vegetarian, you may crave meat because you are not getting sufficient iron from your diet.

As you don't eat red meat, which is the best source of iron, you need to make sure you have plenty of iron from plant sources. Eat lots of whole-grain cereals; mycoprotein (Quorn); green vegetables such as kale and spinach; legumes such as lentils, soy, and kidney beans; and dried fruit such as raisins and apricots.

It also means making sure you can absorb as much of the iron as possible by avoiding drinking tea or coffee until at least 30 minutes after eating, and enhancing absorption by having a vitamin C or protein-rich ingredient at the same time. For ease this means drinking your 150 ml daily citrus juice with your meal, or having tomatoes or peppers in a sandwich or salad.

A dressing made with lemon juice—or chopping a kiwi fruit or clementine into a green salad—will help, too.

STRONGER NAILS

Your nails are likely to be stronger and healthier than ever, due to the hormonal changes that occur during pregnancy.

Since your nails are in good condition, you can simply file them and they'll look nice even without nail polish. If you do decide to have a manicure, make sure it takes place in a well-ventilated room. Avoid using nail polishes that contain dibutyl phthalate (DBP), an ingredient that is linked to birth defects in animals.

Your 18th week

YOU'LL FIND YOU'RE GAINING WEIGHT WEEK BY WEEK, WHICH IS PERFECTLY NORMAL. Not all the additional weight is your baby. In fact, most of the increase is because parts of your body, such as your breasts, are getting bigger and your blood volume is increasing. You might want to think about signing up for prenatal classes now because they fill up quickly. They are a great source of information, as well as a good way to make friends and compare notes with other pregnant women.

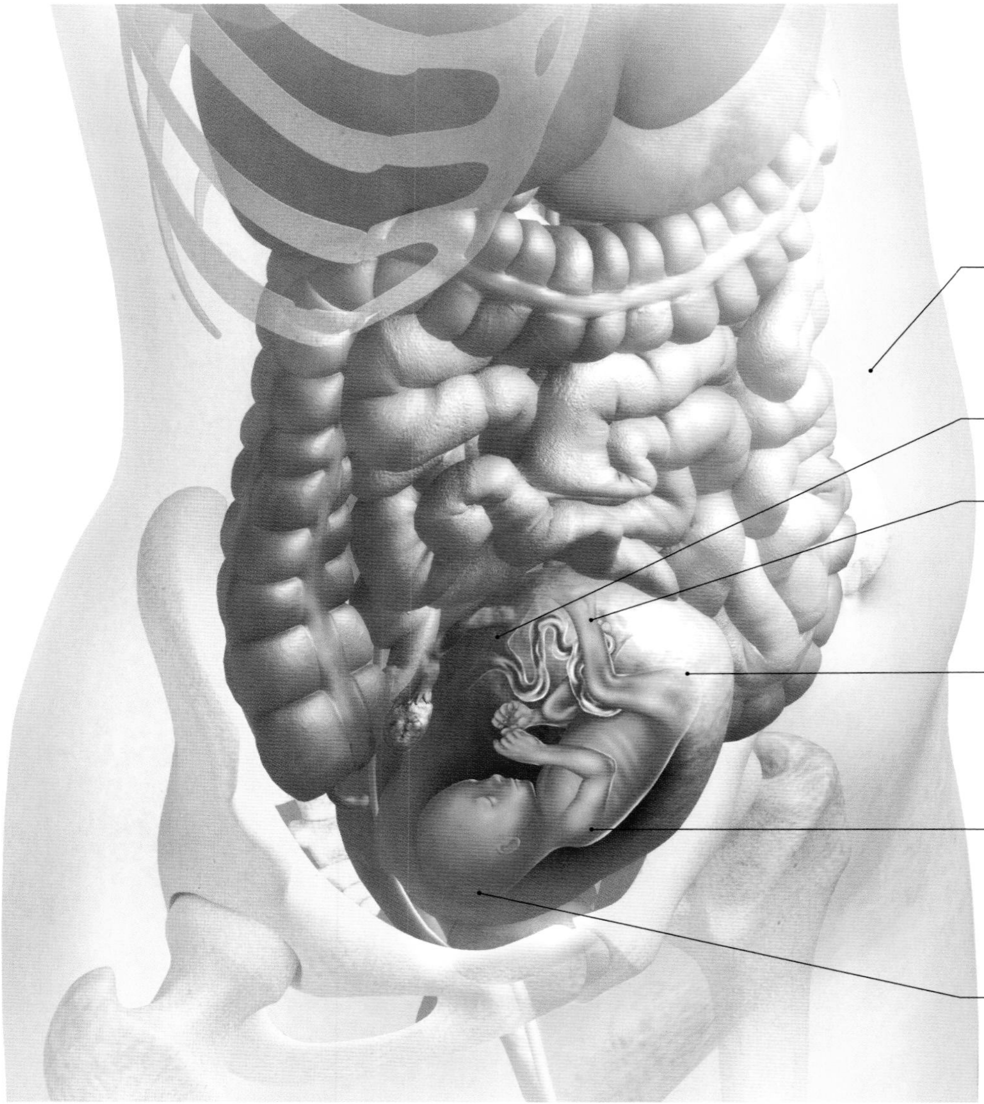
Your uterus is likely to be large enough to give you a noticeably rounded belly.
The placenta is still growing, although not as fast as in earlier weeks. It continues to be a vital supply line for the baby.
The baby's movements are getting more vigorous and you may now be able to feel them.
The sex organs are developing well, both externally and internally. In baby girls, follicles containing immature eggs are already forming in the ovaries.
Your baby is now bigger than the placenta for the first time, and will continue to outgrow it.
At 18 weeks the average crown to rump length is 5.6 in (14.2 cm) and the average weight is 6.7 oz (190 g).

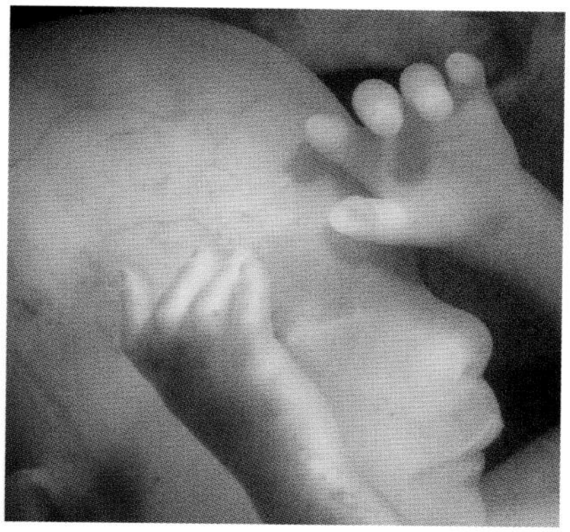

YOU ARE **17 WEEKS AND 1 DAY**

160 days to go

YOUR BABY TODAY

Your baby's jaw continues to grow throughout the pregnancy, but at this time it can still appear to be quite short. The early tooth buds are hardening within both jaws and, just as with the other bones, calcium is being laid down to strengthen their structure.

"Around this time, you may become aware of your baby moving, although for some women first movements are felt much later."

Although your baby is very active, she's not big enough for you to feel any but the strongest kicks on the walls of your uterus. "Quickening" is the term used to describe these first movements, which feel like tiny flutterings or bubbles in your lower abdomen. You may not notice them or not realize that they are the baby at first, since they feel similar to having gas.

If you've been pregnant before, you will be more familiar with the sensation and able to recognize it. First-time moms generally don't feel movements until a bit later, at about 18 to 20 weeks (see p.213), so don't worry if you haven't felt anything yet. The flutterings become more persistent and definite over time, and there will eventually be recognizable kicks and nudges.

Once you can feel the activities, you will become very conscious of them and may become aware of a pattern to them.

Babies move when they are asleep and awake. The reason you are less likely to feel your baby move when you're active is that you are likely to be distracted yourself and miss some movement.

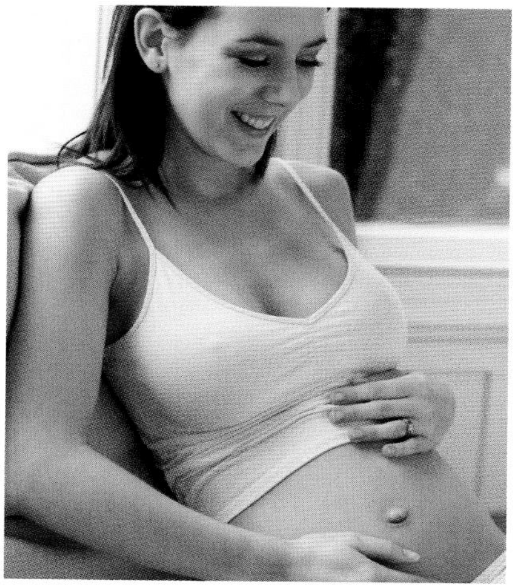

At around this time, you may begin to feel some slight sensations when your baby moves around.

NOTICING FIRST MOVEMENTS

Was it gas, or did your baby move? The first time you notice your baby moving marks the start of a new chapter in the bonding process, and it seems it has always been the case, even in ancient times.

In many cultures, until the advent of pregnancy tests, "quickening" was the first conclusive evidence of pregnancy, and was viewed as the point at which human life began.

According to ancient Egyptian, Greek, American, and Indian beliefs, the first movement marked the moment when the soul entered the fetus. Aboriginals regard the location where the first quickening is felt as highly significant for the baby.

FOCUS ON PARTNERS

It will be exciting when your partner tells you she can feel the baby move for the first time, and this is a great milestone of the pregnancy. However, when you touch her bump, you may be disappointed to find that you can't feel anything at all. Just be a little patient since there will be plenty of opportunities later on in the pregnancy to feel the movements.

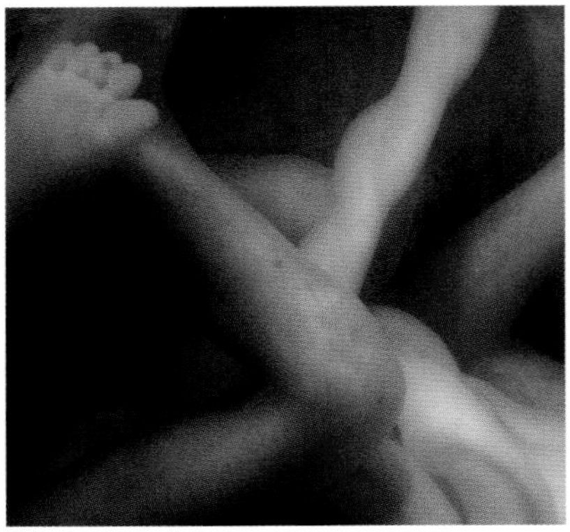

YOU ARE **17 WEEKS AND 2 DAYS**

159 days to go

YOUR BABY TODAY

Here, the baby's legs are in the typical crossed-legs position. The right arm is on the right side of the image. The limbs and umbilical cord appear to be in a tangle, but the umbilical cord is filled with a jellylike fluid and does not become compressed.

" The tiny embryo was once dwarfed by the placenta but now your baby has outgrown it and will continue to do so. "

In the early stages of pregnancy, the placenta grew at a far greater rate than your baby. Your baby has now caught up and from now on will be larger than the placenta.

The structure of the placenta will change over the course of the next few weeks as the second wave of cells move into the spiral arteries in the uterus (see p.172). The placenta is currently at its thickest but as it continues to grow, albeit at a slower rate for a time, it thins out.

Your baby's more rapid growth means that at 5 oz (140 g) she is now heavier than the placenta and by the time she is full term she will be six or seven times its weight. Nutrients supplied across the placenta provide your baby with essential energy for growth, but growth is in part regulated by her own insulin production and insulin-like growth factors.

Although your baby has relatively high concentrations of growth hormone, which is responsible for growth after birth, this does not seem to play an important role in her growth during pregnancy.

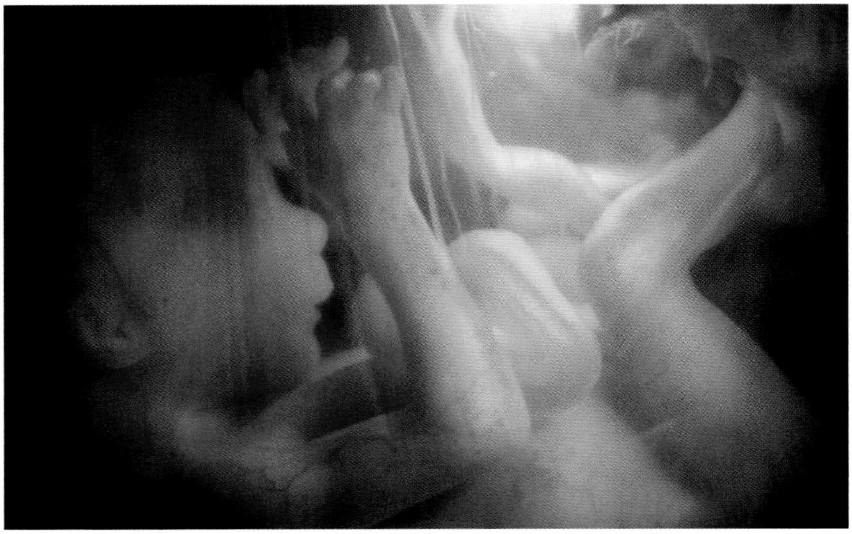

Here, the baby is in a typical position, curled with feet and elbows bent. The well-developed ear is still a little low on the side of the head at this point, and the baby's blood vessels show up well.

TACKLING HEARTBURN

If you're battling heartburn, try these solutions:
Eat smaller meals and chew well
• Avoid spicy, rich, and fatty foods
• Don't smoke or drink alcohol, and avoid carbonated drinks, including sparkling water
• Drink low-fat milk
• Try drinking chamomile tea (check with your doctor first)
• Munch on raw garlic
• Chew gum after eating
• Sit upright after meals
• Don't eat a meal late at night Raise the head of your bed by 6 in (15 cm) and lie on your left side. If these remedies are ineffective, ask your doctor about medication to relieve your symptoms.

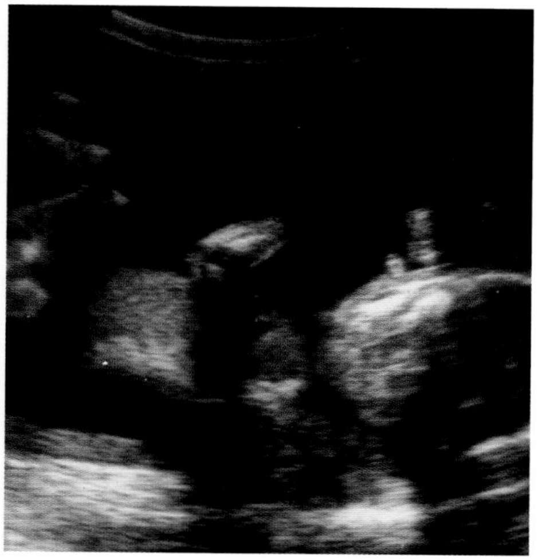

YOU ARE **17 WEEKS AND 3 DAYS**

158 days to go

YOUR BABY TODAY

Although the baby is lying on her side and the face cannot be seen, this image does show the leg and foot particularly well. Because 2D ultrasound only shows a "slice" of the baby, parts may appear to be missing, such as the arm here which stops midway.

While you may have gained little weight in the first trimester, from the second trimester onward you will gain weight each week. On average, women should put on 3–4lb per month from the second trimester to the end of pregnancy, though the weight gain tends to slow down in the last few weeks.

The amount of weight you should be gaining depends on many factors, not least your starting Body Mass Index (BMI) (see p.16). The target weight gains are detailed in the chart below.

Not all of the weight gained is the baby; in fact, the fetus makes up only a small part. The rest of the weight is accounted for by your growing uterus, amniotic fluid, breasts, and increased blood volume and fat (see p.99).

If you have any concerns about your weight, seek advice from your doctor. Your weight may not be checked routinely at your prenatal checkups, but your doctor will weigh you if she's concerned about the amount of weight you're gaining.

" It's normal and healthy for you to gain more weight in the second trimester of pregnancy than you did in the first trimester. "

ASK A DOCTOR

I keep having hot flashes. Is this normal? Many women experience hot flashes during pregnancy as a result of increased levels of the hormone estrogen. This encourages the blood vessels to dilate—suffusing them with blood and heat. What's more, when you're pregnant, your metabolism increases, causing extra heat to be produced. That's not to mention the little heater that you have growing inside you.

Wear layers that can be speedily removed and avoid eating spicy foods and drinking alcohol and caffeine, all of which can encourage hot flashes. Exercise can help by improving circulation, and yoga and other relaxation exercises can help you to keep cool and calm.

WEIGHT GAIN

Your target weight gain for the second trimester (as well as the third trimester) is 12–19lb. If, due to pregnancy discomforts, such as morning sickness, you had a difficult first trimester and did not gain much weight, this is a good time to increase your calories to make up some of the weight gain. If you gained too much weight in the first trimester, focus on staying active and filling your plate with lower-calorie yet nutrient-rich fruits and vegetables.

Keep your target weight gain in mind. The recommended total pregnancy weight gain is 25–35lb for women whose BMI (see p.16) is in the normal range, between 18.5 and 25.

If you were overweight at the start of pregnancy, your recommended weight gain is 11–20lb. Obese women should gain at least 11lb. If you started underweight, the recommended weight gain is 28–40lb. If you're expecting twins, you should aim for a total gain of about 35–45lb.

Weight-gain chart

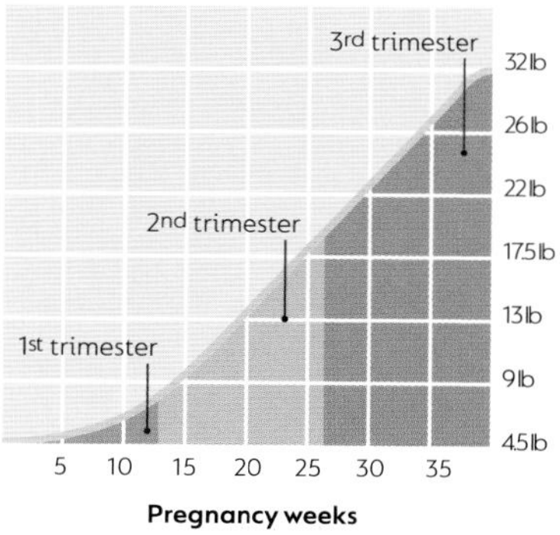
3rd trimester
2nd trimester
1st trimester
32lb
26lb
22lb
17.5lb
13lb
9lb
4.5lb
5
10
15
20
25
30
35
Pregnancy weeks

A safe workout

Alternating upper- and lower-body exercises keeps your heart rate up. Remember to get your doctor's approval before starting exercise programs.

Effective and safe in the second trimester, this workout can be done three to four times a week to maintain tone and fitness. Use 5 lb (2 kg) weights.

Warm up Begin by moving your legs side to side in a step and touch movement for a minute. Continue for another minute but add the arms: each time you step-touch, lift your arms to shoulder height then down. Next, with hands on hips lift your knees up to your stomach. Alternate the legs for two minutes. Stand straight and circle your left arm across the body and back to the side; repeat with the other arm. Continue the sequence for 5 minutes, or until you feel warmed up.

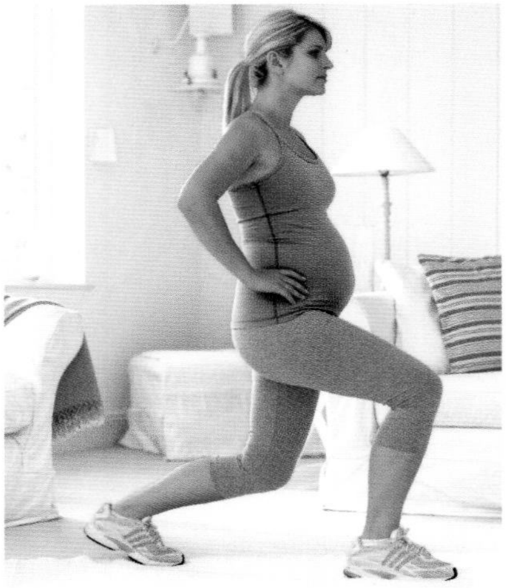

Forward lunge Stand with your hands on your hips. Step your right leg forward, then with the left foot in place, bend your left knee toward the floor until the right knee is nearly at a right angle. Alternate each side until you've done around 30 repetitions. (In the third trimester, you might need to hold the back of a chair.) Keep your stomach pulled in, your back straight, head up, and shoulders relaxed.

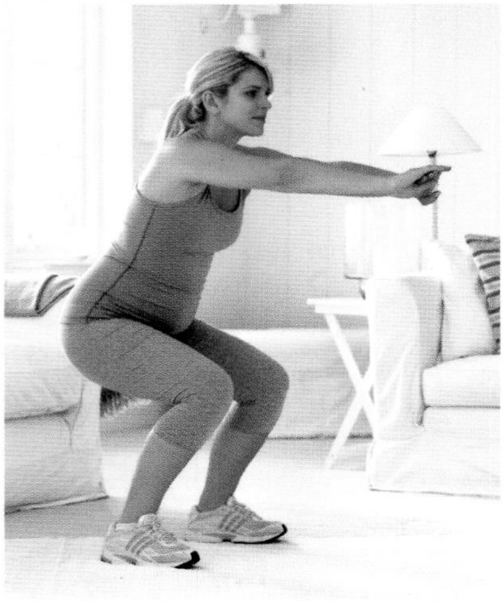

Squats Stand with your feet shoulder-width apart. With your arms stretched out in front of you at shoulder level, squat down, keeping your abdominal muscles pulled in and your feet firmly on the floor. Lower your bottom toward the floor then lift up to the starting point. Breathe out as you lower and in as you lift. Make sure your knees do not go over the end of your toes.

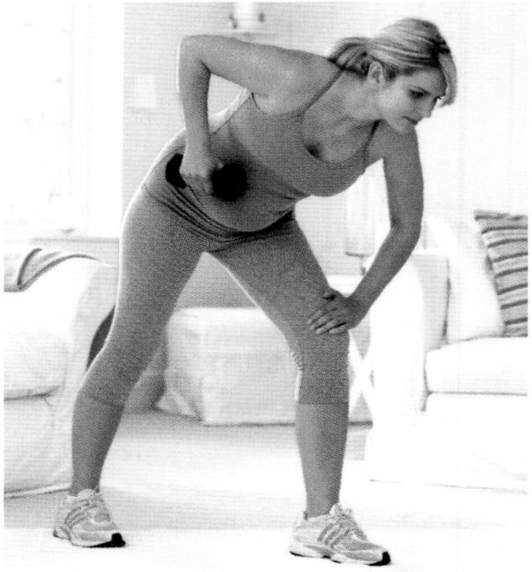

Forward pull-ups Stand with your left leg in front of you and both knees slightly bent; slowly lower your upper body toward your left knee and rest your left hand on the knee for support. Start with your right arm straight down, then lift your arm up. Keep your elbow close to your body. It should end pointing toward the ceiling. Repeat 20 times on each arm.

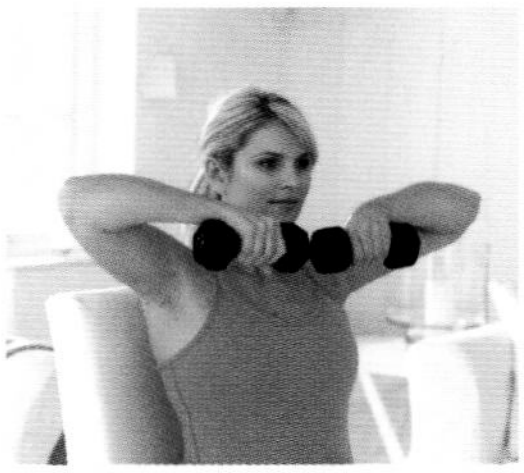

Upright row Sit on an upright chair or stand with legs slightly bent, feet hip-width apart. Hold the weights with your arms down in front of you. Exhaling, slowly lift the weights to chest height, stopping under the chin. Then inhale and lower the weights to the starting point. Repeat 20 times.

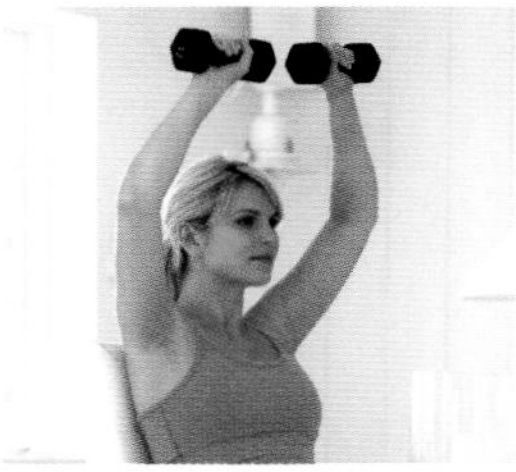

Shoulder press Stand or sit as in the preceding exercise. Holding a weight in each hand, slightly bend your arms at the elbows and hold your hands above your shoulders. Then, while breathing out, slowly lift your arms toward the ceiling until they are straight. Repeat around 30 times.

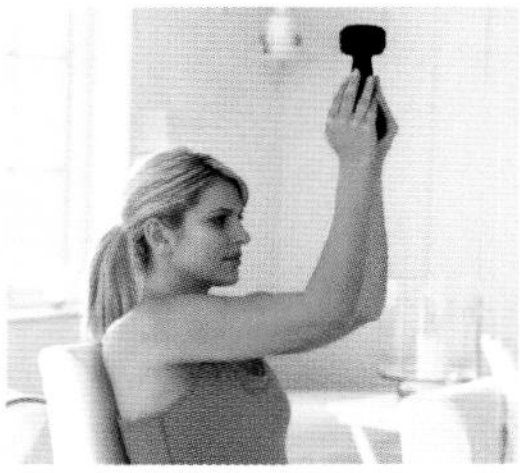

Pectoral lift Sit or stand as before. Hold your arms in front of you at shoulder height while holding a weight. Bend your elbows at a right angle, keeping the upper arms parallel to the floor. Bring your elbows together and then gently lift your arms up and down. Repeat 20 times.

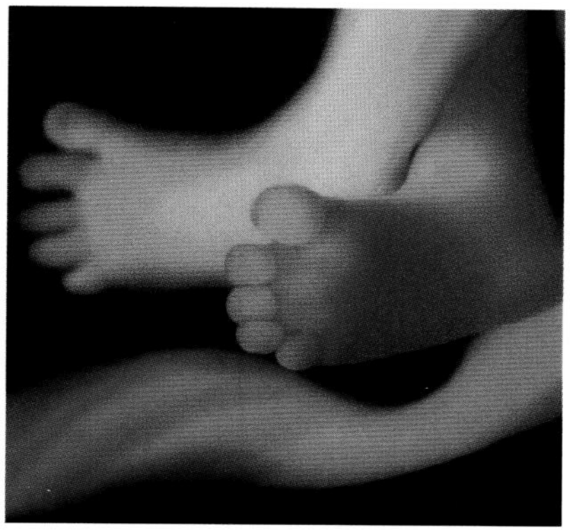

YOU ARE **17 WEEKS 4 DAYS**

157 days to go

YOUR BABY TODAY

Your baby's skin is extremely soft and smooth. The soles of the feet and toes are shown in this image and it is clear they are free from wrinkles. During the next week evidence of fingerprint and toeprint patterns will appear on the skin.

Your baby's complex lung development is continuing. To picture this, imagine the whole of the lungs as a tree: the trunk has developed (the trachea or windpipe), and this has branched into smaller and medium-size branches (bronchi), but the twigs (bronchioles) holding the leaves (alveoli) have not yet formed. It is the alveoli that have walls so thin that they allow oxygen to be absorbed from the air in them and carbon dioxide to leave via the bloodstream.

From now until 28 weeks the "twigs" are forming that will hold the alveoli that will become filled with air after birth. These "twigs" will have a limited ability to transfer gases but the lungs will not be fully effective until the alveoli develop. The growth of the blood vessels that support the lungs closely matches the growth of the lungs themselves. These blood vessels will be essential for the transfer of oxygen after your baby is born.

After birth, all the blood that is leaving the right side of the heart will enter the lung circulation, but before birth, with the lungs filled with fluid and not used for breathing, only a small amount of blood (approximately 10–15 percent) is directed to them.

> "Although changes are taking place, your baby's lungs are still fairly immature and won't be fully developed until week 35."

STRETCHING SAFELY

Only stretch as far as is comfortable because during pregnancy you're more vulnerable to damaging muscles and tendons due to the hormone relaxin. Relaxin is one of the most important pregnancy-related hormones. As its name implies, relaxin relaxes the connective tissue, tendons, and ligaments to allow the diaphragm to expand and create space for your baby to grow. It also loosens the ligaments and tendons enough to facilitate the opening of the birth canal for a vaginal delivery.

Relaxin affects most parts of your body and, as a result, your spine and pelvis and most of your joints will feel less stable. Be aware of your posture and alignment when exercising.

- **When standing,** always keep your hips in a neutral position. Don't move your hips to one side especially when carrying heavy packages and bags.
- **Beware of arching** your lower back and rounding your shoulders.
- **Keep your movements slow** and controlled, and stay in your comfort zone.

The increased flexibility of your muscles and tendons could result in overstretching during activities such as yoga or Pilates, or fast movements in a dance class or weight training.

Relaxin is also responsible for the relaxation of the circulatory system: the walls of the veins are relaxed, which sometimes results in varicose veins (see p.167). Doing cardiovascular exercise will help increase blood flow and can reduce the occurrence of varicose veins.

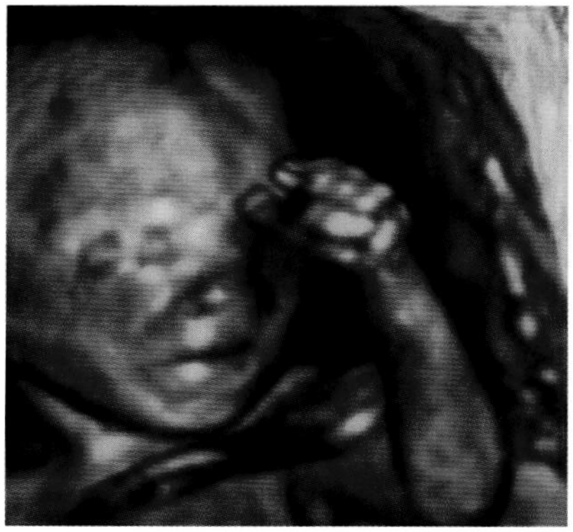

YOU ARE **17 WEEKS AND 5 DAYS**

156 days to go

YOUR BABY TODAY

This image shows how much less obvious the soft spot on the top of the baby's head has become by now. The fingers show up well here, and as your baby increases in size, it becomes easier and easier for ultrasound to show this level of detail.

> "As your belly begins to grow and is more obvious, your pregnancy will become the main focus of people's attention."

Are you getting a little more attention than you would like? Once your belly becomes very obvious, you may begin to feel that it and you are public property. Fascinated by the size of your ever-increasing abdomen, some friends and family, or even strangers, may want to see your belly, touch it, or even kiss it. This can feel very strange because, as a rule, people tend not to go around touching each other's abdomens!

If you're uncomfortable about being touched, then you could politely ask people not to touch the belly, or simply move away. There are, however, some advantages to having people notice that you are pregnant: your belly acts as a warning for people not to jostle you in crowds and people tend to give you a seat on public transportation.

Another unwanted intrusion might be that people feel entitled to ask you intimate questions regarding your medical history and about the baby. This may make you uncomfortable, especially if you tend to be a private person. People you have never met before might comment on your figure, and discuss whether you're having a girl or a boy.

Some pregnant women enjoy the attention, while others feel that people are intruding on a personal experience. If you feel uncomfortable, answer questions vaguely or try to change the subject; ask the person about him- or herself instead. Another way of avoiding the unwanted attention is to wear loose clothing that makes your belly look less prominent and attractive to touch.

SALT INTAKE

Consuming too much salt can lead to high blood pressure. It has been difficult for scientists to study salt intake in pregnancy and advise on whether it should be limited, and if so, by how much. The most sensible route is to be careful not to eat too many salty foods and add salt at the table if you need it.

ASK A DOCTOR

I'm so itchy that I'm scratching to the point of bleeding. What can I do? Most itching in pregnancy, especially on your belly, is due to the skin stretching (see p.255), hormonal changes, and heat. Applying moisturizing cream should help. If you have significant itching, see your doctor to determine whether you have obstetric cholestasis (see p.475), a serious but rare condition that affects the liver and occurs in about 1 percent of pregnancies.

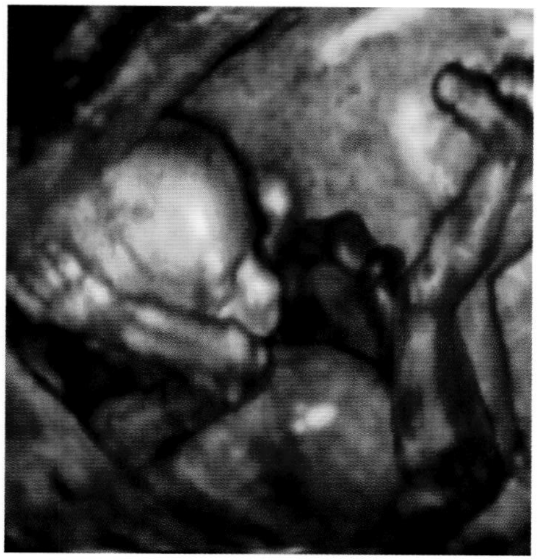

YOU ARE **17 WEEKS AND 6 DAYS**

155 days to go

YOUR BABY TODAY

In this image the whole baby is seen in one view. The legs, held straight, will now be kicking more strongly and, especially if you have had a baby before, you will be increasingly aware of these movements over the next few weeks.

“You might want to think about signing up for prenatal classes now since in many areas they get filled up well in advance.”

Prenatal classes help to prepare you for the birth of your baby. They usually start in the sixth or seventh month. You'll learn about the signs that you're in labor; breathing and relaxation techniques; pain-relief options; and medical interventions. You'll also be given practical advice on caring for your newborn baby, which can be invaluable if you're a first-time parent.

Depending on where you live, there are various types of classes. These range from classes run by a nurse or other certified instructor at the hospital to classes run by organizations like Lamaze International (lamaze.org) or the Bradley Method (bradleybirth.com). Classes are a great way to meet other expectant parents, and by doing so you'll gain an invaluable mutual support system through the rest of your pregnancy and the early weeks of parenting.

By attending prenatal classes with you, your partner can help to prepare for the labor and early weeks of parenting. Classes are also a good way for your partner to meet other expectant partners. The significant role partners can play during labor and in the early weeks of parenting is widely acknowledged, and as a result prenatal classes have become much more partner-friendly.

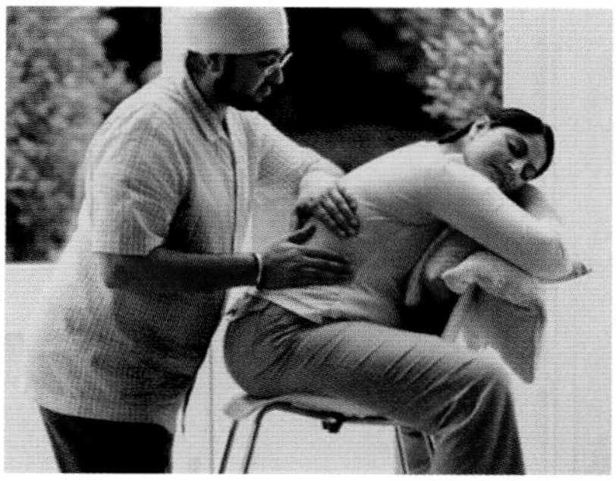

By going to classes, you and your partner can practice and feel more confident about the techniques you'll use in labor.

FOCUS ON TWINS

Since twins are likely to arrive ahead of schedule, you should definitely look into signing up for prenatal classes now so that you can start them early. Besides, your belly could be very large toward the end, and you may feel less mobile and inclined to go to a class. Because twins sometimes need special care, you should arrange a tour of the Neonatal Intensive Care Unit, too.

In some areas, there are special prenatal sessions for those having twins or more, often in the evenings. If your hospital doesn't provide these, a neighboring hospital might. Ask your doctor for information and advice.

FIND A CLASSMATE

If you're single, you don't have to go it alone. There's no reason why you can't go to a class with a friend or relative—preferably the person who will be a birth partner. Alternatively, find out if there are any local classes in your area for single expectant moms. You may feel more comfortable in this environment and you will get the opportunity to meet other women who are in the same position.

Don't skip prenatal classes just because you're single: they're an invaluable way of learning about pregnancy, labor, and parenting.

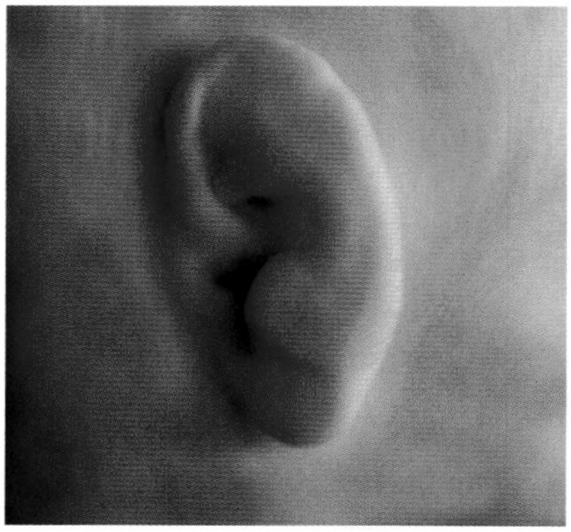

YOU ARE **18 WEEKS EXACTLY**

154 days to go

YOUR BABY TODAY

Like your own ear, your baby's ear is made of soft and flexible cartilage. Although the outer ear is well developed at this stage, inner ear structures will continue to mature throughout your pregnancy.

> "Is it a boy or a girl? You and your partner may want to start thinking about whether you would like to find out."

The sex of your baby should now be apparent on an ultrasound scan, but you may not have this for a couple of weeks yet (see p.211).

Whether your baby develops into a boy or a girl depends on the presence or absence of a Y chromosome. Males are XY and the Y chromosome instructs the reproductive glands (gonads) to become testes. These then produce testosterone and other hormones that inhibit the development of the female organs and in turn stimulate the normal development of the external male genitalia.

If there is no Y chromosome, the gonad becomes an ovary and the internal genitals are female by default; it's not the ovary that dictates that the female reproductive organs will develop but the lack of testosterone. In the female the uterus is formed first and the vagina lengthens upward to meet it.

THINK ABOUT: GENDER

Many women have a strong opinion about whether or not they want to find out the sex of their baby at the 20-week ultrasound, but others are ambivalent. If your partner has strong feelings one way or the other, you can choose to follow his lead. Otherwise, try to figure out your feelings by deciding if you want to choose two names (boy and girl) and get mostly yellow and green baby clothing at your shower, or if identifying with the baby's gender will make these upcoming baby tasks more enjoyable for you.

ASK A MOM

Our 20-week scan is fast approaching. I want to know the baby's sex but my husband doesn't. What should we do? When one person in a relationship wants something that is at odds with what his or her partner wants, tensions can arise.

Like you, I wanted to find out the sex but my partner didn't. We both explained our reasons: I felt that knowing the sex would better help me prepare for the birth; my partner said he wanted the surprise element of discovering the sex when the baby was born. Talk to your partner openly and hopefully you'll be able to reach an agreement.

You may find either one of you doesn't feel as strongly once you start talking. You could agree to find out but not tell anyone else. If you do find out, don't forget the scan result is not 100 percent accurate.

Try not to let the issue get out of hand and consider backing down if necessary. It's important that you feel united at this special time.

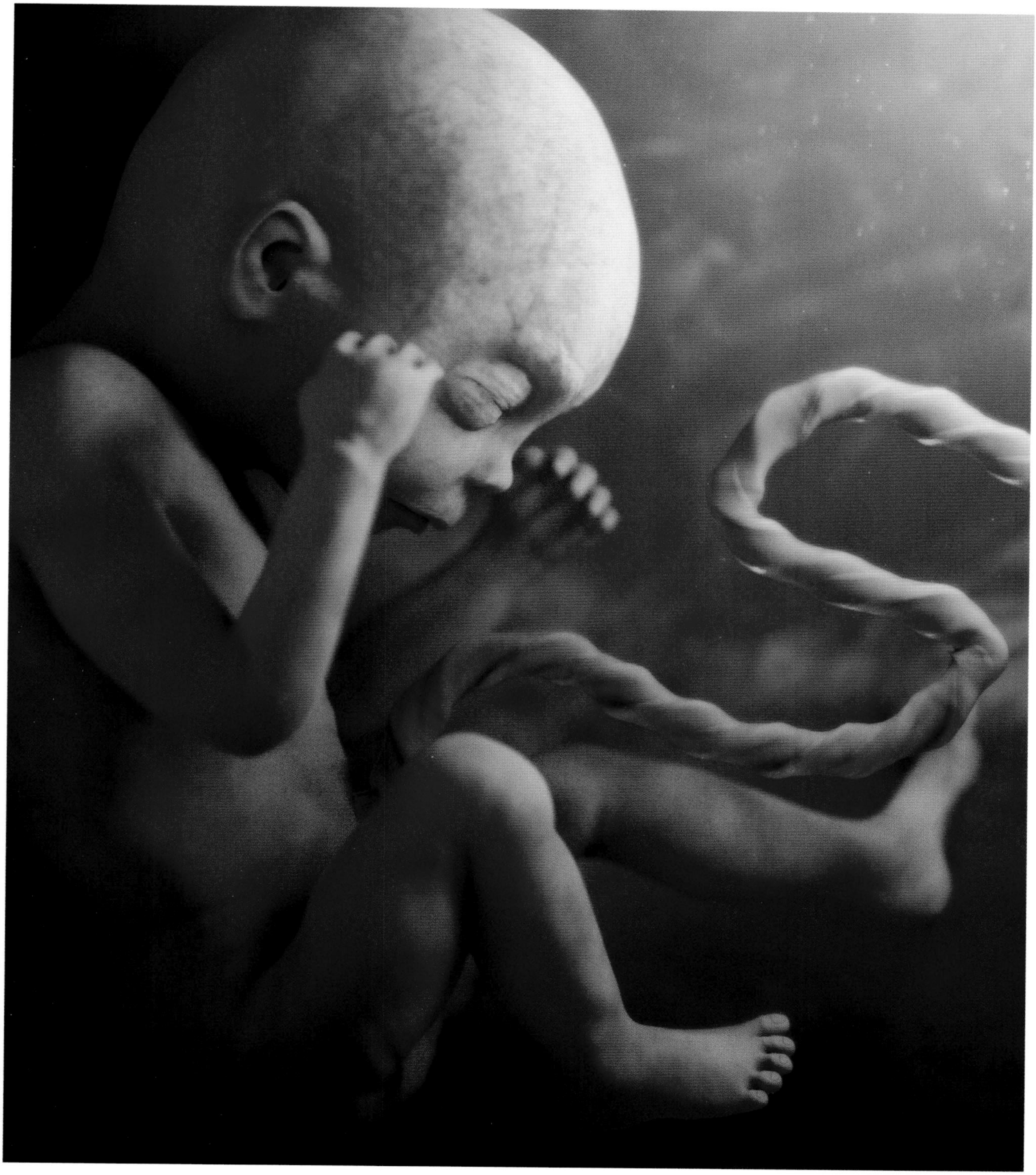

The umbilical cord is growing thicker and stronger as it continues to transport blood and nutrients to your growing baby. Your baby is now bigger and heavier than the placenta.

Your 19th week

YOU'LL PROBABLY FIND YOU'RE BECOMING MORE ATTACHED TO YOUR BABY EACH DAY. It's easier now to think of your baby as a real person, especially if you see him on another scan around this time. He's almost fully formed and the function of his organs is well advanced. You'll be taking your maternal responsibilities very seriously, but don't let anxieties build up. Talk over any worries you may have with your partner and your doctor; many pregnant women also seek comfort and advice from their own mothers.

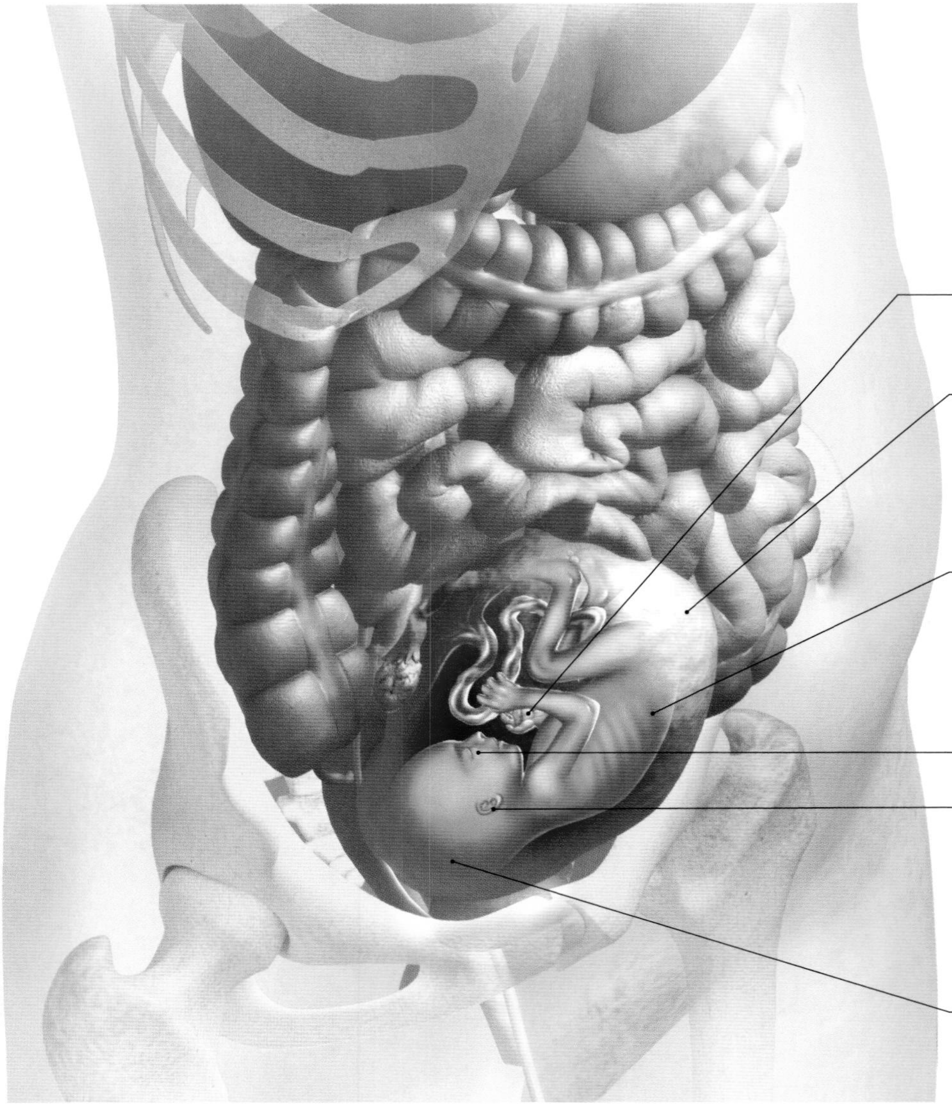

On the pads of the fingers the ridged pattern of the baby's fingerprints, his personal badge of identity, is becoming apparent.
The top of your uterus is now level with your belly button.
A little fat has started to cover the baby's body but he still looks very skinny and his head appears too large for his fragile neck.
The eyes make random movements under the still-closed lids.
The ears have moved up from the jawline to their final position on the side of the head; the eyes, too, are now in their final position, and face forward.
At 19 weeks the average crown to rump length is 6 in (15.3 cm) and the average weight is 8.5 oz (240 g).

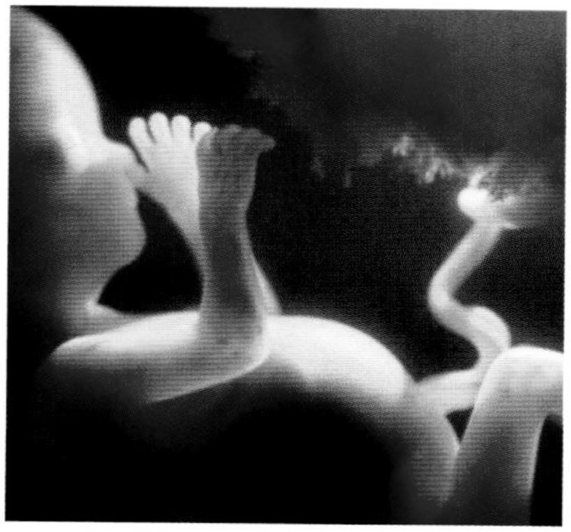

YOU ARE **18 WEEKS AND 1 DAY**

153 days to go

YOUR BABY TODAY

Anchored to the placenta by the umbilical cord, your baby floats in amniotic fluid. Your uterus provides a warm, protective environment for your baby with lots of room to move in near weightless conditions.

“ As you approach the halfway mark of your pregnancy, you’ll continue to be astounded that there’s a baby growing inside you! ”

The further along the path of pregnancy you are, the more attached and protective you’re likely to feel toward your baby. What was once a tiny bundle of cells now looks like an almost fully formed baby—and you will continue to be amazed that you and your partner have made that baby and that this incredible process is happening inside your body.

Once you feel your baby move (see p.213) within the next few weeks, the attachment to them is likely to grow even stronger. While you may have some anxieties at times, try to relax and enjoy your pregnancy—it will be over before you know it.

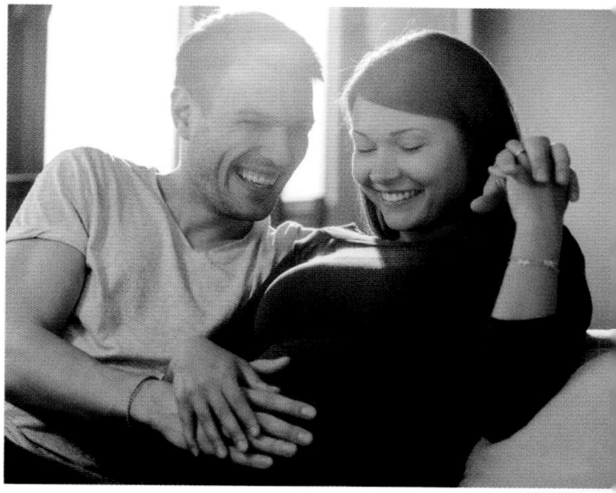

It’s never too early for you and your partner to get to know your baby.

BLURRED VISION

Water retention in pregnancy can affect the eyes. Both the lens and cornea can become thicker, and there can be an increase in fluid in the eyeball, causing pressure and blurred vision. This usually resolves itself after the birth. Exercising to keep the fluid moving, and avoiding wearing contact lenses can help. Notify your doctor if you have vision problems.

ASK A DOCTOR

I have a high-powered career and have hardly had any time to think about the baby since I’ve been pregnant. Will this stop us from bonding? Even if you work full time while you’re pregnant, this doesn’t have to have a negative effect on your relationship with your baby. As your baby grows, you will probably find that you start to develop a relationship with your “belly” as you anticipate your baby’s movements and perhaps talk to him.

Make sure you plan enough maternity leave before your due date since this gives you time for practical and emotional preparations, as well as time to rest.

Full-time working and pregnancy can be a tiring and stressful combination. This highlights the importance of ensuring you have regular opportunities to relax during pregnancy. If your work is stressful, talk to your employer and ask for support.

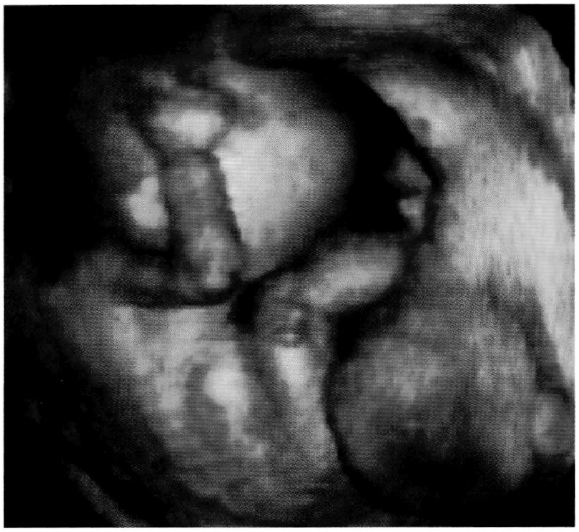

YOU ARE **18 WEEKS AND 2 DAYS**

152 days to go

YOUR BABY TODAY

The sound of your baby's rapidly moving heart muscle can be detected using a simple handheld listening device—the frequency change it produces is converted into a sound that is easy for you and your doctor to hear.

> "You may be able to feel your baby's hiccups as they become stronger and more frequent."

Just like your own, your baby's hiccups are short, powerful, jerky contractions of the diaphragm, causing a sudden rush of air that closes the opening between the vocal cords.

Hiccups frequently follow each other in rapid succession and are often followed by gentle limb-stretching movements. No one is certain why babies hiccup. Perhaps it's due to the immaturity of the nerves supplying the diaphragm, or else to your baby's small stomach quickly becoming overdistended.

Your baby's ears and eyes are now in their final position on his face. The ears have moved up from the jawline and the eyes have moved from the side of the head to lie closer together, looking forward. The eyes move beneath the lids but not yet in a coordinated way. He will open them at around 26 weeks.

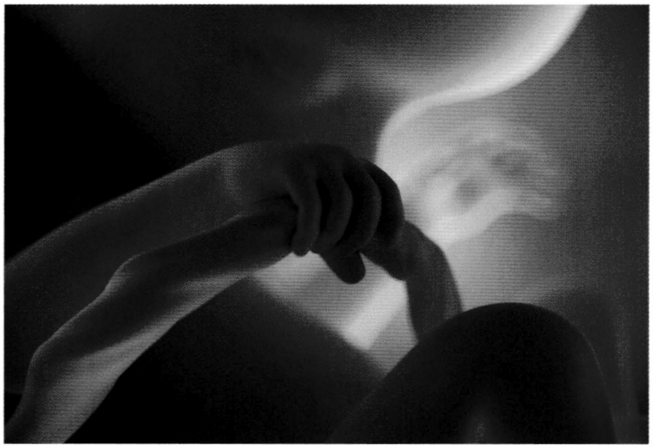

Your baby is looking more human and fully formed every day, with well-developed facial features and limbs—and he may even get the hiccups.

GOOD FATS

Fat is an important nutrient that provides energy as well as vitamins A, D, E, and K. A balanced diet should include fats, but opt for the good fats whenever you can.

Fats tend to be made up of a mixture of different types of fatty acids; some are saturated, others unsaturated. In general, unsaturated fats, which are more prevalent in plant oils and seed oils, are better for heart health than saturated fats. Avocados, nuts, and seeds are a good source of unsaturated fatty acids.

Unsaturated fats are further split into monounsaturated and polyunsaturated fats, and it is better to prioritize monounsaturated fats, such as olive oil, over polyunsaturated fats, such as sunflower or soy spreads, because we have a sufficient amount of these in our diet. Also some polyunsaturated fats called omega-6 compete with the essential fatty acids found in omega-3 (see p.169).

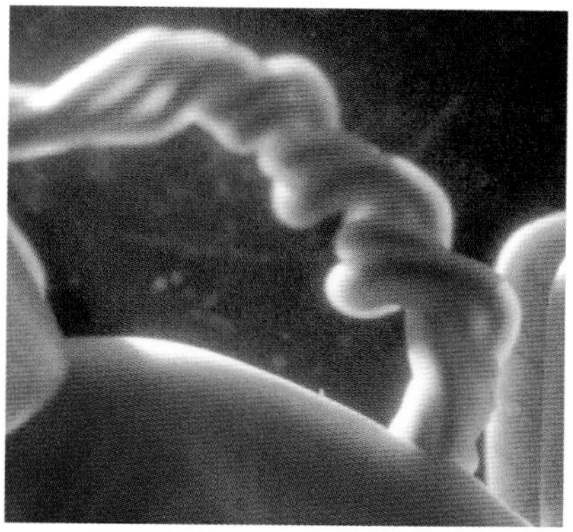

YOU ARE **18 WEEKS AND 3 DAYS**

151 days to go

YOUR BABY TODAY

Coiling is now well established in the umbilical cord. This coiling protects the cord from kinking and from pressing on the umbilical arteries and vein. The coils help ensure that there is a continuous flow of blood both to the placenta and also back to the baby.

“ Wanting to protect your baby is a natural maternal instinct and it's likely to have started already. ”

It's understandable that you want your baby to have the best start in life, but this may lead you to unnecessary anxiety about his health and well-being.

You may find yourself worried about things that previously did not bother you. For example, you may use a computer regularly and only now become concerned about the radiation it might produce (see box, below).

Try to relax and keep concerns in perspective; remember that your baby is very resilient and well-protected inside the uterus. If you have concerns about lifestyle issues or how your baby is developing, your doctor can provide information and reassurance.

Meanwhile, you can take good care of yourself by eating well, exercising regularly, and attending all your prenatal appointments.

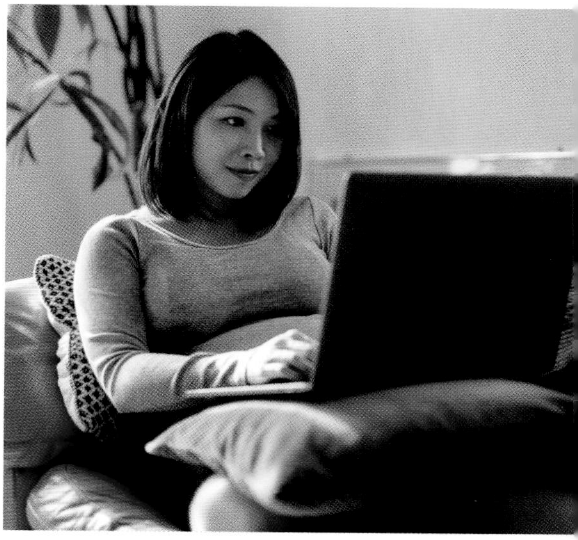

You may want to join online forums to share your pregnancy experience, but be aware of taking health advice from other parents-to-be. Your doctor is the best source of information.

COMPUTER USE

There is no significant radiation from a computer or tablet that can affect an unborn baby. For this reason, they aren't harmful to use during a pregnancy.

ASK A DOCTOR

Are there risks if I gain too much weight? If you gain a lot of weight in pregnancy it can be harder to shift it after the birth, so it's good to remember that you're not eating for two.

If you started pregnancy overweight or have gained a lot of weight, you may be more likely to experience health complications, such as developing gestational diabetes, hypertension (see p.475), and preeclampsia (see p.476), and deep-vein thrombosis (DVT; see p.186).

However, all these conditions can be managed so you shouldn't worry unnecessarily. Most women who are overweight have a straightforward pregnancy and give birth to a healthy baby.

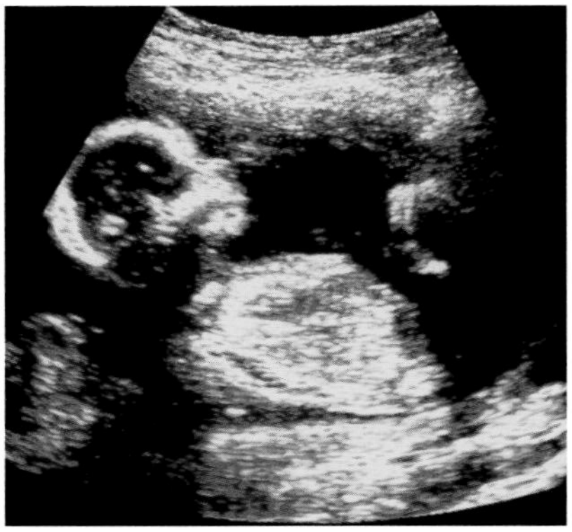

YOU ARE **18 WEEKS AND 4 DAYS**

150 days to go

YOUR BABY TODAY

This is a side view ultrasound scan with the baby's head in the top left. Your baby appears completely human with all fingers and toes fully developed. The skin is now covered with lanugo, fine protective hair.

> "There's no harm in encouraging your baby to move to increase the likelihood of you feeling his wiggles."

ASK A DOCTOR

Can I prompt my baby to move by playing loud music? Your baby cannot hear yet, so playing loud music won't have any effect. By about 22 weeks, they will be able to hear some sounds, by 24–25 weeks they'll be reacting to many sounds, and sudden noises may prompt a "startle" response (see p.256).

If you're waiting to feel your baby's first movements, be patient. Although it's reassuring to feel them wiggling around, becoming stressed about it won't be good for either of you. Remember, many pregnant women—first-time moms especially—don't feel those first flutterings until 18 to 20 weeks or later (see p.213).

It may be that you have been so busy and active that you have been distracted and not felt your baby's movements. So just stop and relax for a little while; when you're resting the movements will be much more obvious. Also remember that the baby does not move continuously and there will be periods when the baby is not moving.

There are a few things you can try to stimulate your baby into action—the more they move, the more chances there are that you'll feel it. It may help to lie down on your side, with your belly supported. If all else fails, sit down and rest while you have something sweet to eat or drink. This may just do the trick, because babies respond to a rise in their mother's blood sugar.

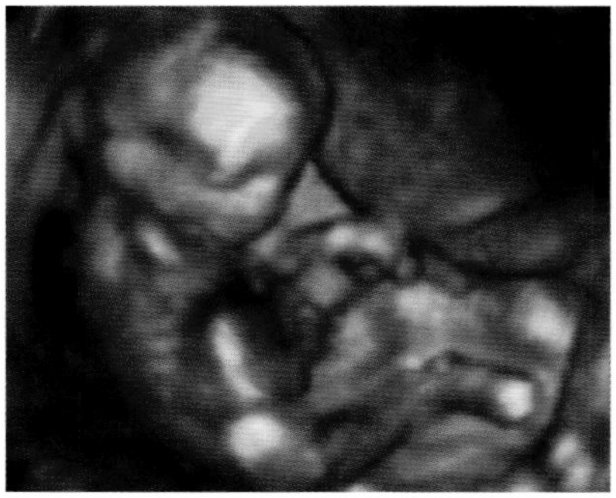

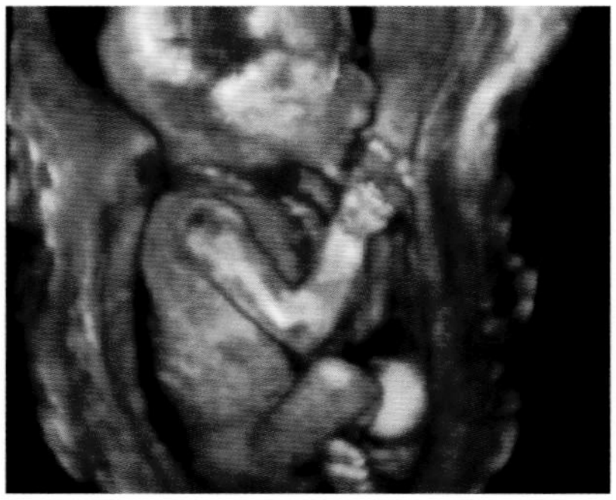

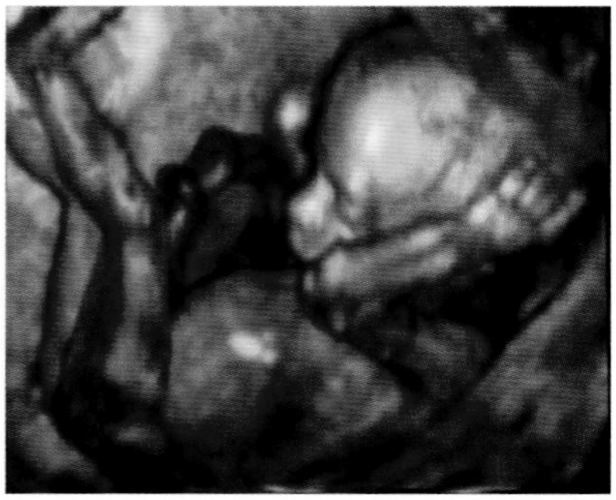

Ultrasound scans reveal a huge range of movement in between inactive periods. You will probably not be able to feel your baby move yet, but they are incredibly active inside your uterus. Somersaults and stretches are part of their daily routine, as are thumb and toe sucking. Your baby moves when awake and asleep; they have no control over their movements at this stage.

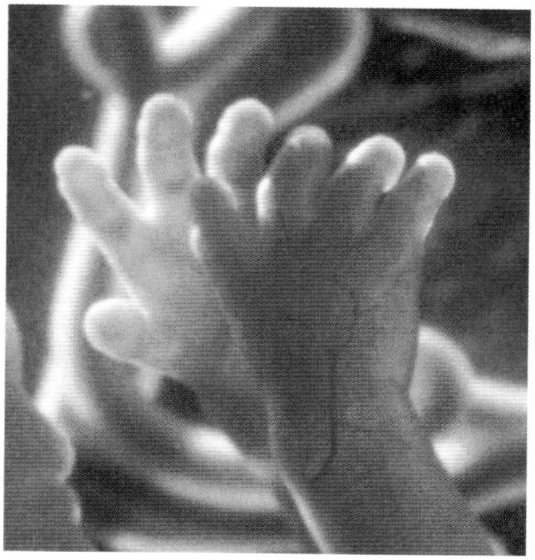

YOU ARE **18 WEEKS AND 5 DAYS**

149 days to go

YOUR BABY TODAY

Your baby's hands—and feet—look quite large at this stage in pregnancy: it is as if your baby needs time to grow into them. The past few weeks have seen rapid changes in the hands and feet and it's now time for the limbs to catch up.

Your baby will be a unique individual and their fingerprints will be proof of this. The ridge patterns in the dermis that will eventually form fingerprints (and "toeprints") are fully developed by this stage of pregnancy. These skin ridges are genetically determined and, as with most developments, are seen about a week earlier in the hands than the feet.

Your baby's sweat glands appeared in their skin in the eighth week, and will continue to increase up to 28 weeks; but they do not function until after birth. The color of your baby's skin is due to melanin, a pigment produced by "melanocytes," specialized skin cells that have now migrated into the skin. Different skin tones are not due to differing numbers of these cells but due to the amount and shade of pigment that each cell produces. Melanin protects the skin from ultraviolet light, which damages DNA.

Although unborn babies produce melanin pigment, they do not achieve their final amount of skin pigment until well into childhood. For this reason, it follows that all newborn babies are particularly vulnerable to sunburn. Dark-skinned babies are likely to have a light skin tone when they're born.

> "Your baby's fingers and toes are fully developed and their unique prints are beginning to form."

ACUPUNCTURE

In acupuncture, certain points on the body associated with energy channels or meridians are stimulated by the insertion of fine needles. The belief is that these conduct vital energy or "qi" around the body. Illness or symptoms are associated with an imbalance of this vital energy.

Acupuncture has been widely and successfully used in pregnancy and regular treatments can help to treat a number of health problems:

- Pain and nausea—a recent study has shown it to be effective in relieving nausea and vomiting or the potentially more dangerous hyperemesis gravidarum (see p.111)
- Heartburn (see p.194)
- Hemorrhoids (see p.470)
- Stress (see p.187)
- Headaches and backaches
- Carpal tunnel syndrome (see p.473).

Acupuncture may be effective in "turning" breech babies (see p.433), and can also be used during labor to boost energy and relieve pain.

Use a licensed acupuncturist with experience treating pregnant women.

VITAMIN E

Eating foods that are rich in vitamin E, especially avocados, boosts your immunity. Vitamin E is an antioxidant vitamin transported in oils and fats. The best known source of vitamin E is avocado, which is a great pregnancy food that's rich in monounsaturated oils (see p.204) and potassium, and is low GI, too (see p.92). Avocados are also great for starting babies on solid food, so get into the habit of buying them!

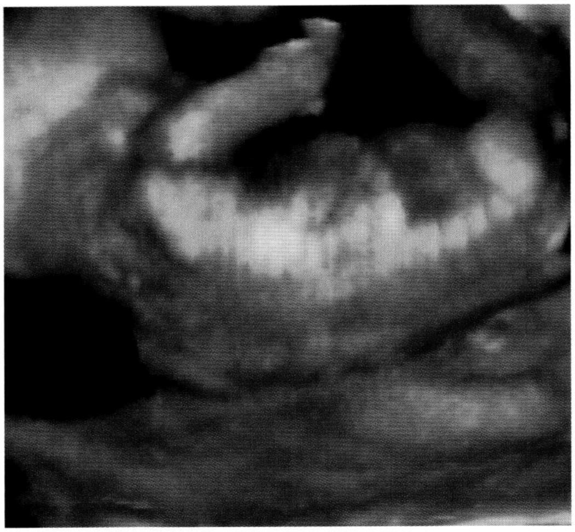

YOU ARE **18 WEEKS AND 6 DAYS**

148 days to go

YOUR BABY TODAY

Your baby appears to be quite thin on early scans. One reason is that fat reserves have not yet been laid down underneath the skin, which looks almost transparent. An ultrasound image also highlights the underlying bony skeleton, enhancing this effect.

> “At around this time you'll have another scan, and your baby will get a thorough health checkup.”

From 18–20 weeks most doctors' offices or hospitals offer a detailed ultrasound scan, which is termed an “anatomy” scan. The scan is used to check the baby's overall development and examine the organs and body systems (see pp.214–5) to check for signs of problems. For most women and their partners, this scan will reassure them that all is progressing well with the baby's development.

The scan can take some time to perform because of the detailed measurements and investigations taking place. The sonographer can do the checks only when the baby is in the correct position—this can be a challenge, given that the baby is likely to be moving around a lot. If the position of your baby makes it difficult to do all the checks, you may be asked to walk around for a little while and then return, or even to come back in a week or two for another attempt.

EXERCISING IN WATER

It's great to work out in water during pregnancy: the added support for your belly and extra resistance will enable you to maintain your fitness and tone. When standing, the water should be just above your waist with your knees slightly bent—too deep and you will not be stable enough; too shallow and you won't get enough support from the water.

- **Running in place:** bring your knees up to just below your waist and push your arms forward and back in a pumping motion under the water. Jog for 3 to 4 minutes, if possible, but always stop if you feel tired. This exercise has cardiovascular benefits, is a great warm up, and will help tone your legs and arms.
- **Bicycle exercise:** stand in the water and place a float under each arm. Lean back slightly and move your legs in front of you, as if you are rotating the pedals on a bicycle. Continue the cycling motion for 3 to 4 minutes, if possible, but always stop if you start feeling tired. This exercise will help you maintain your fitness and help tone your legs. It's also a good way to strengthen your back and arms. Stop if you feel any pain in your back or abdomen.
- **Arm exercises:** stand with your feet apart and knees slightly bent, then crouch to submerge your shoulders in the water. Lift your arms from your sides to the height of your shoulders and back down again. Pull your arms down in the water toward you and push up as hard as you can. Repeat several times. This exercise helps strengthen the muscles in your arms, back, and abdomen. Keep your arms submerged in the water.

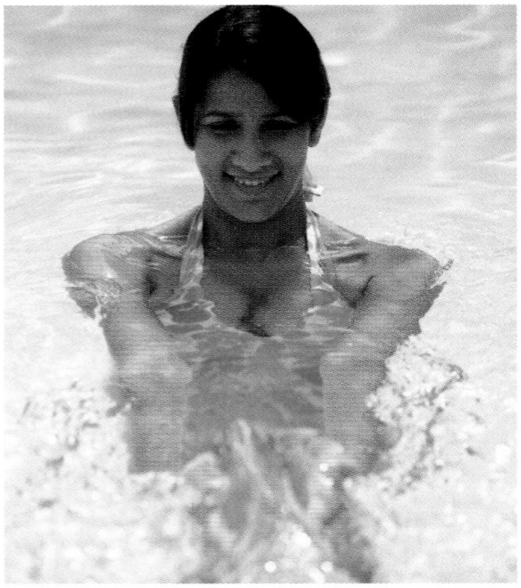

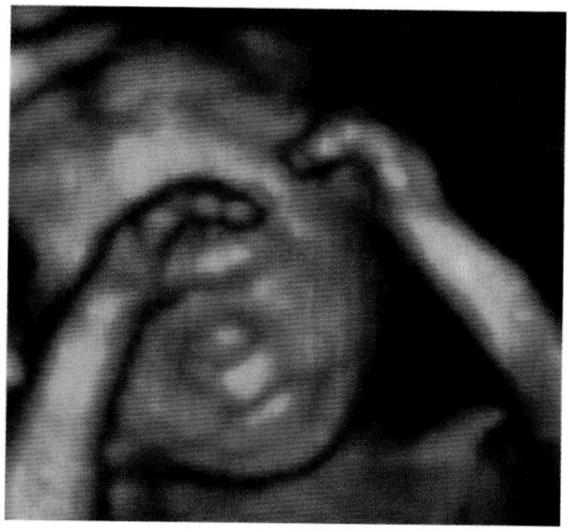

YOU ARE **19 WEEKS EXACTLY**

147 days to go

YOUR BABY TODAY

Your baby has highly flexible joints, enabling her to raise her arms high. This is because her bones are first made of cartilage, which is soft and flexible. Gradually, the cartilage is being replaced by calcium-containing bone.

> "You'll be getting advice from all quarters, but there's one person you might want to listen to—your mother."

Whether or not you're already close to your mother, being pregnant is likely to affect your relationship with each other. Many women feel naturally closer to their mothers as they go through this significant life event, turning to them for help and reassurance during the course of pregnancy and wanting them to be there in the days and weeks following the birth of the baby. It's normal for a mother to respond to her daughter being pregnant by being protective, so do expect more phone calls than usual. Your mother is bound to offer lots of advice. Whether or not you follow it all, listen—you may just find some of it useful.

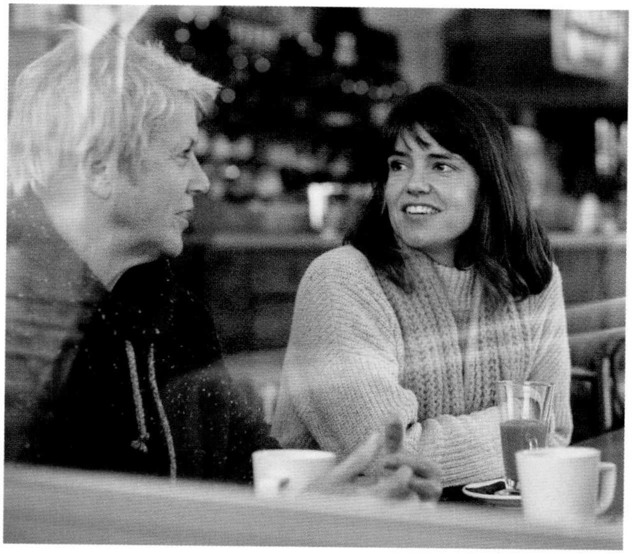

Your pregnancy is bound to trigger lots of memories for your mother of her own pregnancies, so expect to hear many stories of when you were a baby.

TAKING THE STRAIN

There are a number of changes in your body during pregnancy that impact how you can exercise and how your body moves:

- The increased weight of the baby, placenta, enlarged uterus, extra blood, and breast tissue can put stress on your body, especially your muscles and skeleton.
- Postural changes due to changes in the center of gravity can increase your chances of developing hip, back, and knee problems.
- Relaxin (see p.197), a pregnancy-related hormone that affects the ligaments, can increase flexibility and result in improper alignment of the spine and pelvis.

Effective and safe exercises are the most efficient way of maintaining and improving your posture and minimizing the stress on your body. Regular exercise (especially weight bearing such as walking and using weights) generally improves the bone density of your skeleton and your muscle strength.

Your 20th week

THOSE BUTTERFLIES IN YOUR STOMACH MAY BE MORE THAN JUST GAS. In the next few days, you might feel your baby's movements for the first time. The little flutter can be such a tiny sensation that many women write it off as gas. But what a wonderful moment when you realize the truth! If you want to find out the sex of your baby, it could be revealed on the ultrasound scan you have this week.

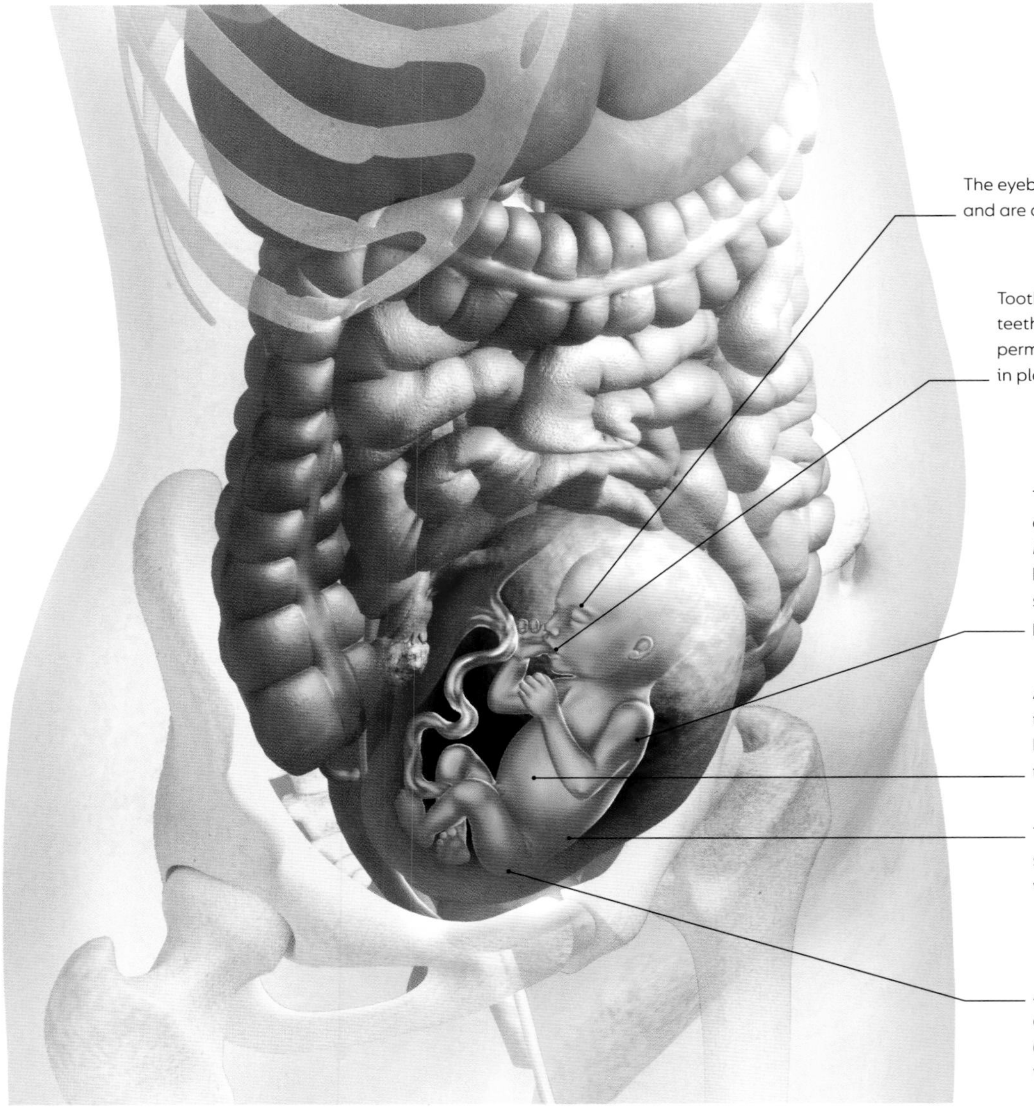
The eyebrows have thickened and are clearly visible.
Tooth buds, for both the baby teeth and the underlying permanent teeth, are now in place under the gums.
The baby's body has a covering of fine hair, called lanugo hair. Most of this hair disappears before birth, although it may still be present in very premature babies.
Abdominal organs, including the stomach, intestines, and liver, are fully enclosed within the abdominal cavity.
The spine is now quite straight. Your 20-week scan will reveal each vertebra.
At 20 weeks the average crown to heel length is 10 in (25.4 cm) and the average weight is 10.6 oz (300 g).

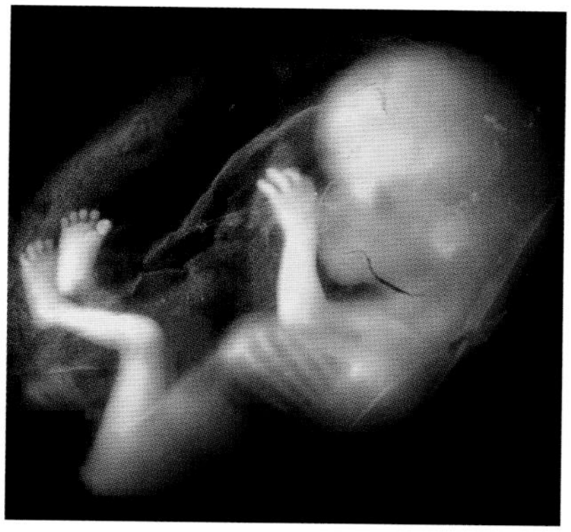

YOU ARE **19 WEEKS AND 1 DAY**

146 days to go

YOUR BABY TODAY

This image shows the entire baby lying within the amniotic sac. Every finger and toe, and even the lower ribs in the chest, can be seen. Although the head is still quite large, the limbs are much more in proportion with the body.

"If you want to know whether you're having a boy or a girl, this is the week you might be able to find out."

You'll have a scan this week and may be given the opportunity to find out the sex of your baby. Identifying the sex is dependent on the position of the baby, particularly the legs, which could obstruct the genitals. Even if all of these factors are favorable and the genitals can be seen, there is an error factor, so the information given is never 100 percent accurate. You may be able to identify the genitals yourself as you're watching the screen, so if you don't want to know, it's advisable to look away.

If you have an amniocentesis, CVS, or NIPT test (see pp.152–153) and want to know the sex of your baby, it can be identified with more accuracy.

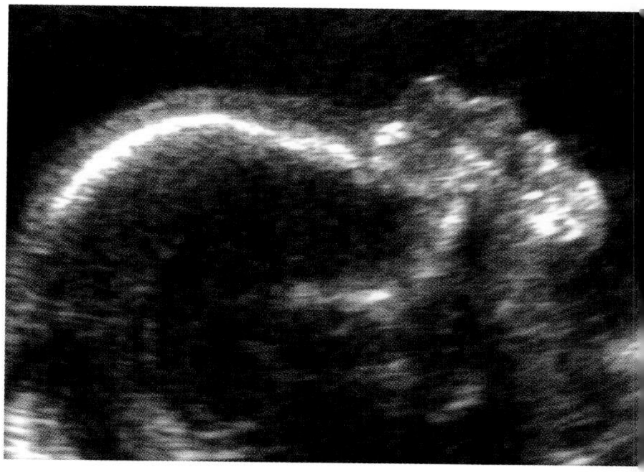

This 2-D scan is a close-up of the baby's profile, showing the bright frontal bone of the forehead, the nose, lips, and chin. The nasal bone appears as a bright area at the top of the bridge of the nose.

FINDING OUT THE SEX

Is it a good idea to find out the sex of your baby before they are born?

Yes...

- **Being able to call your baby** "he" or "she" rather than "it" or "the baby" may help you and your partner to bond with them.
- **Knowing the sex** means you can choose a name before the big day, although bear in mind that it's not guaranteed to suit them.
- **Decorating the nursery** and buying baby clothes may be simpler.

No...

- **Not knowing is a huge motivator** during labor and birth for many women, and the excitement of finding out right at the end can help keep you focused through all the stages of labor and delivery.
- **Unless you had** an amniocentesis, CVS, or NIPT test (see pp.152–153), there's no way of knowing your baby's sex for certain. Occasionally, sonographers can (and do) get it wrong, so don't get too attached to the name you've chosen.

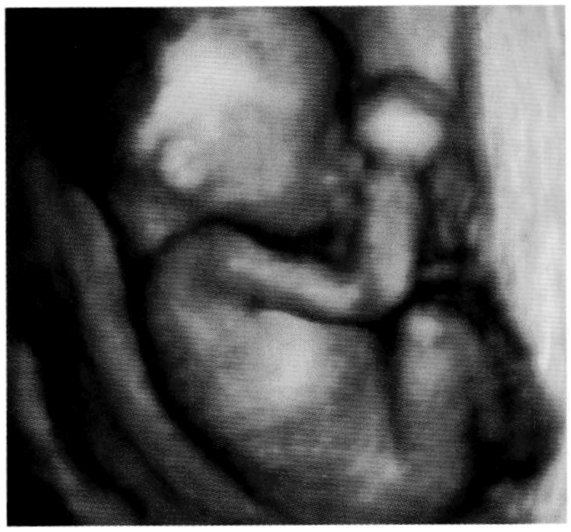

YOU ARE **19 WEEKS AND 2 DAYS**

145 days to go

YOUR BABY TODAY

Your baby is increasingly using their hands and feet to explore their surroundings. All limbs have a full and unobstructed range of movement and the fingertips especially are extremely sensitive. Most of their movements are reflex responses at this stage.

> "Comfortably floating in their fluid-filled amniotic sac, your baby is made up almost completely of water."

Because water can travel through the skin and the baby is floating in amniotic fluid, their water content is really high, nearly 90 percent. As your baby's skin thickens and becomes less permeable, and their kidneys better regulate the amount of water lost in the urine, their proportion of water will reduce to 70 percent at delivery and again to about 60 percent by the age of 10 as kidney function continues to improve.

Fluids conduct sound waves, but the inner ear is still immature and it will be three weeks before a startle response to sounds can be reliably seen on a scan. As both the uterine wall and the ear drums become thinner, they will gradually respond to higher frequencies and quieter sounds.

LOW-LYING PLACENTA

Placenta previa is when the placenta is either partially covering (incomplete) or completely covering (complete) the cervix. In complete placenta previa, the baby cannot be born vaginally. Complete previa poses a high risk of heavy bleeding, either in late pregnancy or during the actual labor, which is treated as an emergency.

If a low-lying placenta is detected at your 20-week scan, you will be scanned again at about 34 weeks; the placenta may "move up" as the uterus grows and no longer be low. In some cases of complete previa, you may be advised to stay in the hospital in later pregnancy in case you have a heavy bleed.

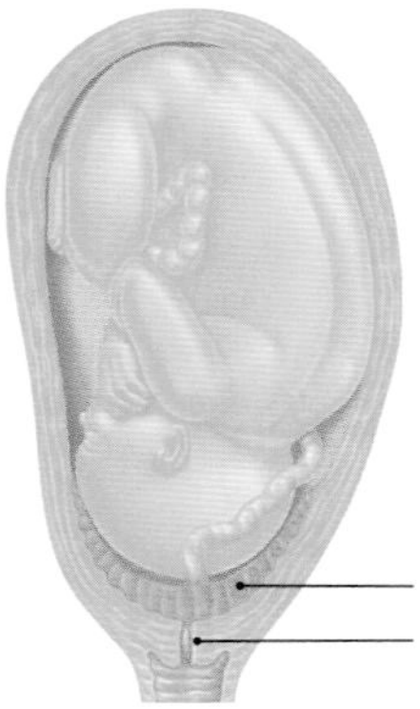
Complete placenta previa
Placenta fully covering cervix
Cervix

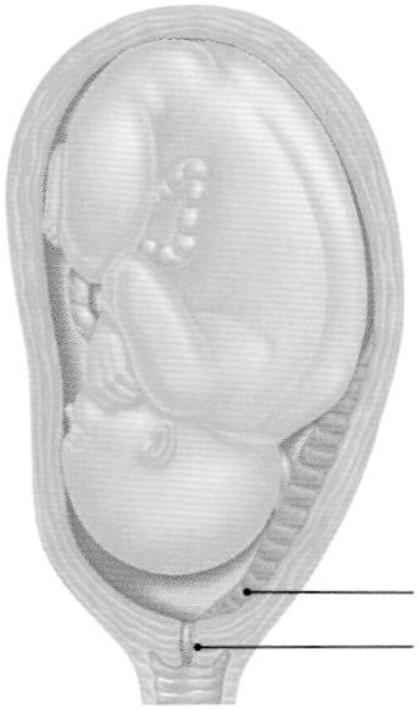
Incomplete placenta previa
Placenta partially covering cervix
Cervix

NUTRITIOUS SARDINES

Canned sardines are a highly nutritious food. A can of sardines provides omega-3, iron, zinc, vitamin B12 and—if you eat the bones—calcium, too. Try having them on toast or add them to a salad.

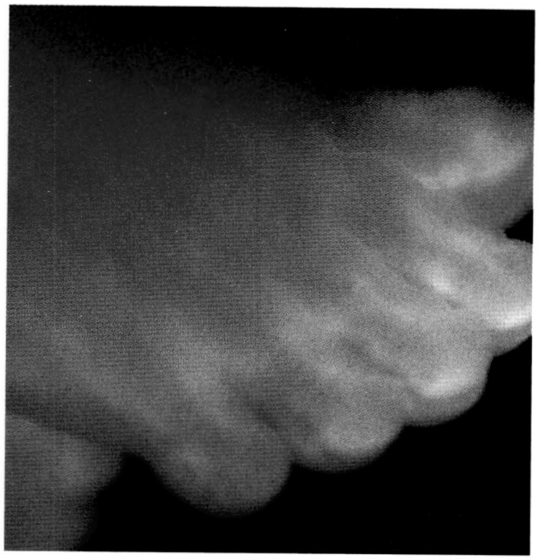

YOU ARE **19 WEEKS AND 3 DAYS**

144 days to go

YOUR BABY TODAY

The toes will wiggle and stretch just as much as the hands and fingers. Your baby is extremely flexible at this time and as likely to bring one or both feet up to their mouth as their hands in order to explore them with her sensitive mouth and lips.

At around this time, you're likely to feel that awe-inspiring first kick. While your baby has been moving in your uterus since around the sixth week of gestation, it's only at this stage that they'll make their movements so definitely felt (although some women do feel movements from around 15 to 16 weeks). When exactly you feel that movement can be affected by your body weight, your baby's position, the location of your placenta, and whether it's your first pregnancy.

Experiencing the first sensation of movement, whether it's a feeling of bubbles, butterflies, flipping goldfish, or even a resounding kick, is likely to be an emotionally charged moment. After all, this is the first time your baby has communicated with you, even though they're not aware of it.

Once you've felt your baby move, you may want to feel it over and over again—just to make sure you didn't imagine it the first time. You may, however, not feel another movement for a few days.

A good time to feel the baby moving is when you're relaxed and resting. Your partner may want to place their hand on your belly to experience those first thumps. It won't hurt your baby.

“ Feeling your baby moving is a wonderful pregnancy milestone and so reassuring! ”

MATERNITY SWIMWEAR

Swimming is fantastic exercise during pregnancy, but you may need to invest in new swimwear as your breasts and abdomen grow.

- **Comfort and support:** maternity swimsuits have additional support. These swimsuits are designed to be higher at the back and have more support in the cups. Maternity swimwear is made with stretchy fabric that is comfortable and will give as you grow.
- **Try a tankini:** this is a two-piece swimsuit that has a tank-style, rather than bra, top. It will flash your belly without revealing too much.
- **If you're self-conscious** about your belly, wear a sarong. If you prefer to bare your belly to females only, go to women's sessions at your local pool.

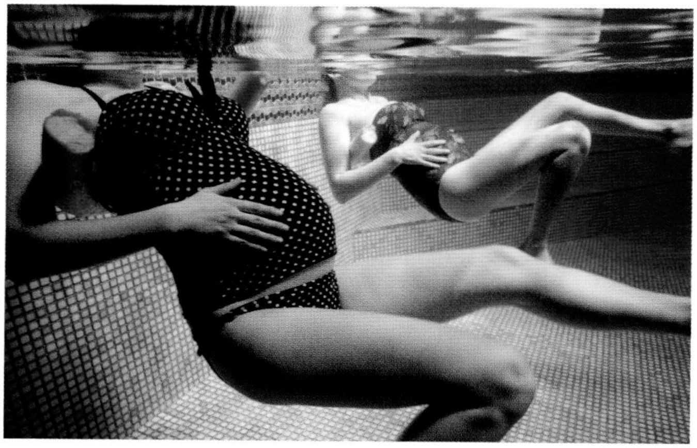

Your 20-week scan

This second-trimester ultrasound, typically done between 18–22 weeks, looks in detail at how your baby's major organs and body systems have developed, as well as checks the placenta and the volume of the amniotic fluid.

What the scan reveals

This scan will be done between 18 and 22 weeks. By this time, your baby's organs and body systems are well developed and can be seen clearly on an ultrasound scan. The sonographer performing the scan will look closely at how your baby's major organs and body systems have formed and whether there are any indications of a problem (see box, below). In the majority of cases, the scan will reassure women that their baby is developing normally.

If your baby is found to have a problem, the sonographer will refer you to a maternal medicine expert who will confirm the findings and offer follow-up ultrasound scans throughout the rest of your pregnancy. She will also talk to a pediatrician to make sure that they have enough information to take care of your baby at birth.

Your due date

If you had a scan in the first trimester, your dates are unlikely to be changed after a second-trimester scan. This is because dating is most accurate in early pregnancy when all babies essentially grow at the same rate. Later on, individual differences in growth start to appear, making it harder to tell if your baby is just big for gestational age or if you are further along than thought.

However, if you didn't have a first-trimester ultrasound, the sonographer may change your dates if your baby is 10–14 days smaller or larger than expected. If your dates have been confirmed by a first-trimester scan, a substantial lag may be a sign of a growth problem (see p.284), although this is rare at this early gestation.

Measuring your baby Because your whole baby no longer fits on the screen, the crown–rump length won't be measured. Instead, your baby's size will be calculated by combining a series of measurements in a mathematical formula. The sonographer will measure the width (biparietal diameter) and circumference of your baby's head, the circumference of your baby's tummy (abdominal circumference), and the length of your baby's upper leg bone (femur length). These measurements help estimate the size of your baby and check that this is within the normal range for this stage of pregnancy.

Placenta and amniotic fluid

The placenta will be examined to ensure that it appears normal and isn't blocking the baby's exit route (the cervix). In early pregnancy the placenta may be low-lying (see p.212). This is more common in subsequent pregnancies. In most cases, the placenta moves up and out of the way by the third trimester as the uterus grows.

If your placenta is low lying, your doctor will arrange a follow-up scan later in pregnancy to check that the placenta has moved up out of the way. If a later scan shows that it has failed to move up, a condition known as

THE ULTRASOUND

The baby's organs are examined in detail and therefore it can take a little longer than previous scans. If the result of your PAPP-A test (see p. 142) was low, or you have other risk factors for preeclampsia, you may also be offered a Doppler scan to look at the blood flow in the uterine arteries. The scan checks:

- **The brain,** including the fluid-filled spaces inside the brain and the shape of the back of your baby's brain (cerebellum).
- **The spine** for spina bifida or other spinal problems.
- **The upper lip** for cleft lip (see p.478).
- **The heart,** and the heartbeat, to rule out any major heart malformation.
- **The stomach** and diaphragm.
- **The kidneys and bladder,** making sure that both kidneys are present and there are no blockages or malformations.
- **The abdominal wall,** to look for a defect, known as gastroschisis.
- **Your baby's limbs,** to make sure there are no hand or feet malformations, such as club foot.
- **The umbilical cord,** to check that this has a normal number of blood vessels.

placenta previa (see p.475), you will be monitored until the birth. The amniotic fluid is assessed. Too little can indicate a problem with fetal growth or the baby's renal tract; it may also be due to early membrane rupture. Too much fluid can be normal but is also seen in diabetic pregnancies and, very rarely, in esophageal atresia, where the baby cannot swallow causing a buildup of amniotic fluid.

Uterine artery Dopplers

If you are at increased risk of developing preeclampsia, you may be offered a Doppler scan to measure the blood flow in the uterine arteries. If there is a resistance to the flow, you may be at increased risk of preeclampsia or growth problems in the baby and will be offered extra monitoring and scans.

Detecting markers

Ultrasound at this stage of pregnancy is not a reliable way to detect Down syndrome—only about 60 percent of babies will have markers or signs of Down syndrome. Some of these markers, for example, a bright spot in the baby's heart, extra fluid in the kidneys, and short arms or legs, can occur even when the baby is not affected by Down syndrome. Some specific abnormalities are linked with a far higher risk of Down or other chromosomal abnormalities. These include certain kinds of heart defects and other major malformations, such as abnormalities in the bowel.

An ultrasound scan can detect almost all babies with Edwards and Patau syndromes (see p.142) since these conditions are associated with very significant abnormalities. However, a diagnostic test will still be required.

HOW THE SCAN IS INTERPRETED

During your ultrasound, a picture of your baby is produced when high-frequency sound waves bounce off your baby's organs and tissues and translate into an image on-screen. In this image, solid matter, such as bones, are white, while softer tissue appears gray. Areas that contain fluid, such as blood vessels or the stomach, as well as the amniotic fluid, do not respond to the sound waves and therefore appear as black areas on the scan. The sonographer will study these details to assess how your baby is developing in the uterus.

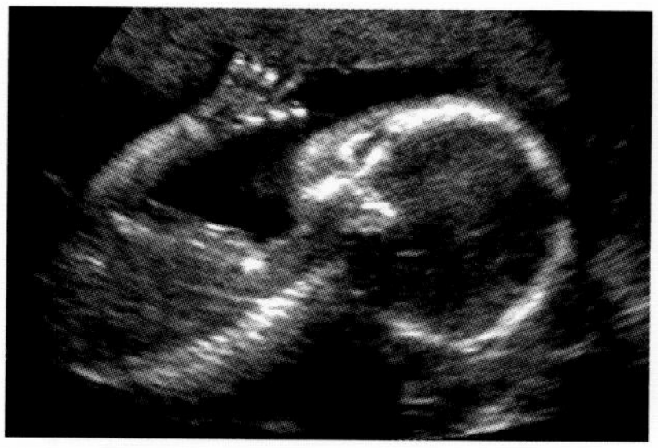

The skull is well developed by now, and features such as the ears are clearly seen.

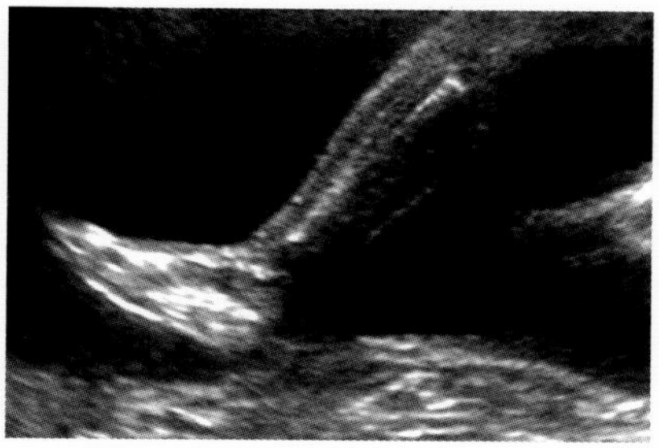

The leg bones are measured to assess how your baby is growing.

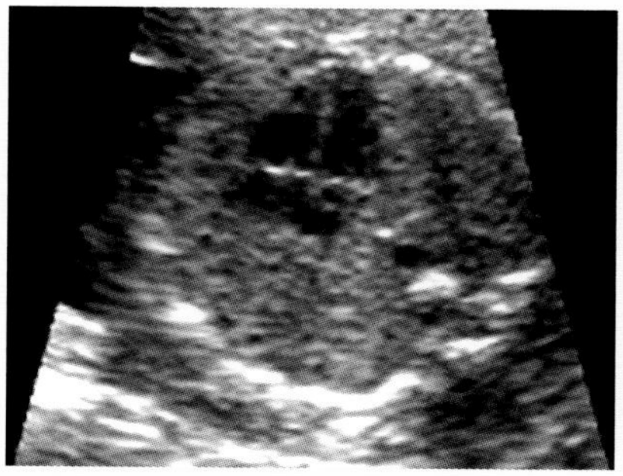

The four chambers of the heart can be identified and certain defects spotted.

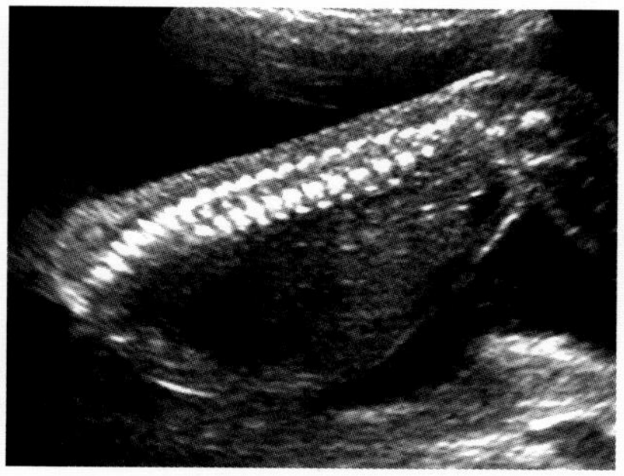

Each vertebra in your baby's spine will be counted to check for spina bifida.

What happens next If soft markers are detected, a diagnostic test (see p.152) may be suggested, especially if you already have an increased risk of Down syndrome. However, an earlier all-clear from a diagnostic test means that you can be confident your baby's chromosomes are normal. If an obvious abnormality is seen, and you haven't had a diagnostic test, this will probably be strongly advised. Whatever your decision, any associated abnormalities will be monitored.

Boy or girl?

Unless your baby is curled up or the legs are closed tight, the sonographer will have a good idea as to whether you're having a boy or a girl. If you don't want to know the sex, tell the sonographer at the start of the scan.

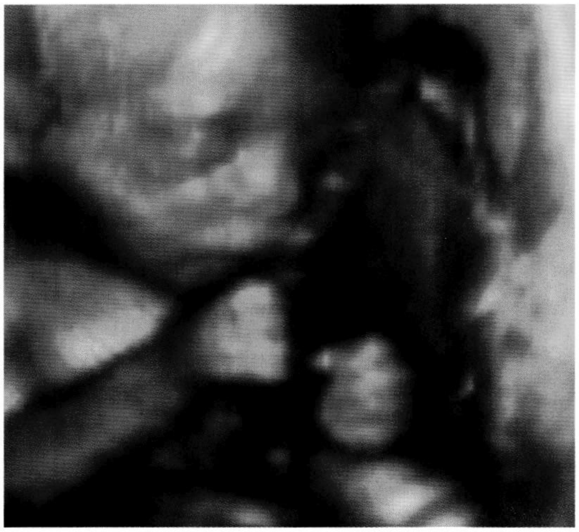

YOU ARE **19 WEEKS AND 4 DAYS**

143 days to go

YOUR BABY TODAY

The appearance of your baby's head is still dominated by a prominent forehead due to the rapidly growing brain. The jaw can seem small but as the tooth buds grow and expand within the jaw, it lengthens and changes proportion.

FEELING FLEXIBLE

Being flexible enables your muscles to work more efficiently, alleviates tightness, helps prevent cramping, and leads to improved balance and posture. Stretching can also help you feel confident and calm, especially if the exercises are combined with deep breathing.

Flexibility can be maintained or improved during pregnancy by doing a series of exercises that stretch your muscles in a safe and effective way.

- **Do not stretch further** than feels comfortable or you risk injuring the muscles and stressing your joints.
- **Ensure that you're stretching** when the muscles are warm, at the end of a workout or after a warm bath.

During the second and third trimester you should avoid any exercises—stretching or otherwise—that require you to lie on your back for extended periods of time.

FETAL ALCOHOL SYNDROME (FAS)

Fetal alcohol syndrome (FAS) is a serious lifelong condition. FAS will affect the behavior, learning ability, and appearance of a child throughout life. The teeth, especially, will be adversely affected.

Although it's very rare for any teeth to have come through by birth (only a 1 in 3,000 chance), your baby's tooth buds that will form the teeth are already in place within the jawbone.

All of the teeth—both the baby teeth and the underlying permanent teeth—start their development beneath the gums while the baby is developing in the uterus. The baby teeth buds began to develop at eight weeks of pregnancy and by this week all of the buds are formed.

The first baby teeth to harden, as calcium builds up, are the central incisor teeth and the last are the back molars, at around 19 weeks. The crown of each baby tooth does not complete development until after birth and root completion takes until your child is more than three years old.

Buds for the permanent teeth begin to form between the 14th and 20th weeks. These lie deeper than those for the baby teeth and closer to the inner edge of the jaw and gum. They remain dormant until it is time for the baby teeth to be lost.

Your baby's baby teeth will start coming through at around six to eight months and she'll have a complete set of baby teeth by the age of 2½.

" The foundations are already laid for your baby's teeth—both the baby teeth and the permanent ones that will follow. "

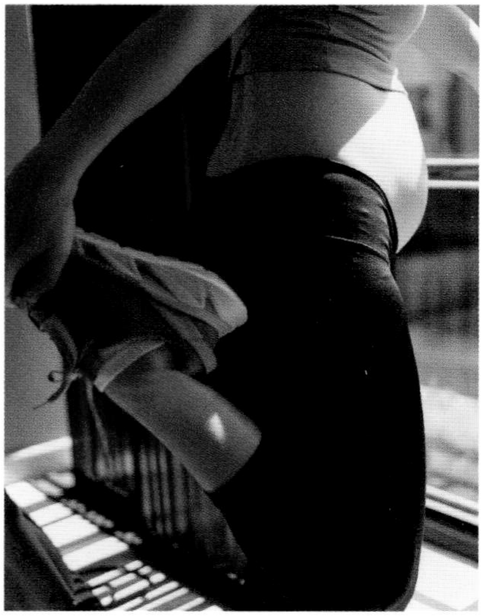

To stretch your calf, lean against a solid support. Keep your front leg bent and straighten the other leg behind you. Hold still for 20 seconds. Repeat with the other leg.

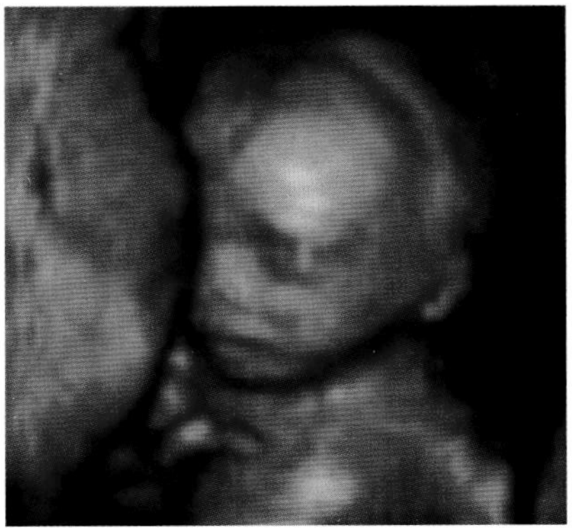

YOU ARE **19 WEEKS AND 5 DAYS**

142 days to go

YOUR BABY TODAY

Your baby often rests against the placenta. This has no effect on the placenta since its surface is protected by the amniotic sac and its composition and blood flow maintain its circulation at all times, leaving your baby free to explore her environment.

By this stage, you may find it tiring to be on your feet for long periods of time. For one thing, the growing weight of your baby and uterus will lead to discomfort, and potentially to muscle strain. Because your center of gravity is shifting, too, you may find that you stand awkwardly, putting pressure on your ligaments, which are, themselves, softened due to hormonal changes (see p.197). What's more, prolonged standing can cause blood and other fluids to pool in your legs, which can cause pain and dizziness.

If possible, take short, frequent breaks, so that you can put your feet up. If you do have to stand for long periods, you may find that resting one foot on a stool or box from time to time can help. Make sure your shoes offer good support (see p.257), and consider wearing maternity hose (see p.225).

Try not to stand for more than three hours at a time. If your work involves standing, make sure you have adequate breaks and walk around when you can.

> "As the weeks go by, you'll find that you'll need to rest more and limit the amount of time you are on your feet."

ASK A DOCTOR

The bigger I get, the more difficult it's becoming to have sex. What should we do? As your pregnancy continues, you will have no choice but to try new sexual positions that will more easily accommodate your growing belly.

You can still use the missionary position but your partner may have to support his weight on his hands instead of lying on you; that way he won't press on your belly. However, you'll find that positioning yourself on top is a better alternative, and as your belly gets bigger you can squat or kneel over your partner. Side-by-side or rear-entry positions are also comfortable during pregnancy. Have fun experimenting to find out what's right for you.

YOUR BABY'S FIRST TASTE

The flavors from the foods you eat will be transferred to the amniotic fluid, which is swallowed by your baby in the uterus. Therefore the types of food you eat can influence your baby before her first exposure to solid foods.

Studies show that prenatal and postpartum (through breast milk) exposure to a flavor enhances a baby's enjoyment of it in solid foods. These early flavor experiences may provide the foundation for healthy choices, as well as explain the cultural and ethnic differences in cuisine. So get your baby started on the road to good food choices by making healthy selections now.

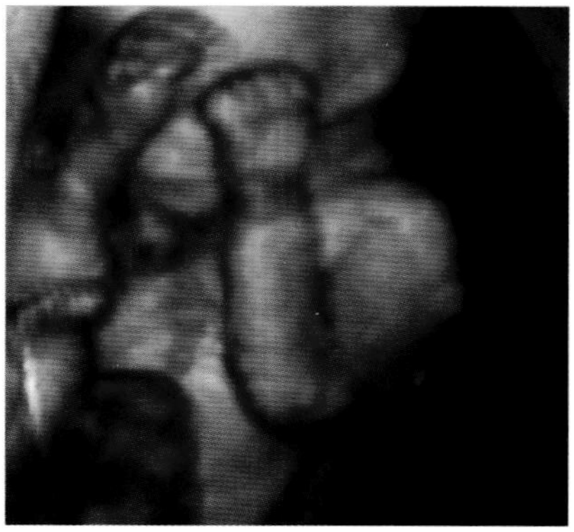

YOU ARE **19 WEEKS AND 6 DAYS**

141 days to go

YOUR BABY TODAY

You will become much more aware of your baby moving as her size and strength increase. You will not be aware of the more gentle movements, or those movements that do not hit the side of the uterus.

“ You’re likely to experience some backaches as your baby grows in size and your body continually adapts to accommodate. ”

The increasing weight of your developing baby, and the fact that your joints and ligaments soften in pregnancy, can cause backaches, but thankfully you don’t just have to put up with this pain. There are many simple ways in which you can ease a backache or even prevent it (see below).

See your doctor to make sure that the problem and its exact location is properly diagnosed. This way you’ll have more chance of stopping it from becoming worse. A common problem, often in later pregnancy, is sciatica (see p.4720)—a sharp pain that travels down the back and leg.

BANISH BACKACHES

To nip backaches in the bud, try the following:

- **Take a warm bath** or use a hot-water bottle on the painful area.
- **Ask your partner** to give you a nice back rub, or get yourself a massage with an experienced prenatal practitioner.
- **Go to yoga or Pilates classes** to strengthen your back muscles.
- **Watch your posture** (see p.249), and raise your legs when seated.
- **Ensure your car seat** is properly positioned to support your back.

FIBROIDS DURING PREGNANCY

In the second trimester, fibroids—which are benign masses of muscle fiber within the uterine wall, or occasionally attached to it—can become problematic. Increased levels of the hormones estrogen and progesterone during pregnancy encourage fibroids to grow along with the uterus.

In some circumstances, the rapid growth of a fibroid causes feelings of pressure, discomfort, or pain. Fibroids may increase a woman’s risk of miscarriage, preterm birth, or having a baby in the breech position. Fibroids that do not cause discomfort do not require treatment.

Fibroids will not usually affect the developing baby, but if a large fibroid is positioned low down in the uterus or near to the cervix, it can prevent the baby from descending into the pelvis, and a cesarean delivery will be necessary.

Once the baby is born and the uterus shrinks, fibroids also usually shrink.

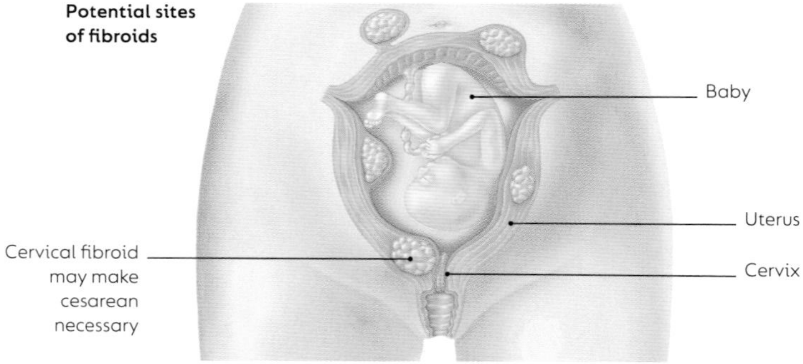
Potential sites of fibroids
Baby
Uterus
Cervix
Cervical fibroid may make cesarean necessary

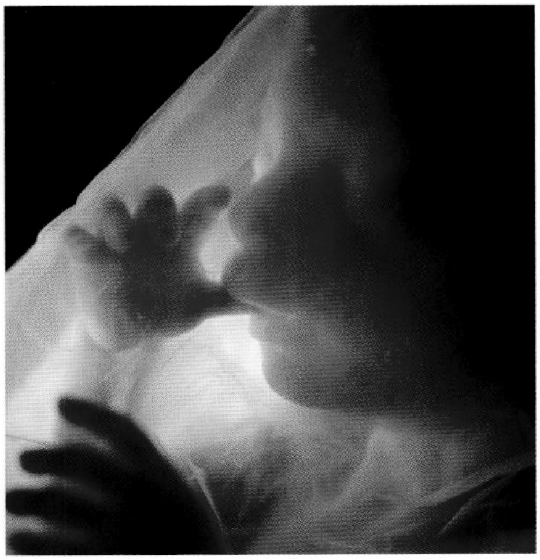

YOU ARE **20 WEEKS EXACTLY**

140 days to go

YOUR BABY TODAY

Although your baby may be sucking their thumb, this is a very complex action that is not fully developed at this stage. For this reason, your baby is as likely to put their fingers or toes in their mouth as their thumb.

Does it seem like a lifetime, or has it flown by? At least from now on, you really will be counting down.

The gestation period for an elephant is 22 months, the longest of any land animal. In addition, the common birth weight for elephants is 265lb (120kg). So, if your pregnancy is already starting to feel long, and your baby a tad heavy, spare a thought for our large-eared friends!

Hopefully, at this halfway point you are feeling fine physically. You're not yet encumbered by a large belly and probably have a reasonable amount of energy. Psychologically, you may still be very emotional, although you will no doubt have gotten used to any mood swings by now (as will your partner).

At this stage you will continue going to prenatal appointments around every four weeks. Remember, your doctor is there to monitor your health and your baby's progress, but also to help, so do get advice on how to cope with some of the discomforts you might experience as you grow bigger.

“ Congratulations—you're now halfway through your pregnancy. In around 20 weeks' time, you'll be a mom. ”

ASK A DOCTOR

I haven't felt my baby move yet. Should I be worried? While you understandably want to feel your baby's movements, there is no cause for concern yet since your recent scan should have shown you that all is well with your baby.

If it's your first baby, you may not notice the early movements since you won't know what to expect. Also, if you're an active person, these slight flutters may be missed. Women with a placenta lying at the front of the uterus may feel movements later, as may larger women since the movement may not be detected through the flesh.

Once you do feel movements, don't become too focused on every one. It's not until after 24 weeks that it becomes important to monitor the pattern. From this stage, the amount your baby moves, as well as the type of movement and when it happens, are relevant since these indicate that the placenta is sustaining the pregnancy and your baby is healthy.

If you're concerned about lack of movement from your baby at any stage of your pregnancy, speak to your midwife or contact your maternity unit as soon as you become concerned.

SITTING CORRECTLY

Good posture can help to minimize pregnancy discomforts, including backaches (see opposite). When seated, make sure your lower back is supported by the back of the chair or a pillow. Keep your feet flat on the floor (see below).

Consider doing pregnancy yoga—it is a great way to learn to keep your spine aligned and your lower back supported.

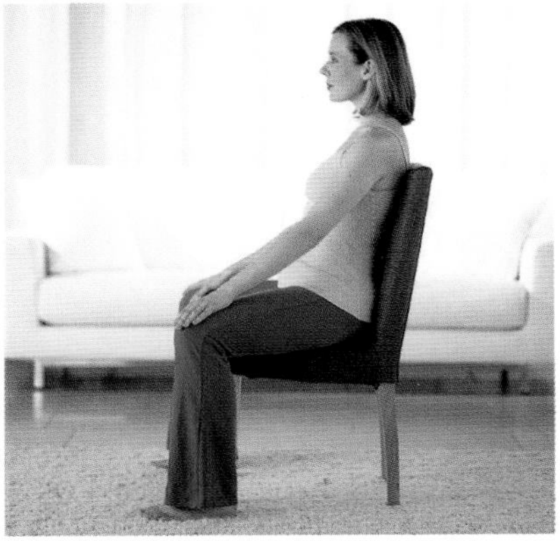

Your 21st week

YOU'RE HALFWAY THROUGH YOUR PREGNANCY ALREADY—IT'S ALL HAPPENING SO FAST. Not all women happily accept their changing body shape, even though they're overjoyed to be pregnant. But a belly "bump" doesn't have to mean frump. You've got a good excuse to treat yourself to a few attractive maternity clothes or to indulge in some pampering, perhaps by having a gentle massage. Keep up your exercise routine, because you'll feel energized and all the better for it.

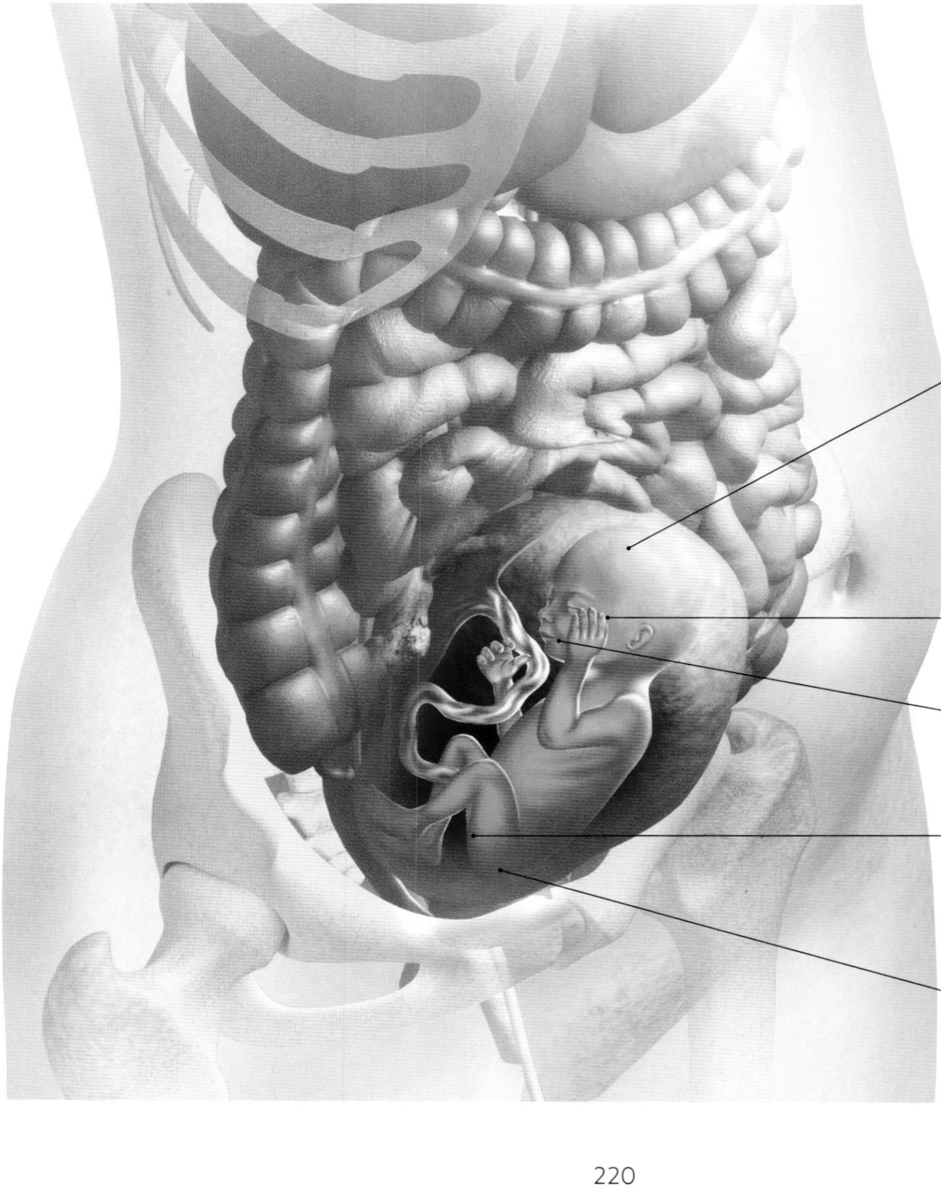
The developing brain is picking up electrical signals from the baby's body about sensations such as pressure and temperature. At this stage, a baby's nervous reactions are not conscious but simply reflexes.
Fingernails are beginning to grow. There's no danger of the baby scratching himself, since his skin is covered in vernix, a protective waxy coating.
The baby is regularly swallowing the amniotic fluid in increasing amounts.
In girl babies the ovaries have descended from the abdomen into the pelvis.
At 21 weeks the average crown to heel length is 10.5 in (26.7 cm) and the average weight is 12.7 oz (360 g).

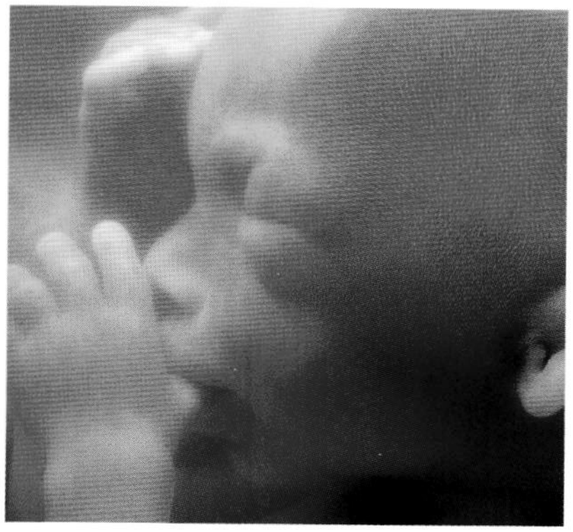

YOU ARE **20 WEEKS AND 1 DAY**

139 days to go

YOUR BABY TODAY

Your baby's movements are still based on a set of reflex actions but this is now beginning to change. As the nerve pathways develop, expand, and mature, your baby gains greater and greater control of their actions.

Your prenatal appointments will become more frequent in the second half of your pregnancy. Even if you are in good health, and your baby has been thoroughly assessed at the 20-week ultrasound scan (see pp.214–5), it can be reassuring to have these regular checkups with the doctor.

The number of appointments you have will differ depending on whether you've had any complications, or whether you are having a high-risk pregnancy for another reason, such as a preexisting medical condition like diabetes. If it's a low-risk pregnancy, you can expect around 14 appointments unless there are complications. As a general rule you can expect to have prenatal appointments from now on: every 4 weeks until you reach 30 weeks' gestation, then appointments at 2-week intervals until you reach 36 weeks' gestation. From then on, you'll have appointments weekly. And if you pass your due date (see p.139), you'll need to see your doctor once or twice weekly However, do contact your doctor if you have any concerns.

If you're expecting twins, appointments will be more frequent and will depend on the type of twins you're having: whether they are nonidentical or identical. If identical, care will depend on whether they share any of their support system (see p.130).

“You're in the second half of your pregnancy and in the months that follow you'll have more regular contact with your doctor.”

MATERNITY CLOTHES

With your usual office clothing feeling very tight, you might have to rethink your work wardrobe. The good news is that, unlike in years gone by, there is now a wealth of beautiful maternity clothing available and much at affordable everyday prices. These are often designed as coordinated sets, which makes putting them together easy.

Remember that you'll be wearing maternity clothing for a few months, and it's easy to become bored by the same items. If possible, designate a little of your wardrobe budget to buy yourself something monthly. If you're tired of your elasticated trousers and smock dress, buy a shirt or jacket to jazz them up; wear them unbuttoned if necessary.

Don't hesitate to accept hand-me-downs; even if they are not right for your office dress code, wearing them at home will enable you to spend a little more on work clothing. And don't forget your shoes; if you were a stiletto girl before becoming pregnant, you'll need to rethink (see p.257).

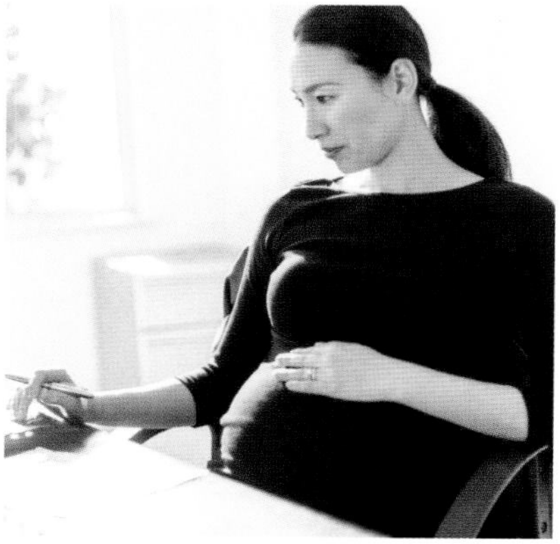

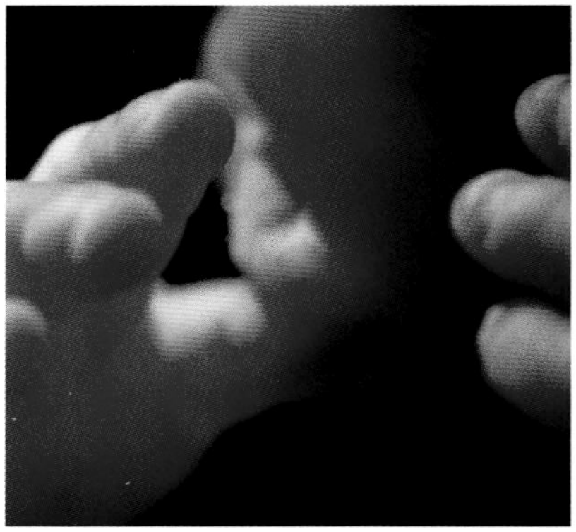

YOU ARE **20 WEEKS AND 2 DAYS**

138 days to go

YOUR BABY TODAY

This close-up of the fingertips shows that the nail beds have formed and the nails are starting to grow. The nails have not yet hardened: this prevents your baby from scratching himself accidentally while he has no control over hand movements.

> “Twin babies have been sharing a home in the uterus for a while now, but how are they relating to each other?”

At 21 weeks, a baby's eyes are still closed, but he'll still be aware of light and dark. Because of this, twins can probably make out their sibling changing position and they're increasingly becoming aware of each other. It's thought that because memory starts developing around now, twin babies may begin to bond at this stage.

As ultrasound scanning has proven, there's plenty of contact between twin babies in the uterus, especially as the amount of space decreases. They have been seen to touch often, kick, and try to grab each other. Each twin reacts to the other's movements.

They may not act in the same way, with one twin favoring different movements than the other one. For instance, one baby may prefer sucking his thumb, while the other likes clutching his cord. Nor do they necessarily have the same body clock, so they may be active at different times.

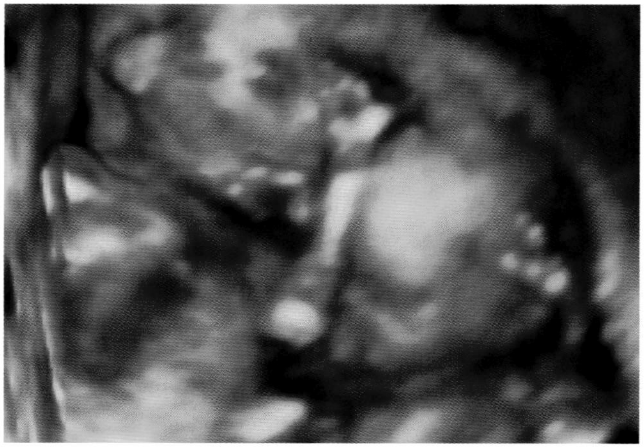

As the pregnancy progresses, contact between your twin babies will increase. Because you'll have more ultrasound scans in a twin pregnancy, you'll have plenty of opportunities to see them interacting with each other.

ASK A DOCTOR

Can my baby feel anything when we have sex? The baby may be aware of some movements when you have sex and of a change in your heart rate, but they won't be harmed by either. You may find that your baby responds to these sensations by moving a lot while you're having sex, or just afterward. Some women find this inhibiting, but remember that it doesn't mean the baby is uncomfortable and, of course, they doesn't understand what you're doing! If you have an orgasm, your uterus will feel tight and you may have Braxton-Hicks contractions (see p.410) but, again, this is not harmful to your baby.

Be reassured that your baby is well protected by the pool of amniotic fluid. Also, the cervix is closed by a plug of mucus during pregnancy so no semen can enter the uterus; this helps to guard against infection.

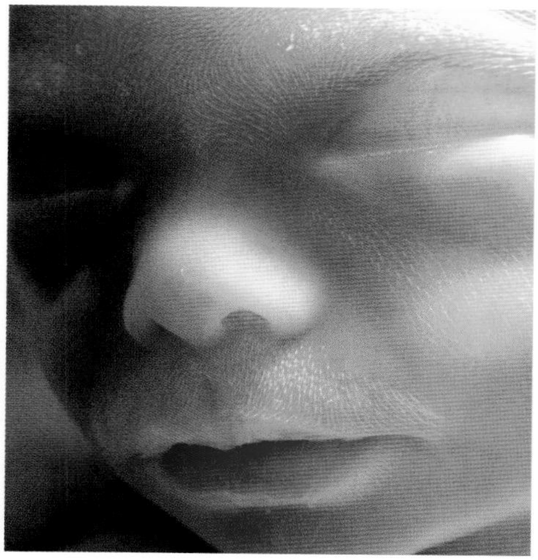

YOU ARE **20 WEEKS 3 DAYS**

137 days to go

YOUR BABY TODAY

The eyelids are still fused shut to protect your baby's developing eyes from prying fingers and toes. Deep within the brain, connections are starting to form to link the senses to those areas within the brain that are able to process information.

> "Part of the fun of not knowing your baby's sex is anticipating what it might be, but be prepared for others to do the same."

If you and your partner decided against finding out the sex of your baby at the 20-week scan, the guessing games will begin and you won't be short of people telling you what they think you're having.

Perhaps your own instinct is the best of all: in one research study that asked pregnant women to guess the sex of their baby, 71 percent of the expectant moms surveyed guessed correctly.

SOME OLD WIVES' TALES

If you like testing a few old wives' tales on gender, consider these:

- **Ask someone to tie a gold ring** on to a piece of string and dangle it over your belly to "dowse" for the sex. If it swings from side to side or back and forth, it's a boy; if it spins around in a circular motion, you're having a girl.
- **Hairier than usual?** Apparently, according to the "old wives," you're more likely to be carrying a boy.
- **If your baby's heart rate** is faster than 140 beats per minute, you're having a girl (but see p.188!).
- **Craving sugar, spice,** and all things sweet: girl. Sour or salty foods: boy.

ASK A MOM

I've found out at the 20-week scan that I'm having my third girl, but I so wanted a boy. How can I feel better about this? It can be enormously disappointing. I felt that I'd let my husband down in some way, especially since I knew he wanted a son.

By the time our daughter was born, we were both over the disappointment and were able to focus on being parents. If we'd waited until the birth to find out, it would have been hard to come to terms with it at the same time as trying to bond with our newborn baby.

At the moment, it may be difficult to imagine loving another daughter, but you will do, in time. Try to focus on the fact that she is healthy and that you're having a beautiful baby.

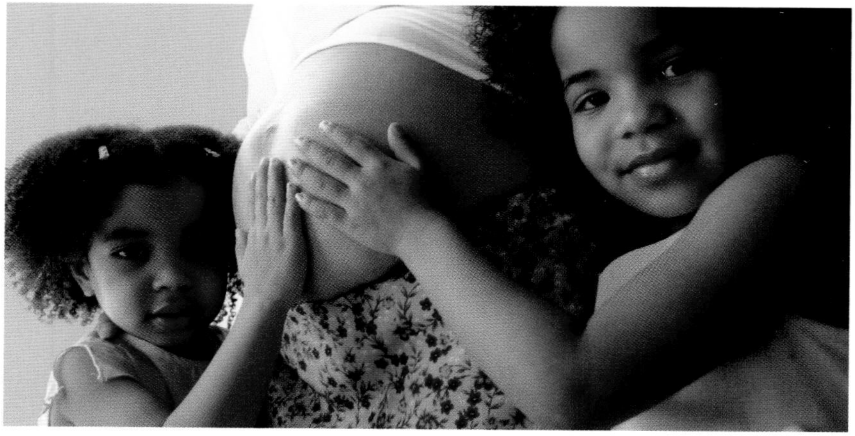

Although you may prefer to have a child of a different gender, you might find that your children are delighted to be having another same-sex playmate.

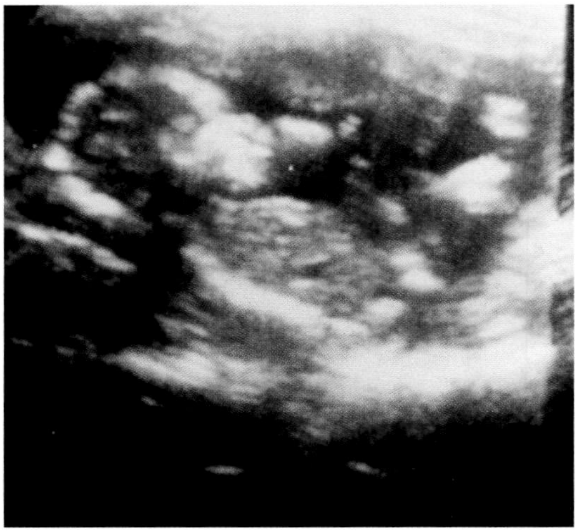

YOU ARE **20 WEEKS AND 4 DAYS**

136 days to go

YOUR BABY TODAY

Shown here is a Doppler ultrasound scan. Your doctor may use a handheld Doppler ultrasound machine to identify your baby's heartbeat; Doppler scanning can also pick up sudden movements and the whoosh of blood through the placenta.

"There are few better ways to relieve those pregnancy aches and pains, and to wind down, than to have a soothing massage."

When you book a massage, make sure you do so with a therapist who is experienced in prenatal massage. Although it's unlikely to occur at this stage, massaging the wrong areas or certain acupressure points can trigger uterine contractions (this can actually make a massage beneficial during labor when you want to speed things up).

Before making an appointment for a massage, check with your doctor that it's okay to have one. Massage may not be recommended if you've had complications such as high blood pressure or diabetes.

Comfort is crucial and most therapists will position you lying on your side with your head supported by a pillow. Don't hesitate to tell the therapist if you're uncomfortable or if any aspect of the massage hurts. An experienced therapist should check that you're comfortable throughout the massage and stop if you're not.

If you don't want a professional massage, you can always call on your partner or a willing friend. It is, however, important that the person who is massaging you is careful and does not attempt to work on the abdominal area.

In addition to making a world of difference to those aches and pains and helping you to relax, a massage from your partner is a good way to be intimate at times when you might not feel like having sex.

If you don't feel up to having a full massage, a foot, hand, or head massage can be very soothing.

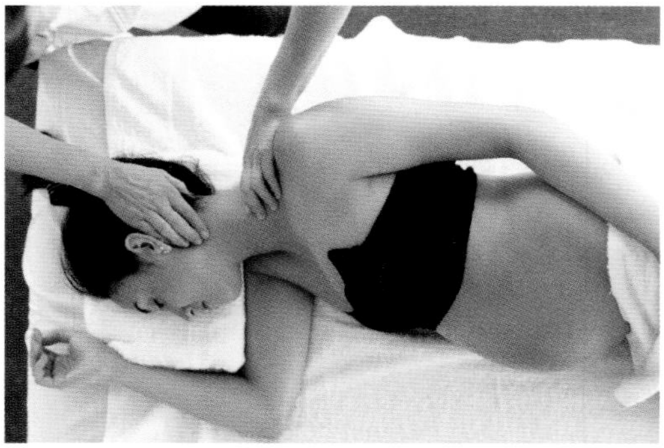

Having a professional massage during pregnancy can be a real treat. Besides feeling blissful, research shows that it eases aches and pains, helps you sleep, and can reduce stress.

ASK A DOCTOR

I'm feeling so down about my size. Will things get better? You're not alone in battling with your self-image in pregnancy. For some women, their changing body shape can create negative feelings.

There's no set emotional response to pregnancy, but in addition to coming to terms with a momentous life and body change, you are under the influence of fluctuating hormones, all of which affects your mood and can add to feelings of negativity.

Feeling a bit down in pregnancy is often helped by reassurance and support from loved ones. Talking over your fears and concerns may help relieve anxiety. If you speak to other pregnant women, you might find that they feel the same.

However, if you think you might be depressed or your sad feelings are affecting your behavior, you must speak to your doctor for additional support with your mental health.

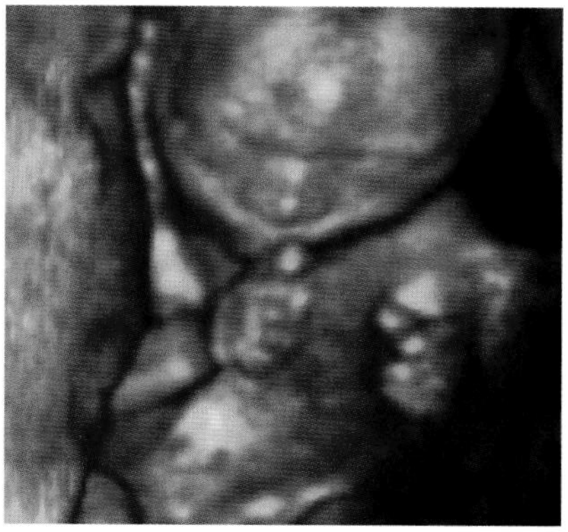

YOU ARE **20 WEEKS AND 5 DAYS**

135 days to go

YOUR BABY TODAY

The skin is less translucent now as your baby is starting to lay down fat reserves, which after the birth will help with temperature control and provide an energy reservoir for your baby to call upon when necessary.

By this stage, your baby can detect a number of tastes and in a few weeks he'll start recognizing and responding to sounds. However, the nerve pathways that carry information about pain, temperature, and touch are only just starting to develop at around 20 weeks, and it will be some time before these sensations can be recognized on a conscious level.

Your baby does have reflexes from an early age—for example, from about 10 weeks he'll close his fingers if they are touched. However, reflexes only require a nerve connection to the spinal cord and do not involve the brain. For information about pain, temperature, and touch to be recognized, it must travel from your baby's body to his spinal cord and then on to the thalamus, which lies in the center of the brain. The thalamus then sends signals to the cortex, the outer surface of your baby's brain, where the stimuli can be recognized and also evoke an emotional response.

These connections are thought to function after 26 weeks of pregnancy, but it may be several weeks later before their electrical activity can be detected on an electroencephalogram (EEG). Many of these nerves require insulation around them to conduct signals effectively, and these do not develop until much later in pregnancy (see p.300).

“ Your baby is becoming more responsive and aware every day as their nervous system begins to work more effectively. ”

ASK A MOM

This is my second baby—does it make sense to go to prenatal classes again? I think so. There were three years between my pregnancies and it helped to have a refresher course; I even found that some of the advice had changed in that time. It's also great to meet some pregnant moms again to share the experience with others.

WEARING MATERNITY SUPPORT STOCKINGS

Maternity stockings promote circulation and the return of blood back to the heart and may be recommended to prevent vein-related problems, particularly if you suffer from varicose veins (see p.167) or spider veins (see p.134).

They help to relieve aching feet, mild swelling in the feet, ankles, and legs, as well as fluid retention. They may be particularly helpful if you have to be on your feet for long periods of time for work.

Thankfully, an element of fashion has been introduced and many brands are sheer and pretty. There is a variety available: some are thigh- or knee-high (see right) and others cover the whole leg. You'll find lighter stockings for summer wear, when the hot weather can lead to more swelling. You can also buy maternity hose that provide support for your baby and uterus, taking the pressure off your back.

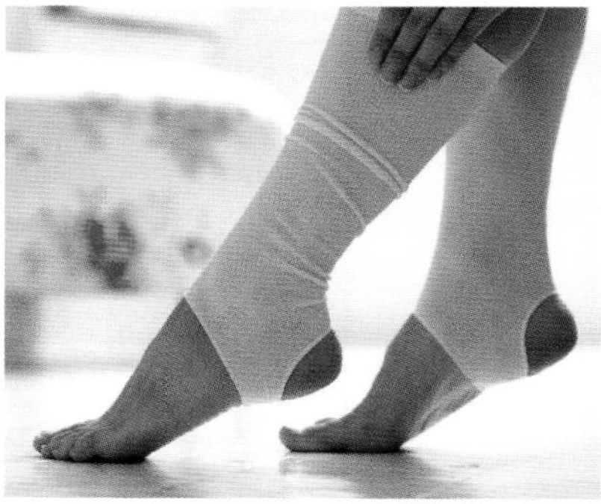

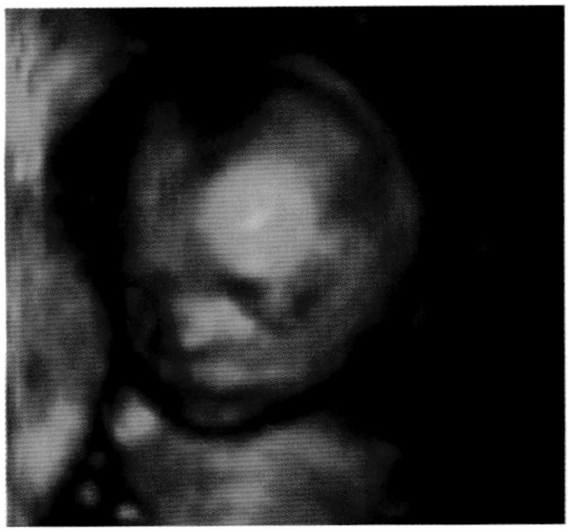

YOU ARE **20 WEEKS AND 6 DAYS**

134 days to go

YOUR BABY TODAY

Your baby is now developing periods of movement and activity and periods of rest and quiet. Soon these periods will become definite cycles of activity, providing something of a daily (and nightly) routine to their movement.

"Your baby's reproductive organs are gradually developing and the differences in the genitals are increasingly obvious."

In the absence of a Y chromosome in a female baby, the reproductive glands become ovaries, which contain 6–8 million follicles at this stage, of which about 1–2 million will remain at birth. The ovaries have now descended from the abdomen into the pelvis. The testes also undergo a similar descent, but have not yet reached the scrotum. Under the influence of the hormone estrogen you produce, your baby of either sex may develop breast buds, although these will disappear after birth.

Whether your baby is a boy or a girl has very little impact. Later in pregnancy, there is a slight weight difference, with boys being slightly heavier than girls on average.

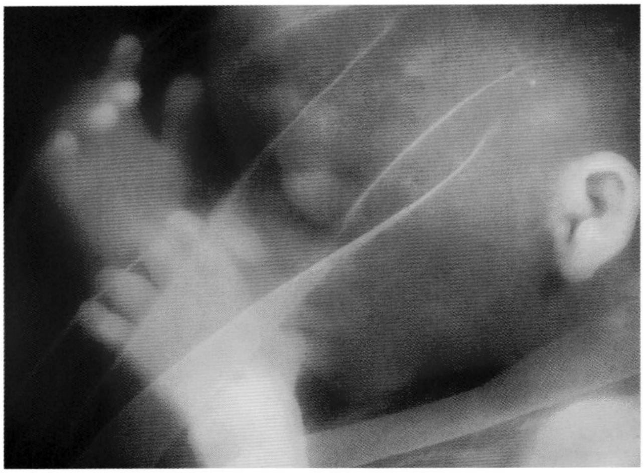

The amniotic sac is sometimes referred to as a "bubble" because of its appearance. It may be transparent, but it's tough and extremely difficult to pierce, so your baby is very well protected in this safe environment.

ASK A DOCTOR

I fell recently. Could I have harmed my baby? Falling during pregnancy is extremely common, as your increasingly protruding abdomen, softening ligaments and joints, and changing center of gravity can cause you to lose your balance. The good news is that your baby is safely cocooned in amniotic fluid, which protects and cushions them when you fall. Your injuries would have to be quite severe to cause any harm to your baby.

The best thing you can do is to monitor your baby's movements after a fall. If they are normal all should be fine, but if you want reassurance, pay a visit to your doctor. If you do experience any discomfort, or unusual discharge or bleeding from your vagina, seek medical help. If you pass water, this is likely to be urine caused by stress incontinence (see opposite), not amniotic fluid.

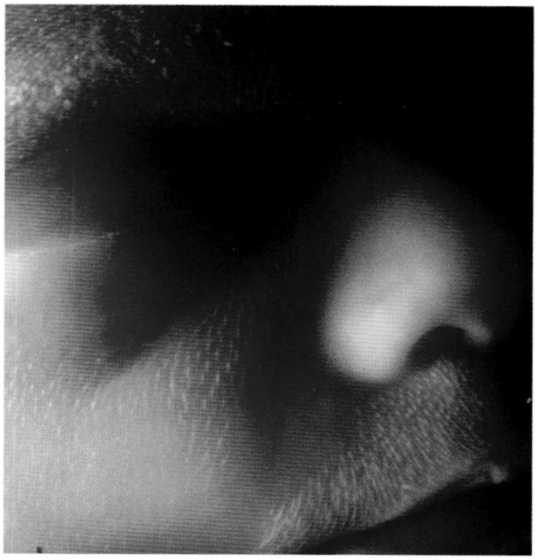

YOU ARE **21 WEEKS EXACTLY**

133 days to go

YOUR BABY TODAY

This image shows the large developing eyes beneath the lids. Babies born with blue eyes have a low level of melanin—and the color may change. Brown-eyed babies will likely keep their color. There are no eyebrows or eyelashes yet, but it is the first adult-type hair to grow.

Maintaining your exercise routine while you're still working can be challenging. The last thing you may feel like doing is exercising after a day at work, especially as your pregnancy progresses. There are ways of exercising without a visit to the gym; it will just take some thought and planning. For example, every now and then, take the stairs, carefully, instead of the elevator, or get off the bus or train at a different stop, so that you walk some of the way. If there's a pool close to work, try to fit in an invigorating lunchtime swim. You'll feel much better in the afternoon.

Walk wherever you can; wear comfortable sneakers and take your work shoes in a bag with you. Remember to take water with you when exercising.

Before you go to bed, try to fit in some exercises to strengthen your abdominal muscles (see p.250), as well as some gentle stretching to ease your tired muscles after a long day.

> **“ Try to find ways to fit in small amounts of energizing exercise every day—you'll feel much better for it. ”**

OFFICE WORKOUT

If your job involves sitting down all day, it's even more important to find ways to keep on the move.

- **Get up from your desk** at least once every hour. Walk to speak to your colleagues instead of calling or emailing them. Volunteer to get coffee for people—this will also make you very popular!
- **Try this exercise while seated:** straighten your leg out in front of you, keeping your thigh parallel to the floor. Then repeatedly bend and straighten your leg to help your circulation. Follow with flexing and pointing your foot from the ankle. Do each exercise at least 10 times with each leg.

ASK A DOCTOR

I seem to have a lot of vaginal discharge. Is this normal? Yes, in the second trimester you may find that you have more discharge than normal. This is usually clear, stringy, or full of mucus and shouldn't smell offensive. If the discharge changes, becoming thick and white, and causes irritation, you may have developed a yeast infection, which is common in pregnancy and easily treated (see p.133).

You should see your doctor immediately if the vaginal discharge becomes yellow or greener, or offensive in smell; see your doctor too if you have burning when you urinate, or your external genitals become sore. These are signs that you have an infection that must be treated. Don't ignore any abnormal discharge since, although it won't directly affect your developing baby, an infection can increase the risk of you going in to premature labor.

You may find that you leak urine, especially when you cough, laugh, or run. This is called stress incontinence (see p.473).

Your 22nd week

DECIDING ON A NAME FOR YOUR BABY CAN BE TRICKY, SO START MAKING THAT LIST. You may not know the sex of your baby but you and your partner can still have fun choosing names. This is a discussion that can run on and on. Some couples don't make up their minds until the baby is born. With such matters to preoccupy you, it's probably hard to stay focused at work. Try to pace yourself without letting standards slip. Eating little and often, and drinking lots of water, will help you stay alert.

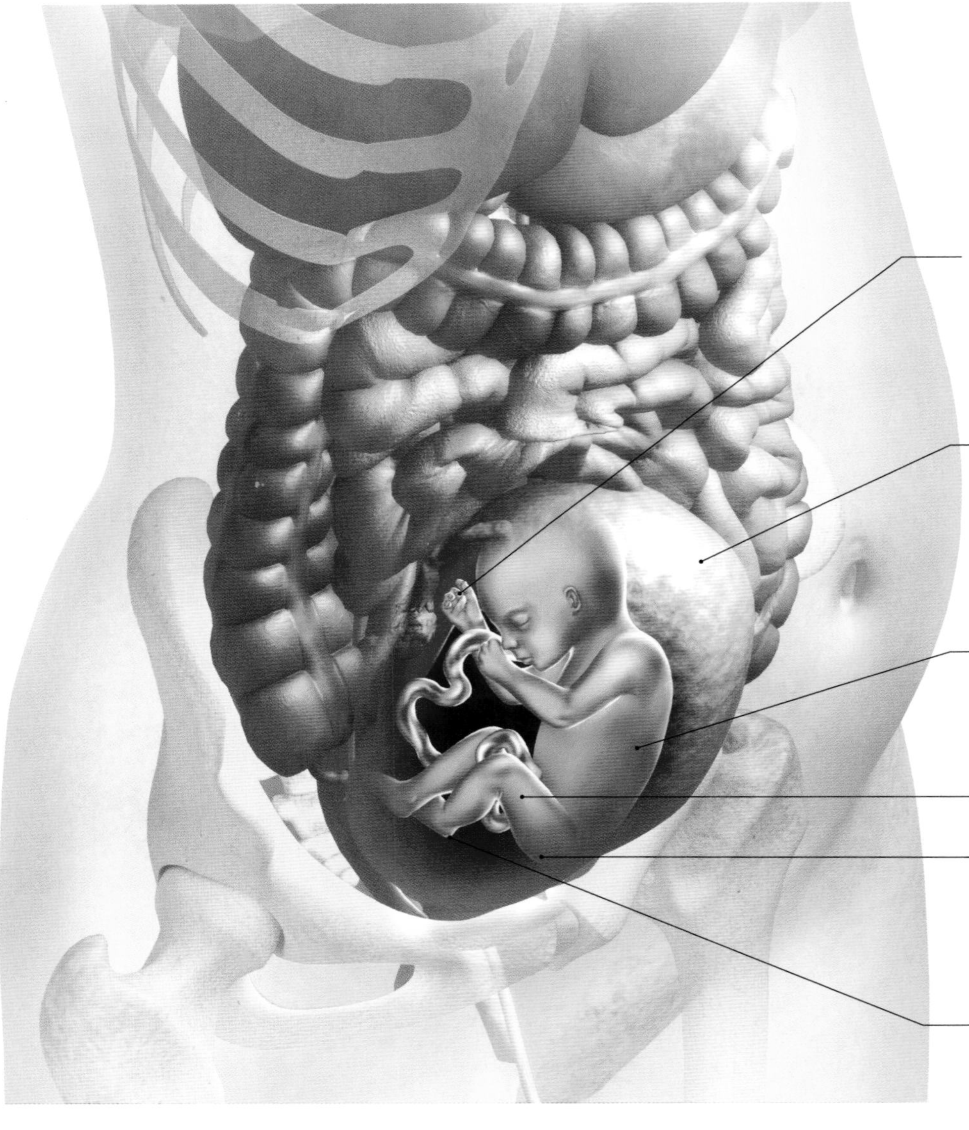

The hands move constantly, reaching out to touch the face or clutch at the umbilical cord.

Your uterus may now reach above your belly button, but there is a wide variation in belly size among women at the same week of pregnancy.

Beneath the skin, layers of body fat are being stored. Fats are essential because they contribute to the full development of the nervous system.

Every bone in your baby's body now contains bone marrow capable of producing blood cells.

In boy babies, the testes are still hidden within the pelvic cavity.

At 22 weeks the average crown to heel length is 10.9 in (27.8 cm), and the average weight is 15.2 oz (430 g).

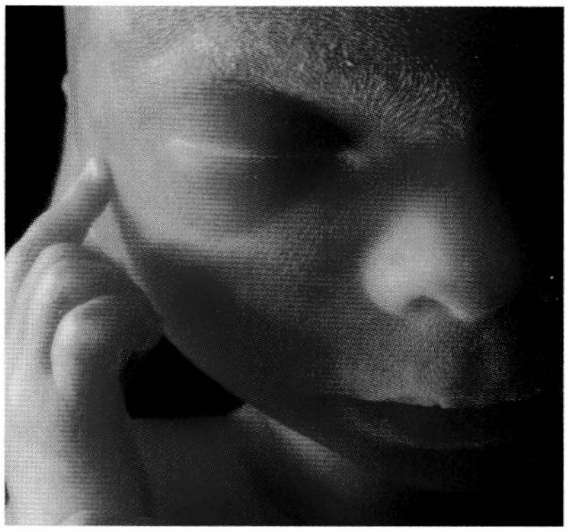

YOU ARE **21 WEEKS AND 1 DAY**

132 days to go

YOUR BABY TODAY

Fine capillaries carrying blood underneath the skin lend a pinkish tone to your baby. Fat deposits are still sparse so the skin is still quite thin. Within the capillaries red blood cells are carrying oxygen to every part of your baby's body.

> " If you often walk into a room and forget why you're there, don't be concerned—you've simply developed "pregnancy brain"! "

Is your mind not feeling quite as sharp these days? Many women find themselves very frustrated by the onset of "pregnancy brain," which makes them so forgetful that they might not remember what they're talking about halfway through a sentence. Your ability to concentrate and pay attention to tasks may also be affected. Doctors are not sure why this happens, but it's likely to be a result of hormonal changes. It may also happen because during pregnancy you're focused internally: you're going through such a major life event, and there are so many changes happening to your body and lifestyle, that you simply pay less attention to other things.

As frustrating as it is, this tendency to forgetfulness is only temporary (although it may last into the first year of motherhood—see below). In the meantime, try making lists at the beginning of each day and check off tasks as you go. Delegate at home and work when you can and, for once in your life, don't try to multitask. Focusing on one thing at a time will help you to remember more and achieve more.

SLEEP DEPRIVATION

"Pregnancy brain" might last until your child's first birthday. This finding is based on research done around the world. After in-depth analysis of the results, the experts concluded that sleep deprivation in the first year of parenting may be a factor.

ASK A DOCTOR

I've always been an enthusiastic walker, but should I cut down now that I'm over halfway through my pregnancy? No, but you might want to take extra precautions. Walking is ideal as it is low-impact and can be maintained throughout your pregnancy. In fact, it's a great exercise in the later months because it doesn't jar your knees and ankles or put any pressure on your lower abdominals, and it will keep your fitness levels up.

If you plan to continue lengthy walks and like to walk briskly, try combining this with a slower, more leisurely pace. It's important to control your body temperature so that you don't overheat and feel uncomfortable. To do this, drink plenty of water to avoid dehydration and wear layers that you can put on and take off as required.

As your belly grows, you may be less stable when walking up hills and over uneven terrain, so be careful. Take frequent breaks if you get breathless. Wear good footwear since your ankles and knees will be more fragile due to the hormone relaxin. Don't carry heavy loads

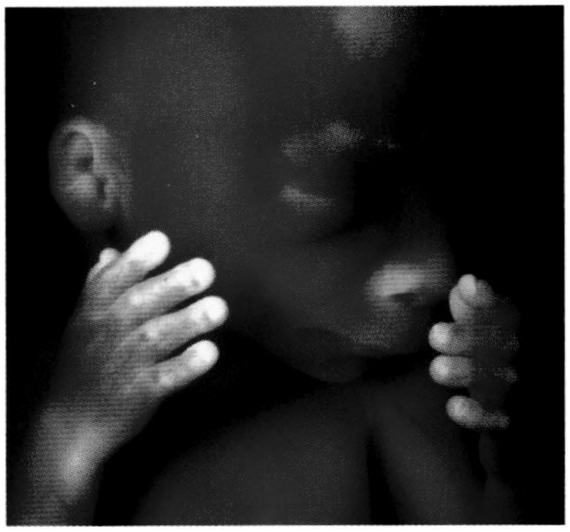

YOU ARE **21 WEEKS AND 2 DAYS**

131 days to go

YOUR BABY TODAY

The next three months are a time of particularly rapid growth for your baby. Cells are dividing, expanding, and maturing in every part of her body. The placenta too is growing and maturing, but this is far less important than your baby's growth from now on.

“ What's in a name? Well, quite a lot actually, as you'll discover when you start trying to choose one for your baby. ”

POPULAR NAMES

Do you want your child to have an original name, or are you influenced by what's in fashion? There are plenty of online resources that tell you the current top 10 or 20 boys' and girls' names, for example, but bear in mind that opting for a popular name may mean your child will be in a class full of namesakes.

Celebrities are known for being particularly creative when naming their babies, but before you follow suit, remember that lots of other people might do the same, making what was an "original" name suddenly very common.

Deciding on a name for your baby is fun but not necessarily an easy task. In addition to finding one that you and your partner agree on, it can feel as though everyone has an opinion. Friends may tell you that they have already chosen a name for their baby, so you can't use it! Your family may have traditions that they want upheld, such as passing on a name that has been in the family for generations.

It's a good idea for you and your partner individually to write down a list of names that you like. Then look at each other's list and talk about which ones you do and don't like. If you're lucky, there will be one or more names on both lists that match.

Factors to consider include: does the name sound right with your last name? Does the middle name go well with the first name? What will the initials be? For example, Robert Anthony Taylor will become RAT! Are the meanings of the names important to you? If so, find out what the meaning is of your favorite names—it can be fun to tell your child what her name means when she's older. Is there a short version of the name that you can use informally or, conversely, do you hate names being shortened? If so, avoid those. If you're feeling obligated to use a family name, perhaps make it a middle name.

It's advisable to come up with a few alternative choices, since you may find that the name you have decided upon just doesn't seem to suit your newborn baby.

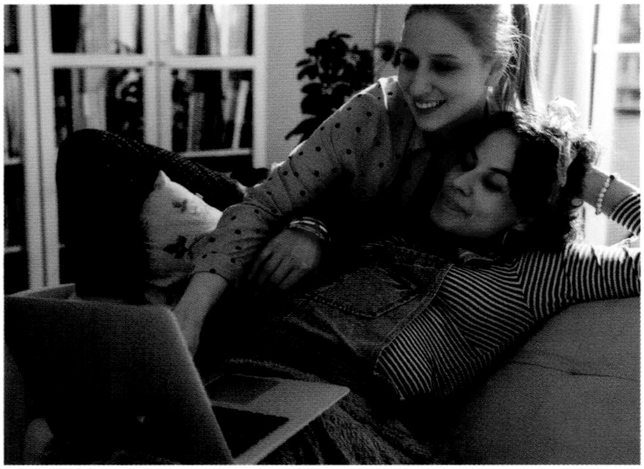

Researching in books or on the internet is a good way to find less popular names, and to discover interesting facts about the origin of names.

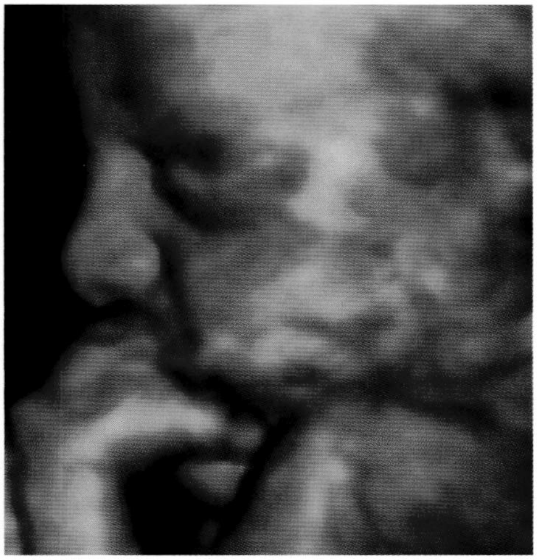

YOU ARE **21 WEEKS AND 3 DAYS**

130 days to go

YOUR BABY TODAY

In this 3D scan the baby's skin looks quite lumpy in parts. This isn't really the case. If the baby suddenly moves during a scan, the image can have difficulty "keeping up" and creates this unusual effect.

Up until this time, your baby has had little opportunity to store fat, because growth has been the most important priority. But now your baby starts to lay down a layer of fat beneath her skin and it becomes less translucent. The placenta is responsible for transferring fats to your baby.

Fat circulates in your bloodstream and within the placenta it is broken down into three free fatty acids, as well as cholesterol, which are passed into your baby's circulation. These fatty acids then recombine to form fats for storage or growth.

Fats are important for adequate nerve and brain development. A layer of fat covers each nerve cell, insulating it from adjacent nerves and improving its connections with other nerve cells.

" In addition to using fat for essential growth and development, your baby is now beginning to store it. "

ASK A MOM

Should we tell people the name that we've chosen? I would advise you not to. We told people at first and found it upsetting to find we had so many negative reactions. People freely told us how they had negative associations with the name or that they knew a cat or gerbil called that—a fact that we didn't need to know! Older relatives told us it was "odd" and went on to give us a list of alternatives.

So I would say keep it to yourself until the baby is born and it's all a fait accompli. It takes a bold person to question your choice once your baby has been named.

FOCUS ON TWINS

Choosing one name can be difficult enough, so if you're expecting twins, start thinking now. If you want to avoid people making jokes at your twins' expense, avoid obvious pairs such as Jack and Jill, and Holly and Ivy. Consider how the names might sound when abbreviated (William and Benjamin, for instance, becomes Bill and Ben).

Finally, it might be a good idea to opt for names of similar length and complexity. For example, young Christopher may be discouraged as he struggles to spell his name, while his twin Jack has no trouble.

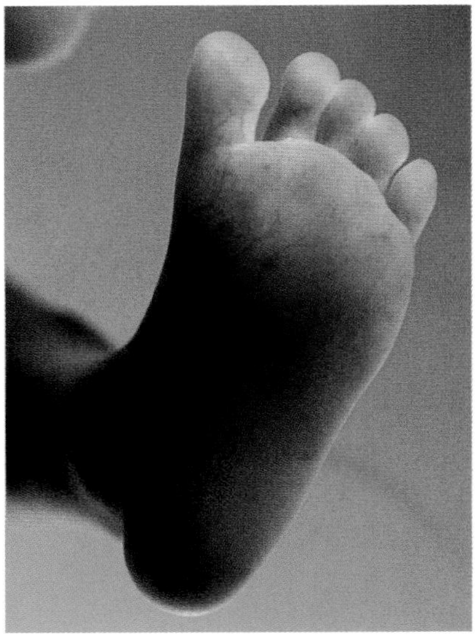

Your baby's veins will become less visible as she gains a layer of fat beneath the skin, making it less transparent than it was in the earlier stages of pregnancy.

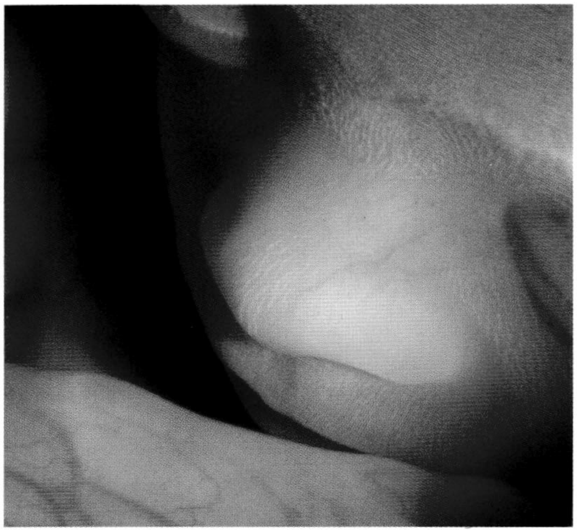

YOU ARE **21 WEEKS AND 4 DAYS**

129 days to go

YOUR BABY TODAY

When looking down on the baby, the nose can look quite wide because the nasal bridge is not yet fully developed. This gives the characteristic "button nose" shape that many babies keep throughout the pregnancy.

> "Your baby is producing essential red and white blood cells at a rate that is greater than your own."

Stem cells in your baby's bone marrow produce red and white blood cells, and platelets—the cells that clump together to form a blood clot. Earlier in pregnancy all of these were produced in the yolk sac (see p.80), then the liver and spleen. Now every bone inside your baby contains red bone marrow capable of producing blood cells. Red blood cells do not last forever and after about 80 days are removed from the baby's circulation. This turnover is higher than your own, where a red blood cell will last for 120 days.

Bilirubin is a breakdown product from red blood cells. It's produced in the liver and removed from your baby's circulation by the placenta. Because your baby's liver takes a few days to efficiently process bilirubin, high levels may lead to jaundice at birth (see p.479).

If jaundice does develop after birth then light phototherapy treatment is capable of breaking down bilirubin into a form that can be more easily excreted in your baby's urine.

Your newborn baby will be protected against infection by white blood cells transferred from you during pregnancy, and by breast milk, especially the colostrum (see p.448). Because of this, breastfed babies are at a lower risk of conditions such as asthma, cow's milk intolerance, and food allergies.

MAKING SENSE OF DOCTOR'S LINGO

Since your prenatal appointments are more regular now, it can be useful to get a handle on the medical jargon used in your pregnancy records:

- **Primagravida:** first pregnancy
- **Multigravida:** subsequent pregnancy
- **Hb:** hemoglobin levels
- **BP:** blood pressure
- **Urine tests:** NAD or nil means that no abnormalities have been detected; P or alb means it contains protein; Tr or + indicates a trace of sugar or protein; G stands for glucose; and "other" is anything else.
- **Heart rate:** FHH is fetal heart heard; FHHR is heard and regular; FMF or FMNF—fetal movements felt or not felt.
- **Your baby's position in the uterus** is usually referred to as the presenting part or lie and there are several terms and abbreviations used to describe this (see p.336). Most babies will be in the correct position by 34 weeks.

Your doctor will check your baby's position at around 36 weeks to ensure that they are vertex, also known as cephalic, or head presenting first in the pelvis. If your baby is positioned breech or transverse, then your doctor may discuss turning your baby so that you can have a vaginal delivery.

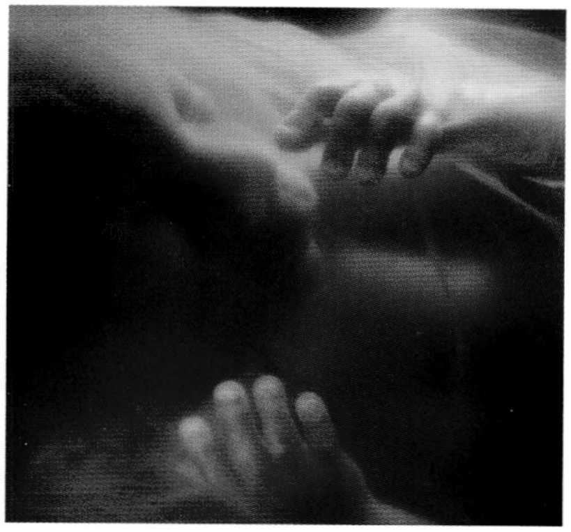

YOU ARE **21 WEEKS AND 5 DAYS**

128 days to go

YOUR BABY TODAY

There is still plenty of room for your baby to move around. Your baby is able to perform complete somersaults and change position several times a day or even several times in a few minutes.

If, like some pregnant women, you are feeling big for this halfway stage, it doesn't necessarily mean that you'll have a big baby. And remember, what you think of as too big can be very different from what your doctor is evaluating.

Being large doesn't mean that all your weight is in your belly and from your baby; you may have put on weight on the rest of your body that doesn't affect your baby's size. Women who are carrying twins or triplets do, of course, show earlier and have much larger bellies than those expecting one baby.

The size of your belly is, however, a good indicator of your baby's growth, so it will be measured by your doctor (see pp.284–285). They will measure from a point on your pubic bone in your pelvis to the top, or fundus, of the uterus. This measurement should correlate with the number of weeks you're pregnant, with an accuracy of within ¾ in (2 cm). So if you're 28 weeks' pregnant, your belly should measure 10/14–11¾ in (26–30 cm). This symphysis fundal height (SFH) will be written in your notes and may be plotted on a growth chart.

If your bump is significantly larger or smaller than it should be for your dates, you're likely to be referred for an ultrasound scan for a more accurate measurement.

> “ Bellies come in all shapes and sizes and your doctor will keep track of how your baby is growing. ”

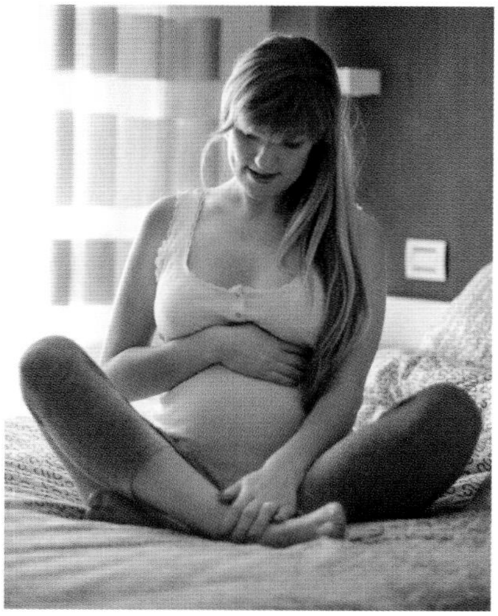

ASK A NUTRITIONIST

I've been told to rest, but will I gain too much weight? It's important to follow the advice you've been given, even though it can feel frustrating. Find out if you can go for gentle walks or a swim, since these activities will help you keep fit and relieve stress.

Remember resting is for a short time and for a good purpose—having a healthy baby at full-term.

If you aren't active, you are likely to gain weight, but you may find that being less active decreases your appetite. Don't be tempted to cut down on food or miss meals, though. Regular meals and snacks are important to continue to nourish yourself and your baby.

Continue to eat a nutritious, healthy diet, including plenty of fresh fruits and vegetables, complex carbohydrates, and lean protein, and take any supplements such as vitamin D.

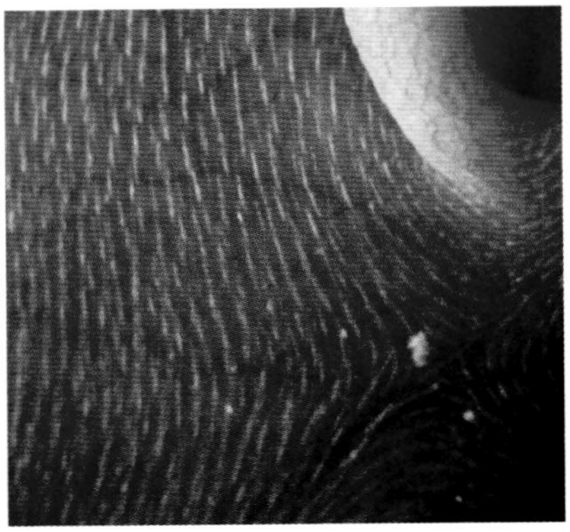

YOU ARE **21 WEEKS AND 6 DAYS**

127 days to go

YOUR BABY TODAY

This is a close-up of the baby's skin just behind the ear. Every part of the skin's surface has small ridges and hollows in a unique pattern. During this week, the dermal ridges—the deeper layers of skin—start to mature, giving rise to finger- and toe-prints.

" Your baby has been filtering amniotic fluid and storing the waste as a substance called meconium. "

At the end of this week, your baby's anal sphincter muscle is fully functional. This should prevent any small particles of meconium from being passed into the amniotic fluid. Meconium is first produced at 12 weeks. It is the greenish/black first bowel movement that 9 out of 10 newborn babies pass in the first 24 hours. Meconium is formed mainly from cells discarded from the lining of the gut as it lengthens and expands, and the waste of any nutrients that have been absorbed from the swallowed amniotic fluid. It is continuously produced, slowly moving down the gut to enter the large bowel (colon) by 16 weeks. Meconium is sterile since there are no organisms inside the gut and no bowel gas is produced.

YOUR BABY'S HANDS

The unborn baby will move their hand to their mouth and even suck their thumb. Research has shown that the baby may even open their mouth in anticipation.

Anything that the baby's hands encounter is firmly grasped and this grip is strong enough to support all of the baby's body weight.

KEEP TONED

Effective strength training during pregnancy, using free weights or a machine at your gym, will help your body deal with the demands of pregnancy. Being stronger will help you carry the increase in body weight and also help you recover after the baby is born. Having more toned limbs will help you look and feel better, too. Always follow these guidelines when exercising with weights:

- **If you've been doing regular weight training,** continue with your program, but do not increase the weight loads or repetitions.
- **If you're new to using weights,** begin with very light ones and few repetitions and build up slowly. Do not increase the weight load until you are confident that you are able to manage the increase.
- **Take a deep breath** to begin and breathe out as you lift the weight, maintaining your posture throughout.
- **Free weights,** rather than machines, are safer to use during pregnancy. If you're using a machine, make sure a trainer has shown you how to use it correctly.
- **If you find standing up while doing strength training too tiring,** sit on a chair to lift your weights (see below).

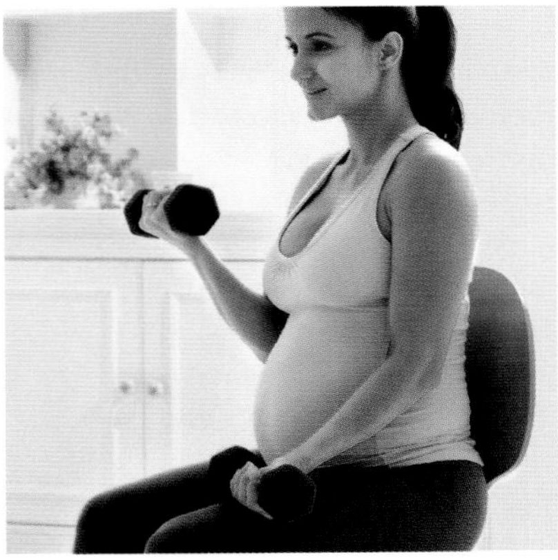

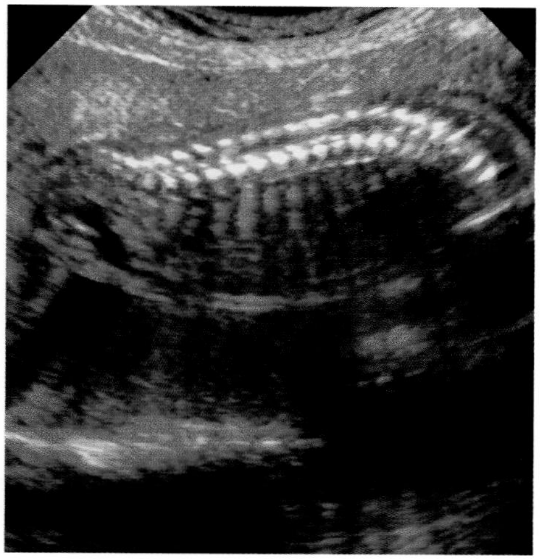

YOU ARE **22 WEEKS EXACTLY**

126 days to go

YOUR BABY TODAY

The vertebrae that make up your baby's spinal column encircle and protect the spinal cord. The vertebrae are seen here on an ultrasound scan, forming a long chain (white areas) that narrows at the base of the spine and ends with a slight outward curve.

"Maintaining a professional manner at work will set the standard for how colleagues treat you during pregnancy."

Chances are that everyone in your office will be aware that you are expecting a baby by this stage, even if you haven't told them personally. Good news does have a habit of traveling fast, and you may have that pregnancy "glow" that makes your condition pretty clear—as well as a fairly prominent belly.

If word of your pregnancy is getting around the office, it might be best to tell your boss now. It's always better and more professional if your boss hears this news before other people in your company.

You may need to adapt your working day a little, but play it carefully. Try to keep up with your work, and act professionally. Your colleagues are, hopefully, thrilled that you're pregnant, but try not to expect special favors or extra attention.

While being pregnant isn't an illness, do take adequate breaks to recharge your batteries, or work flexible hours, if that's an option, so that you can avoid traveling at the busiest times.

Take regular breaks for gentle exercise and to get some fresh air, drink plenty of water, and eat smaller amounts more frequently to keep your energy levels high.

ASK A DOCTOR

My manager said I can't have time off to go to my prenatal doctor appointments. What should I do? You'll be spending a lot of time at the doctor's office for prenatal care during the next several months—every 4 weeks now, but as frequently as once a week at the end of your pregnancy. If you also work full-time, it's a good idea to to schedule your prenatal appointments for the early morning, before you begin work, or during your lunch hour. If your appointments tend to run long or your doctor's office is far from work and your boss isn't understanding, ask if you should use your sick leave or your vacation time for the hours that you'll be away from the office.

VAGINAL BLEEDING

The increased blood supply to the cervix, or inflammation, can produce light bleeding, especially after sexual intercourse.

Heavy bleeding in the second trimester may suggest a problem with your placenta, such as placenta previa (see p.212). Or the placenta may separate from the uterus wall causing pain and bleeding, known as a placental abruption. Light bleeding is common and often it is not possible to determine where it has come from. Always notify your doctor if you have any bleeding.

Your 23rd week

YOU COULD BE FEELING A LITTLE OFF-BALANCE, BOTH PHYSICALLY AND EMOTIONALLY

Being pregnant can have all kinds of unexpected effects. There will probably be days when you just don't feel in control of your emotions and they get the better of you, making you cry for no reason. Or your body feels clumsy and uncoordinated, and you keep walking into the furniture. Just talk to some other moms-to-be and you'll find that these side effects are all a normal part of the pregnancy experience!

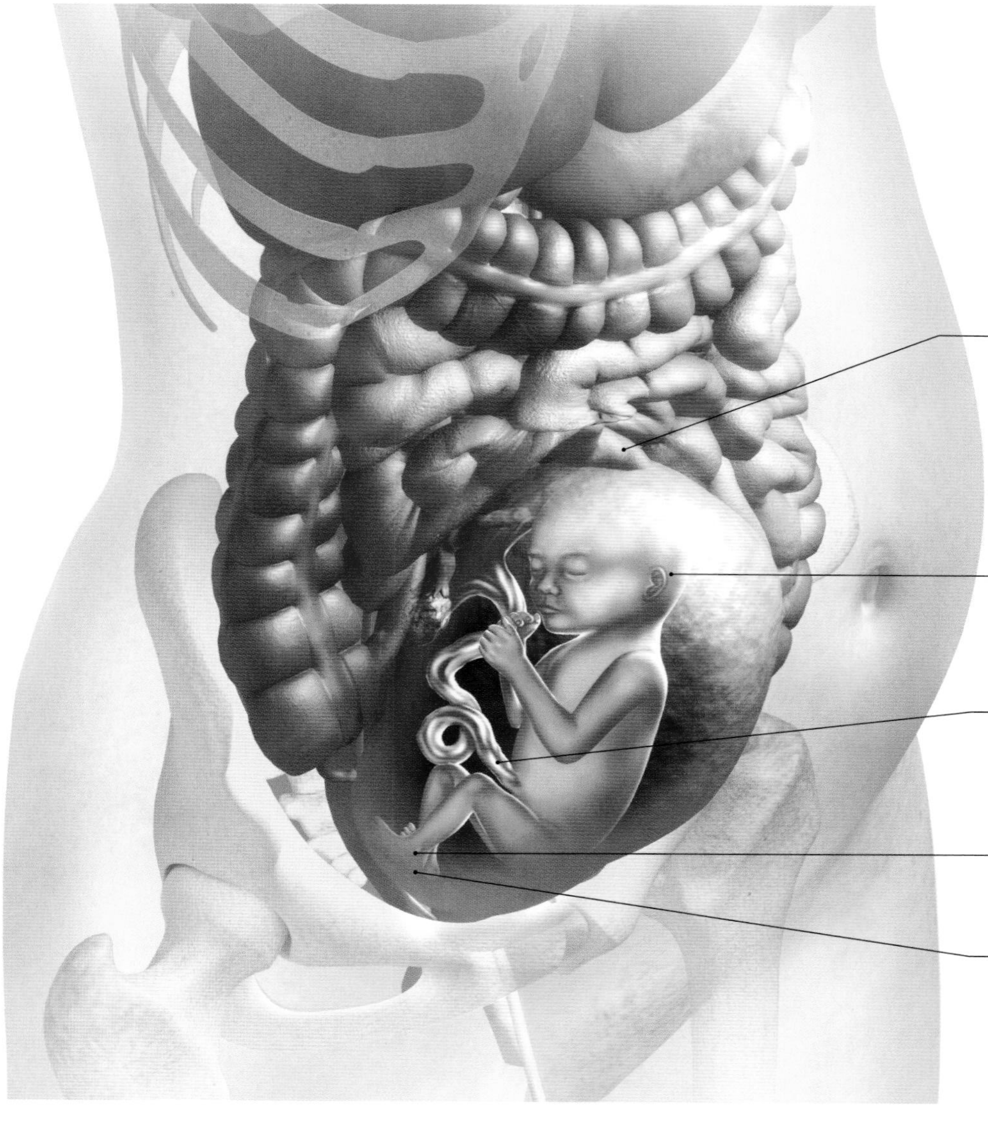

As your abdominal organs become ever more compressed, you may suffer from frequent digestive disturbances, such as heartburn or trapped gas.

The inner ear organs have matured enough to send nerve signals to the brain. Soon, the baby will start responding to many more sounds.

The umbilical cord may be held in your baby's hands as he floats in the amniotic cavity.

Kicks are becoming quite strong and there's no mistaking your baby's movements.

At 23 weeks the average crown to heel length is 11.4 in (28.9 cm) and the average weight is 1.1 lb (501 g).

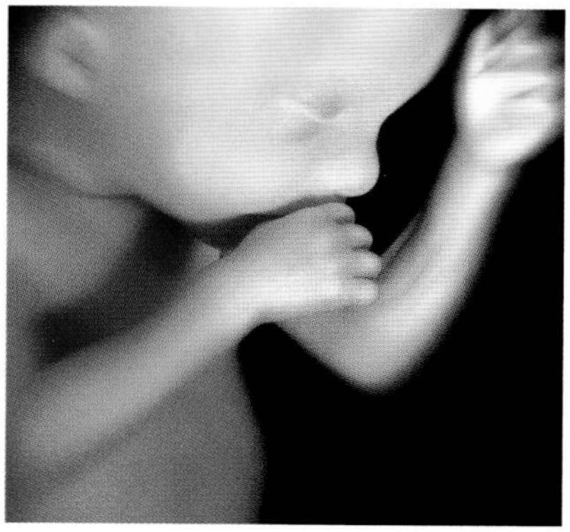

YOU ARE **22 WEEKS AND 1 DAY**

125 days to go

YOUR BABY TODAY

This is a landmark week for your baby's senses: hearing and balance, both controlled by the inner ear, start to mature now. As this image shows, the ears are still not in their final position at the side of the head.

It's normal to feel a bit up and down emotionally. The best way to manage is to give yourself some time out and the low points will soon pass. If you find yourself crying at a commercial yet again, try to see the funny side! Sharing this fact with someone else may also help, especially a pregnant friend or new mom—she more than anyone else will be able to relate to how you're feeling and reassure you.

However, be aware that depression can develop or recur in pregnancy. If the sad feelings persist, you have a history of depression, you are starting to feel very anxious, not sleeping, are feeling irritable, or any combination of these symptoms, you may be have prenatal depression. This can be serious and if untreated, increases your risk of depression postpartum. Speak to your doctor or midwife.

“If your emotions are all over the place, try having a good cry, preferably on someone's shoulder. You'll feel a whole lot better.”

ASK A DOCTOR

I think I may have food poisoning. Will this harm my baby? Some food-borne illnesses, such as salmonella, campylobacter, and E. coli will not directly harm your baby but can make you very ill, causing profuse vomiting and diarrhea that could lead to extreme dehydration. It's important to keep your fluid intake up both to flush out the offending pathogens, and to ensure you're sufficiently hydrated. If the vomiting is so serious that you can't keep any fluid down, contact your doctor's office as you may need IV fluids for rehydration.

Infection with listeria bacteria is the most serious type of food poisoning since it may cause a miscarriage or premature labor. It is, therefore, essential to contact your doctor's office if you believe that you've eaten food that is contaminated (see p.16), so that the relevant checkup can be done and treatment given, if necessary.

Always be especially careful when you are choosing food and follow hygiene rules when preparing it. Avoid eating foods that are commonly associated with food poisoning (see p.16).

FOCUS ON TWINS

If you're having twins, now is the time to discuss your maternity leave with your employers. Some women start their leave toward the end of their pregnancy, while others wait for their babies to be born. Ask your doctor for advice.

You may also want to take off as much time as possible after the babies are born, and your partner will want to take the maximum amount of leave they're eligible for (see p.349). Aside from help from family and friends, which will be essential, consider what you can afford in terms of additional child care.

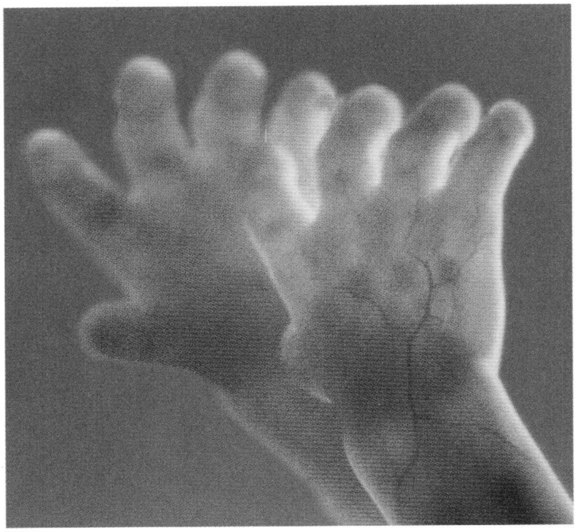

YOU ARE **22 WEEKS AND 2 DAYS**

124 days to go

YOUR BABY TODAY

The hands and fingers are clearly visible and the nail beds have been laid down. The baby's fingers will close if the palm of the hand is touched. The tips of the two bones in the forearm, the radius and the ulna, can just be seen in the lower part of this image.

“ Now that your baby's ears are sufficiently well developed to process sounds, their hearing will gradually improve. ”

Your baby's external ears have been developed for some time but for them to hear, the internal ear structures also need to mature. In the middle ear, three bones—the malleus ("hammer"), incus ("anvil"), and stapes ("stirrup")—conduct sound into the inner ear. These bones are formed initially from soft cartilage and embedded within connective tissue. The bones begin to harden and the connective tissue gradually dissolves. This allows the ear drum to vibrate onto the hammer, which passes the movement on to the anvil, and then the stirrup. The vibrations are then passed to the cochlea, a cavity of the inner ear, where they are translated into nerve impulses to be sent to the brain.

At 22 weeks, your baby's inner ear has matured adequately for sound to be processed into neural signals to the brain. The first part of the cochlea to develop is responsible for receiving lower-sound frequencies. As your baby develops, they will gradually be able to recognize and respond to higher sound frequencies. Over the next three weeks, your baby's responsiveness to sounds will gradually increase. At first the responses are slow and sluggish, but by 25 weeks, they will react to a range of sounds by moving around. In addition to being responsible for your baby's hearing, the inner ear also controls their balance. Small fibers within three semicircular canals of the inner ear are able to sense acceleration in any direction, providing the sense of motion and balance. Floating in the amniotic fluid is similar to weightlessness and, although your baby is very active, they have no sense yet of moving up and down.

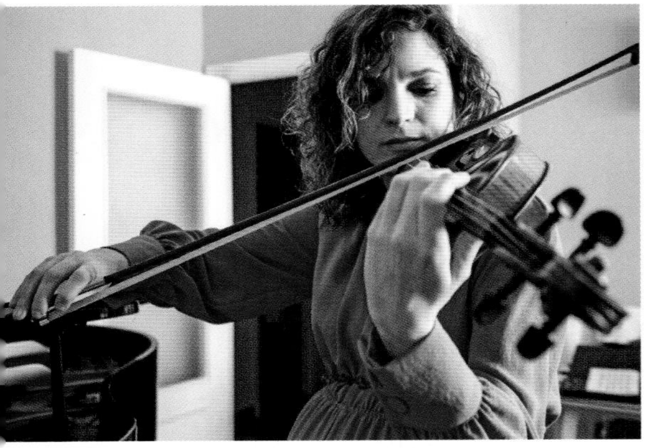

If you play a musical instrument, be reassured that your baby will be tuned in to your performance. As their ears develop, they'll become more responsive to sounds.

RARING TO GO

If, like many pregnant women at this stage of pregnancy, you feel incredibly energized, make the most of it. Here are some ways to direct that energy:

- **Get some exercise,** including doing some gardening.
- **Organize your paperwork** and get your finances in order.
- **Clear out any clothes** that you know you won't wear again.
- **Learn to knit** or crochet. If you already can, get going on knitting some baby clothes or crocheting a blanket.
- **Make time to see all the friends** you haven't been in touch with for a while as you may not feel up to socializing in later months.

However good you're feeling, always try to make time to relax and recharge your batteries.

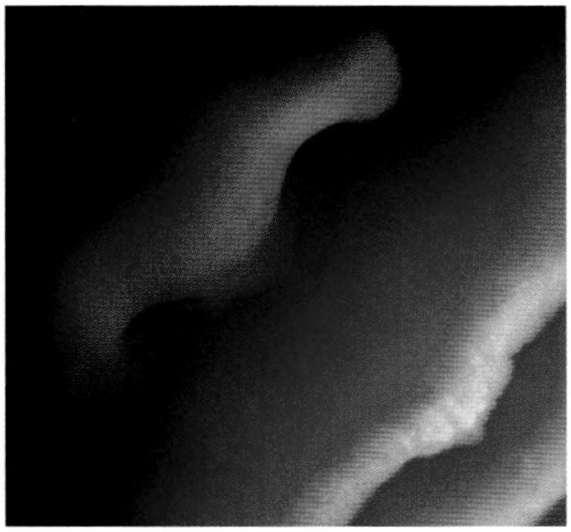

YOU ARE **22 WEEKS AND 3 DAYS**

123 days to go

YOUR BABY TODAY

The baby's mouth and nose are well developed. The nervous and muscular systems are now mature enough for the baby to suck in amniotic fluid, which the kidneys slowly process. Waste is eliminated via the placenta.

> “You'll probably make some new friends, but you may find that some old friendships are affected”

One thing that you may not have anticipated before you were pregnant is how your friendships might change. It's normal to be drawn to other women who are pregnant or who have recently had a baby, and common to make friends at prenatal classes (see p.199). It's natural to want to surround yourself with people who are going through or who have been through the same experience as you, not least because you will have so many questions they can answer. You might also feel closer to female relatives, especially your mother.

You may find that friends who are not pregnant or who don't have children may not be as interested in all the details of your pregnancy. It may be difficult for them to comprehend how all-encompassing pregnancy and then having a child is; it may be literally all you can think about. If these are friendships you value, make an effort to have some “nonpregnancy” chats. It will be good for you not to be 100 percent focused on the pregnancy.

If you find that you drift apart from these friends for a while, don't worry. Good friends will always remain just that, whether or not your lives temporarily go in different directions.

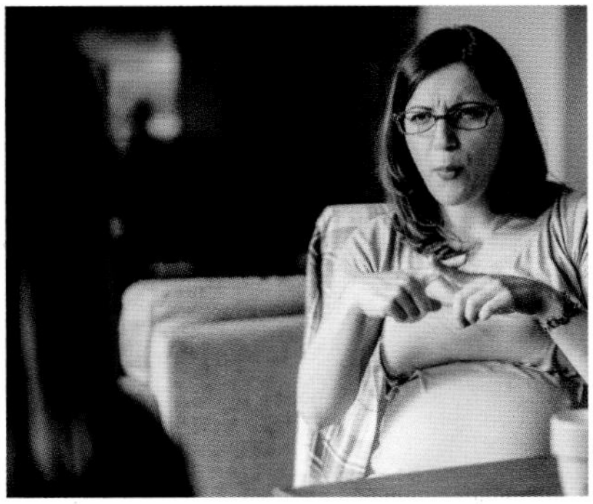

By spending time with women who are also expecting a baby, you can share the ups and downs of your pregnancy experiences.

OLDER MOMS

The number of women over 40 becoming pregnant continues to increase. According to the Centers for Disease Control, the birth rate for women over 40 has risen in recent years. Women over 40 were responsible for more than 10 in 1,000 births in 2016. The average age for pregnancy in the US is between the ages of 30 and 34.

ASK A DOCTOR

I've been told I have carpal tunnel syndrome. What is it? This condition occurs when swollen tissues in the wrist compress the nerves and cause pins and needles and numbness in your fingers. You may also have difficulty grasping and a weakness in the hands. In pregnancy, it's caused by an increase in blood volume and fluid. There are ways to reduce the symptoms, such as circling and stretching exercises to improve circulation and increase wrist mobility. Wearing wrist splints and elevating your hands on a pillow at night can also help. Carpal tunnel syndrome resolves after the birth, once there is no longer excess fluid.

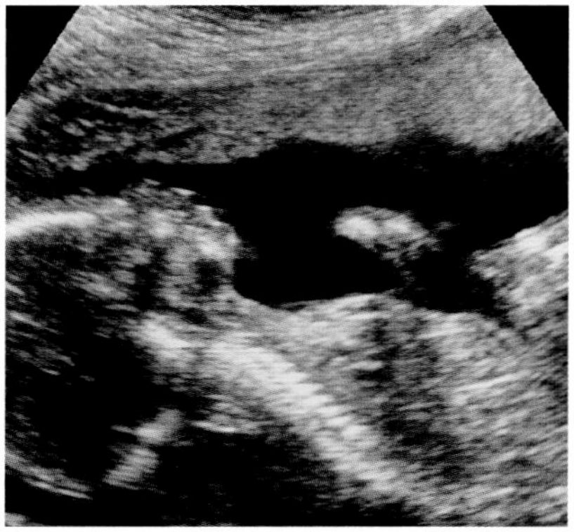

YOU ARE **22 WEEKS AND 4 DAYS**

122 days to go

YOUR BABY TODAY

Seeing your baby on a 3-D or 4-D scan gives you a better view, but most of the information that enables doctors to plan your care comes from looking inside your baby using 2-D ultrasound, which provides the clearest images of internal structures.

“Now that they can hear, your amazing baby is starting to develop the ability to remember things, too.”

As your baby's nervous system develops, and especially once their sense of hearing evolves, they have the opportunity to learn and remember from experience. How this process develops is not fully understood, but experts believe that the first signs of learning coincide with the unborn baby's ability to hear, at around this midstage of pregnancy.

In later months, more sound will reach your baby as the walls of the uterus become thinner. Although babies have been seen to be startled by a noise at this stage, they seem to learn not to react to the sound if it is repeated again and again, gradually adapting to it as it's repeated over time, and eventually ignoring it.

This simple test demonstrates that a fetus can adapt to a repeated stimulus. If, however, the sound pattern is not repeated for some time, your baby will have forgotten it and become startled by it if it occurs again.

Retaining a memory for events is a much more complex function and relies on pathways in the gray matter of the brain. It will be weeks before learning and memory are linked in the last stages of your pregnancy.

At this stage of pregnancy, your baby is likely to be more active and predictable in their movements. Around this time you're likely to start feeling regular, more definite movements and become accustomed to your baby's activities.

UP CLOSE AND PERSONAL

It's possible to see what your unborn baby will look like. Private ultrasound scans enable parents to see their baby up close either in 3-D, as a still image, or 4-D, as a moving picture.

Clear scans of the baby's facial features can be seen from around this week. However, the optimum time to have one of these scans is between 26 and 34 weeks, when your baby still has room to move around easily.

You will be able to see an amazing level of detail that won't be visible on a standard ultrasound scan. Don't forget to inform the ultrasound technician if you don't want to know the sex of your baby, since it is likely to be very clear on these high-tech scans.

Be aware that it could be expensive to have a 3-D scan and if your baby is in the wrong position, you may not get a great result. The position of the placenta, amount of amniotic fluid, and your size are all factors that can affect the quality of the picture.

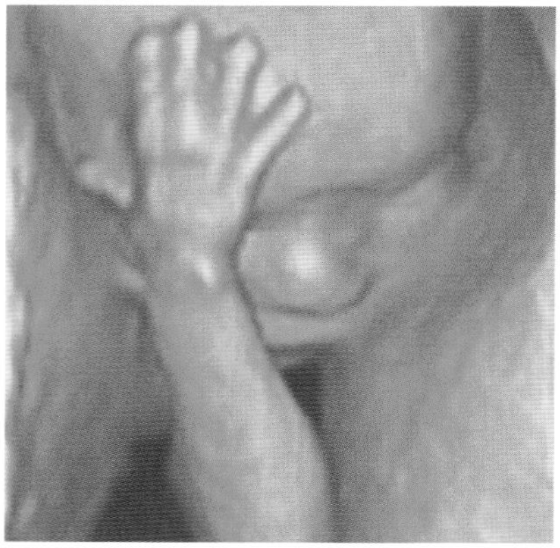

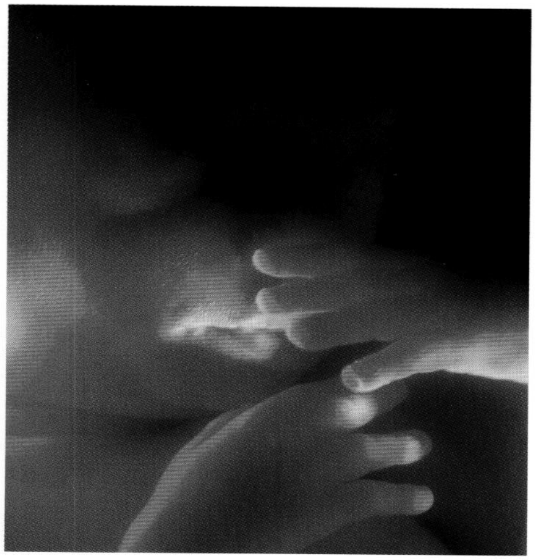

YOU ARE **22 WEEKS AND 5 DAYS**

121 days to go

YOUR BABY TODAY

Extremely fine hairs called lanugo hairs cover your baby's entire skin surface. These are constantly shed and replaced but, during the final few weeks of pregnancy, will be replaced by thicker, permanent hairs. Lanugo cells help insulate the skin.

> "The occasional dizzy spell is common in pregnancy and not a sign that anything is wrong."

As your body works hard to nourish your developing baby, you may find that you have dizzy spells from time to time. It's common to feel dizzy when you stand up suddenly; although your blood supply has increased, getting up quickly causes the blood to rush into your legs. This reduces the supply of blood to your brain, making you feel lightheaded.

Dizziness can also be a symptom of anemia (see p. 474). Although your body produces more red blood cells in pregnancy, your blood volume also increases. This means that proportionally there are fewer red blood cells and your blood count will drop. You may also become low in iron and may need iron supplements.

In addition to dizziness, symptoms of anemia include fatigue and shortness of breath. Low blood-sugar levels (see p.92) can also cause dizziness and can be prevented by making sure you eat regularly.

Although dizziness is likely to be due to the physiological changes in pregnancy, inform your doctor so that you can be examined and have any relevant blood tests done.

If you feel dizzy when you're out of the house, or if you need a seat on a bus, train, or subway because you feel that you might faint, always tell someone—the majority of people will be kind and understanding, and will let you sit down. Wearing "a baby on board" button can help with this.

ASK A MOM

I'm only just over halfway through my pregnancy, but I don't feel up to socializing anymore. Should I force myself to go out? I remember that feeling well! It's normal to feel like battening down the hatches sometimes because you're too tired to socialize.

It's worthwhile, however, to try to make the most of your leisure time before your baby arrives. You may not feel like getting out, but once you do, you'll probably be glad you made the effort and it will help you maintain friendships. When I was pregnant, I chose my activities carefully, opting to meet up in the early evening or on weekends, and I went to cafés rather than bars. I also had friends over for lunch and dinner, but asked everyone to bring a dish to cut down on the work involved.

I realized I might not get to the movies or theater for a while once the baby was born, so I planned lots of great trips. You can always go to weekend matinées if you're too tired in the evening. When I was really too tired to go out, I'd catch up with a friend on the phone.

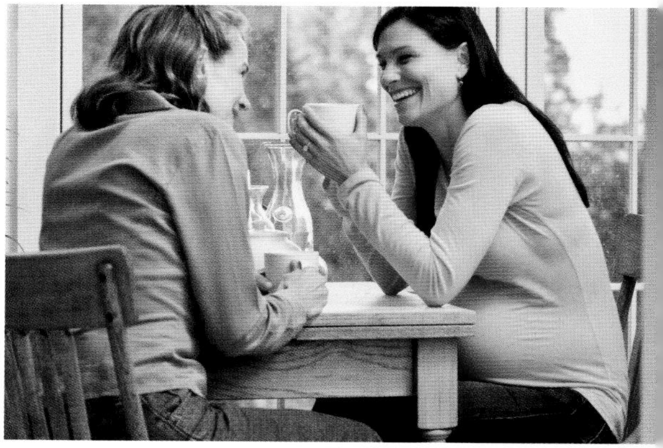

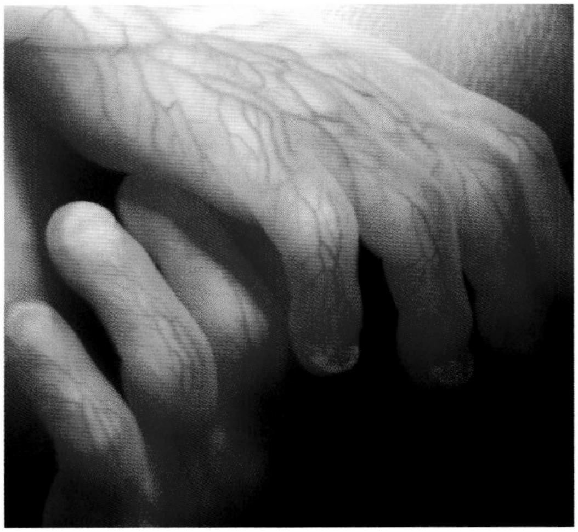

YOU ARE **22 WEEKS AND 6 DAYS**

120 days to go

YOUR BABY TODAY

Your baby's nervous system and muscular coordination are now much more developed. They have a grasp reflex—when the palm is touched, the fingers will close—and are also able to suck their thumb purposefully, rather than through random movements.

> "When clumsiness strikes, something as simple as walking in a straight line may prove difficult!"

If you find that you're often bumping into things and tripping over, it sounds as though you've been hit by clumsiness, a common side effect of being pregnant.

Clumsiness in pregnancy has physical causes: the hormone relaxin causes your joints to loosen, your center of gravity changes as your abdomen expands, and your extra weight shifts you off balance. There are, however, also emotional reasons: if you're preoccupied by being pregnant, your concentration is bound to slip now and then, making you less likely to notice potential hazards in your path.

The good news is that your usual grace will return once you're no longer pregnant, but until that time it's important to avoid situations that might put you at risk of injury. So wear flat shoes rather than heels, avoid wet or slippery surfaces, and be careful on steep staircases. Tape down the edges of loose rugs, and keep the stairs and hallways clear of things that might trip you up. Be particularly careful when you're lifting something because it's very easy to lose your balance if you're leaning forward. Be careful also, getting into and out of the bath or shower, since these are notorious hot spots for pregnancy-related injuries.

It's worth noting that normal clumsiness in pregnancy is not accompanied by visual disturbances, headaches, or dizziness, so if you have any of these symptoms, you should see your doctor.

FOCUS ON PARTNERS

If your partner's nesting instinct has kicked in, make the most of it by figuring out what needs to be done around your home.

- **Decorate the room** your baby will eventually sleep in once you move him out of your bedroom.
- **Take the opportunity** to have a look around and take any unwanted clutter to the dump or charity shop.
- **Make storage space** by putting up some extra shelves and cupboards where you can. Figure out where you'll store large items, such as the carriage.

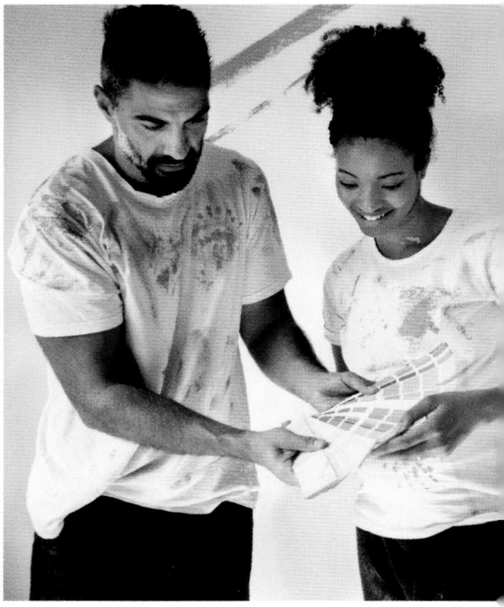

Let your partner do the majority of the decorating and don't attempt to climb a step ladder yourself. Be aware of which paints are safe to use during pregnancy (see pp.24–25).

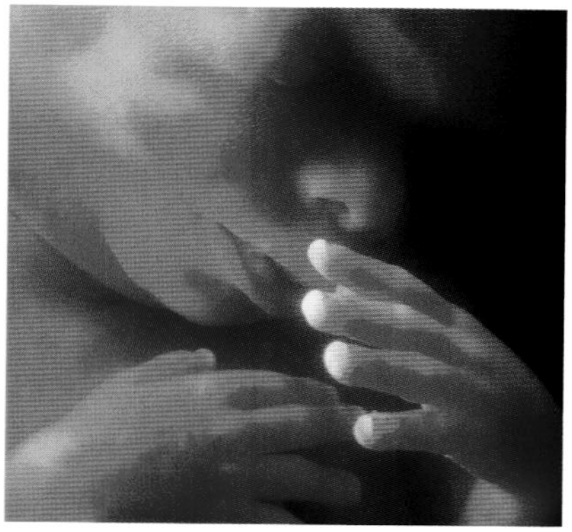

YOU ARE **23 WEEKS EXACTLY**

119 days to go

YOUR BABY TODAY

External appearances are deceptive: although your baby seems very well developed, it's still early in the pregnancy—the state of the cervix and progesterone produced by the placenta both play a part in ensuring that labor does not start for some months yet.

Do you feel as though you're a mom yet? Whether or not you're a maternal person, you'll already have started, instinctively, the process of becoming a mother. You may be taking better care of yourself, eating healthier foods, and making lifestyle changes, not necessarily to benefit your own health but for your baby. You're likely to find yourself being very protective and nurturing toward your growing belly, wanting the best for your baby, and being worried about anything happening to them. It's nothing to worry about if you don't feel this bond: all women are different and it may not be until you're holding and caring for your baby that you experience strong maternal feelings.

The more you involve your partner in the pregnancy, the greater the chance of them developing a strong parental instinct. By reading books or on the internet about how the baby is developing at every stage, and attending some or all of the prenatal appointments with you, they will be able to picture the baby and follow his progress as closely as possible.

"You may be surprised by the strength of feeling you have for your baby, and this maternal instinct will grow stronger each day."

ASK A DOCTOR

I've got the flu. Will this harm my baby?
A mild case of the flu won't harm your baby. The best thing to do to prevent rare but serious complications from the flu is to get your flu shot during pregnancy. If you have a mild symptoms, drink plenty of fluid to stay hydrated, and eat several small meals a day to maintain your energy levels. Ask the pharmacist's advice before taking any over-the-counter medication. Call your doctor if you don't improve after 24–48 hours, or your temperature exceeds 101°F (38°C). If you experience problems breathing, notify your doctor immediately.

CURIOUS TODDLERS

Your toddler will undoubtedly be curious about why you have suddenly got so fat! Keep things simple, along the lines of "Mommy is growing you a baby sister or brother, but they won't be here just yet." Over the coming weeks, explain in more detail what having a new baby means.

There's no need to tell your toddler how the baby got there, or to keep reminding them about it. Just answer their questions when they ask, without showing too much preoccupation with the matter.

Your 24th week

YOUR BABY'S BODY SYSTEMS ARE BECOMING MORE AND MORE EFFICIENT A baby getting prepared for independent life needs all the help you can give her. Keep up your good habits by nourishing the two of you with healthy food; and make sure your own body is in peak physical condition to support your pregnancy. Some minor discomforts, such as feeling too hot, leg cramps, and hemorrhoids may be plaguing you. These annoying problems are only temporary and will disappear once your baby is born.

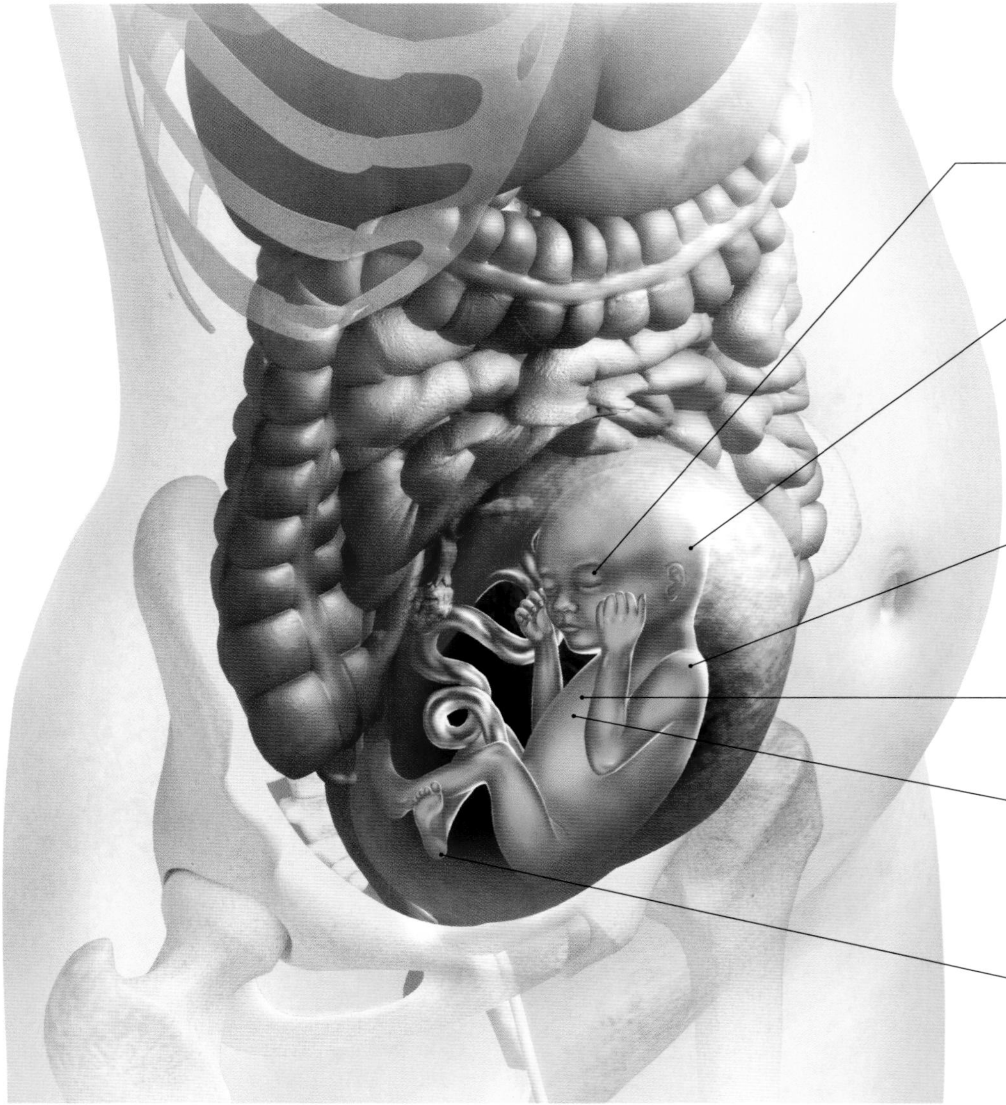
The eyelids are still closed. Beneath them, the eyes are protected by a thin membrane.
The skin is starting to develop a protective outer layer of keratinized cells.
Fine, soft lanugo hairs keep a layer of greasy vernix on the skin.
The lungs are not ready for the outside world but their function is rapidly improving.
The baby's rapid heart rate has slowed down a little. It is usually easy to detect the heart's beating during a scan.
At 24 weeks the average crown to heel length is 11.8 in (30 cm) and the average weight is 1.3 lb (600 g).

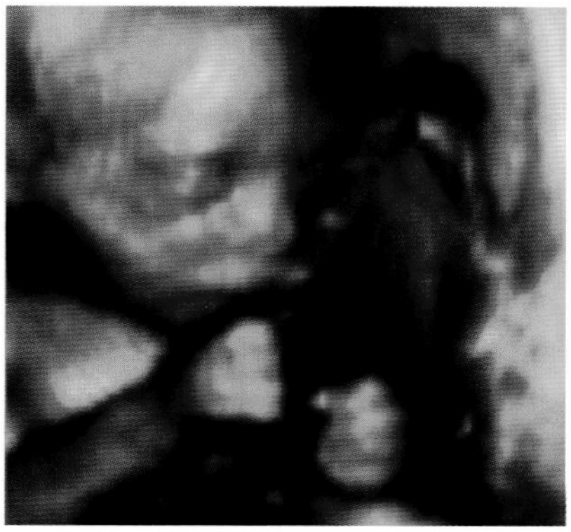

YOU ARE **23 WEEKS AND 1 DAY**

118 days to go

YOUR BABY TODAY

There is no light in the uterus, but 3D ultrasound is designed to produce highlights and shadows to give the same effect as if you shone a flashlight into the uterus. Now your baby may be holding her hands flexed into a fist.

> “ From this point onward, your baby is considered “viable” and would receive life-saving treatment were they born early. ”

Week 24 is considered the age of viability for your baby, and therefore an important pregnancy milestone. Like many women, you may feel relieved to get past this point.

If you went into labor and delivered your baby before this week, they would be unlikely to survive and you would be considered to have had a miscarriage. After 24 weeks, the doctors will to do everything they can to save the baby, although babies delivered this early have an increased risk of long-term disability.

The more advanced you are in your pregnancy before you deliver, the less likely it is that your baby will face the problems associated with being born prematurely.

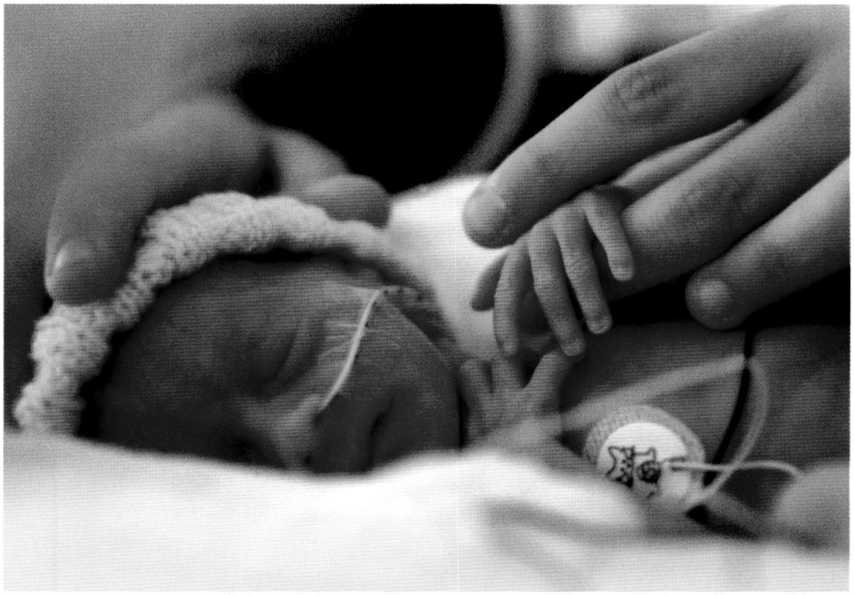

Incredible scientific and technological advancements have meant a huge increase in the survival of premature babies.

NEONATAL INTENSIVE CARE UNITS

Babies who are born prematurely, or newborns who are sick, will receive specialized around-the-clock care in a neonatal intensive care unit (NICU;see pp.454–455). The earlier the baby is born, the more chance there is of complications, such as infections, occurring. If your baby is born several weeks prematurely, they may need to be cared for in a level 3 NICU—this may not be in the hospital where they were born. Your baby may be put in an incubator with monitors attached and receive oxygen through a special ventilator. Some of the equipment looks very frightening, but remember it is there to help them stay warm and nourished and improve their health.

The staff will readily explain what is going on, and they will be eager for you to be involved as closely as possible in your baby's care and encourage bonding.

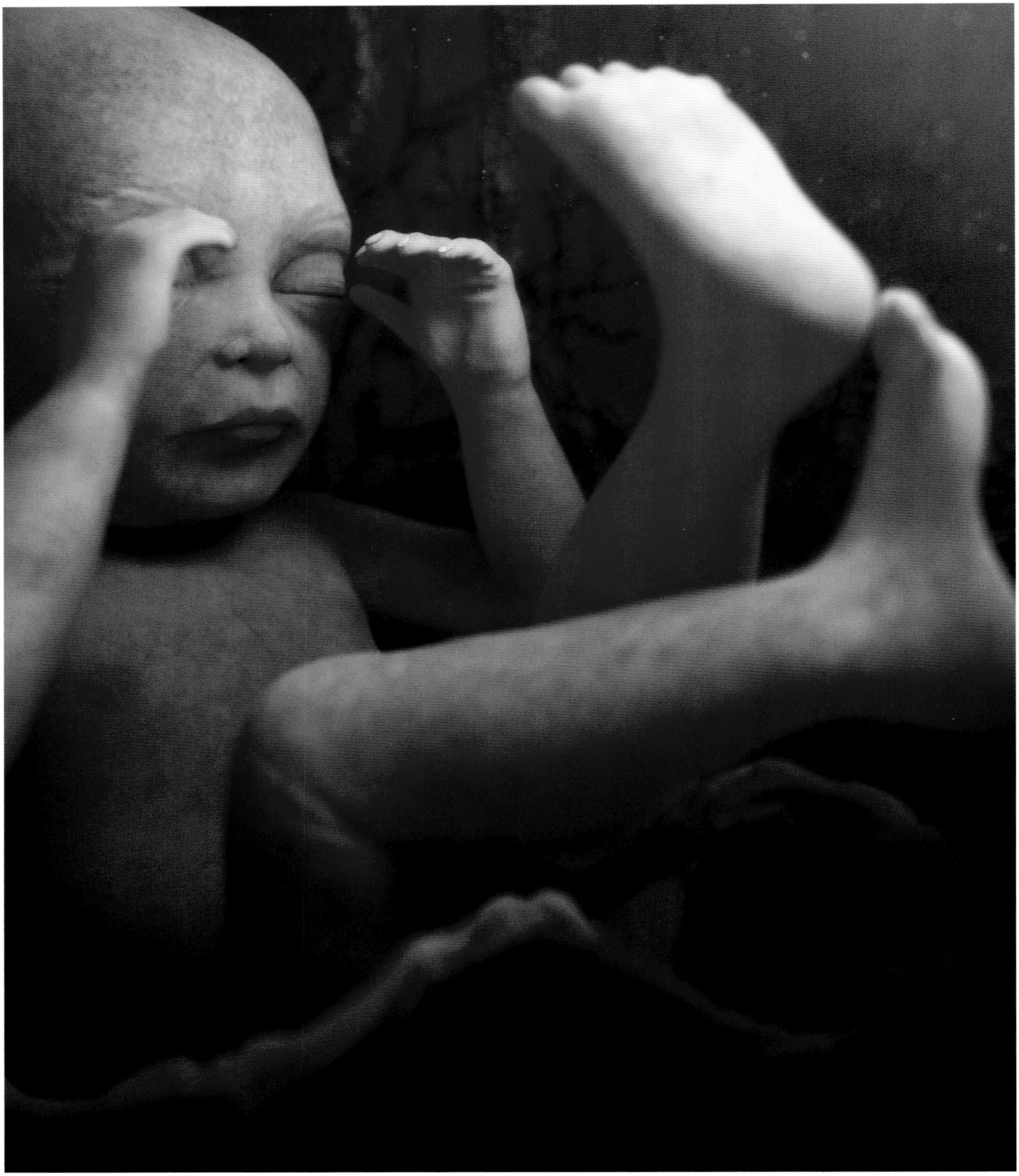

Your baby's bones are hardening and their arms and legs are beginning to flesh out. They bring their hands to their face often. Their skin is starting to develop a protective outer covering of vernix.

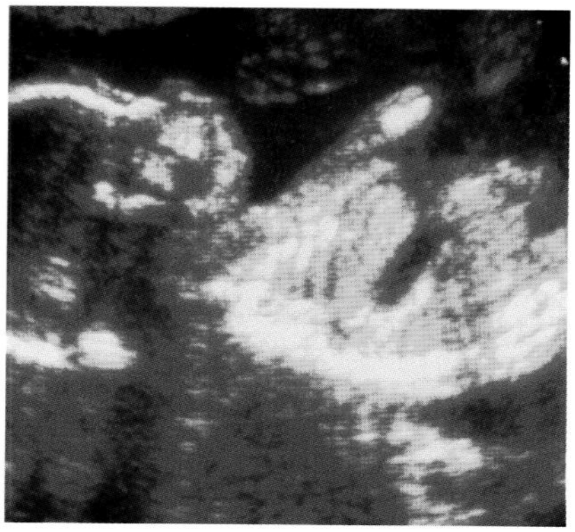

YOU ARE **23 WEEKS AND 2 DAYS**

117 days to go

YOUR BABY TODAY

You will probably be aware of your baby's movements by now: the number of movements and their nature will vary during the day and night and you may notice that they start to form into a particular pattern or respond to your own activity.

> "With a layer of fat and a tough layer of cells, your baby's skin is now becoming more resilient."

Your baby's skin is continuing to develop and has now started to "keratinize." Keratin is the substance that transforms the skin's outer layer into a protective layer of dead cells. Hair and nails also form from keratin.

The outer keratinized layer of skin cells, plus a layer of fat laid down between the skin cells, gives the skin a waterproof covering. This process reduces the amount of water your baby loses into the amniotic fluid. Each new skin cell, made in the deepest part of the skin, matures as it gradually moves up toward the surface and, now keratinized, becomes part of the outer protective layer before it is eventually shed. The cycle takes approximately 30 days.

The thickest layers of keratinized cells are on the palms of the hands and the soles of the feet. The keratinizing process has only just begun. Since the fat layer is very thin at this stage, your baby's skin will still appear translucent, but less so than it did in earlier weeks.

Your baby still has plenty of room to maneuver inside the uterus, and although you're likely to be feeling lots of movements by now this will only be a fraction of the total. This is because the only movements you'll feel are those that cause your baby to kick or bump into the wall of your uterus. You will be unaware of many of the finer movements that are performed close to the baby's body since they won't make any contact with your uterus.

COPING WITH LEG CRAMPS

Getting painful spasms in the leg muscles is common in pregnancy, particularly at night. You may find that you wake up due to the sudden and severe localized pain in your calf muscles. This is thought to be due to the pressure of the uterus on the pelvic nerves.

Some experts believe that leg cramps may be caused by a lack of calcium or salt or an excess of phosphorus, but these theories are as yet unproven.

When you get a spasm, relieve it by flexing your foot or leg (see far right), and gently massaging the affected area. The cramp should resolve itself once you are out of bed and using the muscle.

However, if the pain doesn't recede and there is any reddening or swelling in the leg, you should seek medical advice immediately to eliminate the possibility of a clot (see p.186), since this can be dangerous.

To reduce the incidence or severity of cramping, drink a lot of water to prevent dehydration. Also do leg stretches and ankle exercises regularly, especially before bedtime, circling your heel and wiggling your toes.

Gentle exercise, such as walking or swimming, can also help, as can regularly massaging the calf muscle to improve circulation.

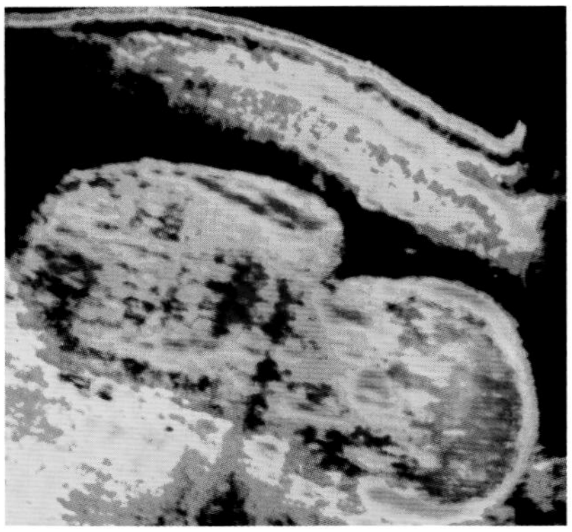

YOU ARE **23 WEEKS AND 3 DAYS**

116 days to go

YOUR BABY TODAY

Ultrasound uses sound waves of a very high frequency, well beyond the audible range of the human ear, so your baby's hearing will be completely unaffected by the sound waves transmitted during these scans that check their growth and development.

" Are you feeling hot? Being pregnant can sometimes feel as though you have your own personal heater strapped to you. "

You may find that you're much hotter and sweating more than normal during pregnancy. This is because you're carrying more weight than usual and you have more blood pumping around your body.

If you're pregnant during the summer, this can be difficult to bear, so find ways to stay cool (see p.324). If you're pregnant in the winter, you may find yourself walking down the street in a light sweater while other people are all bundled up in coats and scarves. You might get into debates with your partner if they want the heating on and you want the windows open!

Drink plenty of fluid throughout the day. You might find that the increased sweat causes a rash in the creases under your breasts or in your groin, so wash frequently and make sure that you dry these areas well.

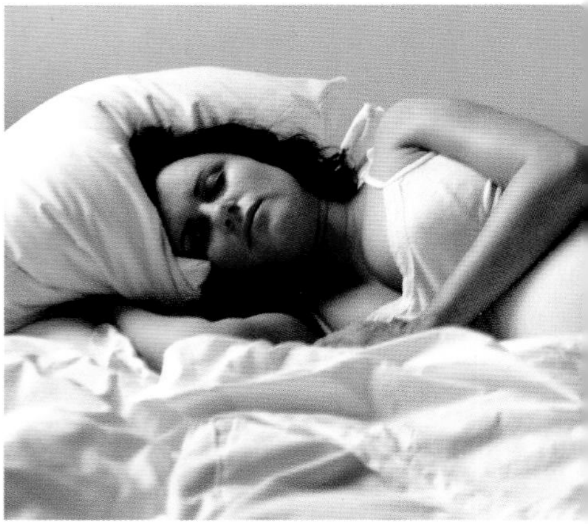

Cotton nightwear and light bedding will help you stay cooler at night and get more restful and restorative sleep.

ASK A DOCTOR

I keep having really strange and vivid dreams. Is this normal during pregnancy? Yes, when you're pregnant, it's common to dream more and to remember your dreams. Experts attribute the vividness of these dreams to all the emotional and physical changes a pregnant woman is going through.

The vivid dreams may be a way for your unconscious to deal with all the hopes and fears you may have about your unborn baby and impending motherhood. It's common to dream that you give birth to an older baby, who is born walking and talking! This is thought to reflect a mother-to-be's insecurities about caring for a tiny, helpless baby. The older the baby, the more self-sufficient they appear. Having more dreams is also believed to be due to hormonal changes in pregnancy: increased levels of estrogen are thought to cause longer periods of REM (rapid eye movement) sleep—the phase of sleep in which we are most likely to dream.

If your dreams are disturbing, try writing them down to get them off your mind.

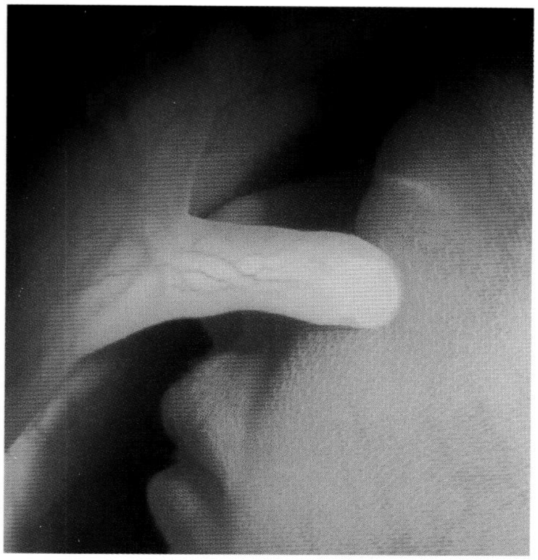

YOU ARE **23 WEEKS AND 4 DAYS**

115 days to go

YOUR BABY TODAY

The joints and bones of the hand are still very soft, although the cartilage skeleton is now gradually being replaced by bone. This image shows well the numerous capillaries supplying blood to the hands, right down to the fingertips.

Your baby's eyelids and eyebrows are well developed at this stage, but the eyelids remain fused. The cells that are destined to become your baby's fingernails were present at 10 weeks, and the cells for the toenails were present four weeks later.

Now, at 23 weeks, the nails are just beginning to make an appearance at the base of the nail bed. The nails will grow continuously throughout life, but it will be several weeks before they have reached the tips of the fingers and then the toes.

Your baby's skin is developing quickly and often appears wrinkled at this stage; it is as if the baby has yet to grow into it. Your baby is now covered in very fine and short hairs, known as "lanugo." This layer of hair will be almost completely lost before birth. The hairs help trap vernix onto the surface of the skin; this is the white, greasy layer often seen in patches on a newborn's skin. It collects in the skin folds and creases and helps protect the skin not only from the water content of the amniotic fluid, but also the waste products within it.

As your pregnancy continues, your baby's kidney function is improving and the amniotic fluid produced becomes increasingly similar to urine in its composition.

> “ Over the next few weeks, your baby will take on more of the appearance of a newborn. ”

PREGNANCY POSTURE

Your posture will naturally change as a result of pregnancy; this is due to the extra weight you're carrying and the softening of your joints.

Prior to pregnancy, your center of gravity was directly over your hips; during later pregnancy it shifts forward to your enlarged abdomen. This dramatic shift in your center of gravity increases the curve of your lower spine, and can result in lower back pain (see p.218). The weight you gain during pregnancy can also put strain on the back.

Exercises can help balance your body and alleviate the aches associated with changes in your posture (see right).

Do abdominal exercises (see p.250), to strengthen the core muscles, as well as back stretches to maintain good posture, enable you to carry your belly well, and avoid back pain later in pregnancy.

Also keep in mind the following:

- **Be aware of** the way you're walking and standing; pull your shoulders down and back, do not arch your lower back, and keep your pelvis in a neutral position.
- **Avoid balancing anything** on your hip, because this can affect alignment.
- **Don't hold a phone between** your head and shoulder because this can result in neck pain.

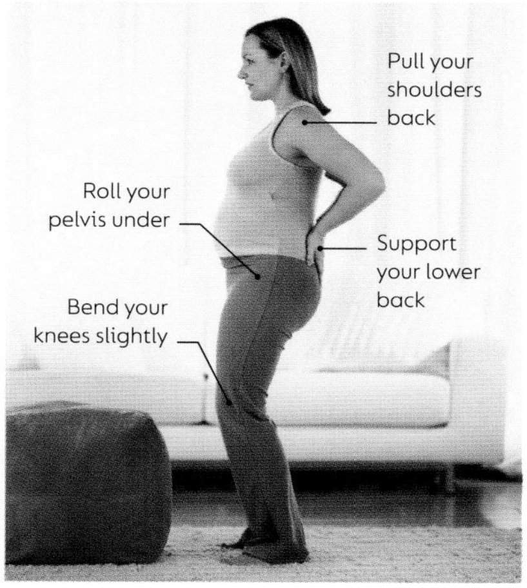
Pull your shoulders back
Roll your pelvis under
Support your lower back
Bend your knees slightly

Abdominal exercises

Strong abdominal muscles will help you carry the weight of your baby and assist you during labor and birth. Try to do the exercises below regularly, but always listen to your body and rest when you need to.

After the first trimester, try to avoid exercises that require you to lie flat on your back. The reason for this is that when you lie on your back, your enlarged uterus presses on one of your major blood vessels, reducing the amount of blood pumped around the body and to the baby. However, the good news is you can strengthen abdominal muscles without lying on your back by using gravity and your body to strengthen and tone the torso.

In pregnancy, you can tone your abdomen with exercises where you adopt an all-fours position or an upright sitting position. Try to do the exercises below around 2–3 times a week.

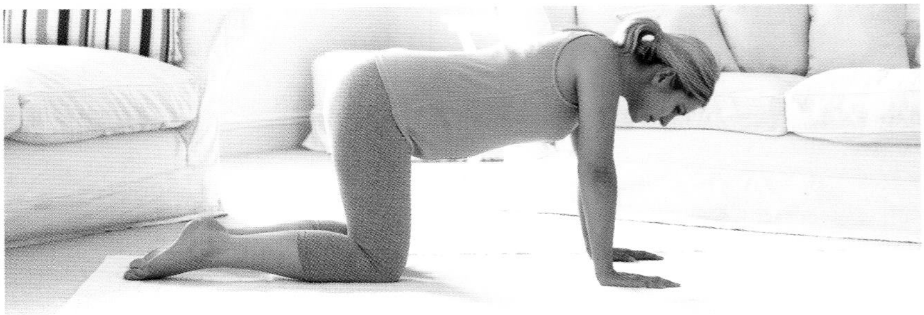

The sling Get down on all fours with your hands on the floor, feet apart, and arms straight. Keep your back flat in a neutral position. Imagine the abdominal muscles as a sling holding your baby. Take a deep breath, then slowly pull your abdominal muscles (the sling) in toward your back, pulling the baby closer to you, and gently release, returning to the starting position. Try to do 20 repetitions. Remember to breathe while doing this exercise, breathing in to start and breathing out as you pull in your belly.

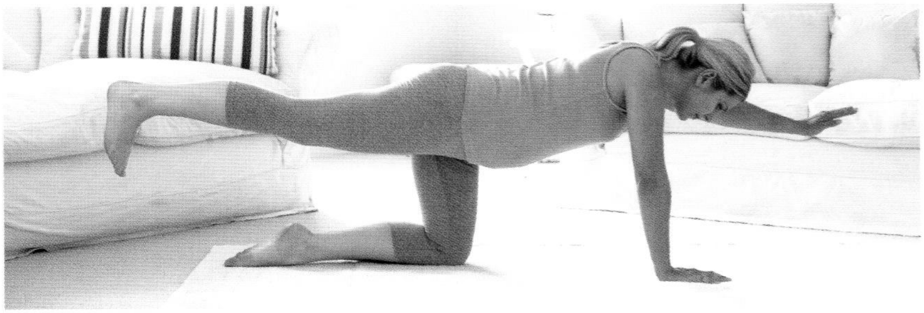

The Superman pose This exercise will strengthen your core muscles, keeping your abdomen and back strong, and helping prevent lower back pain. Start from an all-fours position. Keeping your back in a neutral position, lift your left arm in front of you and your right leg up behind you. Don't arch your back or lift your leg higher than the hips. Hold for a count of five and slowly lower. Repeat with your right arm and left leg. Do 10 repetitions on each side.

Benefits of abdominal exercises
Strong abdominal muscles enable your body to work more efficiently in labor. They also help support the weight of the baby, which takes pressure off the spine, reducing the likelihood of backaches. In addition, keeping your abdominal muscles strong means that you may be less likely to get a condition called diastasis recti, in which the abdominal wall muscles separate, often following childbirth, making it harder to regain your figure.

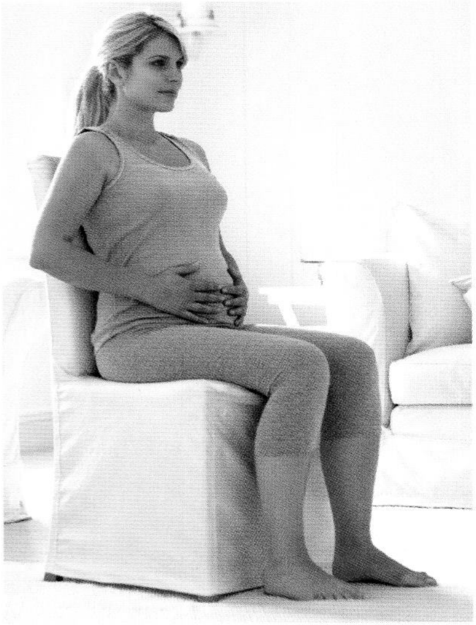

The abdominal pull Sit in a high-backed chair, with your shoulders relaxed and back straight. Put your hands around your belly below your navel. As you breathe in slowly, gently pull in your abdominal muscles for two seconds and then release; repeat 10 times. Take a short break, then start again. Once you've mastered this, move on to the next level. In the same position, pull in your muscles

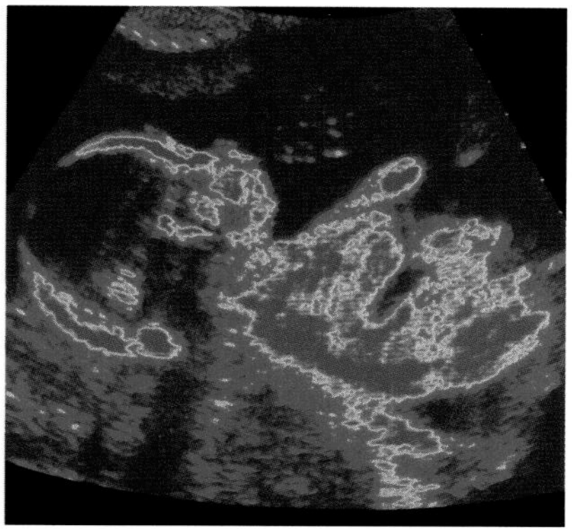

YOU ARE **23 WEEKS AND 5 DAYS**

114 days to go

YOUR BABY TODAY

In this color 2-D ultrasound scan the baby is lying face upward. It is now increasingly difficult to show the whole baby using this type of ultrasound because it only shows a thin slice at any one time. Here, only the upper part of the baby can be seen.

Practicing yoga in pregnancy is safe and can help ease common discomforts. A recent study also found that pregnant women who practiced yoga had a decreased risk of developing pregnancy-induced high blood pressure and of going into preterm labor.

In addition to strengthening and toning muscles, yoga aims to bring about a greater awareness of your breathing. Learning to control your breathing is a great way to relax during pregnancy and an invaluable way to prepare to breathe through the contractions when you're in labor.

Standing poses in yoga focus on achieving core stability, thereby strengthening the abdominal and back muscles. This is beneficial during pregnancy when the additional weight you're carrying can affect your balance and cause unsteadiness. Calm sitting poses that concentrate on aligning your spine help you focus on steadying your breathing and centering yourself. If you feel unsteady doing yoga poses, you can simply lean against a wall.

Pilates is also a good exercise to do in pregnancy because it heightens your bodily awareness, giving you greater control of—and confidence in—your body. Pilates also incorporates Kegel exercises (see p.69).

Whatever classes you're doing, it's important to find an accredited instructor who is experienced in teaching pregnant women. There are now many specialized pregnancy yoga and Pilates classes.

> "Practicing yoga in pregnancy can be hugely beneficial, both physically and emotionally."

ASK A DOCTOR

Why are hemorrhoids so common in pregnancy, and what can I do to relieve them? Hemorrhoids are, like varicose veins (see p.167), dilated veins, but they occur around your anus. The weight of your baby pushes down on your back passage, restricting blood flow and causing the veins to dilate.

Hemorrhoids can be itchy and sore and may cause a throbbing sensation. The discomfort can be relieved with cold packs and creams containing lubricants to help the passage of stools, and/or local anesthetics to relieve soreness. Hemorrhoids can bleed—you may notice bright red blood on the toilet paper after you pass a stool.

If you have hemorrhoids, it is important to try not to get constipated (see p.468) since this means you have to strain and push to pass stools, which increases the pressure on the hemorrhoids and makes them worse. Ensure that you drink lots of water and eat sufficient fiber.

If your hemorrhoids are becoming very problematic and uncomfortable, seek your doctor's advice.

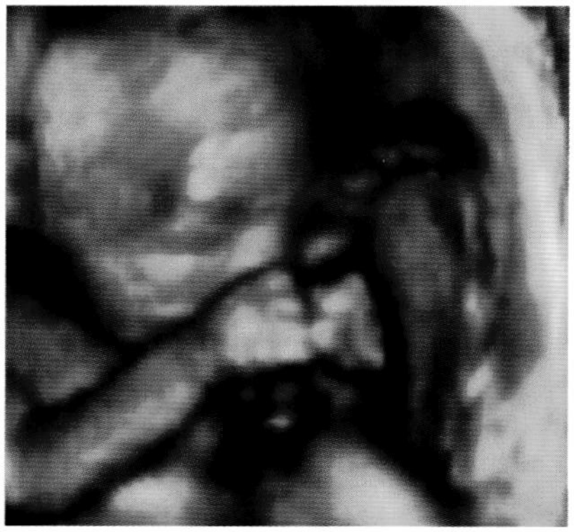

YOU ARE **23 WEEKS AND 6 DAYS**

113 days to go

YOUR BABY TODAY

Your baby is now making regular deep breathing movements. These have been present for some weeks, but not in a sustained and coordinated fashion. These breathing movements are critical for the development and expansion of your baby's lungs.

Your baby's lungs are starting to mature, as the barrier between the bloodstream and what will become air-containing sacs gradually starts to thin. The thinner this barrier, the more easily oxygen and carbon dioxide will transfer into and out of the baby's bloodstream.

The lungs remain filled with fluid during your pregnancy and when your baby practices breathing, the fluid moves out of her lungs into the amniotic fluid.

At 23 weeks, cells begin to line the smallest branches within the lung and start to produce surfactant, which greatly assists lung function. It helps the smallest air sacs to remain open when the newborn baby breathes in and out so gas transfer can continually take place. Without it, the tiny air sacs would collapse after each breath and it would take much more effort to move air in and out of the lungs. The cells that produce surfactant are not, however, fully functional yet.

“Although the lungs are the last of your baby's organs to be fully functional, they are undergoing rapid development now.”

ASK A DOCTOR

Is it true that playing music to my unborn baby will enhance their development? Some research into this claim finds that playing music to an unborn baby will lead to a shorter labor and easier birth, and to the newborn baby crying less, being more relaxed, and, overall, being in better health. At the moment, there doesn't seem to be any significant research to suggest that babies who listen to music in the uterus are more intelligent or develop at a greater speed.

The jury is still out on these findings, but there is anecdotal evidence from pregnant women that their babies move to the rhythm of music. It makes sense that as music relaxes or invigorates you, your baby will respond in kind. Many moms say that music played frequently during pregnancy seems to be familiar to their newborns and soothes them.

So whether your baby is simply experiencing the benefits of your happy state as you listen, or responding to the rhythm, playing music is a good idea.

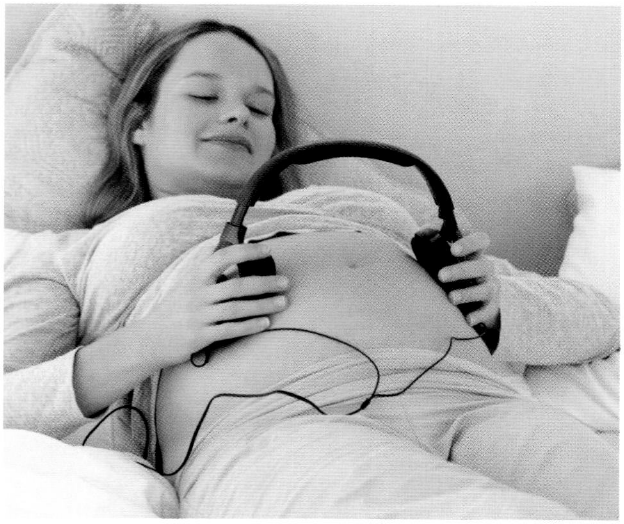

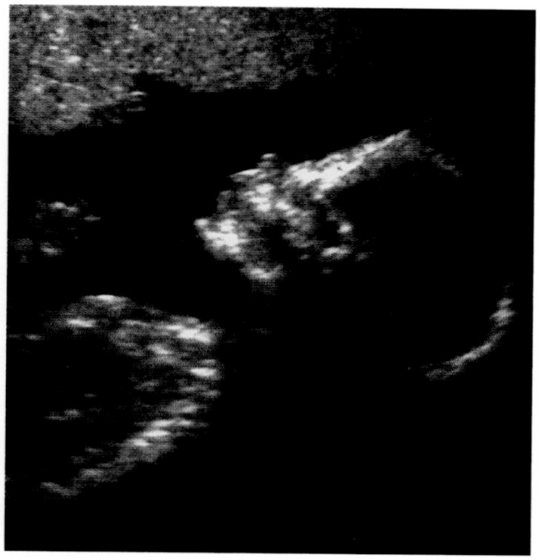

YOU ARE **24 WEEKS EXACTLY**

112 days to go

YOUR BABY TODAY

As your pregnancy advances, your baby's skeleton starts to harden, reflecting more of the ultrasound beam and casting black shadows. In this scan, the forehead casts a shadow, and it is no longer allowing the brain beneath to be easily seen.

> "Even though you're well settled into your pregnancy, ensure you maintain all those healthy lifestyle habits you've established."

You've been pregnant for almost six months and are, hopefully, feeling great in yourself. Don't, however, let this make you complacent. Even though your baby is well developed by this stage, it's important to maximize her health, and your own, by continuing to eat well and taking care of yourself. Changes, such as not smoking or drinking alcohol, will probably be part of your normal lifestyle now as opposed to something that you have to think about and work hard at. If you have not managed to change your lifestyle to become more healthy, then it is never too late to start. Any changes you make now will benefit both you and your baby.

While you'll need to adapt your exercise routine, if you have one, in these later stages, ensure you continue to be active and, ideally, do something physical every day, even if it's just a 20-minute stroll. Also keep up your daily Kegel exercises (see p.69)—once the baby is born, you'll be thankful you did.

FOCUS ON PARTNERS

Don't be afraid to talk to your baby in the womb. After birth, your baby will recognize your voice and this will have a calming effect when they are distressed. So tell them about your day and even read to them—it helps create a bond.

Male partners have a slight advantage over female partners, because to begin with, the baby will recognize lower-pitched sounds, such as deep male voices, more readily than the higher-pitched sounds of female voices.

HOW TO WEAR A SEAT BELT

Research found that over half of pregnant women did not wear their seat belt correctly, positioning it too high across the abdomen and putting the torso strap behind them rather than over the shoulder.

It may feel cumbersome to wear a seat belt while you have a growing bump to contend with, but it is essential, and a legal requirement, and a correctly worn seat belt reduces the risk of injury to the unborn baby by 70 percent.

- **Fasten the belt o**ver your shoulder, as normal, and between your breasts.
- **Position the lower part** of the belt below your belly, and flat over your hips.

If an emergency stop is necessary, be reassured that your baby is very safely cushioned by the amniotic fluid that surrounds her and your strong uterine muscles.

Your 25th week

IT'S THE END OF THE SECOND TRIMESTER, SO YOU MIGHT WANT TO START LOOKING AHEAD

The rest of your pregnancy will pass before you know it. Make sure you have all the practicalities in hand, such as deciding what date to stop work, and you might want to give some thought to the birth. Meanwhile, friends and family will no doubt be monitoring your growing belly with interest. Try to be patient if they bombard you with advice and don't listen to too many "tall tales" about pregnancy and childbirth.

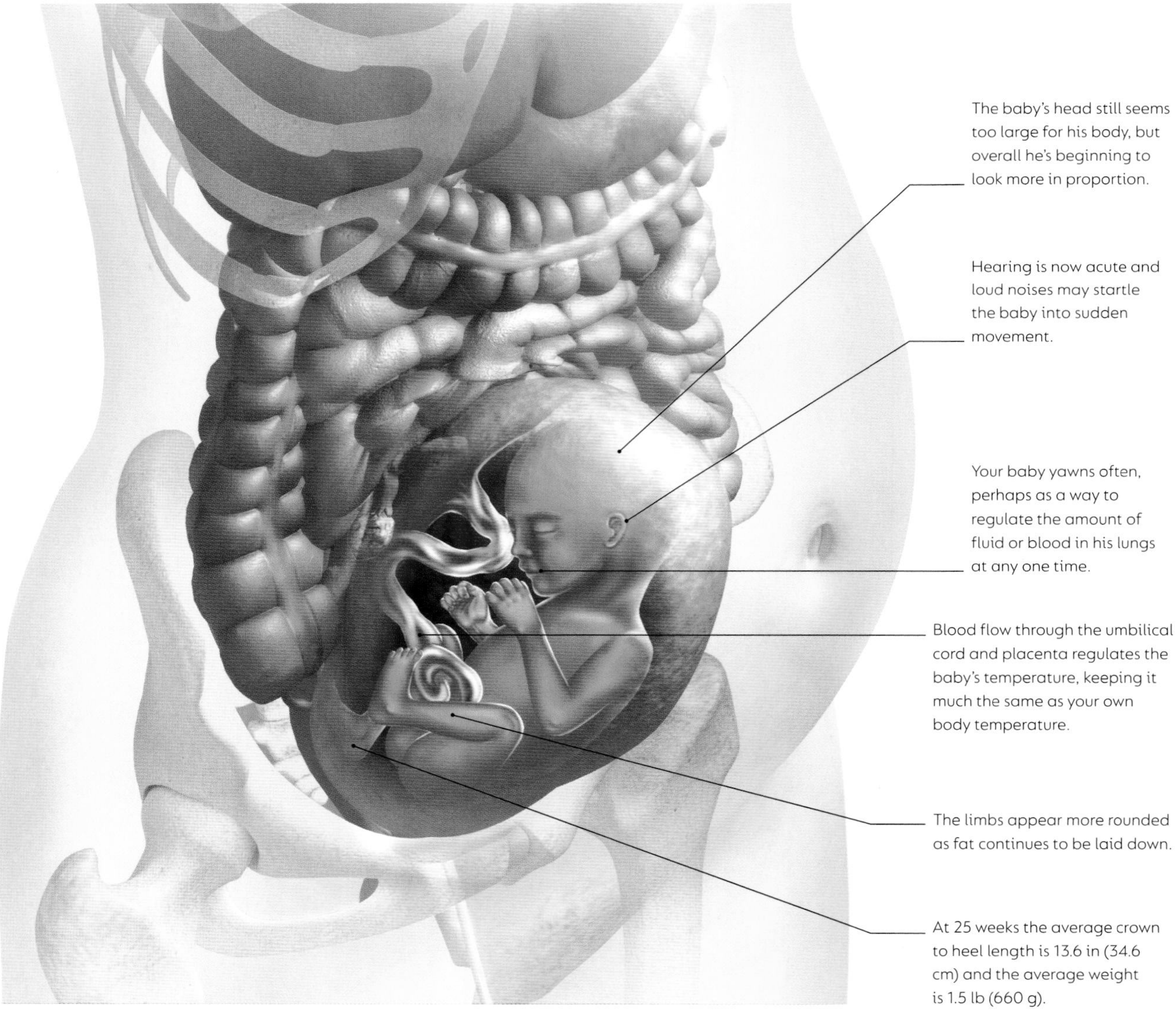

The baby's head still seems too large for his body, but overall he's beginning to look more in proportion.
Hearing is now acute and loud noises may startle the baby into sudden movement.
Your baby yawns often, perhaps as a way to regulate the amount of fluid or blood in his lungs at any one time.
Blood flow through the umbilical cord and placenta regulates the baby's temperature, keeping it much the same as your own body temperature.
The limbs appear more rounded as fat continues to be laid down.
At 25 weeks the average crown to heel length is 13.6 in (34.6 cm) and the average weight is 1.5 lb (660 g).

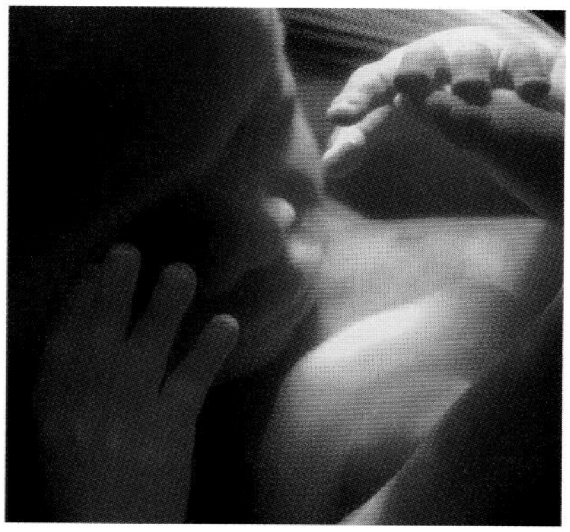

YOU ARE **24 WEEKS AND 1 DAY**

111 days to go

YOUR BABY TODAY

From this week, brown fat is laid down in your baby's neck, chest, and back to be used after birth to produce heat and energy. At the moment, they have no control over their temperature, which is efficiently maintained at a perfect level by the placenta.

> "This week, think about starting discussions with your employer about your upcoming maternity leave."

Since you're more than halfway through your pregnancy by now and are likely showing, you've probably already told your boss that you're pregnant. But just informing your company isn't enough—you need to know all the details that pertain to your upcoming maternity leave and what will happen if you decide to stop working before the baby is born. Every company has different guidelines; some include paid maternity leave while others do not. Talk with a human resources representative to discuss your company's policies on maternity leave and time off. If paid time off isn't available, your company may allow you to use paid vacation days or sick leave, and you may be eligible for Family and Medical Leave Act (FMLA) leave.

To take advantage of the FMLA, you must have worked for an employer at least 12 months (1,250 hours over the past 12 months), and work where the company employs 50 or more people within 75 miles. You may take up to 12 weeks of leave in a 12-month period.

ASK A DOCTOR

What does "small for gestational age" mean? It means your baby appears to be small for your stage of pregnancy, but it doesn't mean there's a problem. You'll be given a scan to accurately measure and check your baby.

Sometimes slow growth is due to fetal growth restriction (FGR), because of a problem with the placenta, affecting the amount of oxygen and nutrients reaching the baby. Preeclampsia (see p.476) can cause FGR, as can lifestyle factors such as smoking, drinking alcohol, and taking recreational drugs.

STRETCHY SKIN

You may have developed stretch marks due to your skin stretching rapidly as you gain pregnancy weight. Initially, these marks are pinky/red and can be itchy. After pregnancy, stretch marks fade to a lighter, silvery color and become less obvious. They generally occur on the breasts, belly, hips, and thighs, and affect the majority of pregnant women.

Stretch marks can be genetic and are more likely to occur the older you are because older skin is less elastic. Moisturizing the skin won't prevent stretch marks but it may help to keep it smooth. A combination of exercising and eating healthily can minimize the rate at which you gain weight and "stretch."

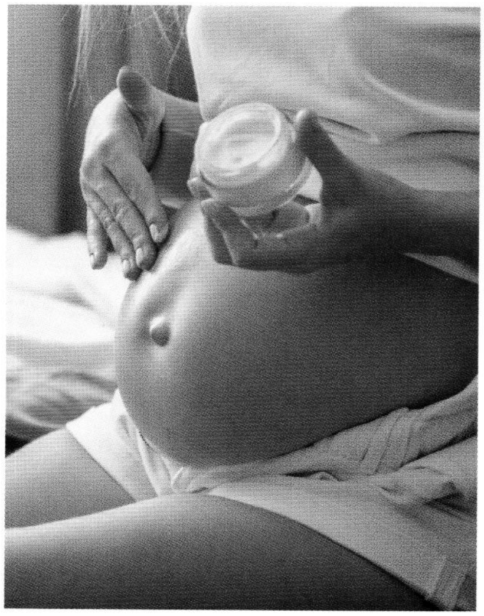

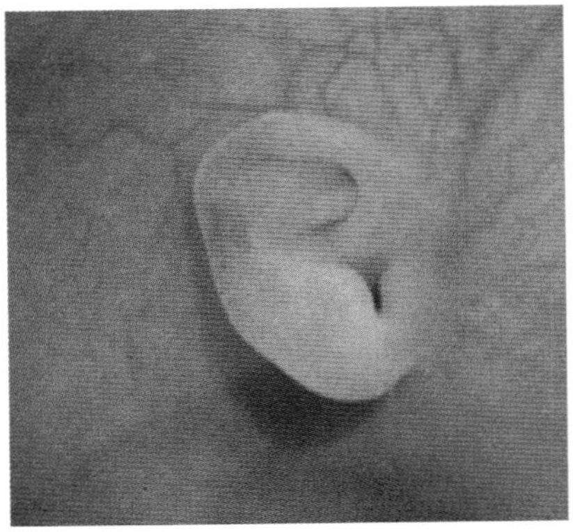

YOU ARE **24 WEEKS AND 2 DAYS**

110 days to go...

YOUR BABY TODAY

In the uterus, your baby's ears have fluid around them and also inside. This is part of the reason that they can hear only certain lower sound frequencies. Yawning may be a way to unblock the ears, and from now on your baby spends a lot of time yawning.

> "If you're feeling tired, you're not alone. Your developing baby has been yawning for some weeks now."

All babies are known to yawn in the uterus, although the reason why they do this remains unclear. Yawning is often accompanied by shrugging of the shoulders or stretching, exactly as you would do when tired. Unborn babies have even been seen to rub their eyes!

Your baby first started yawning at around 15 weeks and has gradually yawned more and more frequently. The precise function of yawning for the baby remains in doubt and there are several hypotheses. While it's difficult to imagine that an unborn baby is actually tired, it has been found that babies who are anemic yawn much more frequently than others. Another theory is that yawning may help the unborn baby to regulate the amount of fluid or blood flow they have within their lungs. Or when the baby yawns, it may simply be a primitive reflex.

Whatever the reason for yawning, the early stage at which this develops, and the fact that all mammals are known to yawn in the uterus suggests that it plays an important, though unknown, role in fetal development.

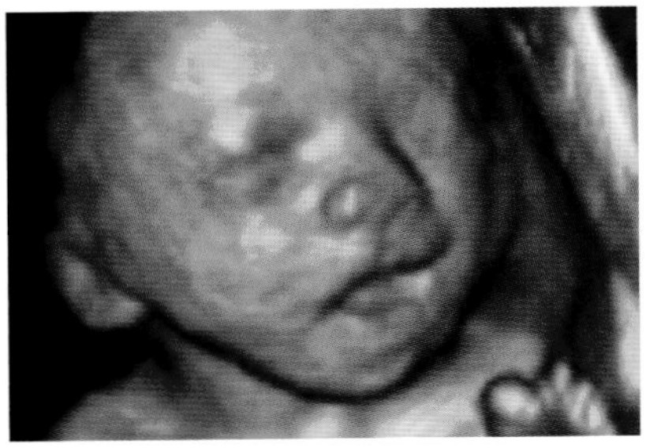

Many unborn babies have been filmed yawning on 4-D scans, which give a very up-close view of fetal behavior.

TALKING TO YOUR BABY

Your developing baby's ears are structurally complete, and studies show that he can hear clearly now. Your breathing and heartbeat and the gurgles of your digestive system provide a constant background rhythm, but he's also aware of other sounds.

In one study, ultrasounds of fetuses showed that they had a "blink-startle" response to loud noises from around 24 weeks.

Talking to your baby will help you to bond: research indicates that newborns recognize—and turn toward—the sound of their mother's voice in preference to other female voices. To begin with he'll hear deeper voices more clearly, but later he'll register higher-pitched sounds. He will, of course, become more familiar with your voice, partly because this is what he will hear most often and because your body is a good conductor of sound vibration.

LEFT-HANDED BABIES

Women aged over 40 are more than twice as likely to have left-handed babies. This is according to a Canadian study and may be related to the fact that older women are more likely to experience complications in pregnancy and have more arduous deliveries. Several studies show a correlation between left-handedness and birth stress.

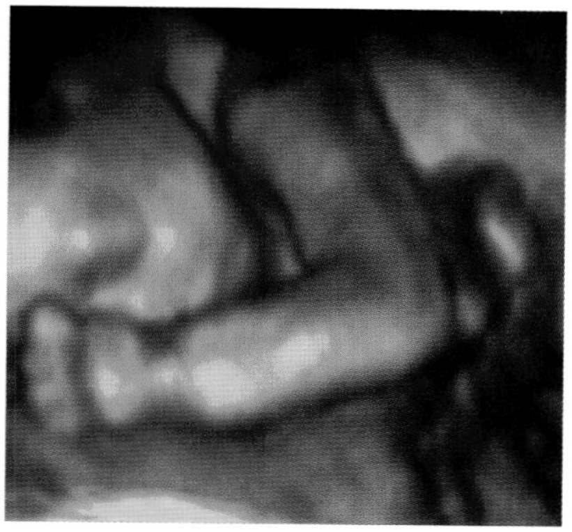

YOU ARE **24 WEEKS AND 3 DAYS**

109 days to go...

YOUR BABY TODAY

Here the baby is lying with an arm up to the face and the face lying on the placenta. The eyes are shut at this time and it will be a couple of weeks before they start to open. The hand is held in the most relaxed position, with the fingers slightly curled.

> "Your body is working hard to grow your baby, so take care of it by enjoying some pampering."

ASK A DOCTOR

I haven't felt my baby move for four hours. Should I be worried? Contact your doctor and explain your baby's usual pattern of movements. They can examine you and provide reassurance. Try lying down—your baby is more likely to sleep when you're active—and have something sweet to eat. Try encouraging your baby to move around (see p.206).

Think of your pregnancy as a time to focus on yourself and your body; once your baby is born, the majority of your focus will be on baby care.

If you have the time and money, treat yourself to a day at a spa and enjoy being pampered in a tranquil environment. Most do special packages for pregnant women. If a spa day is out of the question, create your own at home. Run a bath, add some relaxing music (for a background soundtrack), light some candles, and relax. If you don't want to be disturbed, let your partner know and put your phone on silent.

Getting a pregnancy massage (see p.224), either from a professional or your partner, can be very therapeutic, both physically and emotionally. Another great treatment to have at this stage is a pedicure; you'll increasingly be unable to see your toes, let alone reach them, so it's a treat for someone else to take care of them for you.

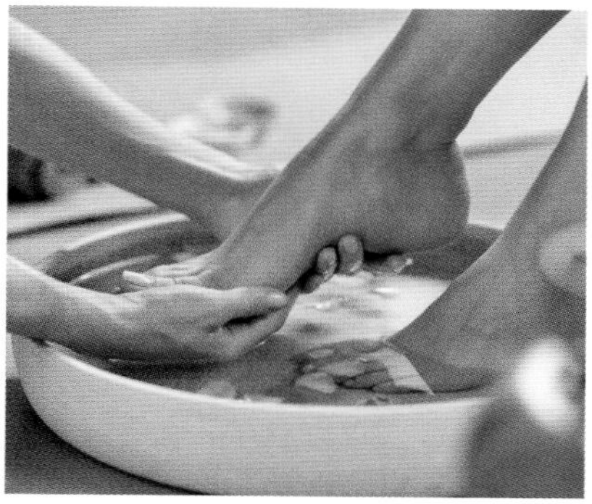

Now is the time to indulge yourself in a little pampering. When booking beauty treatments, always make it known that you're pregnant.

ON YOUR FEET

You may find it harder to be on your feet, especially for long periods of time. Weight gain, changes in your center of gravity (particularly during the second and third trimesters), and hormones can cause foot pain and swelling (see pp.225 and 468). The hormones that relax your joints ready for childbirth can also work to loosen the ligaments in your feet and hips, which can cause some discomfort. To minimize foot discomfort:

- **Wear athletic shoes** that have a good arch support to help reduce strain on your spine. They may also prevent a condition called plantar fasciitis—this is where the large ligament that connects the heel to the ball of the foot becomes inflamed.
- **Avoid wearing high-heeled shoes.** In addition to being uncomfortable, they may make you unsteady on your feet and cause you to fall.
- **Ensure that your shoes fit** correctly and invest in new ones if not. Some pregnant women's feet expand by a size and never return to their normal size after pregnancy.
- **Get regular exercise,** and avoid standing for long periods. Take regular breaks if your job involves standing.

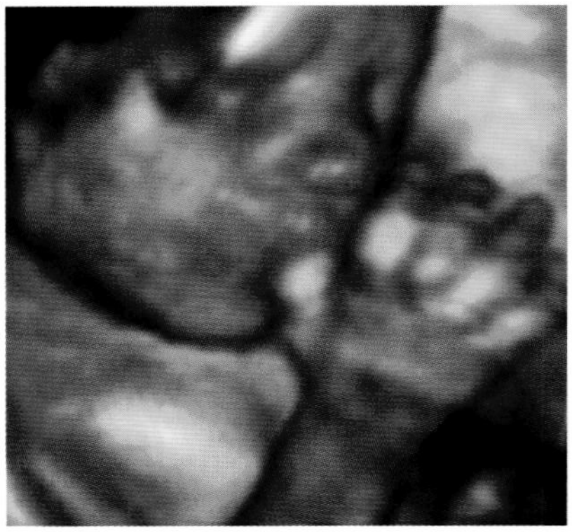

YOU ARE **24 WEEKS AND 4 DAYS**

108 days to go

YOUR BABY TODAY

This 3-D scan shows the baby thumb sucking. The technique uses several routine 2-D images, linked together to give the 3-D effect. In a 4-D scan, a series of 3-D images are shown in quick succession to give almost real-time movements: the 4th dimension is time.

> "A natural temperature-regulating mechanism within the uterus means your baby never gets cold."

The temperature inside the uterus is between a third and half a degree higher than yours. Because your body temperature is so closely controlled, your baby never becomes cold so never needs to shiver. They've started to lay down a special form of brown fat, particularly around the neck, chest, and back. After birth, metabolism of this fat produces both energy and heat. In the uterus, however, the baby cannot use this fat to raise their temperature. Some temperature control occurs as heat is lost from the baby's skin into the amniotic fluid through the uterine wall and then into your body tissues.

However, the regulation of temperature is predominantly achieved by means of the blood flow to the placenta. The large surface area of the placenta allows it to act as a heat exchange, keeping the temperature of the blood leaving the baby in the umbilical arteries constant with that of the oxygenated blood returning to the baby through the umbilical vein.

After birth, babies lose heat quickly. They are still unable to shiver and cannot maintain their temperature, cooling rapidly if they're not wrapped up warmly or held skin-to-skin shortly after the birth.

SENSIBLE SNACKING

As your pregnancy progresses, you may find that you can't eat large meals and that you prefer smaller meals and snacks. If you are on the go, try:

- Unsalted nuts or seeds.
- Pretzels, oatcakes, rice or corn cakes, and breadsticks.
- Dried fruits, which are a good source of iron, so try dried peaches figs, and prunes, as well as raisins and apricots. Opt for unsweetened versions when possible.
- An apple or clementine.

If you're at home, other nutritious mini meals or snacks can include eggs, cheese, or soup. A slice of whole-wheat toast makes a great partner for chicken salad, nut butters, cheese, or eggs. Try to include a vegetable with each snack, such as grated carrots, slices of red bell peppers or celery, a few cherry tomatoes, or some arugula.

To make healthy snacking easier, keep your fruit bowl well stocked with a variety of different fruits, and keep a supply of grapes and berries in the fridge.

Yogurt, whether dairy based or not, can be an easily digested quick snack. Opt for sugarless versions, and add chopped fruit or nuts, or a small handful of granola. In summer, yogurt-based ice creams can be very refreshing.

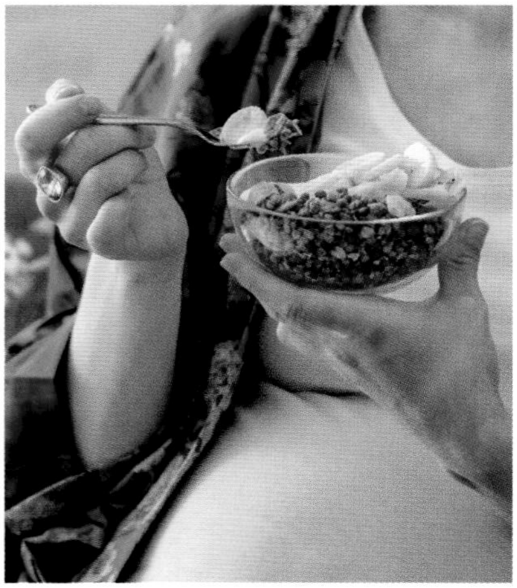

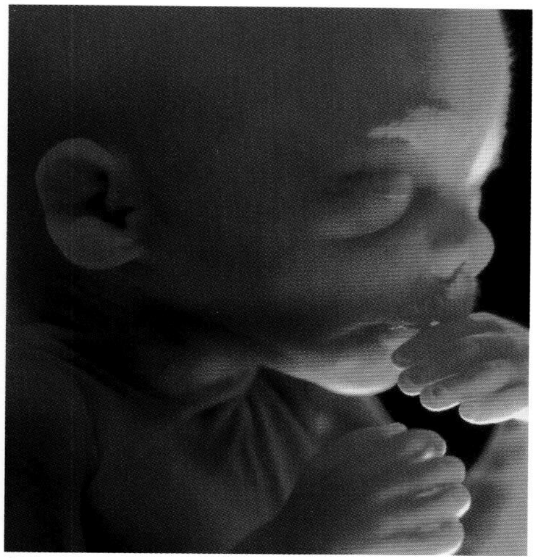

YOU ARE **24 WEEKS AND 5 DAYS**

107 days to go

YOUR BABY TODAY

Here the skin looks almost loose around the neck as the baby has turned their head slightly. This is normal at this stage: the lack of fat beneath the skin and the need to grow rapidly can make your baby appear as if they need time to "grow into" their skin.

While you may be enjoying your food, you could be paying the price with indigestion. The pregnancy hormone progesterone relaxes the muscles in the entire digestive tract. This slows digestion and the sphincters, or rings of muscles, at each end of the stomach become less effective. This can cause heartburn and indigestion as acidic juices from the stomach leak back into the esophagus. In addition, as your pregnancy progresses, your growing baby is squashing your stomach so that you have a smaller space to digest food.

To relieve indigestion, eat little and often, eat slowly, don't eat late at night, and cut down on fatty or spicy foods. Check with your pharmacist before taking any over-the-counter medicine. You could also try natural remedies, such as peppermint, which is beneficial in its fresh or dried herbal form. Peppermint contains menthol, which has been shown in studies to be an effective digestive muscle relaxant and an effective remedy for gas, nausea, and indigestion. It has a "carminative" effect, meaning that it works specifically on the digestive system. Try drinking tea or sucking on peppermint candy, especially if you've eaten a big meal. If these simple remedies do not work, speak with your doctor about other treatment options.

> "Some meals may be followed by an uncomfortable bout of indigestion, but you can take steps to prevent and relieve this."

ASK A NUTRITIONIST

What can I eat to relieve my constipation? Increase your intake of fiber, with high-fiber breakfast cereals, whole-wheat bread, and oatmeal. Eat legumes, such as lentils, beans, and peas too.

Include whole grains in your diet every day, as well as vegetables and fruits. The humble prune not only contains fiber, but also a natural laxative called sorbitol.

Fiber bulks out the stools, but you will need to drink plenty of water to pass them with ease. And don't forget that being active helps, so exercise gently when you can. Don't be embarrassed to ask for help—about one-third of pregnant women get constipated, so your doctor has heard it all before.

FOCUS ON PARTNERS

You may be eligible for paternity pay and leave if you are the father, the husband or partner of the mother, including same-sex partners, the adopter, or the intended parent (if it's surrogacy). The amount of leave and pay will depend on your company policy and how long you have worked there (see p.349). Speak to your human resources department now to find out your rights and whether your company offers additional perks. To maximize the time you can take off once the baby is born, figure out how much vacation you have left and consider saving up days.

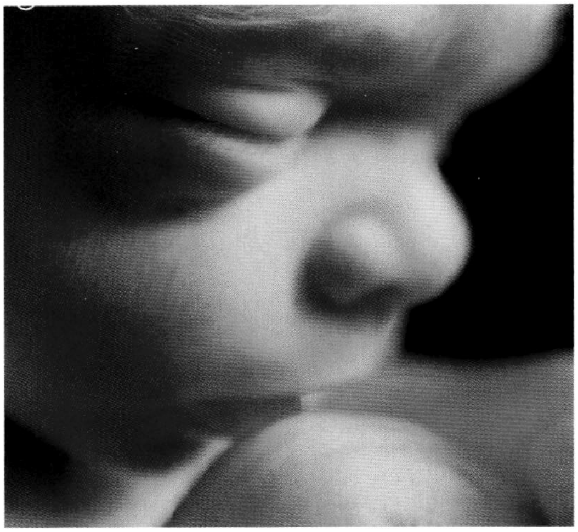

YOU ARE **24 WEEKS AND 6 DAYS**

106 days to go

YOUR BABY TODAY

The nose is well defined and in addition to regularly swallowing the amniotic fluid your baby is breathing it in and out through each nostril. Just as adults do, your baby will tend to favor breathing more through one nostril than the other.

> "The proportions of your baby's body are becoming much closer to those of a newborn baby."

Up until the third month, your baby's head accounted for almost half of their overall length. Now their head, torso, and legs account for a third each. At birth your baby's head will still be large in proportion compared to an adult's, but it will be just a quarter of their overall length.

Still very skinny, your baby is now starting to fill out more as fat reserves continue to be laid down. Until about 14 weeks, most babies are approximately the same size and weight. After this point, genetic and especially environmental forces increasingly come into play, influencing how quickly your baby can grow and whether his full growth potential is eventually reached.

Because babies increasingly vary in size as the pregnancy progresses, ultrasound dating becomes less accurate at determining the due date. The best time to do so is during the first trimester, by ultrasound, measuring from the top of the baby's head to their bottom (the crown-rump length; see p.138). The 20-week scan (see pp.214–215) also dates the pregnancy very accurately from the head and abdominal circumferences and the bone measurement in the leg.

If your first scan is at this late stage, it is only possible to estimate roughly the stage of pregnancy and age of the baby. It is never appropriate to change your due date if an earlier, more accurate scan has been performed.

OLD WIVES' TALES

It is often said that if you're carrying your baby low, you're having a boy, if you're carrying high, then it's a girl. But the way you carry is probably determined by the tone of your abdominal and uterine muscles and the baby's position.

According to those "old wives," there are other physical clues: if you've gained weight on your face and it's round and full, you're having a girl. If your right breast is larger than your left, it's a boy—and if your partner gains weight, you're "definitely" having a girl!

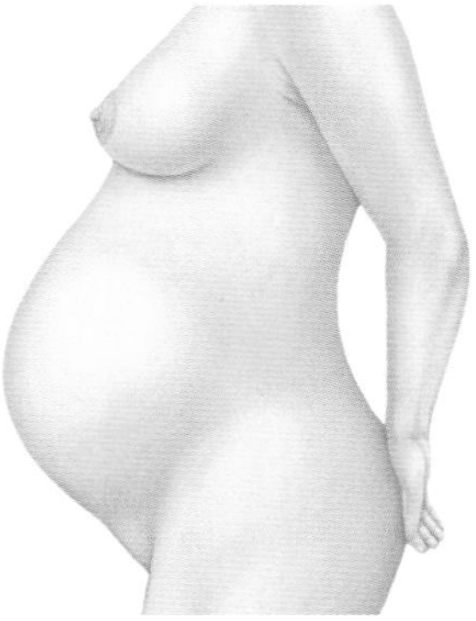

Woman carrying baby low

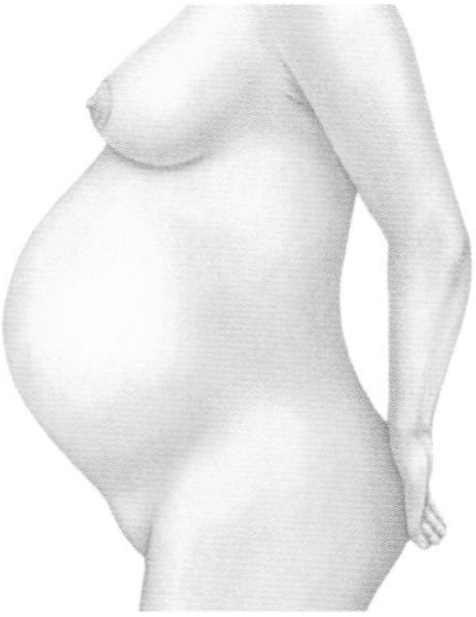

Woman carrying baby to the front

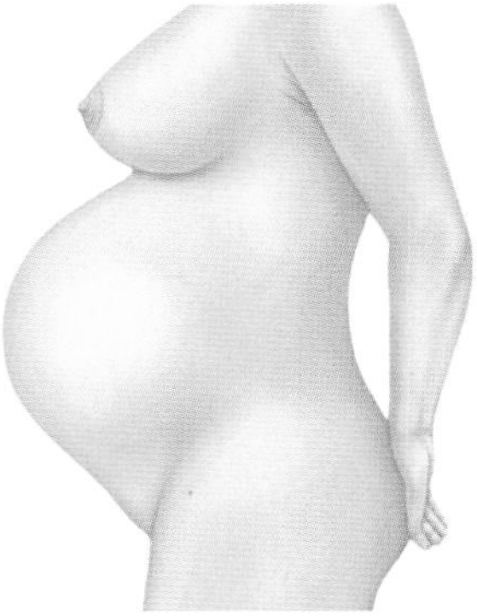

Woman carrying baby high

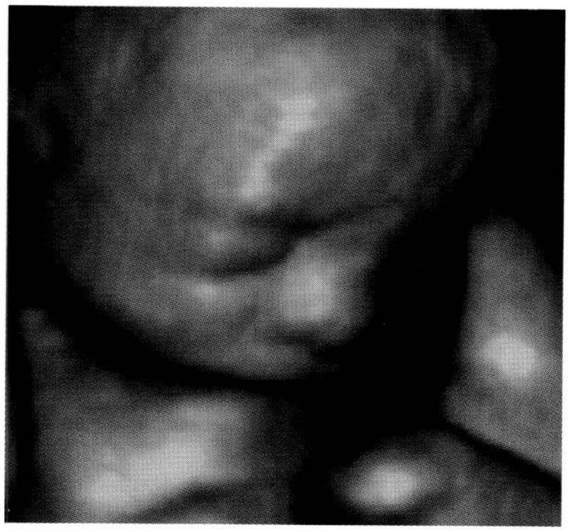

YOU ARE **25 WEEKS EXACTLY**

105 days to go

YOUR BABY TODAY

Here the baby's head is looking down toward the chest. The right arm is bent at the elbow to lie across the neck, the left arm is only just visible as it is partly in shadow, and finally the tip of a knee can be seen tucked up just below the right forearm.

" You can expect to be subjected to a few unwelcome birth stories, whether you want to hear them or not! "

It appears to be a rite of passage for some women to describe the birth of their babies in minute detail, literally giving an hour-by-hour account. For these women, it appears to be part of the recovery process and they like nothing better than a new audience, and, especially, a woman who is pregnant for the first time. So you'll no doubt find yourself on the receiving end of a few birth horror stories—sometimes from complete strangers!

These women may feel it's their duty to "warn" you about the "reality" of childbirth, and what you should and shouldn't do—for example, "definitely have an epidural; otherwise, the pain is horrendous." Remember that every woman's experience is different, so stay focused on your own birth plan.

Childbirth is undoubtedly difficult for some women, while others have straightforward deliveries, without complications. Politely let the storyteller know that you'd rather not hear the gory details but promise to book a date for a joint debrief once your baby is born!

MOTHER'S HELP

The prospect of giving birth and then taking care of a newborn can be daunting. For some new moms, hiring a doula is the perfect way to ensure a gentle progression from pregnancy into motherhood.

Doulas are women who "mother the mother" by providing emotional and physical (but nonmedical) support before, during, and after childbirth. Widespread research shows that the presence of a doula can help you have a shorter, easier birth, making it less likely that you'll need pain relief or medical intervention (including an epidural or cesarean). To find out more about hiring a doula, visit dona.org/mothers/find_a_doula.php.

BIRTH PARTNERS

The benefits of having a supportive birth partner are indisputable, so it's a good idea to think about it now.

- **Research shows that** women who receive continuous emotional and physical encouragement during labor are less likely to need pain relief or medical intervention such as an epidural (see pp.404–405), assisted birth (see pp.436–437), or Cesarean (see pp.438–441), and should experience a shorter labor.
- **Women who feel their birth partner** was supportive are more likely to view their birth in a positive light, and to take to motherhood and breastfeeding easily, and are less prone to postpartum depression.
- **Your birth partner** doesn't have to be the baby's father (although he may be there as well); in fact, studies indicate that a woman may do the job better. A close female friend who's had her own children could be ideal; your mom is another option.
- **You could consider** hiring a doula (see left).

Welcome to your third trimester

WEEK 26 | WEEK 27 | WEEK 28 | WEEK 29 | WEEK 30 | WEEK 31 | WEEK 32 | WEEK 33

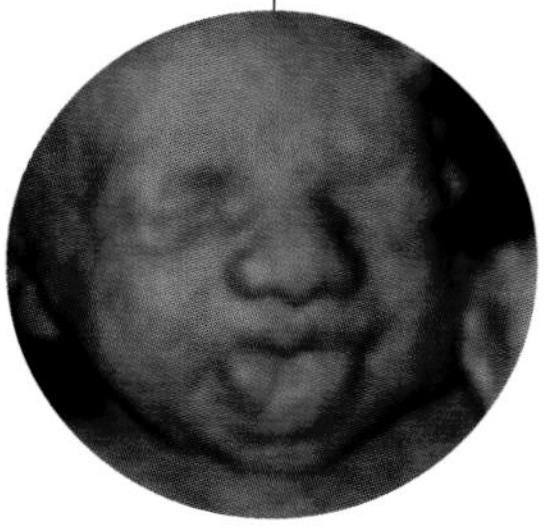

Your baby will often stick their **tongue** out, especially after swallowing a **big gulp** of amniotic fluid.

WEEK 26: START PRENATAL CLASSES

For many women and their partners, going to prenatal classes signals the start of their labor and birth preparations. Meeting other parents-to-be, and sharing this amazing life experience can be the start of new and long-lasting new friendships.

WEEK 30: WRITE YOUR BIRTH PLAN

As you imaging what your delivery might look like, it can help to create a birth plan. This can help organize conversation about your preferences, such as pain-relief options, with your doctor. The plan is useful, too, for your birth partner, who may need to advocate for you once you are in labor.

Although your baby often sleeps, the **eyes** will open for **short periods** of time.

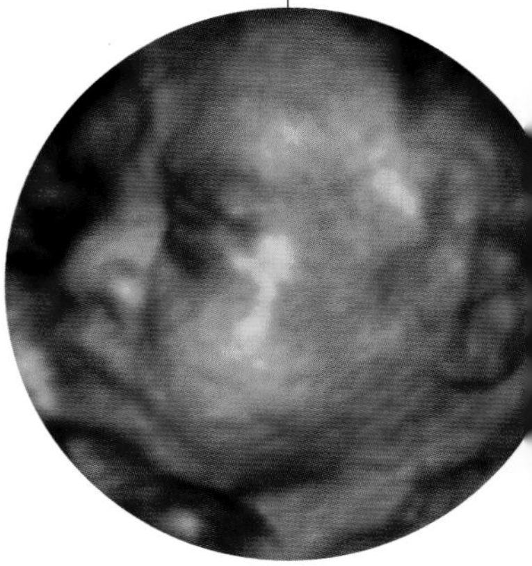

“ Excitement and anticipation mark this trimester, as you prepare for labor and count down to meeting your baby. ”

WEEK 34 | WEEK 35 | WEEK 36 | WEEK 37 | WEEK 38 | WEEK 39 | WEEK 40

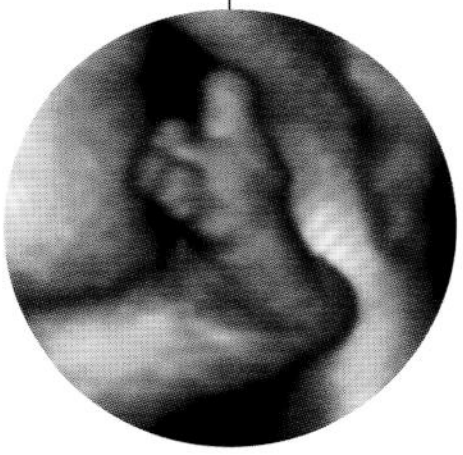

You will become increasingly aware of your baby’s **limbs**. The less space there is, the more **kicks** and **punches** you will feel!

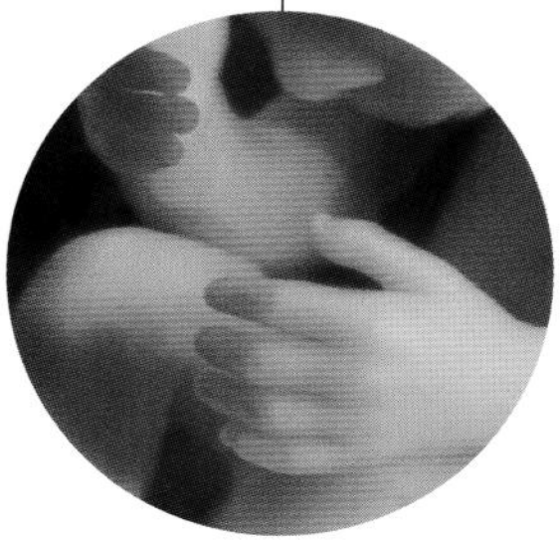

At **37 weeks,** your baby is considered **full term** and will continue to grow and gain **weight** until delivery.

WEEK 36: PACK YOUR HOSPITAL BAG

As your due date approaches, you’ll feel more prepared if you get your hospital bag ready, so start gathering essential items for both you and your baby. You will find a useful checklist of things to bring on p.358. You may also want to prepare things at home so you are ready for when your baby arrives.

YOU AND YOUR BABY **AT 40 WEEKS**

Your baby is engaged in the pelvis, hopefully head down, ready to be born. The skull bones are separated by membranes that allow for movement and easier passage of the head through the birth canal. As you reach your due date, it’s normal to expereince a wide range of emotions as you await your baby’s arrival.

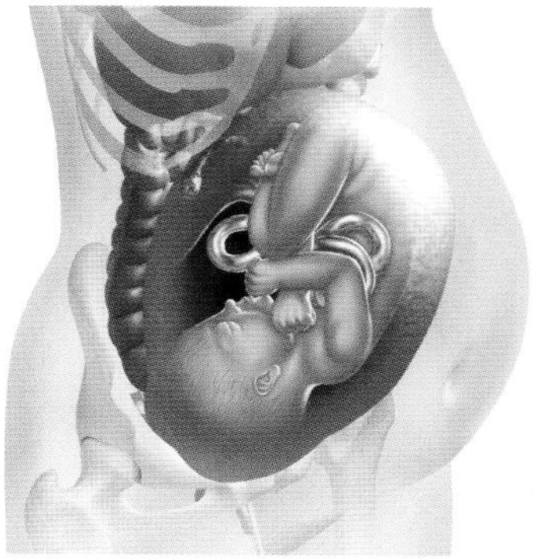

Your 26th week

YOU'VE REACHED THE THIRD AND FINAL TRIMESTER. You're in the last lap and, although your belly is probably big, you've still got a lot more expanding to do. Your baby will be moving around quite vigorously and may even respond to loud noises and music. Nerve cells in her brain are beginning to connect and her coordination is improving. Keep your own brain stimulated by going to prenatal classes for fun, company, and information.

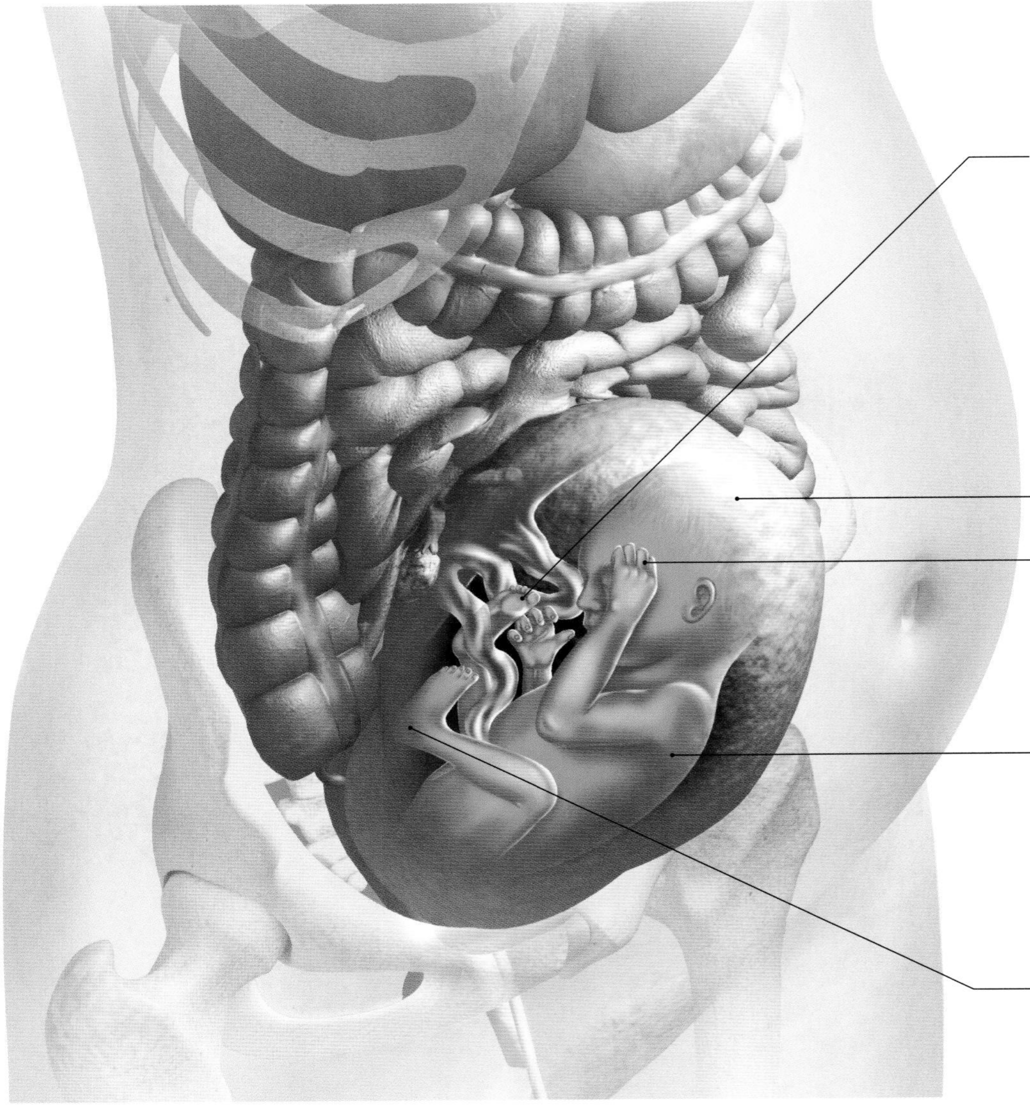
The toes are often grabbed by the baby's hand and may even be brought up to her mouth.
All the nerve cells that make up the outer surface of the brain are in place. They will gradually branch out to form neural connections.
Hand coordination is improving and your baby often brings her hands to her face, and especially her mouth.
Your baby's body is very flexible and she can double herself up with ease. As she gets bigger, her movements become stronger.
At 26 weeks the average crown to heel length is 14 in (35.6 cm) and the average weight is 1.7 lb (760 g).

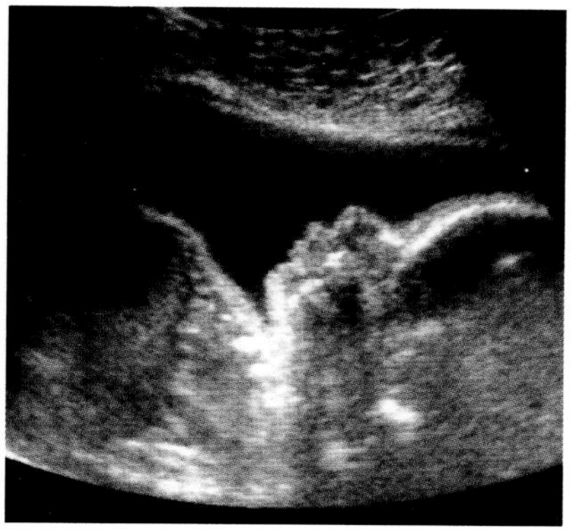

YOU ARE **25 WEEKS AND 1 DAY**

104 days to go

YOUR BABY TODAY

Here the baby is looking directly upward. The profile is nicely detailed with the nose, lips, and chin clearly outlined. The neck is still quite short so, as this image shows, the head is still held quite close to the chest.

> "Your prenatal classes will give you a chance to learn about labor, birth, and life with a newborn, and make new friends."

If you arranged them earlier in your pregnancy (see p.199), you may be starting prenatal classes, also called childbirth education classes. The Lamaze Method and The Bradley Method are common classes. Ask your health-care provider, friends, and staff at the hospital where you're giving birth about classes near you. In the class, you may be taught, for example, relaxation or breathing techniques, or be told about the different types of pain relief available. You'll also be given advice on topics where you'll learn all the basics: How to diaper, dress, feed, carry, and generally take care of your baby when you bring them home from the hospital. It's common to feel excited about the classes and eager to learn about what's going to happen. But prenatal classes are not just about gathering information; they're also about meeting others, which is difficult for some people. You'll likely find a lot of common ground with your classmates. Just talking about your symptoms or worries can help. It can be reassuring to know that you're not the only person to feel a certain way.

If you do make friends in your prenatal class, this support group can also be very helpful after you all have your babies.

RIB PAIN

As the uterus expands, the rib cage is pushed outward to make room for it, and this can lead to rib pain or discomfort. It is more likely if you have a smaller than average body frame or in a multiple pregnancy. It can be made worse if your baby kicks a lot or spends a lot of time in the breech position since her head will push against your diaphragm and rib cage.

Sitting may make the pain worse since it compresses your internal organs more. When you have to sit for long periods, you may find that you have to keep adjusting your position for comfort. Get up and move around as often as you can.

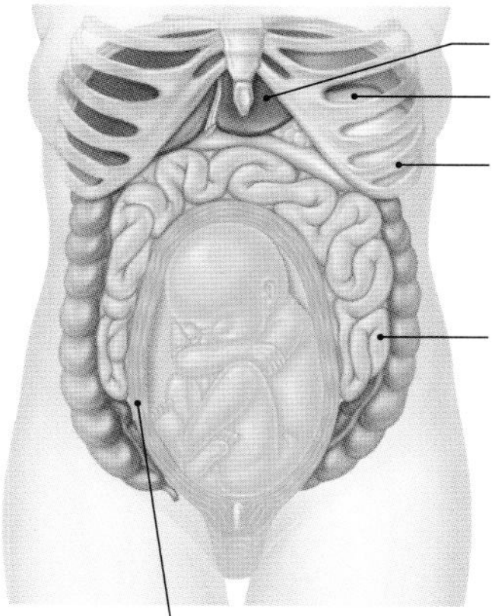
Liver
Stomach
Rib
Intestines

Expanding uterus reduces space for stomach and intestines

VAGINAL INFECTIONS

I think I have a vaginal infection. Will this harm my baby? It is unlikely to harm your baby since the mucus plug around the cervix stops infection from reaching them. The symptoms of an symptoms—itching, irritation, and a discharge with an unpleasant odor—are uncomfortable. Your doctor will test for an infection by taking a swab from your vagina and will prescribe medication if necessary.

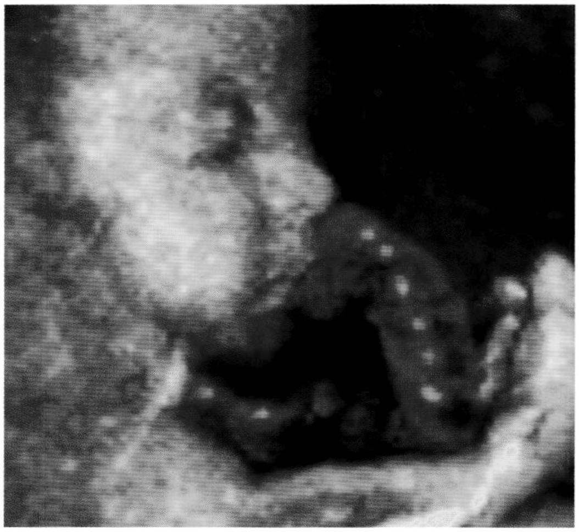

YOU ARE **25 WEEKS AND 2 DAYS**

103 days to go

YOUR BABY TODAY

This image shows the baby in profile, this time in 3-D. The coils of the umbilical cord are just seen in the background passing behind the baby's head. The eyelids can be seen, still firmly closed. Fat reserves are now giving the face a much more rounded contour.

“ Two tiny glands control your baby's growth and development, and enable them to face up to life's stresses. ”

ASK A DOCTOR

I have lumps in my breasts. Should I be worried? Breast lumps can be normal in pregnancy, especially in the third trimester as the breasts get ready for breast-feeding. These lumps are generally soft and may move around; they may also be tender. If you are feeling a new lump, let your doctor know. They will be able to confirm whether this is pregnancy related. .

Relative to body size, your baby's adrenal glands are 20 times larger than your own. The adrenal glands are roughly triangular in shape, with their base wrapped over the top of each kidney. They have an outer layer, or cortex, which releases steroid hormones such as cortisol, and an inner layer, or medulla. Adrenaline and the related hormone noradrenaline are secreted from the medulla in response to stress.

Adrenaline prepares the body for a “fight or flight” response, increasing the availability of glucose, speeding up the heart rate, and maintaining or raising blood pressure. These are vital adaptive responses for your baby that will help to maintain a stable environment within the uterus and prepare them for the stresses of life later on in the outside world.

It is the outer cortex, however, that needs to work hard, producing many hormones that help to coordinate your baby's growth and development. The cortex produces three types of hormones: mineralocorticoids that regulate salt balance; glucocorticoids that help to control the availability of sugars, fat, and amino acids in the bloodstream; and androgens, male-type sex hormones, such as testosterone. It is the cortex that accounts for the large size of your baby's adrenal glands. After birth, in the first couple of weeks, the adrenal glands rapidly reduce in size.

HOW IDENTICAL ARE TWINS?

Twins from the same egg have the same DNA. They will certainly look very similar and have the same hair, eye, and skin color. They will also have the same blood group and tissue type.

However, the environment isn't the same for each baby, even prebirth. Small differences in blood flow, and in location in the uterus, can have far-reaching effects.

- **There may be recognizable differences** in the weight, height, and head shape of identical twins.
- **Each twin** has unique fingerprints and iris patterns.
- **Identical twins** can have different personalities too, partly because of subtle dissimilarities in their very early environment.

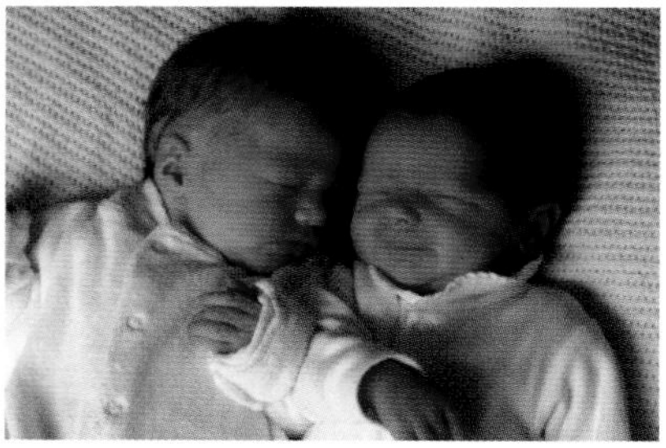

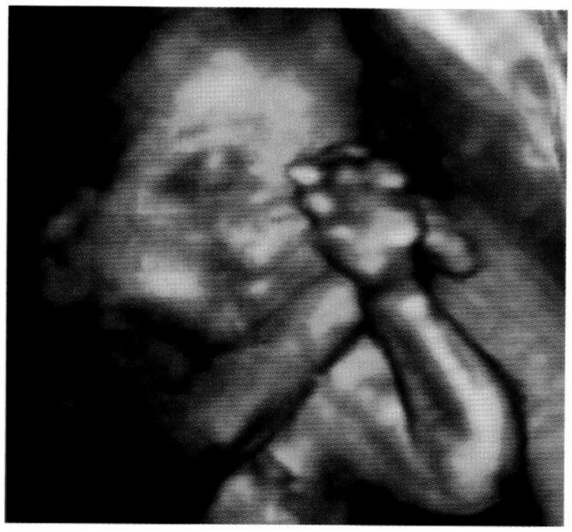

YOU ARE **25 WEEKS AND 3 DAYS**

102 days to go

YOUR BABY TODAY

The hands are held up in front of the face. In the top right-hand corner is the inner lining of the uterus. Shadows in the image give the impression of hair, but ultrasound is not detailed enough to show hair—even if there was any to see at this stage.

Not all partners are eager to go to prenatal classes. They might not feel the classes apply to them, and may fear that they will be asked to do exercises that they find embarrassing.

If your partner is reluctant, discuss their concerns. You can review what the classes are for and why you need their support. You could explain that you want them to be informed about labor so that they are not anxious in the delivery room. Your partner may find it useful to chat to other friends who attended classes when they were having a baby.

Classes may include some sessions just for partners and others where the pregnant women attend on their own, for example, to practice breathing techniques. If time off work is an issue for your partner, ask for a list of what topics will be covered each week and pick those sessions that you think are the most relevant. When your partner is well informed, they will feel more involved in the pregnancy and more confident in helping you during labor and birth.

“ Going to prenatal classes together is a good way for your partner to stay closely involved with your pregnancy. ”

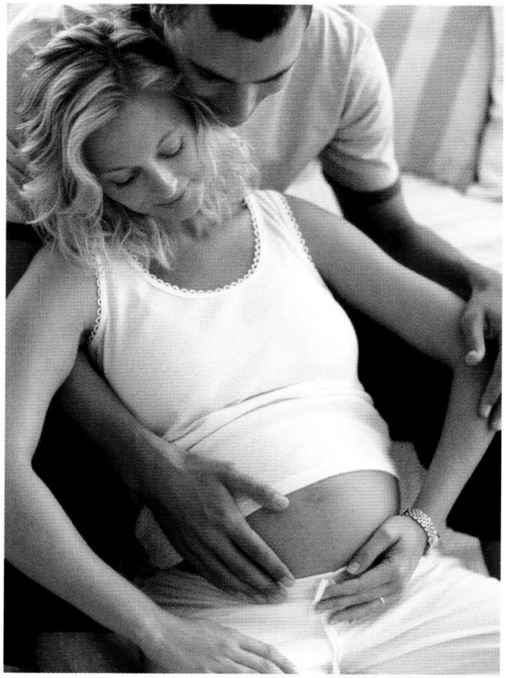

RELATIONSHIP CHANGES

Once your baby is born, your relationship won't just be about you and your partner any more. Suddenly a tiny new person is around, who wakes during the night and has their own needs. By necessity, after your baby is born you and your partner will pay less attention to each other. There may also be less physical intimacy between the two of you, not least because you both will be very tired.

It's best to talk about, and acknowledge, these issues before the birth. This way, you and your partner will better accept that these factors are a normal part of making the life change from coupledom to being a family.

MATERNITY RIGHTS

Thanks to the Family and Medical Leave Act (FMLA), most companies must give employees (men and women) up to 12 weeks of unpaid family leave after your baby is born. The rules: If your company has fewer than 50 employees, they don't have to offer FMLA. Also, you must have worked for the company for at least one year. It's a good idea to ask your human resources department about your company's policy about leave and have your partner do the same.

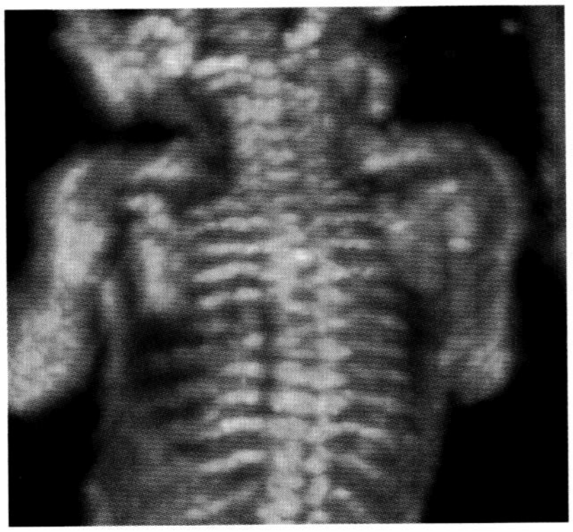

YOU ARE **25 WEEKS AND 4 DAYS**

101 days to go

YOUR BABY TODAY

This 3-D image is taken using an ultrasound setting that enhances the reflections from the skeleton. The back of the spine, ribs, and shoulder blades are clear. This technique has opened up new possibilities for visualizing the baby's development.

> " All the nerve cells are now on the surface of your baby's brain; what they need to do next is make connections with each other. "

ASK A DOCTOR

I love swimming but am getting quite big now. Should I adapt my swimming style? Yes, you may find that in these final couple of months, you need to change your swimming style to one that is more comfortable; many women opt for breaststroke, which can also help to get the baby in to an optimum position (see p.329).

If you don't feel up to swimming laps, just relax in the pool instead. Being in the water will relieve pressure on your abdomen and help to ease lower back pain.

Your baby's brain is so complex that it needs the entire length of your pregnancy not only to grow, but also to mature. It is continually forming new connections and sensory pathways.

The nerves that make up the brain's gray matter started in the center of the brain on the outer surface of the lateral ventricles (there is one ventricle in each hemisphere of the brain). The lateral ventricles contain the part of the brain known as the choroid plexus, a loose, seaweedlike structure that produces the fluid that bathes your baby's brain and spinal cord. Constantly circulating around the brain, this fluid protects and buffers the brain from the harder structure of the bones of the surrounding skull.

The gradual, wavelike, outward movement of nerve cells in the gray matter, which started more than 12 weeks ago, is now complete. Coming to rest close to the brain's surface, these cells need to mature, branching out to make multiple connections, or "synapses," with other nerve cells.

The surface of your baby's brain is very smooth at this stage but as the cortex matures, beginning to form six clear layers, it takes on its familiar wrinkled appearance.

SHOWING YOUR BUMP

Whether you want to clothe your belly in figure-hugging fabrics and proudly show it off, or choose looser styles that may fit you longer and obscure just how pregnant you are, is a personal choice.

- **If you're fine showing your belly,** you may feel comfortable in stretchy fabrics that can expand as your belly does. The downside to wearing tight clothing is that your skin may be sensitive to anything snug. Tight-fitting tops may become less comfortable as your breast size increases.
- **If you feel more comfortable** not showing the profile of your belly, choose baggier clothes, such as tunics, smocks, and overshirts. These may be more comfortable and will cloak your belly longer.
- **If you want to bare your belly,** do so when the weather is warm enough. One advantage is you may find you can wear some prepregnancy tops.

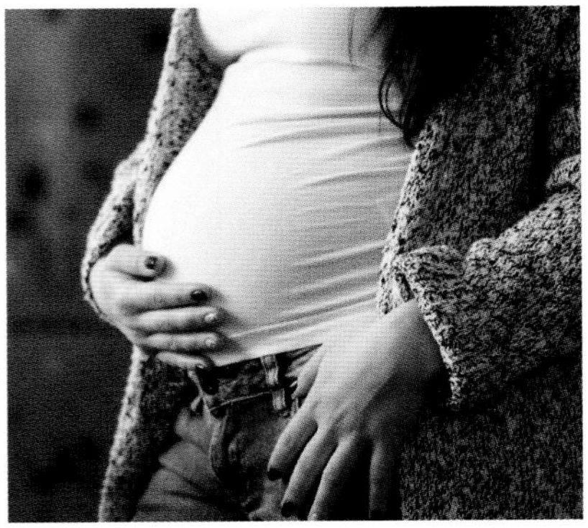

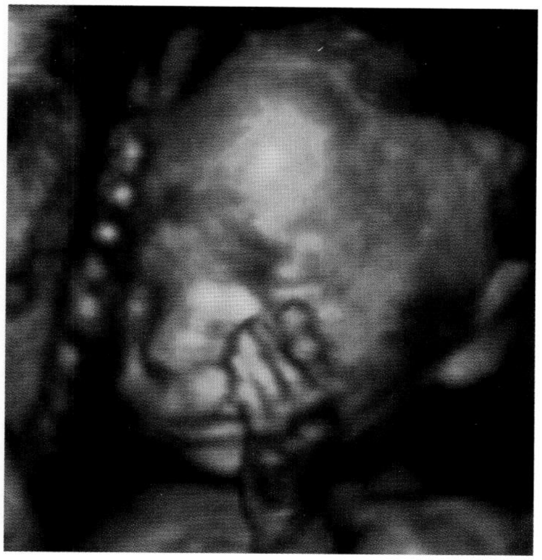

YOU ARE **25 WEEKS AND 5 DAYS**

100 days to go

YOUR BABY TODAY

With fingers held up to the cheek, eyes closed, and the ear just visible in the background, this image shows a very peaceful baby. To the left, the umbilical cord is visible on its way to the placenta, seen further to the left.

As your baby continues to grow you may find yourself wondering what they're going to be like: easygoing or demanding? Funny or serious? Happy playing alone or social? Boisterous or quiet? You may believe that babies are born with their personalities already developed, or that they are born with a personality that is further shaped and developed as they grow. The nature versus nurture debate rages on and, in all likelihood, it's a combination of the two: some aspects of your child's personality may already be decided before birth, some may be developed later in childhood, or even adulthood.

You may already have noticed that your baby has certain likes or dislikes, for example, they may kick or move in response to loud music or to a certain genre of music, though it's difficult to tell whether the increased movements mean your baby is enjoying it or not.

Your baby is very stimulated inside the uterus. By the third trimester, they can feel vibrations and hear not just sounds from inside your body, such as your heartbeat, but also sounds from outside, such as people talking. Your baby is aware of when you're being active or still and you may notice a pattern of movements and more "communication" when you're resting.

As part of their development, your baby will continue practicing for life after the birth, with breathing movements and swallowing—and they may even suck their thumb.

“It will be some years before you'll know your child's personality, but even in the uterus your baby has some likes and dislikes.”

BUYING FOR YOUR BABY

Preparing for your baby's arrival doesn't have to break the bank. Here are the things that your baby needs:

Milk: if bottle-feeding, you'll need bottles, nipples, formula, and a sterilizing system.

- **Diapers:** you'll need to decide between disposables, reusables, or a combination of the two (see p.291). Whichever type you choose, you'll also need to use wipes.
- **Somewhere to sleep:** your baby can sleep in a crib from birth if you don't want to buy a bassinet. Even if you buy a secondhand crib, you should always buy a new mattress.
- **Lots of onesies:** don't buy too many newborn size.
- **Transportation:** a stroller (with a lie-down option until your baby can sit up), or a sling or frontpack to carry your baby.
- **Car seat:** this is a legal requirement for car travel. Don't buy secondhand.

Here are things your baby can live without:

- **Changing station:** a mat (or towel) on the floor is cheaper and safer.
- **Bottle warmer:** heat the milk in a jug.
- **Designer wardrobe**
- **Pack-n-Play:** borrow one if necessary.

Save money by shopping online. Scour secondhand shops and garage sales. Swap clothes and toys with other parents.

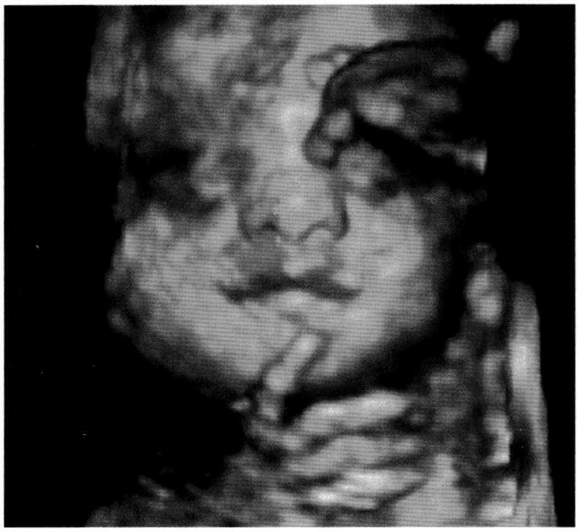

YOU ARE **25 WEEKS AND 6 DAYS**

99 days to go

YOUR BABY TODAY

A 3-D scan can be colored in different ways. This image demonstrates that by this stage your baby's lip shape is clearly defined. The lips are the most sensitive part of the entire body and your baby's hands are often held up toward them.

> "Your baby can make coordinated movements with their hands and feet, make a fist, and grab hold of their toes."

Your baby's hand coordination dramatically improves now and they constantly brings their hands up to their face, particularly their mouth. The face, and especially the lips, are extremely sensitive, and this heightened sensitivity provides strong positive feedback as your baby successfully coordinates smooth, purposeful movements between hand (and foot) and mouth. There is still plenty of room in the uterus for all sorts of movements and your baby is extremely flexible. It is quite easy for them to adopt a doubled-up position, with their feet up by their mouth or even on top of their head, and do full somersaults.

Your baby's bones are hardening from the inside out—the outer edges are still formed of soft cartilage.

BIRTH WEIGHT

Weight gain during pregnancy influences the baby's birth weight. High birth weights have been associated with an increased chance of health problems in the baby's future. Thus, pregnancy is a balancing act, in which women need to take in just enough, but not too many, calories.

Health experts are concerned that fetal overnutrition is resulting in more babies being born with a high birth weight. This is thought to predispose the baby to an increased risk of poor health in childhood and beyond. Being overweight already, or putting on excessive amounts of weight during pregnancy, increases the chances of gestational diabetes (see p.475), needing a Cesarean delivery, or complications during the birth.

It is also important to try to return gradually to a healthy weight when you've stopped breastfeeding and before you try for another baby.

ASK A DOCTOR

Why do I get so hot when I'm exercising? During pregnancy, your core body temperature rises due to the effects of the hormone progesterone, your increased weight, and the greater demands on your body. Exercise generates heat and raises your core temperature even further.

You'll also sweat more easily while you are pregnant. This is because pregnancy-related hormones cause dilation of blood vessels and thus blood flow to your skin (this explains the rosy "glow" some women get), allowing your body to lose heat through the skin more readily. This means that, although you get hotter while you're exercising, you'll cool down more quickly than usual. When you're exercising, always remember to:

- **Drink room temperature water** before, during, and after a workout.
- **Wear loose clothing** that will allow your skin to breathe.
- **Avoid exercising** when conditions are hot and humid.

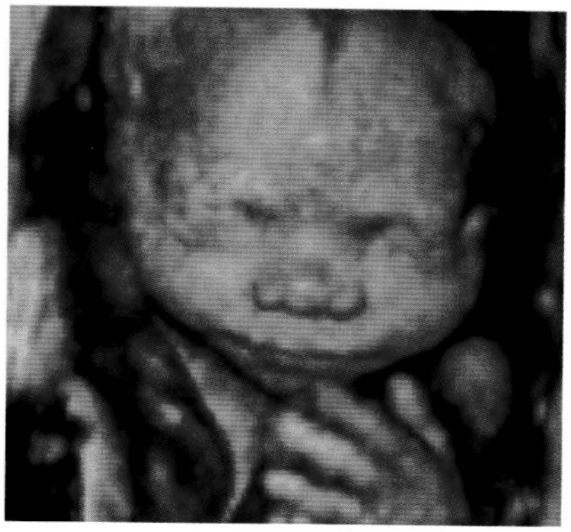

YOU ARE **26 WEEKS EXACTLY**

98 days to go

YOUR BABY TODAY

The space between the two frontal bones of the forehead (the dark line) has now nearly closed. The bones on the left and right sides come to lie very close to each other with a small gap to allow for further growth of the head and brain.

Vivid dreams are common in the third trimester. You may, in fact, not be dreaming more than usual, but difficulty in finding a comfortable sleeping position and waking often to go to the bathroom may mean that you remember your dreams more than usual (you normally would not wake during the dreaming phase of your sleep cycle, so often do not recall your dreams in the morning).

It is common to dream about stressful situations like babies in distress or danger. While these dreams can make you feel very anxious, know that they are in no way insights into what is in store for you. Dreaming is a way of filtering any negative emotions so that you do not have to experience them at first hand. Although disturbing, these dreams will help you cope with your natural concern for your baby's welfare.

> " Dreaming is a natural and healthy part of your sleep cycle, but at this stage of pregnancy unsettling dreams can be common. "

GOING ON A HOSPITAL TOUR

As part of the buildup to your baby's birth, you may be offered a tour of the hospital. Not only will you be able to see firsthand where you'll be delivering your baby, but you can also figure out the practical details, such as parking, admission procedures, what to bring, and what facilities there are, such as cafes and shops for visiting friends and family.

Ultimately ,a hospital tour offers you a reassuring chance for you and your partner to prepare yourself mentally for the big day and what will follow your baby's birth.

Use the opportunity as a fact-finding mission. Ask how the hospital uses birth plans, and when and why they might have to be adapted. Ask how many other moms there will be in the unit, and, if you want, how you can arrange a private room. There is usually a fee for this. Find out what support you'll have in the first 24 hours. Most hospitals now expect the mother to keep the baby with her during the night. Ask about visiting hours, the number of visitors you can have at any one time. You could also ask how many babies are born at the hospital each year, and how many of these are born by Cesarean (emergency or otherwise). Request information about how long the shifts are and what nurses and doctors do to provide continuity of care during labor and birth. Ask to see a delivery room and the nursery.

Are birth pools or baths available? Do they have TENS machines or other form of pain relief you may be considering? What support is there for breastfeeding; are breast pumps available?

Finally, although you hopefully won't need to use it, you may want to see the neonatal intensive care unit (NICU; see pp.452–453). If your baby needs this type of care, it can help to have toured the unit and to have seen the equipment so you can gain a basic understanding of what it's used for.

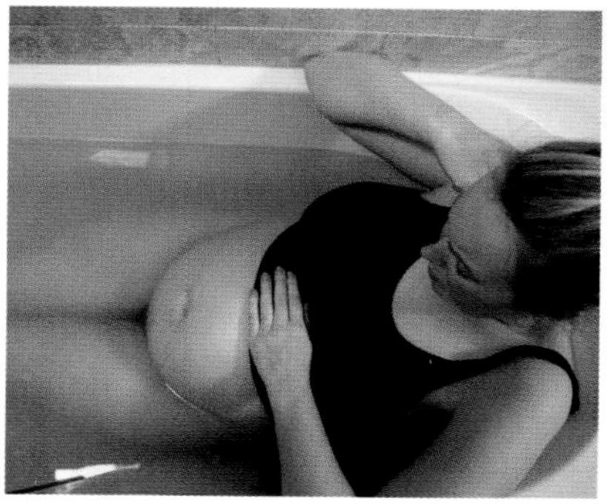

Your 27th week

YOU MAY FIND IT DIFFICULT TO SLEEP DUE TO YOUR BABY'S ACTIVITIES. Space is now getting tight in your uterus. The baby is likely to give you a few sharp jabs with their feet and fists as they stretch and turn. However uncomfortable the kicks may be, you'll find them a welcome reassurance that the baby is thriving. Relax in bed or in the bath and watch your belly—you'll be amazed and amused at how it pops up and down and moves around.

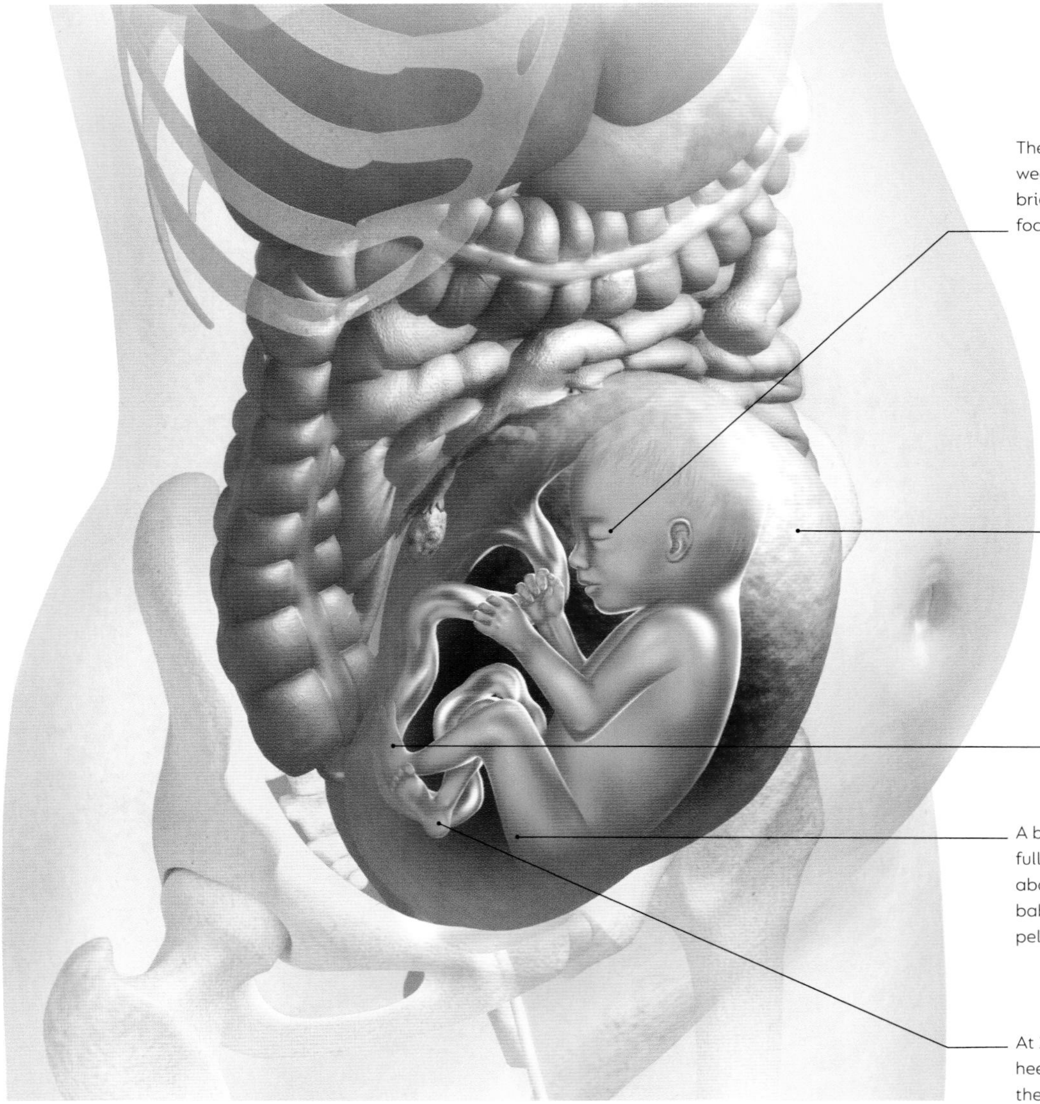

The eyelids are fully open this week. Your baby responds to bright light, although he cannot focus, and he can blink.

The baby is taking up a lot of space in the uterus and there is less amniotic fluid surrounding him.

The baby kicks often and a large kick against your ribs may take your breath away.

A boy baby's testes often descend fully into the scrotum around about now. However, in some babies, the testes remain in the pelvic cavity until after birth.

At 27 weeks the average crown to heel length is 14.4 in (36.6 cm) and the average weight is 1.9 lb (875 g).

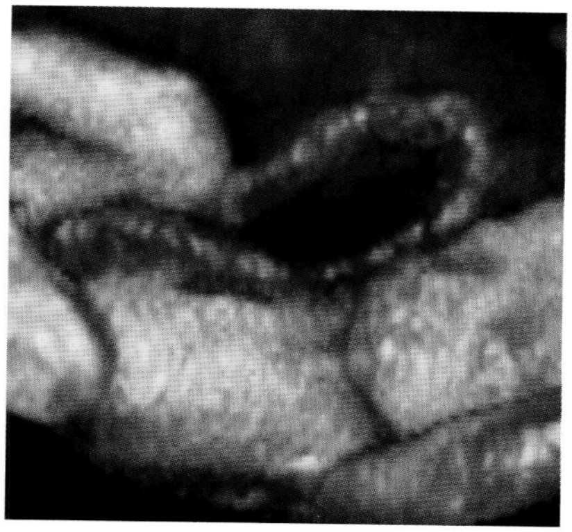

YOU ARE **26 WEEKS AND 1 DAY**

97 days to go

YOUR BABY TODAY

The coiling umbilical cord is very clearly seen in this image. The umbilical cord grows as your baby grows and will be about the same length as your baby at this stage of your pregnancy: about 14.4 in (36.6 cm).

You may have noticed that your baby is more active at some times than at others, often when you're trying to relax or sleep! This is likely to be because when you're busy or distracted, you're less aware of your baby moving.

Babies have different cycle of waking and sleeping, and there are no rules as to when your baby should be kicking and when they should be still.

If you're familiar with your baby's pattern of movements and are concerned that you haven't felt them move, or the pattern of movements has changed, you should let your doctor know and do fetal kick counts. Have a snack and glass of water, and lay down on your side with your hands on your stomach. Try to relax and focus on your baby's movements.

If you are not able to notice your baby's movements, then you will need to be evaluated at your doctor's office or at the hospital. When you go to the hospital, they will monitor your baby's heart rate by performing a nonstress test. They may offer an ultrasound to demonstrate fetal movement to you so you can feel more reassured when you go home.

Remember that while most of the time not feeling your baby move well is a false alarm, you don't want to ignore this as it can be the only sign that something catastrophic has happened.

> “When you settle down for a nap it can be frustrating if your baby starts exercising, but take this as a sign that all is well.”

ASK A DOCTOR

Why am I being told I need to have a glucose tolerance test? In pregnancy, some women develop a form of diabetes known as gestational diabetes (see p.475), which disappears when the baby is born.

Certain women are more likely to develop gestational diabetes, including

- those with a family history of it
- those who have had a previous pregnancy with gestational diabetes
- those with a high BMI

If you are at high risk, you will take an oral glucose tolerance test (OGT) between 24 and 28 weeks of pregnancy.

BLOOD VOLUME

During pregnancy, your total volume of blood is 50 percent higher than normal. The amount of blood pumped with each heartbeat increases by about 40 percent and you make around 20 per-cent more red blood cells than normal.

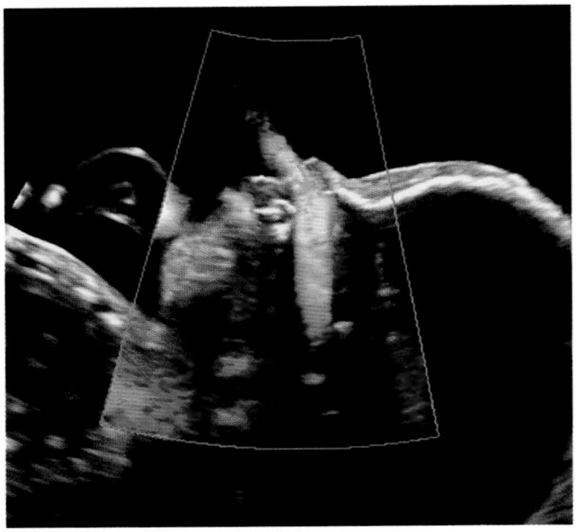

YOU ARE **26 WEEKS AND 2 DAYS**

96 days to go

YOUR BABY TODAY

This color ultrasound shows the baby breathing the amniotic fluid (red, flowing toward the ultrasound beam) in and out. The baby is breathing a stream of fluid out through the nostrils and, at the same time, a smaller amount through the mouth.

> “As the development of your baby’s eyes and sense of sight continues, they reach another milestone: the eyelids open.”

Although your baby’s eyelids formed at nine weeks of pregnancy, they have remained fused together until this week. Your baby is not in complete darkness, however, because as the uterus grows, its wall thins, allowing in increasing amounts of light.

Even with the eyelids open, the delicate structures of the eyeballs are protected by a fine membrane that will completely disappear during the final month of pregnancy.

It’s too early for your baby to respond to light in a fully coordinated way, but they may turn toward very strong lights or, if startled by a sudden loud noise, they will often respond with a blink.

The retina has just started to be lined by light-receptive rods and cones. The cones are responsible for color vision and develop later than the more numerous rods. The rods transmit an image in black and white and are used for nighttime vision and for peripheral vision. Connections form between the retina and the optic nerve, that then transmits the information it receives to be decoded in the visual cortex at the back of the brain.

Your baby will often bring their hands to their face, but because their limb movements are now so well coordinated, they won’t touch their eyes.

ASK A DOCTOR

I’ve got inverted nipples. Will I be able to breastfeed? Babies breastfeed rather than “nipple feed” and if your baby latches onto your breast correctly (see p.450), inverted nipples shouldn’t cause difficulties. About 10 percent of women have flat or inverted nipples. The best way to find out whether you can breastfeed is simply to try once your baby is born. There are various techniques that may help: consult your doctor if you’re having problems or contact a lactation consultant. Your doctor or hospital may recommend one or the La Leche League can help (see p.482).

FOCUS ON TWINS

In these last three months, you’re likely to get very big. As you’d expect, the more babies inside, the greater the challenge for your body to provide enough space as well as the perfect conditions for growth.

To check that the babies are growing normally, you will have regular growth scans. From around 28–29 weeks, the growth of twins and other multiples slows down compared with that of singletons. They do, however, still move and kick as much as possible, cushioned by amniotic fluid, which continues to increase in volume until 36 weeks.

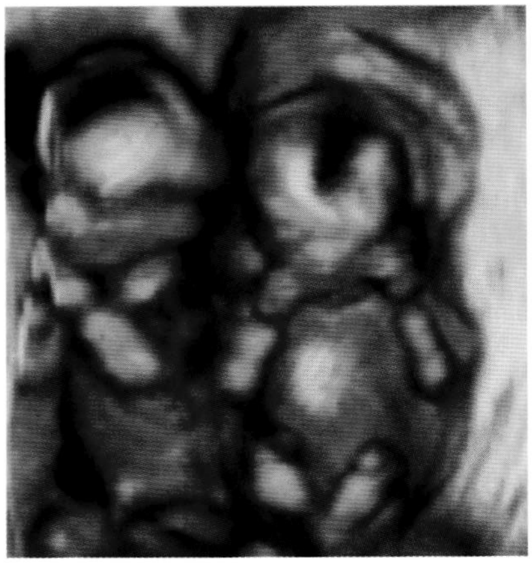

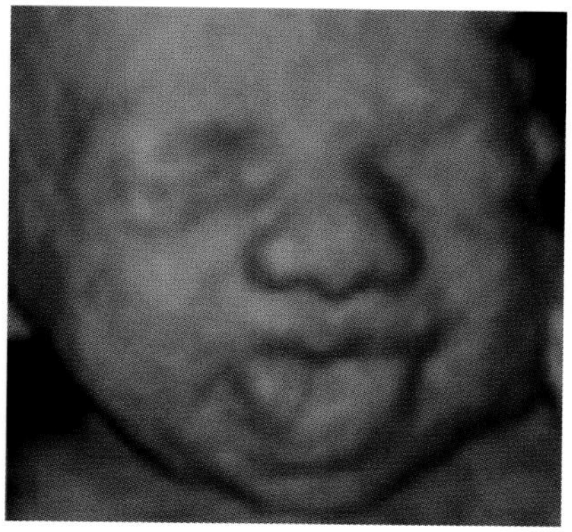

YOU ARE **26 WEEKS AND 3 DAYS**

95 days to go

YOUR BABY TODAY

Your baby sticks their tongue out often especially before or after a particularly large gulp of amniotic fluid. Fluid doesn't enter the lungs but is swallowed into the stomach. Your baby is completely unaware of the ultrasound scan, so is not reacting to the scanner.

You may be feeling very protective of your belly and baby. The belly almost acts as a beacon to other people, making them aware that you're pregnant. It's not unusual to feel quite vulnerable, for example, in a jostling crowd or when you're out shopping. When this happens, make it clear to people that you're pregnant and, hopefully, they'll give you more space and give up their seat, if necessary.

When you're driving, you may find you're doing so even more carefully than normal, or becoming a very nervous or critical passenger. You may become more irritated than usual by people who you feel are driving without concern for your safety.

This protective instinct is a natural part of becoming a mother. It's the desire to protect and nurture your child, even before yourself.

Rest assured, though, that your baby is in the safest possible environment inside your uterus. Your body is providing your baby with warmth, food, and oxygen. The baby is cushioned and protected by the amniotic fluid in which he floats, and this acts as a buffer to any shoving or bumping by crowds of people.

> " It's a natural instinct that parents are fiercely protective of their children, and not unusual for this to start well before the birth. "

HYPNOBIRTHING

Giving birth in such a relaxed state that you barely feel pain sounds too good to be true. But the research extolling the benefits of hypnobirthing is impressive. Several studies have shown that self-hypnosis helps women feel less anxious about labor and birth. They also tend to require minimal pain relief and medical intervention and many succeed in giving birth at home. Look online for classes or ask your doctor.

- **You will learn a series of self-hypnosis,** relaxation, visualization, and breathing techniques that help you approach childbirth in a calm, positive frame of mind.
- **You should feel in control** of your body and able to manage the pain of labor.
- **The key is to practice frequently,** and a supportive birth partner is invaluable for helping you perfect the techniques and use them in labor. .

ASK A DOCTOR

My partner and I had sex last night and this morning I noticed a small amount of fresh bleeding. Is this anything to worry about? Post-coital bleeding is common in pregnancy and usually nothing to worry about, as long as you are not having any cramping or abdominal pain and your baby is moving.

However, you should notify your doctor and explain what happened as you may need an examine to confirm the source of the bleeding. .

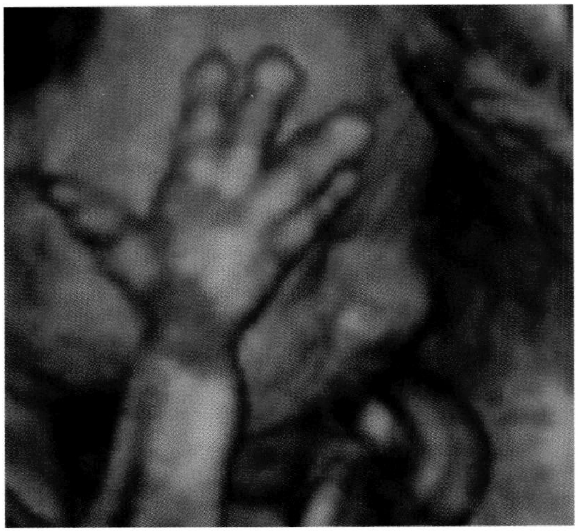

YOU ARE **26 WEEKS AND 4 DAYS**

94 days to go

YOUR BABY TODAY

On this 3-D image each finger is held outstretched. Holding the fingers in this way for any length of time is tiring, so most of the time the hands are held with the wrists slightly flexed and the fingers bent, ready to grasp any object that floats into reach.

“Your baby’s reproductive organs are now in place; a boy’s testes have descended and a girl’s ovaries have all their follicles.”

If your baby is a boy, it’s at about this time that the testes complete their descent into the scrotum. This is often associated with a small amount of fluid around each testis called a “hydrocele.” This fluid will disappear naturally either before or after birth.

The cremaster muscle, part of the spermatic cord, is able to raise the testes back into the groin. This helps to regulate the temperature within the testes after birth, relaxing when cooling is needed. If your baby is slightly cool when examined, the cremaster muscle retracts the testes giving the impression of an undescended testes in your newborn baby.

Temperature control is not required in the uterus and the testes slowly move down into the scrotum. It is by no means unusual for one testis (or both) not to have descended at birth. Your doctor will check for this as part of the routine baby development checkup and confirm that both testes can be brought down into the scrotum.

Unlike the ovary, which already contains all of the egg-producing follicles that it will ever make, the testes do not start to make sperm until puberty.

Differences in the speed of growth and weight gain become more apparent now, and boys tend to be slightly heavier than girls at birth.

ASK A MOM

Is it normal to argue all the time when we should be happily looking forward to our baby’s arrival? It can be. Concerns about having a healthy baby and adjusting to parenthood were at the heart of most of our arguments. We found we had conflicting opinions about big child-rearing issues. I was sensitive, irritable, and moody and often snapped when I didn’t mean to.

We sat down and talked calmly and agreed to avoid areas of contention and compromise when it didn’t really matter. In the throes of a disagreement, I’d stop and think: I love this man, we’re having a baby together— is this really important? We also made time to do positive things together that we had enjoyed before I was pregnant, and tried to find opportunities to laugh, to reduce stress, and to put things into perspective. By the time the baby arrived, we were both much more relaxed.

WEIGHT GAIN IN THE THIRD TRIMESTER

In your third trimester, gaining weight steadily is important. If you were a healthy weight before your pregnancy, you should gain 3–5 pounds in the first trimester and 1–2 pounds a week the rest of your pregnancy, for a total of 25–37 pounds. Keep in mind that the largest contributing factor to your overall weight gain will be your baby, followed by extra fat, which you will need to sustain your pregnancy and when breastfeeding.

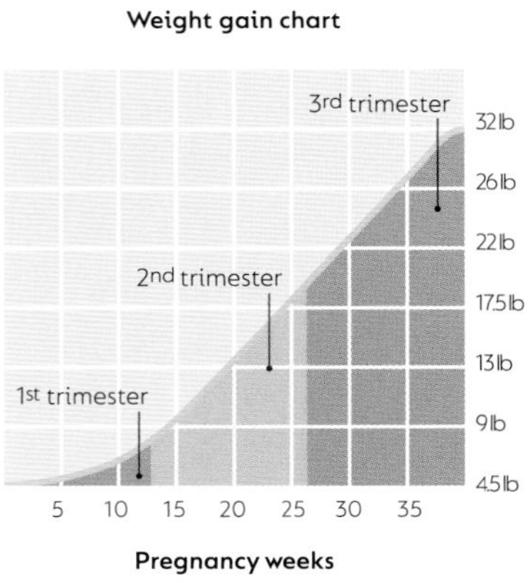
Weight gain chart
3rd trimester
2nd trimester
1st trimester
32lb
26lb
22lb
17.5lb
13lb
9lb
4.5lb
5
10
15
20
25
30
35
Pregnancy weeks

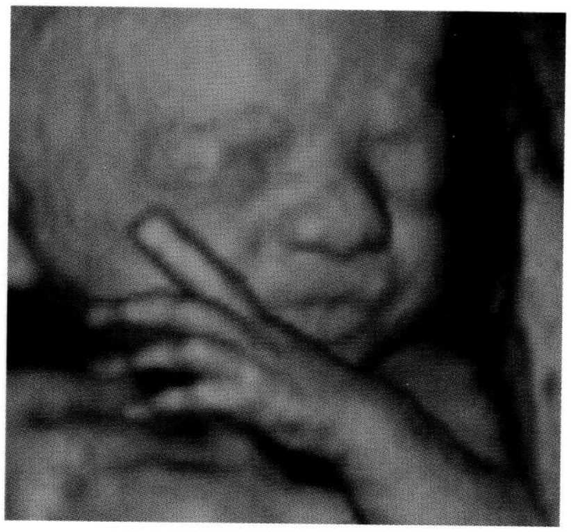

YOU ARE **26 WEEKS AND 5 DAYS**

93 days to go

YOUR BABY TODAY

Although some babies open their eyes, this happens only very briefly, so it is difficult to capture on an ultrasound scan. Some light is reaching your baby, but they haven't developed a sleep-wake cycle that corresponds in any way with day and night.

As wonderful as it is to feel your baby move inside you, sometimes it can be uncomfortable. As your baby grows, there is less and less room for him to move around, especially as he kicks or stretches against the walls of your uterus. These movements can vary from gentle paddling motions to feeling as though the baby has hiccups. Sometimes the baby will kick hard; if it's under the ribs, it can take your breath away and leave you feeling quite sore. The kicking can also wake you when you're sleeping, and many women say that their babies are more active at night. If you're sitting or lying in a position that the baby doesn't like—for example, if you spend too much time on one side—your baby may well kick until you move.

Although sometimes these movements can be uncomfortable or take you by surprise, most of the time they're just a gentle reminder of your growing baby and, as such, are something to look forward to feeling.

" As each day passes, your baby is getting bigger and bigger and you will be more conscious of his body and movement. "

ASK A DOCTOR

If I went into labor now, would my baby survive? Until relatively recently, babies born before 28 weeks' gestation often did not survive. Today, with medical advances in neonatal intensive care units (NICU), babies of 22 weeks' gestation have survived outside the uterus, although this is still very rare. At many hospitals, doctors won't resuscitate a baby under 24 weeks, because there is little chance of survival.

Extremely premature babies have an increased risk of disability, even with the best medical care, and often the delivery itself can put an enormous strain on the baby. Very experienced doctors and nurses are involved in the care of extremely premature babies.

If possible, the delivery should take place in a hospital with a neonatal intensive care unit (NICU; see pp.452–453). If this isn't possible, babies are often transferred to a special center when they are stable enough to be moved. Very premature babies take a long time to "catch up" and meet developmental milestones.

Each day and week of pregnancy is a milestone, and the closer to full term (37–42 weeks) you deliver, the better it is for your baby.

BUYING BEDDING

Your baby doesn't need a blanket or pillow—in fact, experts advise against them. To reduce your baby's risk of sudden infant death syndrome (SIDS), put a fitted sheet on a firm crib mattress (don't use a second-hand mattress), and keep blankets, pillows and stuffed animals out of the crib. If your baby sleeps in a Moses basket or bassinet, you should buy sheets designed specifically for these. Keep the room at a temperature that feels good to you. If you're concerned that your baby is chilly, consider a sleep sack. Many parents find them to be comfortable for their baby.

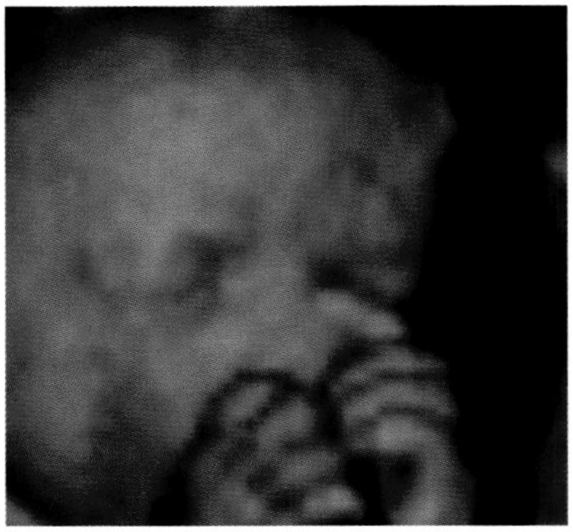

YOU ARE **26 WEEKS AND 6 DAYS**

92 days to go

YOUR BABY TODAY

Thumb-sucking is becoming much more coordinated as the sensitive lips and fingers meet. On scans most babies look as if they enjoy it, and there's no doubt that it provides important sensory feedback and perhaps reassurance to your developing baby.

“ The thought of being off work in the last months of pregnancy is tempting, but it will give you less time off with your baby. ”

As long as you're feeling in good health, try to work into the last month of your pregnancy. It can be particularly frustrating if you finish two months before, only to find that your baby is born later than expected. Working as late as possible may also allow you to spend some time with your replacement. If you're finding work tiring, try to adapt your working day and avoid traveling during rush hour, if possible. Whenever you start your leave, colleagues may hold a party and want to buy gifts for your newborn. If you're asked what you want, suggest gift certificates since these will allow you to purchase some of the more expensive baby equipment, and prevent duplication of gifts. Many stores also offer baby registries, which are a good way to choose the items you want.

BACK PAIN IN THE THIRD TRIMESTER

One of the most common pregnancy complaints, back pain is generally a reaction to your increased weight and the laxity of the joints that are an integral part of pregnancy. You can alleviate this, and evidence suggests that women who exercise are far less likely to suffer from extreme back pain than those who don't.

Do exercises to strengthen your abdominal muscles, which will give your belly and your back support, and keep your legs and arms strong too. See p.250 for an effective abdominal workout.

Carrying does not end when you have your baby. You will have a car seat, diaper bag, and perhaps groceries or older children to carry, as well as your newborn. So it's best to keep your muscles strong to prepare for this. Here are five tips to avoid back pain in the third trimester:

- **Stay strong:** strength training for all parts of your body (see p.196) will help you deal with the weight you are gaining throughout pregnancy.
- **Support:** invest in a support belt that will give your back a break from bearing the load of your belly. It will also support your sagging belly and may relieve the pressure in your legs. This can be particularly useful if you're carrying twins or more.
- **Sleep:** place a pillow between your legs to ease the stress on your back. Buy or borrow a shaped pillow that gives your belly and back support at the same time.
- **Stretch:** flexibility will help your back to relax and avoid your muscles getting tense.
- **Sit:** use a pillow to increase the support in your lower back. If you work at a desk, make sure your chair adequately supports your back or take frequent breaks to stand.

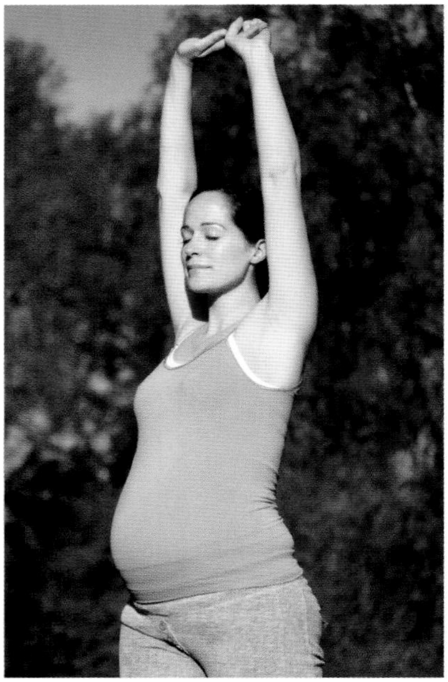

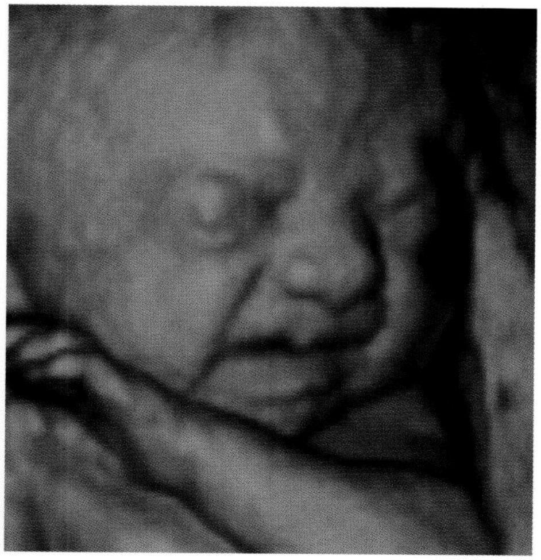

YOU ARE **27 WEEKS EXACTLY**

91 days to go

YOUR BABY TODAY

This baby looks quite upset. Your baby often makes strange and funny faces in the uterus. It's as if he is practicing every type of facial expression in preparation for after the birth when these will be one of the tools he uses to communicate his needs and emotions.

Your belly is a marvelous thing. It's already changed so much over the last 27 weeks and will continue to grow until you give birth.

Inside that belly your growing baby is moving around. When your baby is kicking and turning around, take the time to look down, and you may be able to see him move or even see the imprint of a foot as it kicks you.

While you're taking a bath is a good time to watch your belly—you may find that your baby is more active around this time because you're relaxed—and you can take the time to observe his movements.

Keep your partner involved when your baby is active by encouraging them to touch your bump and talk to the baby.

“ As you soak in a relaxing bath, it's an amazing sight to look at your baby moving and stretching your belly. ”

FOCUS ON PARTNERS

Being pregnant is more tiring than most women anticipate. In the third trimester, your partner's bladder is under increased pressure, and this can cause her to wake frequently during the night to use the bathroom. The size of her belly starts to become cumbersome, and it can be difficult to find a comfortable sleeping position. Other changes, including shifting internal organs and changes in hormone levels, can contribute to her restlessness. And if she's having trouble sleeping, you are likely to be disturbed too. The end result is that both of you may feel tired much of the time.

Unfortunately, there is no easy answer. Going to bed earlier can help, but having some time to relax together before bed is just as important. The bottom line is that disrupted sleeping patterns will continue to be the norm for both of you, and this may be nature's way of readying you for the many sleepless nights ahead!

ASK A DOCTOR

My belly measurement has not changed in two visits. Why isn't my baby growing?
In pregnancy, your abdomen is measured to establish the height of the top of the uterus, which indicates how the baby is growing. There is an element of subjectivity depending on the technique the doctor uses. In early pregnancy, measuring is not necessary because this doesn't give an indication of fetal growth, but after 26 weeks, growth can be assessed this way. However, the estimation of your baby's growth may still not be 100 percent accurate. If there are any concerns, your doctor may order an ultrasound.

Your 28th week

EVEN BEFORE BIRTH, YOUR BABY IS ESTABLISHING A PATTERN OF BEHAVIOR. They are beginning to have regular sleep–wake cycles and their breathing, yawning, and swallowing are taking on a more definite pattern. However, your own life may seem less rhythmical. You may find things are slightly different at work and, perhaps, be seeing less of some friends because you don't always feel up to socializing. Don't become isolated, though—if nothing else, stay in touch by phone, email, and social media.

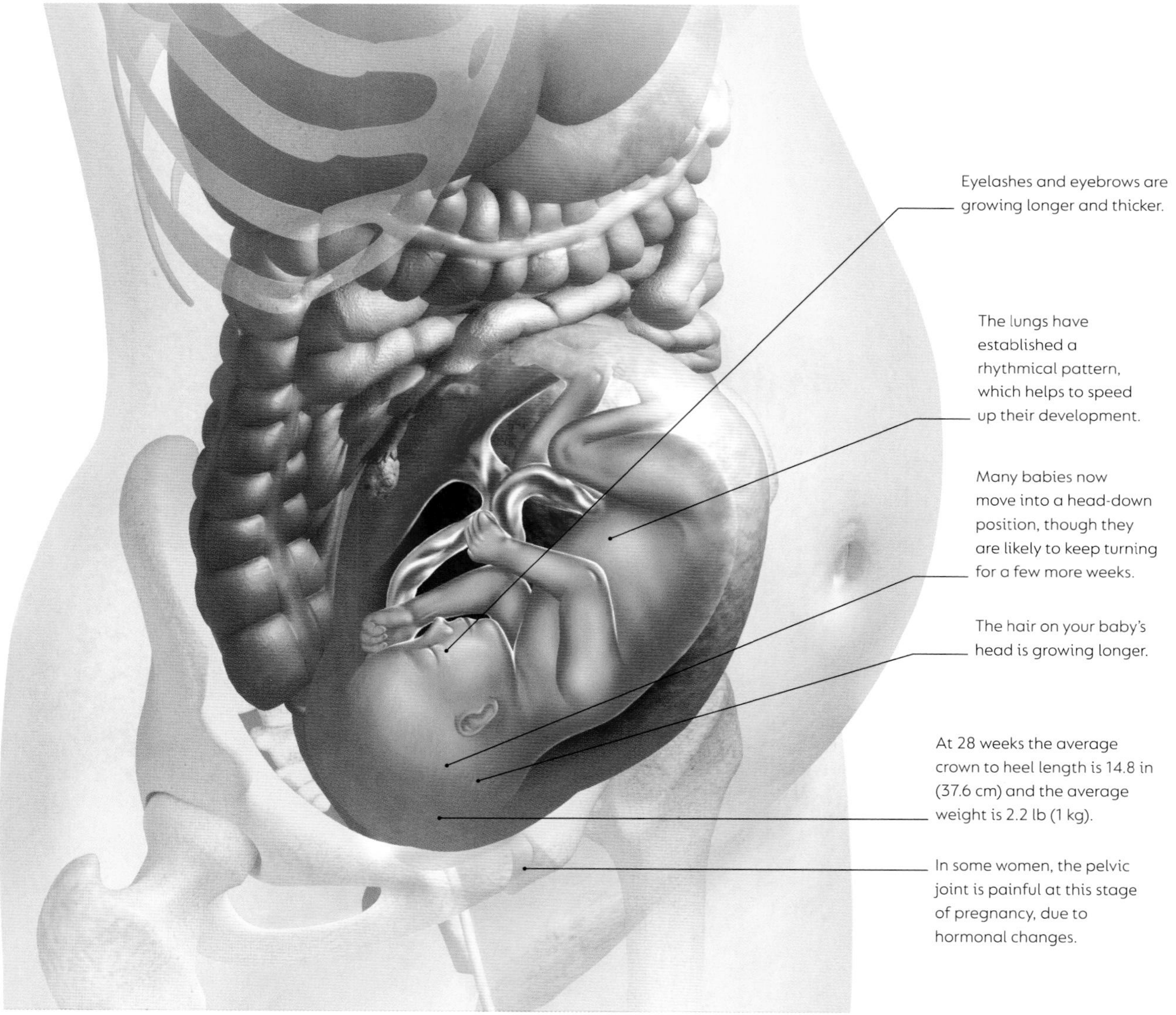

Eyelashes and eyebrows are growing longer and thicker.
The lungs have established a rhythmical pattern, which helps to speed up their development.
Many babies now move into a head-down position, though they are likely to keep turning for a few more weeks.
The hair on your baby's head is growing longer.
At 28 weeks the average crown to heel length is 14.8 in (37.6 cm) and the average weight is 2.2 lb (1 kg).
In some women, the pelvic joint is painful at this stage of pregnancy, due to hormonal changes.

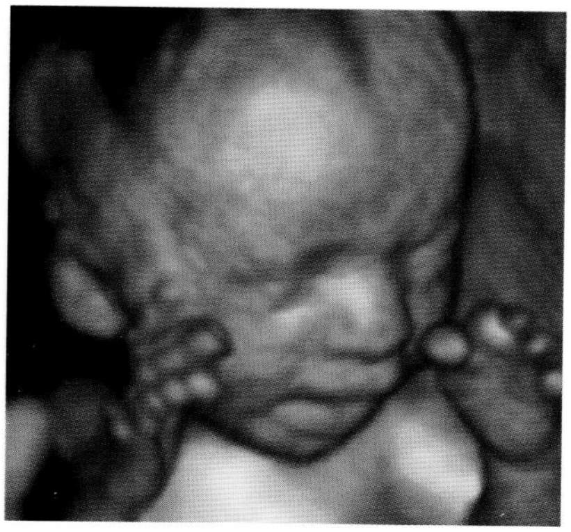

YOU ARE **27 WEEKS AND 1 DAY**

90 days to go

YOUR BABY TODAY

The space between the frontal bones of the forehead appears as a dark line on the top of the head. This is not a line on the skin: instead where there is no underlying bone, more of the ultrasound beam passes through rather than being reflected.

" Do all you can to stay involved with medium- and long-term plans at work so that you continue to feel part of the team. "

The difficulty of balancing motherhood and a career can crop up already while you're pregnant. You may find yourself excluded from long-term planning as colleagues assume that you won't be around, or won't come back after your maternity leave. Some colleagues may treat you differently just because you're pregnant, assuming you can no longer do your job in the same way. You may feel that your ideas are disregarded since you will not be there to implement them. This can be compounded by the fact that it can be difficult to motivate yourself if you know you won't be there to see a project through to the end. No one can be certain of being in a job in six months' or a year's time, but you have the advantage of knowing how much longer you're going to work and you may even have a reasonable idea of when you're intending to return to work. Continue to do your job and make it clear by your actions that you want to provide input on all projects. If at this point in time you're intending to return to work after your maternity leave has ended, make this clear to any colleagues who may doubt your long-term commitment.

You can also help plan for your maternity leave by, perhaps, dividing up your workload or helping to search for a replacement to cover your role. Being organized now will make the countdown to going on maternity leave much easier in the coming weeks.

BREATHE EASY

As your uterus grows, your diaphragm is compressed with the result that you may find it difficult to breathe deeply. In fact, you're actually taking in more air. It's important not to fight the natural tendency to hollow your back. This opens up your rib cage to let in more air, and also helps balance the excess weight of your belly.

ASK A MOM

Should we buy a baby bath or can the baby use our bath? I thought a baby bath was an optional extra, but having bought one found it really useful. A huge advantage is that you can use it in any room (though if the room doesn't have a water supply, you'll need to transport water).

I was a bit apprehensive the first few times we bathed the baby, then experienced parents told me even they found it tricky to hold a wiggling baby safely in a bath of water. Using a smaller baby bath is less daunting and helps you develop confidence. However, a baby outgrows a baby bath by around six months and, once not in use, the bath can take up a lot of storage space (unless you can recycle it to a pregnant friend). Many parents choose a bath seat designed for newborns in the family bath. Alternatively, enjoy a bath together, although you must keep the water tepid for the baby and you may find this too cold for you.

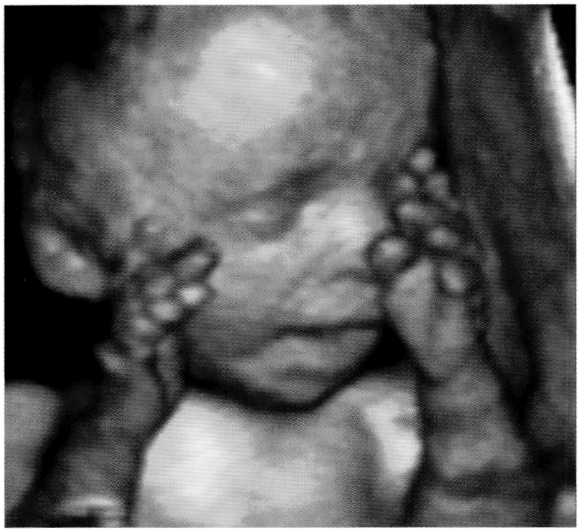

YOU ARE **27 WEEKS AND 2 DAYS**

89 days to go

YOUR BABY TODAY

Your baby may be looking happy today. Babies smile and grimace, wrinkle their foreheads, and stick their tongues out. Many of these behaviors are only becoming more apparent now as 3-D ultrasound has provided a unique opportunity for their study.

“Your baby has developed a sleep–wake cycle very similar to the one they will have in the days and weeks after birth.”

Your baby's yawns have, until this point, occurred only occasionally as a single event but are now becoming more repetitive, with several yawns following one another. Your baby's swallowing reflexes were developed at 25 weeks but still need to become much better coordinated.

The baby's breathing movements are vital for the normal development of the lung tissue. Your baby does not breathe amniotic fluid into their lungs; The lungs are filled with fluid produced by the lung tissue itself, and as breathing movements are practiced, small amounts are expelled. With each breath, the diaphragm pushes down, and the chest wall moves in as the larynx relaxes, allowing fluid to escape. Only a tiny proportion (0.5 percent) of the fluid in the lung escapes with each breath. This compares to a fifth (20 percent) of the air in the lungs moving in and out with each breathing movement.

Your baby has been breathing for some weeks, but the pattern up until now has been somewhat random. Now, their breathing patterns start to reflect their better developed sleep–wake cycle and becomes more rhythmical.

PRENATAL CARE

You'll have prenatal appointments this week and at 32 and 36 weeks.

At each one, your blood pressure will be measured, and your urine tested for protein. The doctor will also check the size of your baby by measuring the height of your uterus and will listen to any concerns and offer you advice.

EATING A LITTLE MORE

You may feel hungrier now than you did earlier in pregnancy. This is to be expected as your developing baby is increasing rapidly in weight.

At this late stage of pregnancy, you need to increase your energy intake by about 200 calories per day; try to do so with healthy snacks and light meals. Here are a few suggestions:

- 2 tbsp of Greek yogurt with 1 banana.
- 10 oz (300 g) tomato soup with a slice of whole wheat toast and low-fat spread.
- ¾ oz (20 g) raw almonds with 1¾ oz (50 g) dried apricots.
- 2 rice cakes, 1¾ oz (50 g) grapes, and a 1 oz (30 g) piece of Cheddar cheese.
- A slice of whole wheat toast and 5 oz (135 g) of hummus.

Being active at this stage continues to be important, especially since it will help prevent you from becoming constipated.

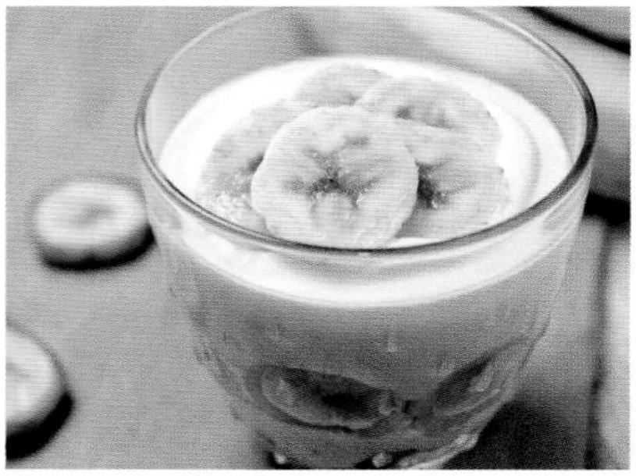

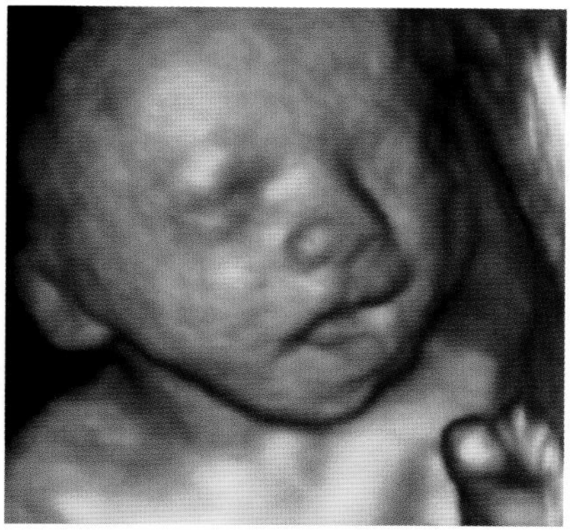

YOU ARE **27 WEEKS AND 3 DAYS**

88 days to go

YOUR BABY TODAY

This baby is at the end of a yawn. Your baby is yawning in a more coordinated way now with one yawn often following another. It may look as if this image shows the fingertips in the bottom right but in fact it is a foot, nearly brought up to the mouth.

> "Pregnancy is a subject about which everybody has an opinion they want to share with you, whether you like it or not."

Although you may have become very proud and protective of your belly, it can be extremely irritating if other people become overprotective of you. It may seem like everyone has an opinion on your pregnancy, and what you should and should not be doing to stay healthy. Some women find all the attention comforting, but others find it frustrating or suffocating. If you're someone who finds all the advice difficult to handle, try to remember that people mean well.

Of course, it's your body, and you'll do what is best for you and your baby. If it's all getting too much, then try talking to the main offenders, often a partner, mother, or mother-in-law. Explain that you're trying your best and that you're aware of what you should and shouldn't do while you're pregnant and are following the advice of your doctors. Politely thank them for their input and reassure them that you're taking good care of yourself and your baby.

BLOOD-PRESSURE CHECKS

About 8 percent of women have problems with high blood pressure in pregnancy. High blood pressure can be caused by preeclampsia (see p.476), a serious condition that also leads to protein in the urine. Preeclampsia can affect the liver and kidneys and, if untreated, lead to eclampsia or seizures.

If you have preeclampsia, your doctor will closely monitor your blood pressure. High blood pressure can also affect your baby, so medication may be recommended. Don't stop the medication without your doctor's okay.

SMELLING GOOD

Are you wafting through pregnancy smelling as fresh as a daisy? It's rarely discussed, but being pregnant may make you feel less fragrant than usual, not least because you will sweat more than before—although it's unlikely that anyone else will have noticed.

An increase in vaginal discharge is also nothing to worry about, but if it has a strong odor or is yellowish or greenish in color, you could have an infection so see your doctor. To stay smelling sweet:

- **Shower or bathe like usual** and apply deodorant. Carry handy wipes with you.
- **Switch to body sprays** and lotions; they tend to be lighter than perfumes and are less likely to cause headaches.
- **Avoid wearing tight clothing:** wear loose clothes in natural fabrics, which absorb sweat and allow your skin to breathe.
- **Wear cotton underwear,** and change it more often, if necessary.
- **Use disposable panty liners,** if needed, to stay feeling fresh.

Assessing fetal growth and well-being

In addition to monitoring your own health and well-being throughout your pregnancy, the doctor will also assess how your baby is growing, and will refer you for further tests if she has any concerns about your baby's well-being.

Measuring your baby

In a low-risk pregnancy, your doctor measures your abdomen at prenatal visits to assess the baby's growth. The measurement in centimeters from the top of the uterus, the fundus, to the top of the pubic bone should be the same as the number of weeks of pregnancy with an allowance of up to 2 cm either way. For example, if you are 26 weeks' pregnant, you should measure between 24 and 28 cm. Your fundal height can be measured from 24 weeks until about 36–37 weeks. If there is a variation of 3 cm or more, your doctor will arrange for an ultrasound to check your baby's growth (see opposite) and the amount of amniotic fluid. If the scan indicates a problem, the doctor will arrange for scans every two weeks since analyzing growth patterns over time gives a more accurate assessment of whether your baby's growth is normal.

In certain cases, for example if a woman is obese, in twin pregnancies, and where there are large uterine fibroids, the only accurate way to measure growth is by ultrasound.

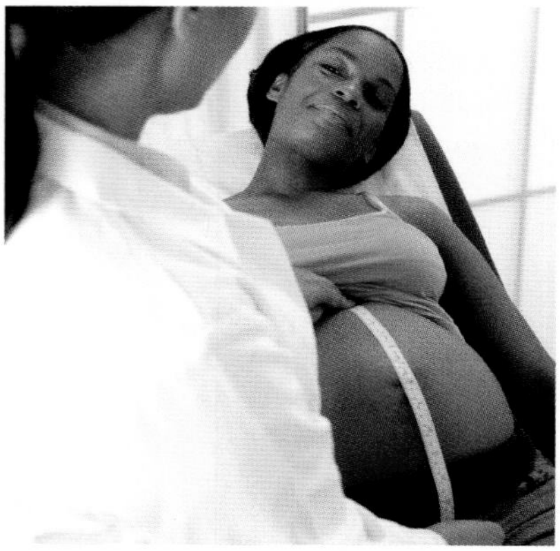

Measuring your abdomen helps the doctor monitor your baby's growth.

GROWTH CHARTS

If your doctor has concerns about your baby's growth later in pregnancy, they may arrange for scans over a period of time to plot and monitor your baby's growth. Individual measurements will be taken of the head, abdomen, and limbs. Measurements of the head and abdomen are most important since an unequal growth pattern in these areas may indicate a particular problem.

The three lines on the graphs here represent different growth rates. The red line in the center, referred to as the 50th percentile, shows an average pattern of growth. The thinner lines above and below, the 90th and the 10th percentiles, show the top and bottom ranges of normal growth. Since the head and abdominal circumferences are measured over time and plotted on a graph, a pattern of growth becomes clear. Here, the head is growing normally, but growth has slowed in the abdomen, possibly due to a placental problem that in itself may be caused by a condition in the mother. For example, conditions such as high blood pressure (see p.283) can affect placental blood flow. If the blood flow to the baby is restricted, this can result in the oxygen and nutrients carried in the blood being diverted to the baby's most vital organs, the brain and heart, rather than to the abdominal organs, which results in unequal growth patterns in the head and abdomen.

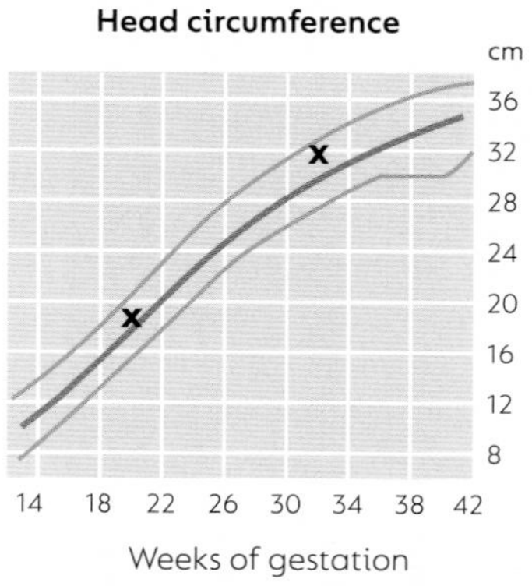
Head circumference
cm
36
32
28
24
20
16
12
8
14 18 22 26 30 34 38 42
Weeks of gestation

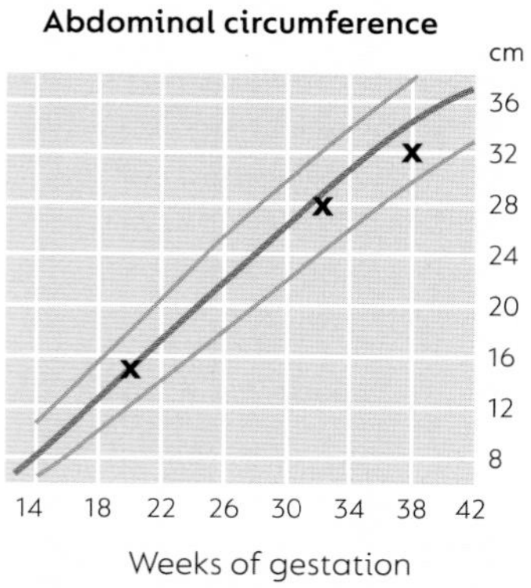
Abdominal circumference
cm
36
32
28
24
20
16
12
8
14 18 22 26 30 34 38 42
Weeks of gestation

Measuring growth with ultrasound

By late pregnancy, the length of your baby can no longer fit on the screen, so your doctor will calculate their size by combining several measurements in a mathematical formula, as is done at the 20-week scan (see p.214). Measurements include the width of the head (biparietal diameter), circumference of the head, and the abdominal circumference, which are plotted on a graph over a period of time (see box, opposite page). The length of the upper leg bone (femur length) may also be measured. If your baby is smaller than the 10th percentile or has a small abdomen, you may have more tests to assess their well-being (see below). A measurement above the 90th percentile can be a sign of gestational diabetes (see p.475) and will need investigating. Also, if your baby is thought to weigh over 11 lb (5 kg), your doctor will discuss with you the option of a Cesarean section.

If there are concerns over your baby's growth, you may be referred for fetal heart-rate monitoring and/or biophysical profile testing, which observe how your baby responds to stimuli and whether there are signs of distress. If you have a known condition that can affect your baby's growth (see opposite), your doctor may arrange for you to have one or both tests once or twice a week after about 32 weeks. Some doctors perform Doppler scans (see box, right) to assess placental blood flow when the baby is small for gestational age.

A nonstress test This test assesses your baby's well-being. An external transducer is placed on your abdomen to listen for accelerations in your baby's heart rate that last about 15 seconds. You may or may not notice any fetal movement during these accelerations. The test result is said to be "reassuring" if the heart accelerates twice over 20–30 minutes and no large decelerations occur. About 10–20 percent of babies have a test with less than two accelerations. This doesn't necessarily mean a problem exists; your baby my just have been asleep, and the test may be repeated.

A biophysical profile (BPP) If, after the nonstress test, your doctor still has concerns, a BPP may be done. A BPP combines the results of a CTG reading to evaluate four factors: the volume of amniotic fluid, fetal movement, fetal muscle tone and posture, and fetal breathing. Two points are given for each part of the test, so a "reassuring" BPP result would be eight points.

DOPPLER SCANS

A Doppler scan analyzes blood flow through the placenta. If the placenta is functioning well, the blood flows easily. If there is a problem, the placenta is resistant to the blood flow and the baby's heart has to work harder to pump blood. In extreme cases, there are periods between your baby's heartbeats of no blood flow or reversed blood flow and an early delivery may be suggested.

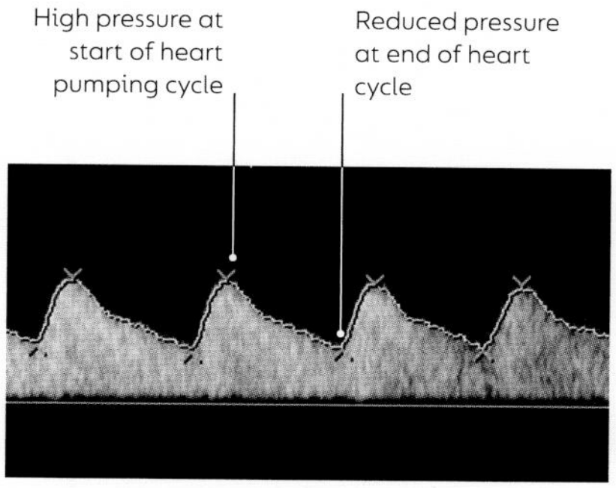
High pressure at start of heart pumping cycle
Reduced pressure at end of heart cycle

A normal Doppler reading shows the continuous blood flow to the baby via the placenta. At the beginning of a heart cycle, the pressure is high; it then dips at the end of the cycle, but doesn't ever stop.

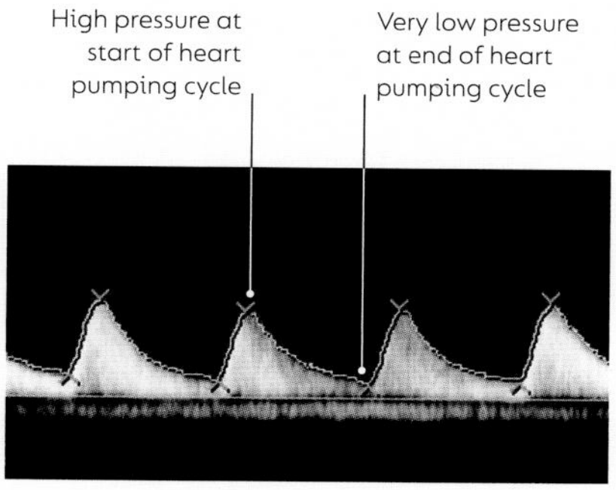
High pressure at start of heart pumping cycle
Very low pressure at end of heart pumping cycle

An abnormal reading indicates that there is resistance to blood flow in the placenta, resulting in very little or no flow at the end of the cycle. The baby may not receive sufficient oxygen, which can affect growth.

QUESTIONS AND ANSWERS

I've heard about "kick counts." Should I be doing these? You may be advised to count how many times your baby moves over a period of time. However, it can cause undue worry to moms, and other indicators of movement, such as noting a change in the pattern of movement and inactivity when your baby is normally active, are important. Your doctor may ask you to note your baby's normal movement and contact them immediately if there are any changes in the pattern.

Can my baby move too much?
Usually, the more movement, the better, even if this keeps you up at night or causes discomfort. An active fetus is not a sign that you'll have a restless baby or a hyperactive child.

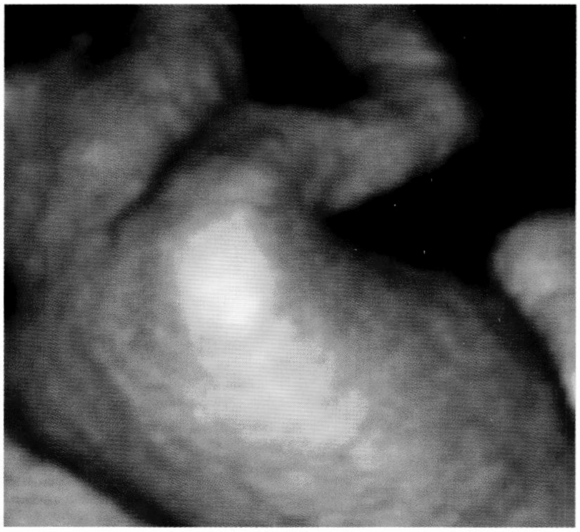

YOU ARE **27 WEEKS AND 4 DAYS**

87 days to go

YOUR BABY TODAY

This baby's back is turned and is facing away from the ultrasound scanner. The skin is much less transparent than before since your baby is constantly laying down fat reserves beneath it. This fat accounts, in part, for much of your baby's weight gain from now on.

" Your baby is growing eyebrows and eyelashes—and hair on their head—and making good use of all the space in your uterus. "

Your baby's eyes are now open, and both the eyebrows and the eyelashes have grown. The hair on your baby's head continues to get longer.

It's quite likely that your baby is making use of all the space available and may well be in a breech position (bottom down), at least some of the time. This is the case in a third of pregnancies at this stage, but your baby's position is unlikely to stabilize until after 36 or 37 weeks of pregnancy. Because the shape of your uterus naturally favors a head-down position, only 3 to 4 percent of babies remain in the breech position after 37 weeks. It may be quite difficult for you (and your doctor) to tell your baby's position at this stage. For example, just because the feet kick you in a particular place doesn't tell you much about your baby's position. Babies are very flexible and a scan might show that they are doubled up with their feet on their head.

PELVIC GIRDLE PAIN (PGP)

Hormonal shifts lead to changes in your bony pelvis, which can be extremely painful. You know you've got PGP when sneezing hurts, you waddle when you walk, and turning over in bed is a major task. Formerly known as SPD, or symphysis pubis dysfunction, PGP affects one in five pregnant women. Try the following if you have PGP:

- Keep your legs together when getting in and out of bed or the car (place a plastic bag on the seat to help you swivel).
- Sleep on your side with a pillow between your legs.
- Wear comfortable shoes.
- Avoid tasks that hurt.
- Relax in warm water.
- Ask your doctor for a support belt to help ease the pain.
- Studies show that physical therapy and acupuncture may help symphysis pubis dysfunction.

BLOOD TESTS

Some time between 26 and 30 weeks your blood will be tested to check that you aren't anemic. If you are found to be anemic your doctor may prescribe iron pills for you. Because of an increase in the fluid content of your blood, your hemoglobin count is likely to fall later on in your pregnancy, so it's a good idea to address this issue now.

Iron pills can cause digestive problems, such as constipation or diarrhea, so if this happens to you, ask your doctor if your prescription can be changed. The liquid medications available over the counter are kinder on the digestive system than pills, so ask your doctor if one of these is appropriate for you.

If a previous blood test has shown that you're Rh negative, you'll receive an injection of Rh immunoglobulin (RhIg) at around 28–34 weeks. You'll get another shot after the baby is born.

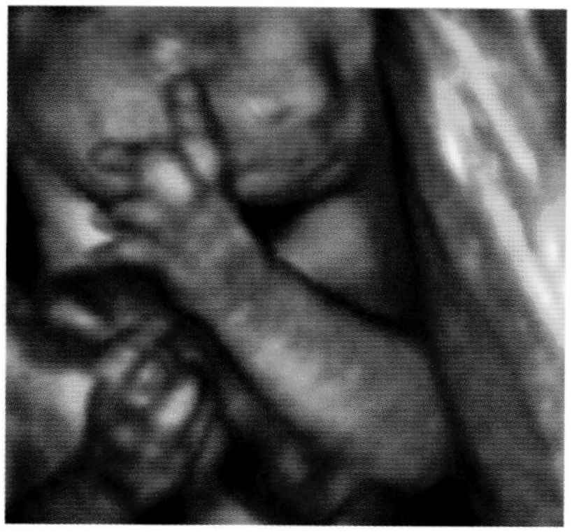

YOU ARE **27 WEEKS AND 5 DAYS**

86 days to go

YOUR BABY TODAY

A finger is held close to the eye in this image. The eyes are shut for most of the time but also a simple reflex action will prevent a stray finger (or toe) from touching the eye. Furthermore, the fingernails are still well away from the fingertips at this time.

It's reassuring to know that many women have babies on their own and do not find life an endless struggle. Although it would be wrong to pretend that parenting alone is as easy as it is when you share the care, with additional support it is possible. Even if you are in a relationship, you may feel you are going it alone at times. You may have very strong reasons why you want a baby, for example your increasing age, and this determination will give you strength and focus.

It is helpful for all pregnant women to find someone to talk to and confide in. This could be your mother or a close friend or relative. As you are making far-reaching decisions about your future, it's important that you have support, accurate information, and time to think things through without fear, panic, or pressure from others. Finding somebody you really trust and whom you know can give you support when you need it—especially in labor and in the first days and weeks with your baby—may help relieve any pressure you are under. It will also enable you to think more calmly and clearly about your situation and make plans.

It's worth, even at this early stage, starting to think about who you would like to ask to be your birth partner: this is a big decision that should not be rushed.

> “ Deciding to go it alone is never an easy option, but with the right support, you can look forward happily to your baby's birth. ”

BUILDING A SUPPORT NETWORK

It's important for all pregnant women to have emotional and practical support, and this is especially true if you're single.

- **Make sure you go to all your prenatal appointments** and build a relationship with your doctor; they are an invaluable source of information.
- **Sign up for prenatal classes.** If you're single, you may find that daytime courses are less populated by "couples"; this gives you a chance to build up a network of female friends. Also try to go to exercise classes, such as yoga and water aerobics.
- **Give plenty of thought** to choosing your birth partner: a trusted friend, or perhaps your own mother, who is likely to be thrilled to be asked to share this experience with you.
- **Don't be too proud to accept offers of help** from friends and family—most will genuinely want to be involved now and after the birth.

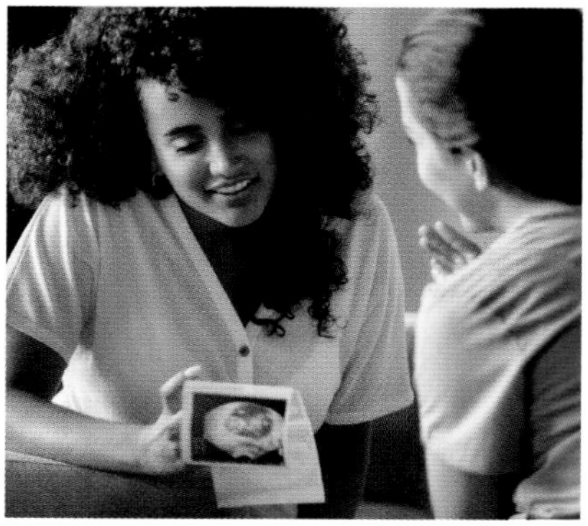

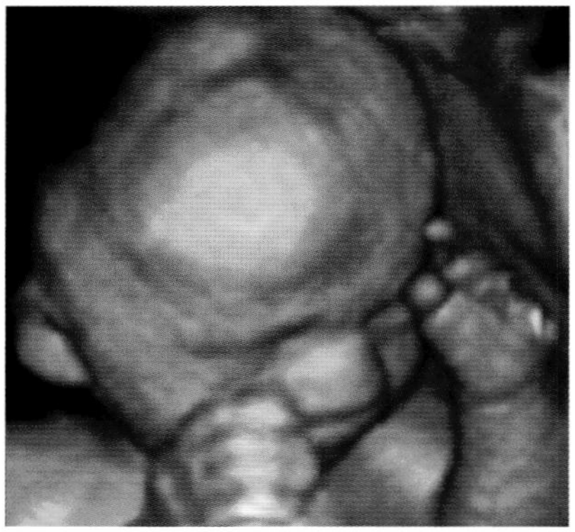

YOU ARE **27 WEEKS AND 6 DAYS**

85 days to go

YOUR BABY TODAY

Although ultrasound cannot show it, there is now some hair on your baby's head and their eyelashes and eyebrows have grown. The pattern and color of hair growth has a significant impact on the overall look of your baby, but this is not apparent on a scan.

> "While women who are pregnant in the summer may find it hard to stay cool, being pregnant in the winter is also challenging."

Most women are understandably reluctant to buy a winter coat that will see them all the way through pregnancy and may well never be worn again. The good news is that you probably won't need one at all! You are likely to feel very warm toward the end of your pregnancy, and may find it more comfortable to wear plenty of layered knits rather than one warm coat or jacket. Layers can also be easily discarded if you become overheated while you're traveling.

You can also probably hijack some of your partner's wardrobe, and borrow a coat or jacket that will fasten over your belly if you're planning to be outside for extended periods. Alternatively, go to a local second-hand shop—you may well find a larger coat or jacket for a bargain price that will carry you through the final few weeks of your pregnancy.

Also consider wearing your own coat unfastened, with a long scarf hanging down to fill the gap.

Think about purchasing a large shawl or wrap, which will see you through the winter months, and keep you and your baby warm after the birth. Shawls and wraps are ideal for keeping you warm when your baby is in a sling, and also for unexpected breast-feeding sessions outdoors.

You'll need to be extra careful in the winter, when you're in icy conditions. Make sure you wear sensible flat shoes when you're out and about to reduce the risk of slipping and falling.

FOCUS ON TWINS

If you're having two or more babies, you'll need to consider making some adjustments to your living space. To reduce the risk of crib death, it's best for babies to sleep in the same room as their parents but you don't need two cribs. You can put both your newborn babies to sleep in one crib (see p.335), but this isn't recommended after they're three months old.

It's a legal requirement for each baby to have an individual car seat if you plan to drive them anywhere, including home from the hospital

ASK A NUTRITIONIST

I've heard that I need more vitamin B1, thiamine, in the last trimester. Is this true? Thiamine is one of the B vitamins that helps in the metabolism of carbohydrate foods (see p.14), releasing energy to the body, which you definitely need in this last trimester of pregnancy.

Women who have had really severe vomiting can sometimes become deficient in thiamine and may need a supplement. Because it isn't stored in the body, having a regular supply of this vitamin is important.

For meat eaters, pork is an excellent source of thiamine, so try making a stir-fry with a lean pork loin or a ham steak.

For vegetarians and vegans, oats, brown rice, yeast extract, and fortified breakfast cereals are all good sources of thiamine.

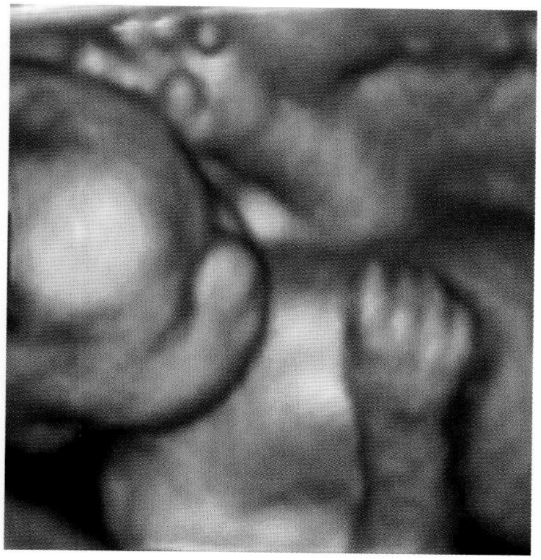

YOU ARE **28 WEEKS EXACTLY**

84 days to go

YOUR BABY TODAY

The amniotic fluid is approaching its maximum amount at this time and your baby will have plenty of space in which to move. Here the baby is down toward the level of the umbilical cord. Your baby is still likely to change position several times a day.

Some friendships change as you go through different life stages. You'll probably have had different groups of friends through school, college, and different jobs, with one or two close friends throughout. Friendships often develop with people when you're at a similar stage in your lives. This means that during your pregnancy and when you have young children you may feel most comfortable with other women in similar situations. You'll meet new friends at postpartum classes or postpartum groups, or in situations such as toddler swimming or music classes.

As you make new friends, you may find your old relationships begin to change. Friends without children may find it difficult to understand your new role as a mother, and the intense love that you have for your child, and you may start to drift apart. Of course this is not always the case; some friendships are unchanging, irrespective of whether your lives go along different paths.

" If you're the first among your friends to have a baby, be prepared for friendships to evolve and change. "

CHOOSING ORGANIC

Opting to eat organic food is a personal choice, dictated by your beliefs and whether or not you can afford the higher price. Organic fruits and vegetables are grown with almost no pesticides, synthetic fertilizers, and herbicides. Organic meat, poultry, eggs, and dairy products come from animals that have high standards of animal welfare, without the routine use of antibiotics. For these reasons, organic foods should be lower in pesticide residues. However, all food in the US has to stay below pesticide residue tolerances.

Despite years of research, there is no consistent evidence from large-scale studies that organic food contains more nutrients than nonorganic foods. Some studies suggest that some fruits and vegetables may contain more antioxidant vitamins. This may be because organic vegetables contain less water, so the vitamins are more concentrated. One study found that organic milk provided more omega-3 fatty acids than nonorganic.

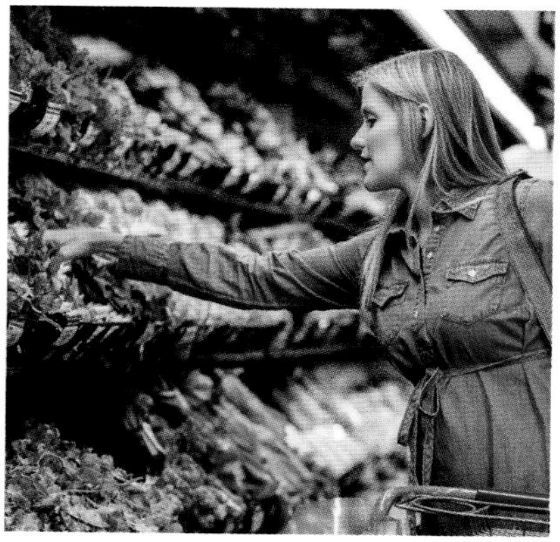

ASK A DOCTOR

I've seen a secondhand car seat advertised. Is there any reason why I shouldn't buy it? Don't use a secondhand car seat unless you can be absolutely certain of its history because it may have been in an accident or damaged.

If you must use a secondhand seat, only accept one if you are absolutely certain that you know its history and that it hasn't been in a bad accident. Don't use a seat that cracked, that doesn't come with the original instructions, is missing parts, was recalled, or is too old. Don't purchase a car seat for your baby at a secondhand store or through classified ads, or on the internet.

Your 29th week

USE THIS THIRD TRIMESTER TO GET ORGANIZED BEFORE YOUR BABY IS BORN. You may feel a little bored and back-achey at this stage of pregnancy, but there are plenty of positive ways to take your mind off things. For example, you could start to make inquiries about breast-feeding classes, plan your maternity leave, and draw up shopping lists of baby essentials, such as diapers, a changing mat, onesies, bibs, and baby wipes, and perhaps buy a couple of items each week.

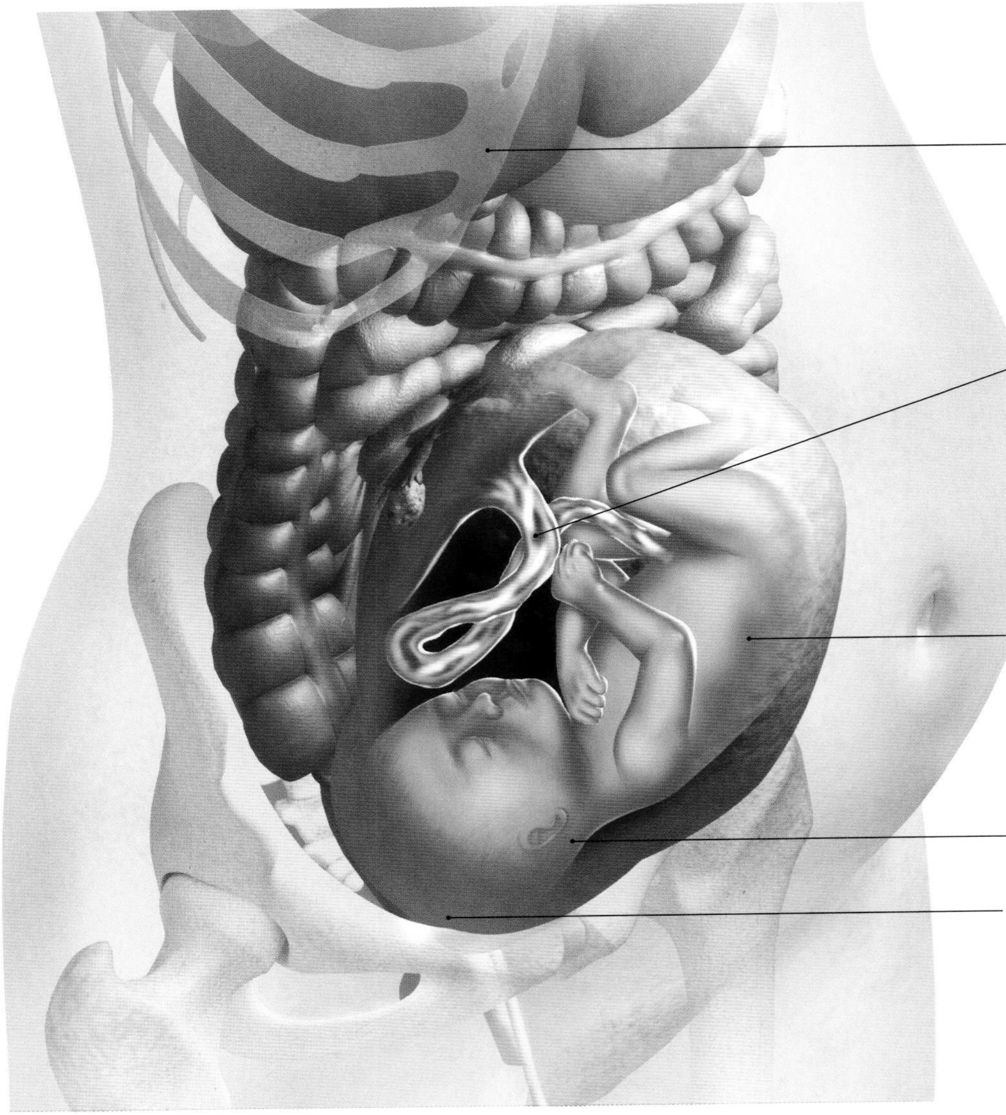

As your belly continues to get bigger it may put pressure on your ribs and diaphragm.

A jellylike fluid in the coiling umbilical cord prevents it from becoming compressed as the baby twists and turns.

Fine lanugo hairs cover the baby's body. Most will disappear before the birth, but a few may still be seen on the baby's back when he is born.

The brain continues to get bigger and its surface is beginning to take on the creases and folds seen in mature brains.

At 29 weeks the average crown to heel length is 15.2 in (38.6 cm) and the average weight is 2.5 lb (1.2 kg).

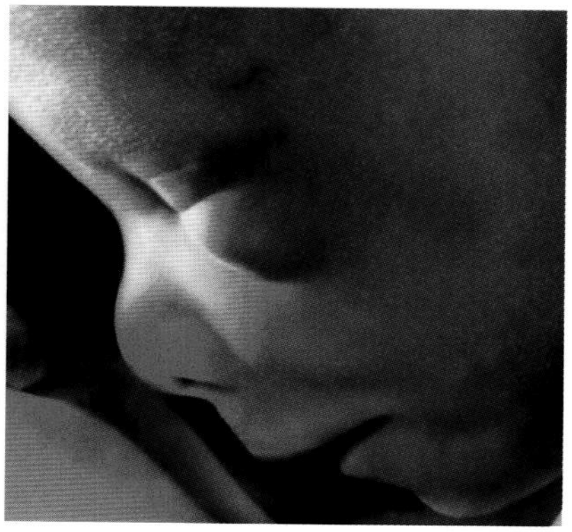

YOU ARE **28 WEEKS AND 1 DAY**

83 days to go

YOUR BABY TODAY

This week marks a milestone in your baby's development. Although a baby born at this stage would still need help with breathing, the lungs have matured to an extent that survival chances outside the uterus are significantly better than earlier in the pregnancy.

> " It's never too early to start thinking about the financial implications of maternity leave, and whether to return to work. "

When you're on maternity leave, it may be the first occasion that you haven't worked for a long time. This change can be quite daunting, even though you know you'll soon be busy taking care of a baby. Depending on your employer, you'll be entitled to varying amounts of pay during your maternity leave. Every company has a different maternity leave policy. You may get paid or unpaid leave for a specific number of weeks or you may be able to use sick days or vacation days. Ask a human resources representative about your options. Depending on your partner's employer, he may be eligible for the Family Medical Leave Act (FMLA), which means he could get 12 weeks of unpaid leave. Some companies are more generous than others, offering a percentage of your salary during your maternity leave. Going on maternity leave may cause a significant drop in your income. You should talk to your partner about how much money will be coming in and going out and how you will manage a change in your finances.

Even though it's a long way in the future, you might also start thinking about plans for working after the baby is born. You may think that you have no real option financially and have to return full time, but explore the possibilities of working more flexibly, or part time, or from home one or two days a week. You may also want to start thinking about your child-care options (see p.332).

CHOOSING DIAPERS

Should you opt for disposables (use once, then throw away) or cloth (wash, dry, and use again)?

- **Disposable diapers** are slim fitting, super absorbent, and will keep your baby dry, even overnight. However, they cost more (by some estimates, up to $1,000 per child by the time you start potty training) and there's the landfill factor to consider. Eco-friendly diapers use no polluting bleaching agents and fewer chemicals are used to produce them.
- **Cloth** costs less—although the initial investment is greater. They also provide a softer landing for toddlers who topple over. However, all that soaking, washing, and drying could get you down (plus this has an environmental impact). You may opt to use a diaper-laundering service each week (at a cost) Cloth diapers need changing more often than disposables. They are slightly more difficult to put on and take off.
- **Using a combination** of reusable and disposable diapers can work well: buy the occasional package of disposables for when you are out and about or for if you have to leave the baby with a babysitter, but opt for cloth the rest of the time.

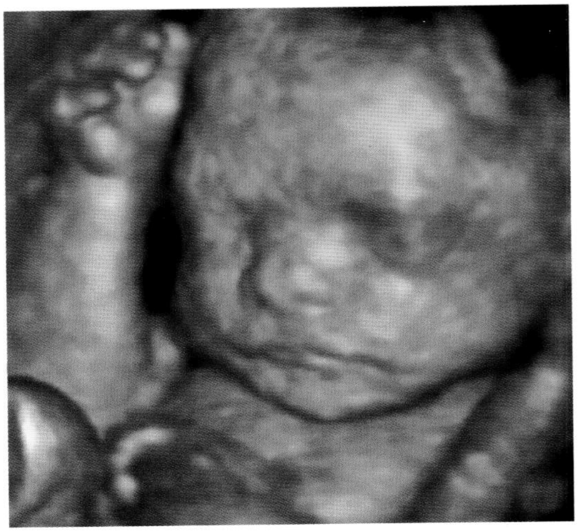

YOU ARE **28 WEEKS AND 2 DAYS**

82 days to go...

YOUR BABY TODAY

This image shows a chin-on-the-chest position with an arm held up to the side of the face. A knee is just visible to the left of the image with a loop of umbilical cord above it. Your baby now is likely to be in a head down position but there's still time to change.

" The coiled umbilical cord connects your baby to the placenta, their life-support system until birth. "

Most umbilical cords grow to be about the same length as the baby (although there are exceptions), reaching a final length of 20–23.5 in (50–60 cm). The umbilical cord has up to 40 turns along its length. These turns are seven times more likely to twist to the left than the right. The coiling pattern was in place nine weeks after conception, with more coils at the baby's end than the placental end; this may be a response to your baby's movements. The cord contains three blood vessels: two arteries taking deoxygenated blood and waste from your baby to the placenta and one vein carrying oxygen-rich blood from the placenta to the baby. The cord diameter is usually less than ¾ in (2 cm) and the blood vessels are embedded in and protected by a layer of jelly. The watery composition of the jelly, and with the cord's coiling pattern, prevents compression of the cord.

At the 20-week scan (see pp.214–215), they will check that the umbilical cord has three vessels. In 1 percent of pregnancies, there is only one umbilical artery. When this happens, you'll need extra scans to monitor your baby's growth

ASK A DOCTOR

If my baby has a low birthweight, will he have health problems? A low birthweight is less than 5½ lb (2.5 kg) and although the majority of small babies thrive, some do have difficulties. Most low birthweight babies are small because they are premature. There are many ways you can reduce the risk of your baby being a low birthweight: eating adequate amounts of healthy food to gain the right amount of weight (see p.99), not smoking or drinking alcohol, reducing stress, and attending all of your prenatal appointments.

RESTLESS LEGS

Some pregnant women experience restless legs syndrome (RLS), whereby they have an irresistible urge to move their legs. It most commonly happens while resting, so can be very disruptive to sleep.

The exact cause of RLS isn't known but it may be related to an imbalance of a brain chemical called dopamine. The level of dopamine can be affected by a lack of iron. Restless legs syndrome will pass once you're no longer pregnant. To minimize the effects of restless legs syndrome:

- **Ensure your diet** includes an adequate intake of iron (see p.154).
- **Take steps to get a good night's sleep**. Keep your bedroom cool, quiet, comfortable, and dark. Don't watch television, use a laptop, talk on the phone, or do any work in bed, and keep a consistent sleep schedule. Also, try doing something to challenge your brain before bed (a crossword puzzle, word jumble, or Sudoku puzzle). This may help ease your restless legs. Avoid exercising close to bedtime.

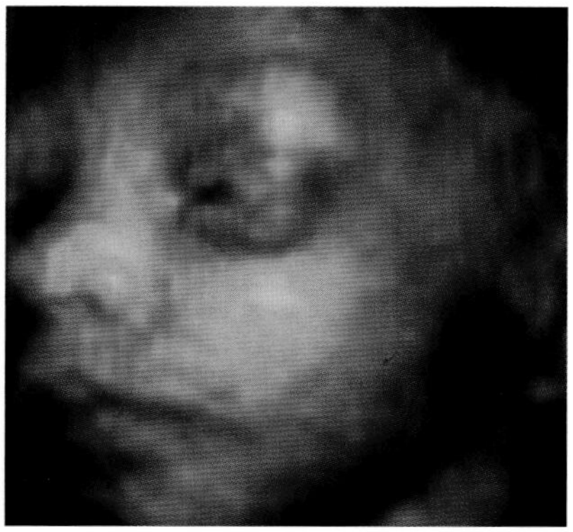

YOU ARE **28 WEEKS AND 3 DAYS**

81 days to go...

YOUR BABY TODAY

This image offers the first view of the eye opening. The lids have separated and the dark pupil can be seen. There is no true reflection of color on ultrasound so the white of the eye is colored the same as the eyelids and face. The "eyebrows" are in fact shadow.

> "If you're starting to feel that you've been eclipsed by your belly, it's time to do something just for you."

Like many pregnant women, you may feel that you've disappeared behind your belly; that the essence of who you are has been lost in the guise of "pregnant woman." People may no longer ask about how you're feeling, or what's going on in your life. Instead of "How are you?" they might ask, "Is everything OK with the baby?"

It can be difficult for people, and even for you, to remember that you still exist in a role that is separate from pregnant woman or mother. If during your pregnancy you are feeling very frustrated by this, consider doing something just for you, maybe some pampering or a dinner for two, to make you feel special again.

GRAZING THROUGH THE DAY

You need to eat plenty of good-quality protein to encourage your baby's growth and keep you in glowing good health, so try to eat either eggs, cheese, lean meats, fish, legumes, or whole grains at every meal. Add to that lots of fruits and vegetables, nuts, seeds, and some complex carbohydrates (see p.92).

Break the food down into a plan of five to seven small meals and snacks each day. If you usually have soup and a sandwich for lunch, try a vegetable soup midmorning, and have the sandwich later; prepare snacks such as raw vegetables, cheese, nuts, and fruit and graze on them through the afternoon. Perhaps have a bowl of oatmeal early in the evening, followed by fruit later.

ASK A DOCTOR

I have a sharp pain in my lower back and leg. What causes this? This sounds like sciatica, a sharp pain that travels down the back and leg when the sciatic nerve—the longest nerve in the body—is trapped in a joint in the lower back. This is not related to your pregnancy, although it can get worse in pregnancy. For lower back pain, warm baths and a warm compress can help, as can gentle massage by an experienced practitioner.

Exercise such as yoga or water aerobics classes can help strengthen back muscles, but check with your doctor before embarking on a new exercise regimen. Watch your posture (see p.249) and wear comfortable, supportive shoes.

If you have sciatica, ask your doctor to refer you to a physical therapist. You'll be shown exercises to help relieve the pain and minimize the risk of it recurring.

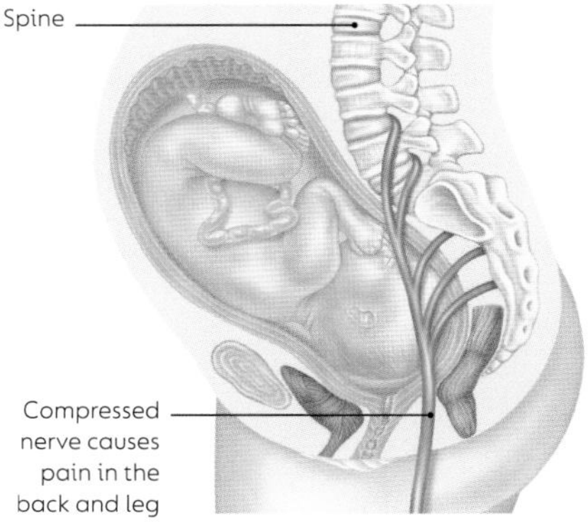
Spine
Compressed nerve causes pain in the back and leg

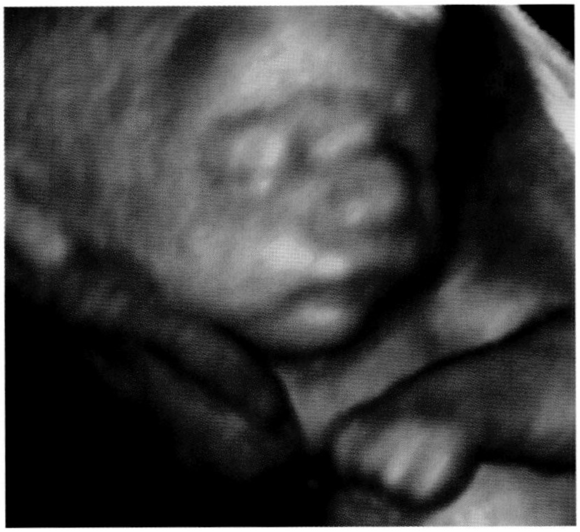

YOU ARE **28 WEEKS AND 4 DAYS**

80 days to go

YOUR BABY TODAY

The sleep-wake cycle is now more established, however, just because your baby is moving, you cannot assume they are awake. They spend little time fully active with their eyes open, so many of the movements you are feeling are happening while they are asleep.

> " Your baby's growth depends on many factors and its rate varies through the course of your pregnancy. "

The growth of your baby relies on a steady stream of nutrients. Most nutrients are transferred unaltered across the placenta, but some substances are made by the placenta itself and a few are produced from scratch by your baby. These include the hormone thyroxine, the production of which depends on iodine from the mother crossing the placenta. Thyroxine has several functions and its level needs to be controlled very precisely. The placenta forms a nearly perfect barrier to thyroxine, enabling you and your baby to adjust thyroxine levels independently of each other.

In the early stages of pregnancy, genetic factors largely determined the size of your baby, but by now environmental factors are becoming more important. Overall, your baby's final birthweight is determined about 40 percent by genetic factors and 60 percent by environmental factors. Your baby grows at a steady rate from 24 weeks until the last 2–3 weeks, when growth continues but more slowly. (If you're expecting twins, your babies grow as if alone in the uterus up until 28 weeks but from this point there is a reduction in their growth rate.) Your baby's internal organs account for much of his current growth

The liver and brain, in particular, continue to enlarge and muscle mass increases. Later, fat will be deposited under the skin, rounding out your baby's contours.

IDENTICAL TWINS

The incidence of identical twins has been stable for some years. Identical twins represent about a third of all twin pregnancies, regardless of race, maternal age, or geography.

FOCUS ON TWINS

The clothes you buy for your twins should be easy to put on and take off, and, of course, machine washable. You'll probably be given outfits as presents, so just buy the basics.

For each baby, you're likely to need at least::

- Six undershirts
- Six onesies
- Two jackets
- One or two hats (sun hat for summer)
- Several burp cloths and bibs.

Keep in mind when choosing diapers that twins are often smaller on arrival than a single baby, and you may therefore get through a wide range of sizes in the first few months.

It's advisable to buy a good-quality double stroller, since it will be used for quite a while. When choosing a stroller, a side-by-side model is preferable to a tandem stroller, so that your babies can see each other and communicate as they grow older.

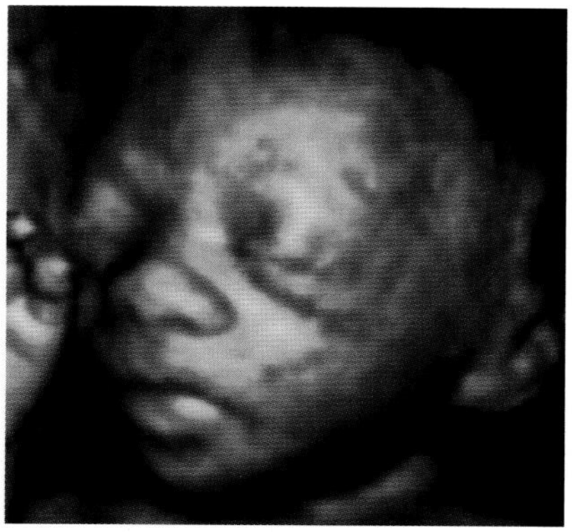

YOU ARE **28 WEEKS AND 5 DAYS**

79 days to go

YOUR BABY TODAY

Although many babies look similar on 3-D ultrasound, particularly strong features, such as those affecting the shape of the ears, lips, or nose, are easy to see. From now on, these features will become more and more individualized and recognizable.

There is a lot of expectation on women to breastfeed because breastfeeding has health benefits for both you and your baby and it helps with bonding. People may already be asking you whether you intend to breastfeed or not, and it's reasonable that you don't yet know the answer. After all, you haven't tried!

Most women want to try breastfeeding, but some feel uncomfortable with the thought of doing it, especially in public. There will likely be a lactation consultant in the hospital or you may be able to hire one. In some areas, you can go to classes during pregnancy, which will explain the benefits of breastfeeding and aspects such as positioning the baby so that you're both comfortable and the baby is latched on (see p.451).

The expectation of breastfeeding is that, because it's natural, it's easy. The reality is that until you get the hang of it, it can be difficult. Ask your delivery nurse to show you how to position the baby. Most importantly, keep an open mind and try it. Once breastfeeding is established, it can have enormous benefits to your baby's health, can help you to lose some of the pregnancy weight, and, best of all, it's a wonderful way to be close to your baby.

> “Breastfeeding may be natural but it can be tricky to get started, so try to go to a class or two now while you have the time.”

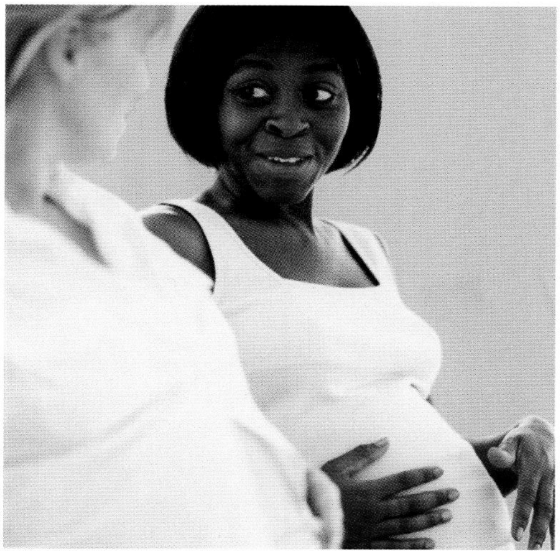

Talk to pregnant friends about breast-feeding now, and you can support each other once you start feeding your babies. Also get your partner involved research shows that partners who are aware of the benefits of breastfeeding are more likely to be supportive.

LEAKING BREAST MILK

Some pregnant women experience some leakage of breast milk, perhaps when their breasts are massaged or sexually stimulated, and sometimes for no apparent reason. Some discharge in pregnancy does mean that things are working properly, but women who don't experience this symptom are perfectly able to produce and provide milk for their baby.

CULTURED FOODS

Probiotics—such as in some yogurts, kimchi, vegetable pickles, sauerkraut, and miso—contain enzymes and bacteria that help your body digest food, and build up friendly bacteria in the gut. If your digestion is sluggish and you're finding constipation a problem, try some of these foods but be aware that they are salty, so eat them in moderation.

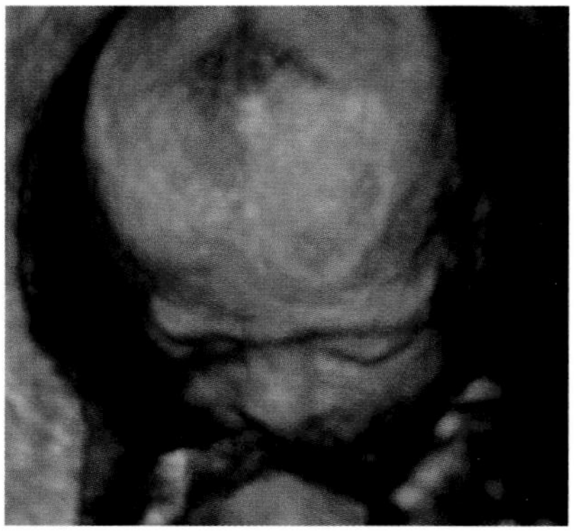

YOU ARE **28 WEEKS AND 6 DAYS**

78 days to go

YOUR BABY TODAY

Your baby's external appearance is fully formed but inside there is still a great deal of activity as many of the organs are continuing to mature. Even after pregnancy further development occurs, especially of the brain and lungs.

> “ Back pain is not an inevitable part of being pregnant: there are lots of things you can do to help prevent and relieve it. ”

Yoga and other stretching exercises are great during pregnancy, since they strengthen key ligaments while relaxing areas that are tight and painful. Although it may seem easier to rest when you experience pain (especially back pain), and to avoid exercise, gentle stretching and movement often decreases muscle spasm and improves the function of the spine, resulting in less pain. Exercise also boosts energy levels and contributes to an easier labor, delivery, and postpartum recovery. Try stretching and relaxation techniques as a first resort for back pain.

If the pain is severe, ask your partner to massage the area. Ask your doctor if you can safely take any painkillers or if acupuncture might help ease your pain. If the area feels inflamed and painful, try placing a cold pack on the affected area for 5–10 minutes, several times a day.

ASK A MOM

I'm bored with being pregnant! How will I get through the next couple of months? I felt the same at about six months but found the last three months passed quickly because more was happening. Along with more prenatal visits and classes, there was planning when to start maternity leave, then finishing work, then getting the nursery ready, and buying things for the baby. And I made an effort to see all my girlfriends—it all made the time pass quickly.

MINIMIZING THE STRAIN ON YOUR BACK

As the weight of your baby strains your abdominal muscles, and pregnancy hormones soften your ligaments, your abdominals give less support to your spine. This results in your muscles straining to keep you upright and can cause back pain. Lifting and bending can exacerbate back pain, so try these strategies to help avoid added strain.

- **To lift something from the floor,** stand close to the object with one foot in front of the other. Bend your knees, then straighten them, so that you use your thigh muscles to lift. Avoid locking your knees: always bend from the waist with your knees bent. If you need to pick something up, consider sitting, kneeling, or squatting to reach it to avoid putting your lower back under stress.
- **If you have to move a heavy object** (try to avoid this if you possibly can), push it rather than pull it: that way, your legs, not your back, take the strain.
- **To get into and out of a car,** or bed, keep your hips, pelvis, and back aligned in the same direction. To get out of bed, roll on to your side, and use your arms to push yourself up.

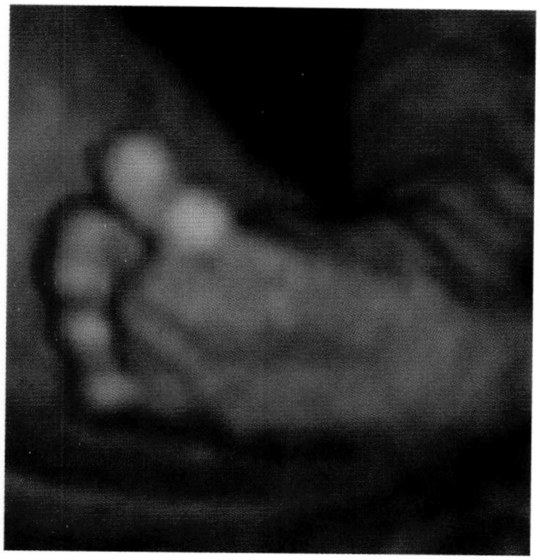

YOU ARE **29 WEEKS EXACTLY**

77 days to go

YOUR BABY TODAY

This is a close-up of how your baby's foot is looking now. Your baby will easily put their feet on top of their head one minute only to bring them down the next, so just because your baby is kicking you at one end it doesn't mean the head is at the other.

In today's society women are simply overloaded with information about pregnancy, from newspapers, magazines, books, and the internet. Photographs of glamorous pregnant celebrities, who look as if they don't have a care in the world, abound in the media. Two sources on the same topic can offer conflicting opinions.

Although the internet can be a wonderful source of useful information, it has drawbacks: you don't know who has written an article on a website, it may not have been written by a health professional, and some recommendations may even contradict standard medical advice. This means that constantly scouring the internet and reading everything you find can be confusing and scary.

Articles telling you that you risk the health and well-being of your baby by doing something can make you feel inadequate. Keep telling yourself that women have been having children for centuries without the aid of the internet! If reading lots of information makes you feel empowered and better able to make informed choices, then read away, but if it makes you feel confused then don't. A sensible course might be to pick just one reliable book or information source to read instead.

> “ Pregnancy can be a time of information overload, and sometimes it's difficult to know which sources are reliable. ”

NUTRITIOUS BLUEBERRIES

According to a US study, blueberries topped a list of more than 40 fruits in terms of antioxidant activity. They are also a source of fiber, which is great during pregnancy, especially if—like many women—you suffer from constipation. Blueberries also contain nutrients that can prevent or repair damage to the body's cells. This may strengthen your immune system and ability to fight infections.

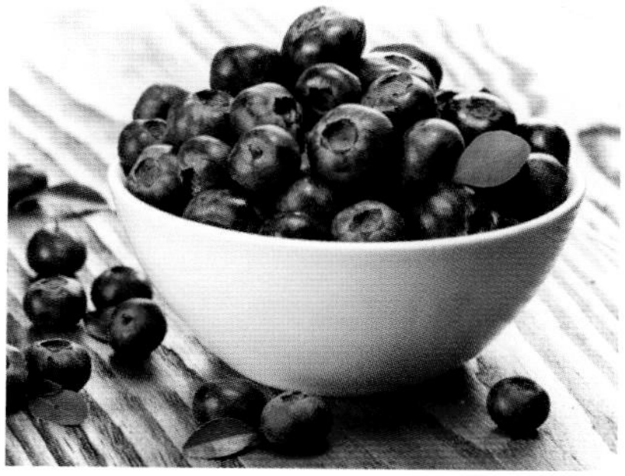

ASK A DOCTOR

I plan to bottle-feed. What do I need to buy in advance? You'll need plastic bottles (nipples are included), a sterilizing unit or kit (see p.451), which often has everything you need, and your preferred formula. Each comes in a range of options, so you need to decide what works best for you.

As you get to know your newborn baby, you may have to change the type of nipple and/or formula, so it's not advisable to buy too many before the birth.

Your 30th week

YOU'RE GETTING TIRED MORE EASILY BUT THAT PROBABLY WON'T STOP YOUR NESTING PLANS. The nest-building instinct often kicks in as a woman approaches her due date. You may be overwhelmed with the urge to clean and decorate, but although it's natural to want a perfect home for your baby don't wear yourself out. Work, traveling, and a constant round of prenatal appointments are probably all much more of an effort these days. If you need to keep stopping to rest, listen to your body and do just that.

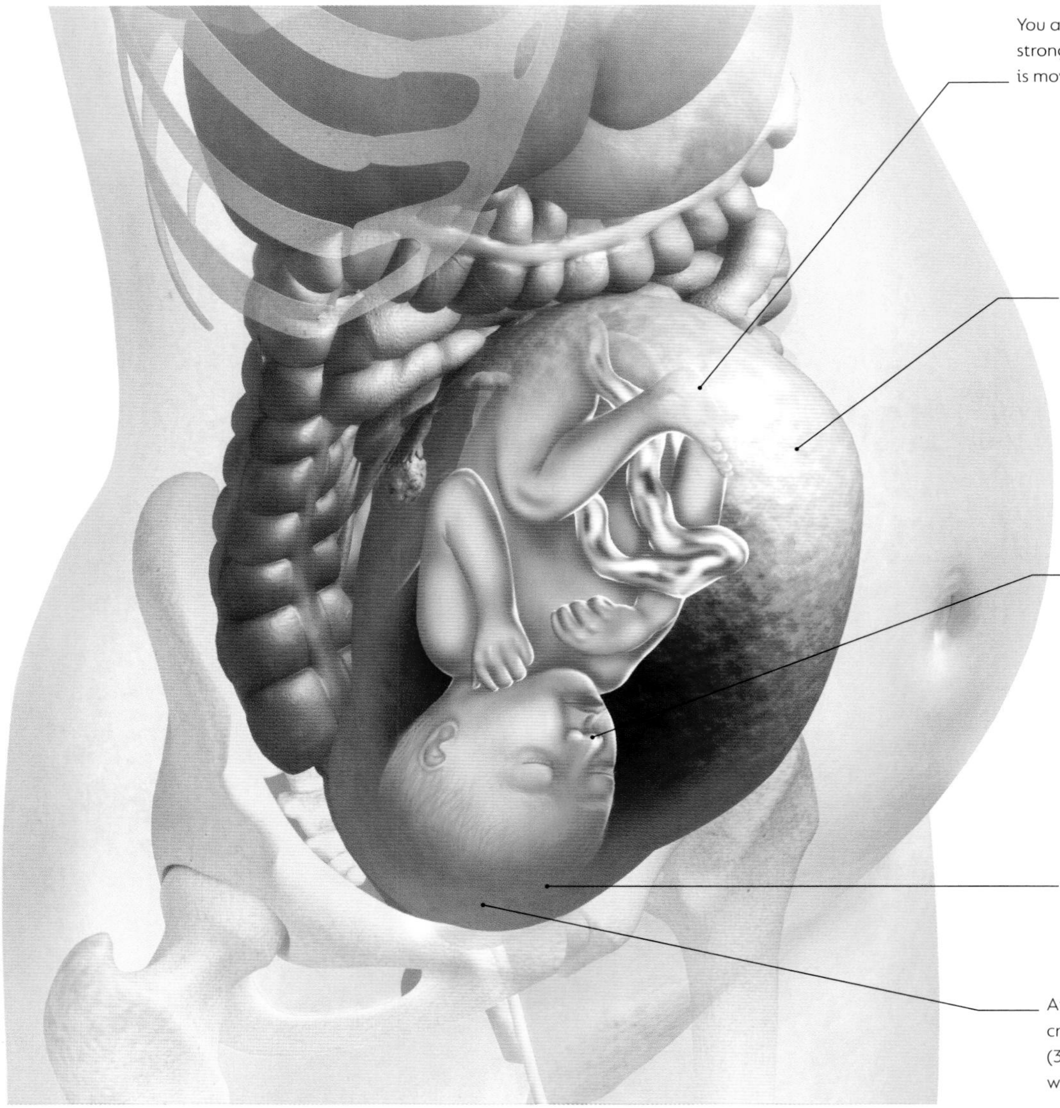
You are still feeling a lot of strong kicks, although the baby is moving around less.
The amniotic sac has finished growing and is no longer forming new cells. Because the membranes of the sac are highly elastic, they keep stretching as the baby gets bigger.
The tip of your baby's nose is still upturned and the bridge is becoming more evident.
In the brain, nerve cells are developing into distinct areas that will eventually control specific functions such as memory and coordinated movement. As yet, the neural network is very immature.
At 30 weeks the average crown to heel length is 15.7 in (39.9 cm) and the average weight is 2.9 lb (1.3 kg).

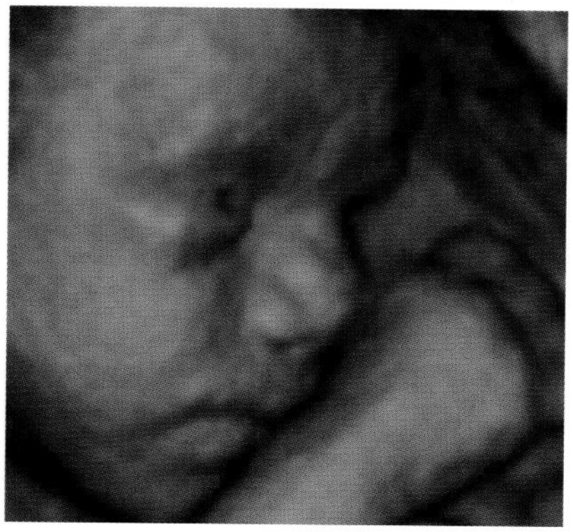

YOU ARE **29 WEEKS AND 1 DAY**

76 days to go

YOUR BABY TODAY

The image shows the eyes are open once more for a brief look around. It's not completely dark within the uterus and the more advanced your pregnancy, the more light can penetrate inside. Your baby will gradually be assimilating this information.

> "Be prepared to spend more time in waiting rooms from now on, as your care providers ask to see you more often."

Remember that your pregnancy is a natural, healthy process. With more regular prenatal appointments, and a lot of time spent sitting in a waiting room at the doctor's office, sometimes surrounded by people with various medical conditions, you may start to feel that you have a medical problem.

At this stage, your blood pressure will return to prepregnancy levels. If it starts trending upward, you may be asked to leave a urine sample, which is checked for protein. If you have difficulty trying to reach around your belly to catch your sample in the tiny cup, don't worry. Only a small amount of urine is needed, so if you can't see anything, just start to urinate and then move the cup underneath the flow to catch some. Urine is sterile (unless you have a UTI) so don't worry about getting some on your hands—just wash them thoroughly afterward.

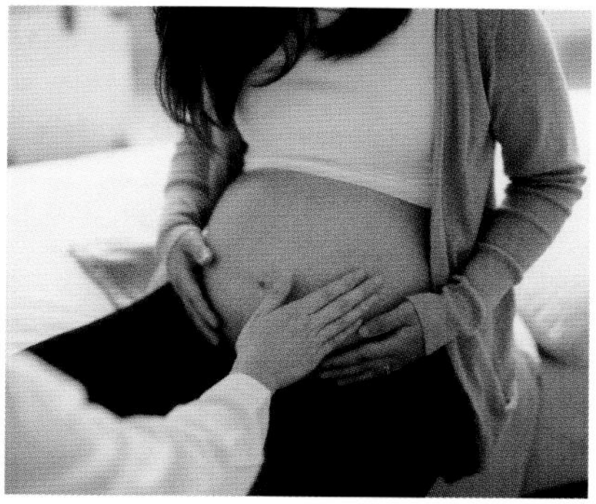

Regular appointments with your doctor take time out of your day, but they offer reassurance that all is well with your baby.

ASK A DOCTOR

We know our baby has Down syndrome. How can we prepare ourselves? Knowing now will give you time to come to terms with the fact that your baby will have Down syndrome. You won't need any special equipment or toys when your baby is born, but you will need emotional support, so turn to the people now who you think will best give you this.

Contact the Down Syndrome Association (see p.482) for information and support, including getting in touch with parents of children with Down syndrome through your local support group.

FREEBIRTHING

Giving birth without medical assistance from a midwife or doctor might seem a little crazy, but a small minority of women believe that so-called freebirthing is the ultimate way to welcome their baby into the world. Some moms-to-be plan an unassisted home birth after having a negative experience during a previous labor; others want their birth to be "natural," "private," and devoid of medical intervention.

- **Freebirthing is not against the law,** but it is radical. The American College of Obstetricians and Gynecologists and the American Medical Association oppose home births because of the potential for complications, even in low-risk pregnancies. Complications such as the baby needing oxygen can and do happen.
- **Some women have an unplanned DIY delivery**—usually because of a short labor—and in these instances the mothers and babies are usually fine. But actually choosing to go it alone is definitely not something that should be considered lightly.

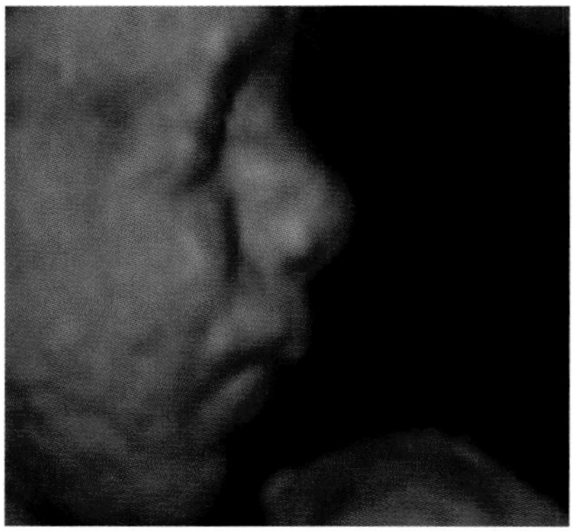

YOU ARE **29 WEEKS AND 2 DAYS**

75 days to go

YOUR BABY TODAY

Now the bridge of the nose is more apparent than earlier in the pregnancy. The tip of the nose can still look slightly upturned at this stage adding to the "button nose" appearance. As the face lengthens, the tip of the nose does move downward slightly.

> "Your baby's nerve cells are developing, but they are still not mature enough for them to feel pain, temperature, or touch."

Electrical activity can be detected in the increasingly convoluted folds of gray matter, the part of your baby's brain that controls the higher functions, such as memory and consciousness, as well as muscle control and sensory perceptions, such as seeing and hearing.

The neurons of the cortex—the outer layer of gray matter—have started to develop into six distinct layers with separate functions, a process that will be completed in about five weeks, although further maturing will be needed. Your baby is born with almost a full complement of neurons, but there is further growth in early childhood.

For nerves to function effectively and signals to pass along them faster, they need insulating. In a process known as myelination, the nerves are insulated with myelin sheaths of fat. Although all of the components of the nervous system are present from an early stage of development, the peripheral sensory and motor nerves, spinal cord, and brain need the entire pregnancy to develop and function as a unit.

The nerves of the brain and spinal cord carry the sensations of pain, temperature, and touch. However, the process of myelination will not be complete until the final few weeks, so the baby does not recognize pain, temperature, and touch at this stage.

ASK A DOCTOR

The reality of having to give birth is hitting me now! How can I avoid getting too anxious? A little way into your third trimester, the reality of childbirth may sink in. You may be experiencing some pregnancy discomforts, including Braxton Hicks contractions (see p.410), which give an indication of what is to come.

First of all, remember that the calmer and more relaxed you are, the easier your birth will be. Try to use a little positive visualization—your baby coming out easily in a "whoosh" of fluid and contractions being "positive pain" to bring your baby into the world. Remember that your baby will be fine, however long she takes to arrive, and that your pain and discomfort are all controllable. In other words, even if you decide on a natural birth now, you can get help and relief when you need it.

Try to relax and enjoy the last few months of pregnancy. Redirect any anxious thoughts you may have about childbirth and focus instead on welcoming your baby into the world.

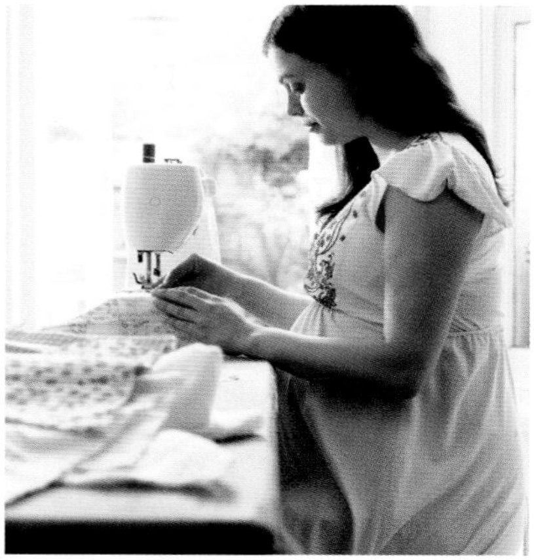

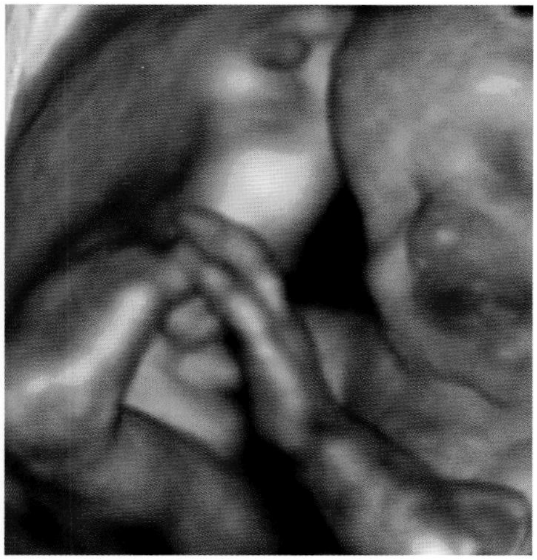

YOU ARE **29 WEEKS AND 3 DAYS**

74 days to go

YOUR BABY TODAY

Your baby often grasps one hand with the other or, as this image shows, grasps a foot. This helps with important sensory feedback to the brain as the nerves within the brain start to mature and become insulated along their length to carry signals more effectively.

It's recommended that your baby sleeps in the same room as you for the first six months, but many parents-to-be still like to prepare the baby's bedroom. This room can still be used for the baby's clothes and any newborn gifts you're given. You might also want to set up feeding and diaper-changing areas in there.

Check out garage sales and online for secondhand baby equipment. This can be a good opportunity to buy some bigger items at a reduced price. If you do buy a secondhand crib, make sure it's certified by the Juvenile Product Manufacturers Association and that the slats are no more than 23/8 in apart. Hand-me down clothes, sheets, and towels also save money. If this isn't your first baby you may find that you have more or less everything you need, except for disposables, such as diapers (unless you are using cloth diapers—see p.291).

Although it's good to be prepared (and sometimes babies do arrive early), remember you won't be trapped in your house forever so you don't need to prepare as if for a siege. If you don't have something you need or you run out, you can always get it after your baby is born.

" Start getting your baby's room ready now, while you still have the energy for shopping and helping with decorating. "

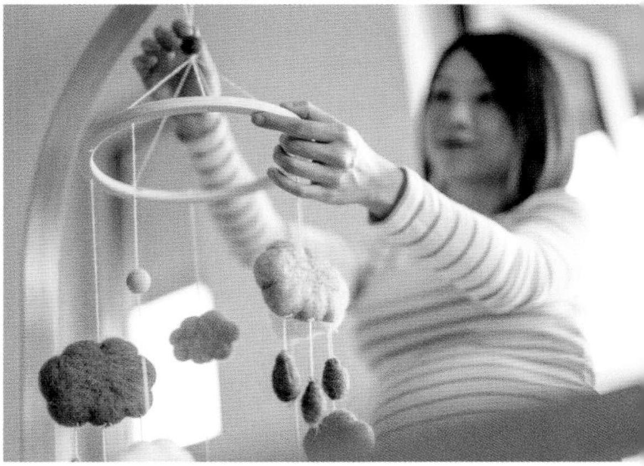

If possible, get the baby's room ready before the birth. It will be one less job to do in the busy first months of parenthood.

ASK A DOCTOR

Do I need a travel system/stroller? Most parents-to-be are unsure about the type of stroller they'll need for their baby and, since there are a number of options and types available, this can make choosing the right item difficult. You will need to buy some type of travel equipment for your baby and what you choose will vary depending on your circumstances.

If you mostly drive a car, you may want to consider a car seat that attaches to a stroller, or a car seat and separate travel crib. If you intend to walk a lot, you may find a lightweight stroller more appropriate than a stroller. Keep in mind how long your baby will be in the stroller: it must be comfortable, have a lie-flat option for the first six months, and adjustable seat options as your baby grows. The stroller must also be weatherproof.

If you do a lot of "around town" travel, you might consider a lightweight option in addition to your main system. It's a good idea to take a look around in stores and online to compare different models and get the best price.

Planning for your birth

As your due date approaches, you may start to think in greater detail about how you would like to manage your labor and birth. Being informed will help you feel more confident about the choices you make.

Your choices for birth

When planning the type of birth experience you would like to have, you'll need to consider a number of factors. One of the most important decisions is where you would like to give birth. You may also want to think about the details of your birth, such as which positions you would like to adopt during the birth, and what type of pain relief you might choose to use (see pp.396–407).

It's important to be flexible. You may have preferences as to the type of birth you want, but accepting that your choice may be limited or advised against because of a preexisting medical problem, or because a problem arises in labor, will help you prepare mentally and curb disappointment if events don't go as planned. It is generally accepted that the care of healthy women in labor who have had a straightforward pregnancy should be monitored and managed by their doctors at the hospital, with support given by the nursing staff throughout the process.

The place of birth Earlier in pregnancy, you'll probably have thought about where you would like to give birth and discussed the options with your doctor. Although you may have already stated a preference, it's important to know that you can review your choice and change your mind toward the end of the pregnancy.

Where you give birth may be influenced by factors such as whether you've had complications in pregnancy, such as gestational diabetes (see p.475) or high blood pressure, that would make a hospital birth preferable. On the other hand, if your pregnancy has been straightforward and you have become more informed about labor and birth over the course of your pregnancy, your confidence may have grown and you may decide to look into a home birth in familiar surroundings, or to investigate midwife-run birthing centers in your area.

An active labor In childbirth classes, you'll learn a range of techniques to help you cope with pain during labor. Most methods center around breathing and relaxation techniques that help you focus during labor and birth and don't inhibit movement. Maintaining mobility and an upright position during labor is thought to help you deal with contractions and to

HOME BIRTH

In the United States, the number of home births rose by 22 percent in 2019–2020 to more than 40,000. Approximately 1.3 percent of all births in the US occur at home. Although having your baby at home can certainly be appealing, it is associated with two times the risk of perinatal death, and three times the risk of neonatal seizures than planned hospital births.

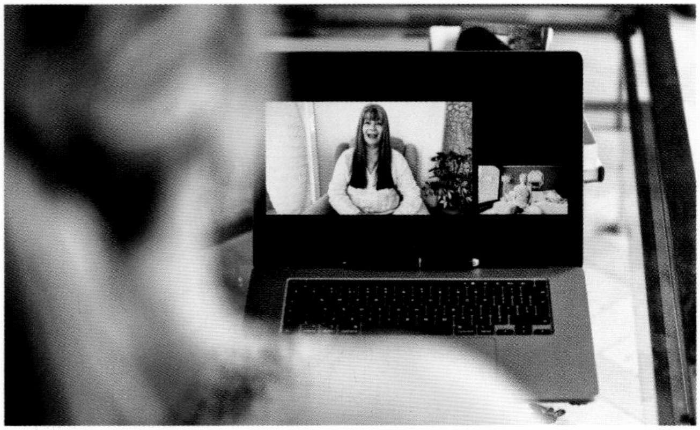

use gravity to help push your baby down the birth canal.

If you want an active birth, this may influence how you feel about the type of pain relief you want to use (see below) and about monitoring in labor. For example, continuous monitoring (see p.418) can limit your movement. If the doctor wants to monitor your labor continuously, talk to them about how you can maintain some mobility; for example, by sitting on a birthing ball, or adopting an all-fours position on the bed or on a mattress on the floor.

Most units now use wireless technology, so you can move around as you wish without being constrained by the wires hooking you up to the machine.

Your pain relief options Factors that may influence the type of pain relief you would like include how active you want to be (see left); what effect different drugs may have on how you experience labor, and how drugs can affect the baby.

Natural methods, such as breathing techniques, laboring in water, and TENS (see p.399), and some medical pain-relief options, such as analgesics (see pp.402–403), allow an active birth because you won't lose all feeling or muscle movement. However, systemic (IV) analgesics cross the placenta and can affect the baby's breathing at birth. Regional anesthetics, such as epidurals (see p.404), limit movement and can mean that you won't feel when you're pushing.

Making a birth plan

Writing your preferences in a birth plan helps consolidate your thoughts and to pass this information to your doctor. A birth plan is useful, too, for your birthing partner, who may need to advocate for you in labor. Birth plans also allow you to state any special needs, such as the help you will need if you have a disability.

Try to make your birth plan straightforward and accessible. Working with your caregivers as a team will help you feel involved in decision making, whatever the outcome.

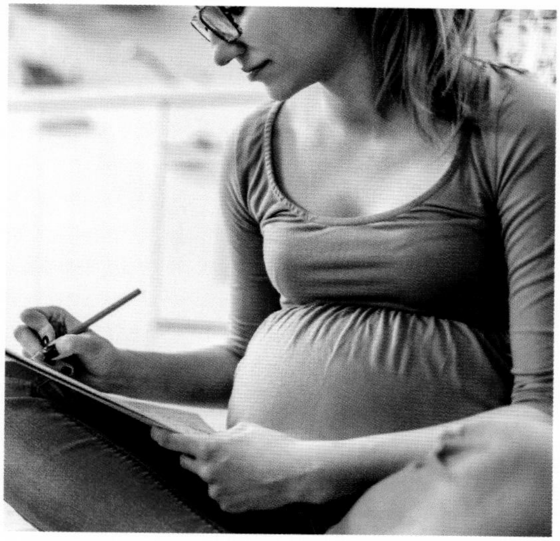

Focusing on your birth preferences helps you to consider your options and feel mentally prepared for labor.

QUESTIONS TO CONSIDER

When planning where and how you ideally want to give birth, you need to consider both what you would prefer and what the hospital or birthing centers can offer. The following questions may act as helpful prompts.

Questions to ask yourself

- Who would you like to have with you during the labor and birth?
- Do you want an active labor?
- What pain relief do you want?
- If you have an assisted birth, would you prefer vacuum or forceps?
- Do you want your partner to be present if you have a cesarean?
- Do you want the third stage of labor to be managed naturally or assisted with drugs?
- How do you want to feed your baby?

Questions to ask the hospital

- What is the policy on induction? Will the hospital monitor your baby before labor if you don't want to be induced?
- Will the choice of pain relief and the place of birth change if you're induced?
- Are there tubs or birthing pool facilities?
- Will you be able to bring in aids such as massage oils or music?
- How much privacy will you have?
- How many people will you be allowed to invite into your labor and delivery room?
- Will your baby remain with you throughout your stay in the hospital?
- Does the hospital have facilities for sick babies, or are babies transferred?
- Can you go home when you feel ready, or is there a set discharge time?

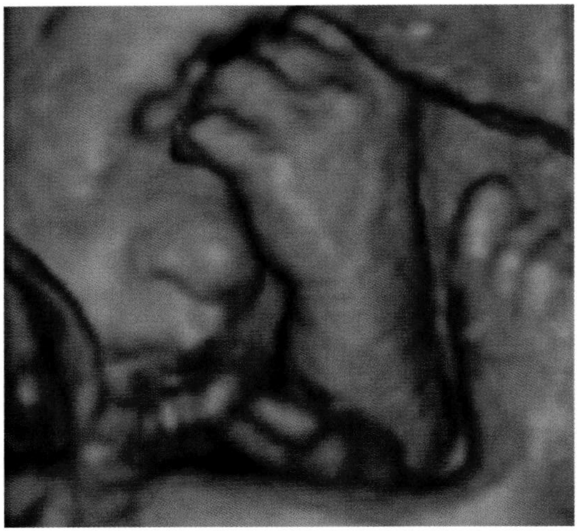

YOU ARE **29 WEEKS AND 4 DAYS**

73 days to go

YOUR BABY TODAY

In this image a hand is held up to the forehead and, to the right, part of a foot can be seen. The groove between the nose and the upper lip is visible and the nose has the characteristic "button" shape. It looks cramped in there but there is still room to move.

"Your baby is cushioned in a sac of amniotic fluid, which surrounds them until your water breaks and you go into labor."

As your uterus has enlarged throughout your pregnancy, the amniotic sac has expanded to accommodate both your baby and the amniotic fluid. From now on, however, the sac will grow by simply stretching rather than forming new cells.

The amniotic sac is formed from two distinct layers or membranes, an inner "amnion" and outer "chorion." The chorion originally had a blood supply of its own, but this has now been lost. The thinner amnion is able to slide over the chorion as your baby pushes against it. Neither layer contains nerve cells: this explains why it's not painful when your membranes rupture or "water breaks." Combined, the layers are only 0.5 mm thick. Collagen fibers in each layer allow for a great deal of stretch—this is vital in these final months to avoid early rupture of the membranes. Indeed, the membranes may be so resistant to rupture that they don't break until the final stages of your labor (see p.411).

In addition to holding in the amniotic fluid and providing a barrier to possible infection through the cervix, the membranes contain substances that form prostaglandins. Prostaglandins play an important part in the initiation of labor. This is one of the reasons why labor often starts when the membranes have ruptured.

THE SEX OF THE BABY

There is no test that will guarantee the sex of your baby, unless you are having an amniocentesis or CVS for some other reason (see pp.152–3).. An ultrasound scan can get it wrong, and, despite the old belief, the size and shape of your belly are not good indicators of the gender. The new NIPT (see p.142) is the best noninvasive way to determine the sex.

FOCUS ON PARTNERS

By now, it's possible to see and feel your baby moving, often with kicks and punches. This may happen more often in the evenings, when your partner finally gets to sit down and relax. Watching your baby's movements can be a great way to bond with them, and with your partner.

Your baby will respond to your voice, to music, and may even jump at unexpected noises (see p.256); it's impossible to say whether this is because these noises are enjoyed or because they're irritating.

Your baby will also hiccup sometimes (see p.204) and you have a better chance of feeling them moving while they are hiccuping than during any other form of movement. This is because hiccups occur over prolonged periods of time, while kicks and punches can be fairly random.

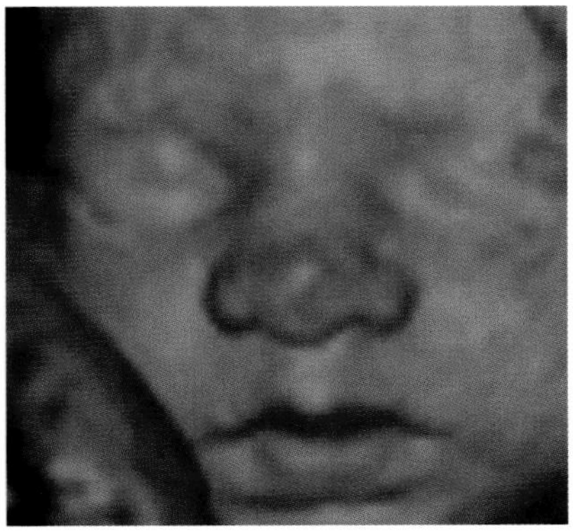

YOU ARE **29 WEEKS AND 5 DAYS**

72 days to go

YOUR BABY TODAY

The lip shape and groove between the nose and upper lip are particularly well shown here. If you or your partner has a prominent groove, or philtrum, above the upper lip, your baby may too, or may inherit characteristics that are somewhere in between.

The size of your hips is not always a good indication of the size of your pelvis, so having narrow hips doesn't mean you'll have a difficult birth, and having larger "child-bearing" hips doesn't mean you'll have an easy birth.

Your baby's growth and development is determined genetically, although women do have an extra influence on the size of their babies while they are in the uterus. So, even if your child ends up being tall, if you're small you'll limit how big they develop in utero. If you're small, you may not be able to deliver a hefty baby, so your body limits the baby's size at delivery. Your baby will then catch up on their expected growth after the birth.

There's a condition called cephalo-pelvic disproportion in which the baby is too big or the pelvis is too small for the baby to engage. You'll only know for sure whether your baby will pass through the birth canal when you're in labor.

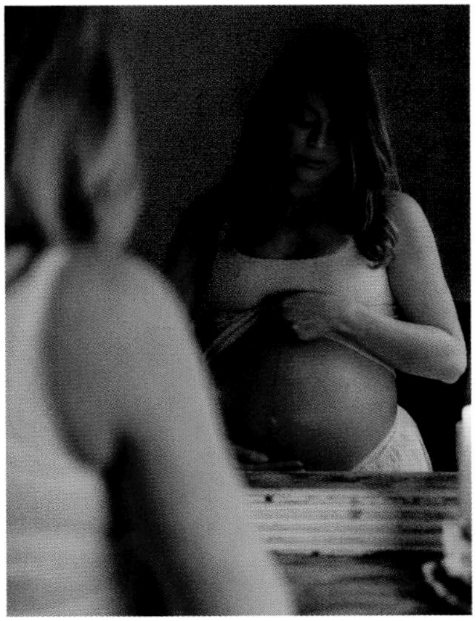

As you marvel at the size of your belly, you may be concerned about how you'll ever deliver your baby. But don't worry—nature is on your side.

> " Regardless of your size—and your baby's—nature won't let them grow too large for you to be able to give birth. "

ASK A DOCTOR

What will happen when I go for a gestational diabetes screening? You'll be given a very sugary drink and asked to wait for an hour, after which your blood will be tested. If your levels are high, you'll have to take a glucose tolerance test, which is similar, but longer. If you do have gestational diabetes, you will be taught how to test your blood sugar at home. You'll likely be able to control your condition with diet and exercise.

It's reassuring to know that most women who have sugar in their urine have normal blood-sugar levels in the glucose test.

PLANNING AHEAD

There will not be as much time for household chores once the baby is born. If you don't like living in a mess, act now to prevent resentment (and the laundry) from building up in a few months' time.

- Talk to your partner now about how you're going to split the chores once you have a newborn.
- Your "job" will be to nurture your baby, so you'll need domestic backup, if possible, particularly during the first few weeks. Recruit helpers (family and friends; or pay professionals if needed). Delegate so that you won't have to think about shopping, cooking, or cleaning.
- New parents need their own space, so it's never too early to arrange for some babysitters for a few weeks after the birth. If you're breastfeeding, you'll need to express your milk.

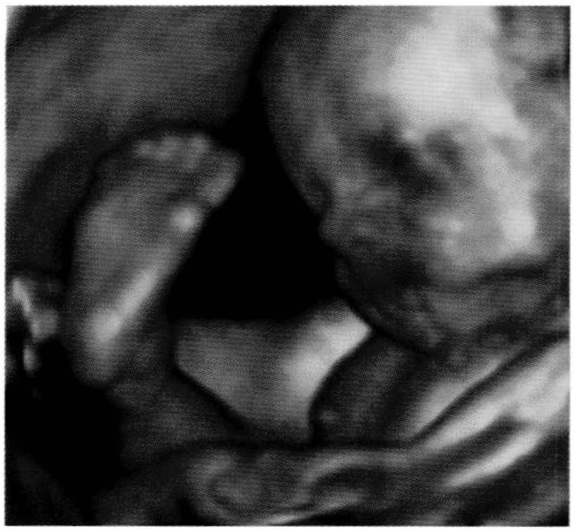

YOU ARE **29 WEEKS AND 6 DAYS**

71 days to go

YOUR BABY TODAY

Increasingly sounds enter the uterus and your baby will respond to some of the loudest. The fluid all around them can have quite an effect on the sounds that they can hear—the effect is similar to how you might feel when you swim with your head under water.

> “Your maximum blood volume won’t be reached for a few weeks yet, but your circulation is working harder than ever at this stage.”

Your blood volume is likely to be nearly a gallon and a half between weeks 25 and 35—an increase of about 25 percent. This increased blood volume means that your heart is pumping harder and faster. Your blood vessels are as relaxed as they can be by this stage of pregnancy, and will not stretch any further to accommodate this extra blood flow. You may notice that you sweat more, and that your skin feels hotter (this gives a rosy glow to some women). In addition to this extra blood, there is also a lot more fluid circulating around your body, which can cause you to feel swollen.

It’s common and normal for your face, fingers, and ankles to be puffy or swollen (see pp.468–469). However, since puffiness is also a sign of preeclampsia (see p.476), it’s important to have your doctor to check this out.

ASK A DOCTOR

I’ve noticed that I get short of breath very easily. Should I be concerned? No, when you’re pregnant, your lungs have to work much harder to meet your body’s increased oxygen needs. To help you take in more air, your ribs spread sideways and your lung capacity increases dramatically. This can make you feel short of breath, particularly from midpregnancy.

In the third trimester, most women find they get breathless even during mild exertion, which happens as the expanding uterus pushes up against the lungs. However, being breathless can also be a sign of anemia (see p.474), which may need to be treated. Your breathing may start to get easier when your baby engages (moves down into your pelvis ready to be born, see p.361).

FOCUS ON TWINS

If you’re pregnant with twins, it’s recommended that you don’t do any vigorous or aerobic exercise in the third trimester. The last three months are particularly tiring so you probably won’t feel up to doing much anyway. You’ll also get bigger sooner than someone who is having a single baby, and your size may preclude you from doing certain activities.

If you do want to be active, go for a gentle walk or swim, or to a pregnancy yoga or Pilates class. If you want to do any exercise in the third trimester, check with your doctor first.

Your doctor will be monitoring your babies’ progress and she may advise you on your level of activity if there is any slowdown in the babies’ growth and development.

Whatever activity you’re doing, always follow the guidelines for safe exercising (see p.18).

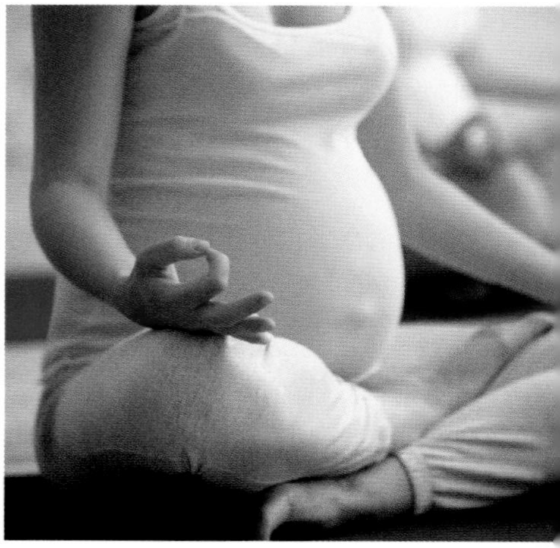

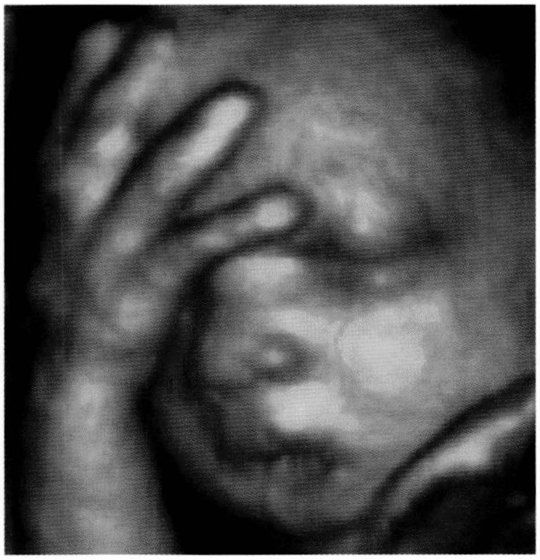

YOU ARE **30 WEEKS EXACTLY**

70 days to go

YOUR BABY TODAY

Does your baby start to feel tired? Certainly on some scans it can look as if they are. In fact, your baby actually spends most of the time in a state of sleep rather than full wakefulness: it seems that during pregnancy your baby does need to spend most of the time asleep.

Later on in the third trimester you may begin to feel more tired than usual. The strain on your body may begin to show itself—you may find yourself uncomfortable and easily fatigued. Things that never bothered you previously, such as standing for long periods of time or walking a lot, may get increasingly difficult. For example, your trip to and from work may tire you much more than it did previously. If that is the case, find out whether you can alter your hours to avoid traveling at the busiest times of the day and, if you find yourself traveling during rush hours, don't be shy about asking someone to give up their seat on the train for you. If there is a room in which you can rest at work, you may be able to take a short nap in the middle of the day or early afternoon, which might help to alleviate your fatigue a little.

You may want to discuss with your employer ways to make your job less physically demanding, or ask for help, for example if you need to carry heavy files or your job involves walking long distances. With a few adjustments you should be able to keep going until the start of your maternity leave, but above all, listen to your body: if you're tired, rest; if your feet and legs hurt, sit down.

“ You probably won't want to stop working just yet, but you may need to make some adjustments if you're feeling very tired. ”

USING A BIRTHING POOL

Laboring and giving birth in water can induce relaxation and reduce blood pressure. Research shows that warm water on the lower back (the area of the spinal cord that receives the nerves from the lower abdominal region) can reduce labor pain, while the level of endorphins, or natural painkillers, rises in the same environment.

Although it can be beneficial to labor in water, there is no known benefit to water births and there is an increased risk of infection for your baby. Due to these risks, it is not recommended that you deliver in the tub or pool. You should speak with your doctor about the use of water in your birth plan so that you can make an informed decision, especially if your pregnancy is considered high risk.

FOCUS ON TWINS

You're more likely to deliver twins by Cesarean. Many of these are schedule, meaning the decision is made in advance, and the mother doesn't go into labor. It is a major surgery, but for the babies it's often the best way to arrive and the small risk for the mother is worth the benefit..

A vaginal birth can be complicated for twins, especially for the second twin, who may develop complications after the birth of the first twin and require urgent delivery.

Your 31st week

EVEN IF YOU HAVE A BIRTH PLAN IN MIND, BE PREPARED TO BE FLEXIBLE. You may have firm thoughts about what you consider to be the ideal birth experience. However, keep an open mind because many factors can influence where and how your baby is born. There's nothing unusual in a woman changing her mind, even after her labor has actually started. Your health-care team will expect you to ask a lot of questions about childbirth, so take advantage of their experience and expertise.

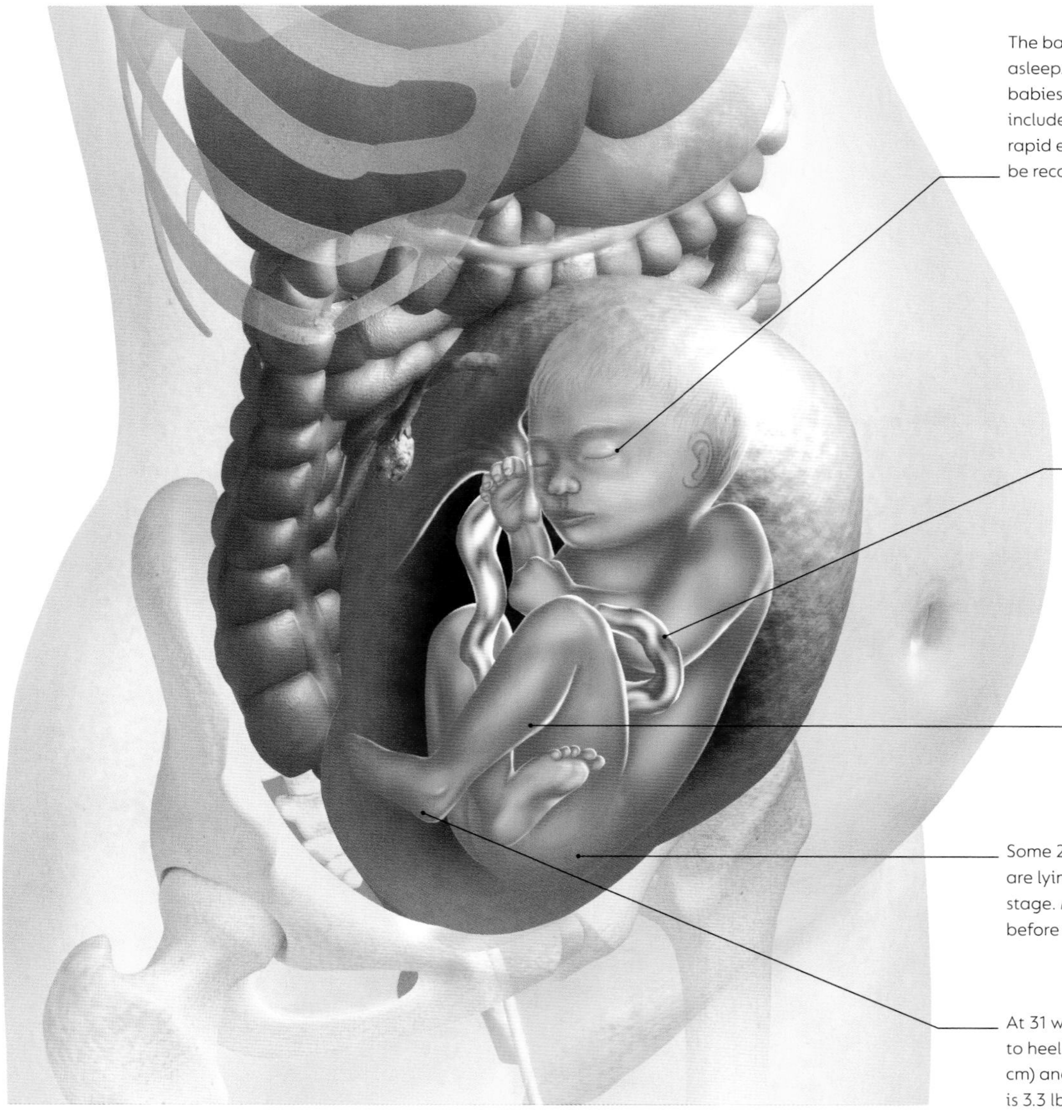

The baby spends much of his time asleep. Like children and adults, babies have a sleep pattern that includes a "dreaming" stage, when rapid eye movements (REM) can be recorded.

The blood in the umbilical cord contains stem cells, which have the ability to develop into specific body cells such as those forming blood, or brain, or muscle tissues.

The legs may be crossed or even curled up on top of the head at times but there is still space for them to be stretched out fully.

Some 25 percent of babies are lying bottom first at this stage. Most of them turn before the end of pregnancy.

At 31 weeks the average crown to heel length is 16.2 in (41.1 cm) and the average weight is 3.3 lb (1.5 kg).

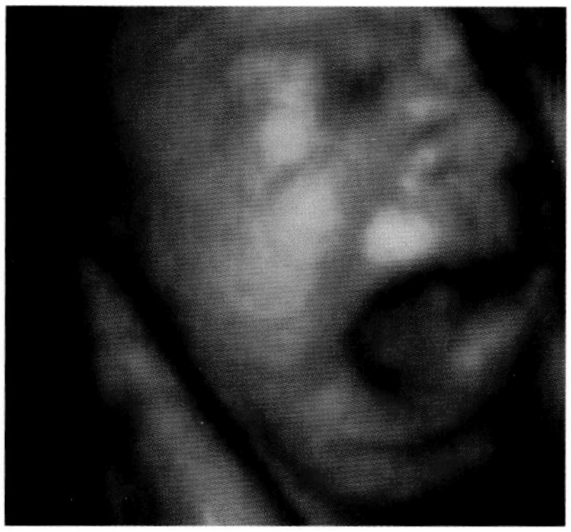

YOU ARE **30 WEEKS AND 1 DAY**

69 days to go

YOUR BABY TODAY

From this point in the pregnancy your baby will yawn just as often as during the first few weeks after birth. Exactly why babies yawn before birth remains unknown, but seeing your baby yawn on a scan is quite likely to make you yawn as well.

“It’s well worth giving some thought to where your baby is going to sleep before you actually bring them home from the hospital.”

SHOULD YOU CO-SLEEP?

You may want to put your baby into your bed with you, and yet you may be concerned that you might roll over on them. For this reason, the American Academy of Pediatrics does not recommend co-sleeping. It can be especially dangerous if either of you smoke or use alcohol or drugs that make it hard to wake up, or if you sleep with the baby on a waterbed, couch, or in a chair. The safest place for your baby is in a bassinet near your bed.

It’s recommended that your baby sleeps in a crib in your bedroom for the first six months. See the box, below left, if you’re considering co-sleeping. With your baby in your bedroom, you’ll be close by when they cry at night and able to attend to them easily. This is especially useful if you’re breastfeeding your baby.

Remember that babies are not necessarily quiet sleepers: they may wiggle, grunt, and move around and these noises may disturb you or your partner. If your partner has to go to work the following day, this extra disturbance may affect them. It will affect you, too, but you may have a chance to “catch up” on some sleep, or at least rest, when your baby naps. You should do what is best for your family, even if that means your partner spends some nights in the spare room. Some parents find that they are so exhausted by life with a newborn that they sleep, regardless of whether their baby is snuffling or not.

If the baby is in their own room you may worry that you may not hear them cry, but you will if you use a baby monitor. When they do cry, yet again at 3 a.m., be aware that a short trip along the landing can seem like a mile.

BREAST CHANGES

In the third trimester, your breasts will begin to prepare themselves for feeding your baby, and you may experience some discomfort and changes that you had not anticipated. Your breasts will become fuller, and may actually feel very heavy; your areolas (the area around your nipples) will become darker, and you may feel lumps and bumps in your breasts, as the first milk, colostrum, begins to be produced. This may leak out a little (see p.295).

The small glands on the surface of your areolas (known as Montgomery’s tubercles) will also become raised bumps. You may have darkened veins along your breasts, due to their increased blood supply. Your breasts may also feel more tender and sensitive than usual, especially if touched.

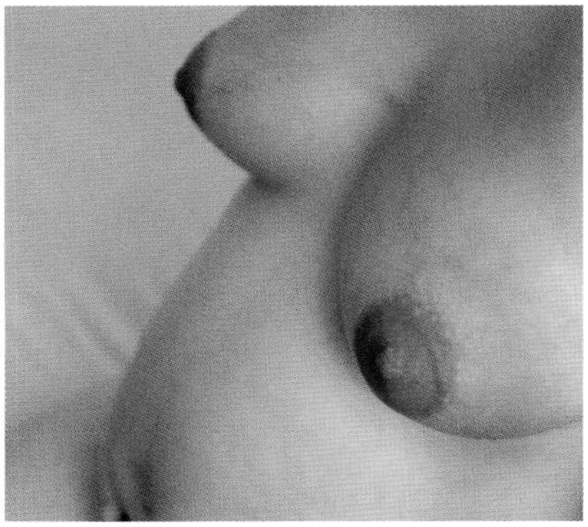

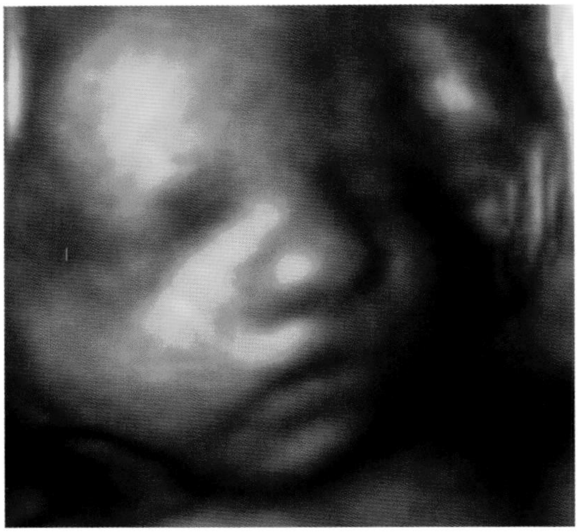

YOU ARE **30 WEEKS AND 2 DAYS**

68 days to go

YOUR BABY TODAY

You will be aware of times when your baby is especially active and times when they are more quiet. There is still a lot of space for your baby to move within the uterus but it is likely that there will be a favorite spot that receives more kicks than any other.

> "Your baby has now developed a clear rhythm of sleeping and waking that may mimic your own or be personal to them."

Exactly when and how your baby develops a cycle of sleeping and waking before birth remains a bit of a mystery. It's not known whether your own rhythms influence your baby's sleep–wake cycle or whether your baby develops his own internal clock. Indeed, such a clock might be triggered in response to the small amount of light that is able to penetrate through the uterus during the last few weeks of pregnancy. It's apparent from brain scans, however, that by this stage of pregnancy, your baby does have very separate periods of activity.

There is a clear cycle, alternating between periods of quiet rest, sleep with rapid eye movements (REM), wakefulness with activity but no eye movement, and wakefulness with lots of activity and eye movements. During this sleep–wake cycle, the baby's actions become more coordinated as periods of activity are linked to rhythmical breathing and increased heart rate, and eye movements.

By this stage of your pregnancy, electrical activity in your baby's brain shows patterns reflecting periods of sleep or wakefulness. An EEG of your baby's brain would show that the quietest period, deep sleep, takes up almost half of the time. The next most common state is REM sleep (the sleep stage during which children and adults dream). This is a time of great electrical activity within your baby's brain. During REM sleep the baby may be quiet or making lots of movements, so it's not possible to tell whether your baby is truly awake at this time or if they're dreaming. Paradoxically, the least electrical activity happens when your baby is most awake—in fact, less than 10 percent of your baby's time is spent truly awake at this stage.

STEM CELL COLLECTION

The blood in your baby's umbilical cord contains "cord blood," which is rich in stem cells. These cells are the building blocks of organ tissue, blood, and the immune system. Some parents save these cells and store them (in a private facility at a cost) in the event that their child or another family member needs their healing benefits.

Studies have found that they are very effective in the treatment of more than 70 diseases, including juvenile arthritis, cancers, heart disease, and brain injury.

However, recent studies have demonstrated that the chances of the blood being used are 1:5,000 to 1:20,000, and it is very expensive to store. Consider, instead, donating the cord blood to a public cord blood bank. Donated blood is used to treat patients who need it the most.

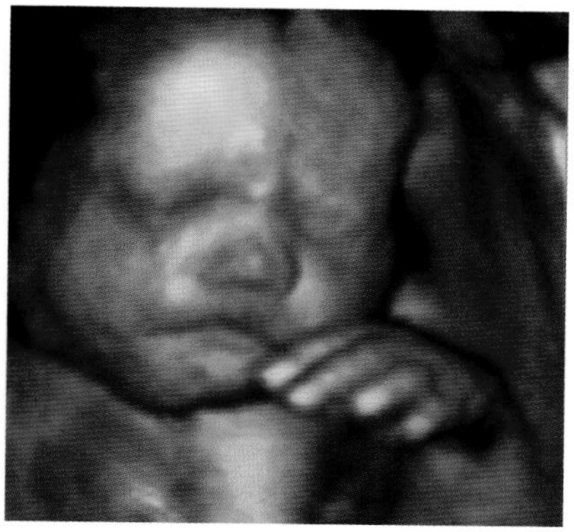

YOU ARE **30 WEEKS AND 3 DAYS**

67 days to go

YOUR BABY TODAY

It can come as quite a surprise to see that your baby will be increasingly making all sorts of expressions. Here the baby had their mouth turned down but the next minute will be yawning, grimacing, or peacefully sleeping.

Giving birth naturally is for some reason perceived as the "best" way, and to do otherwise means that you somehow "failed." This pressure can cause women to feel guilty or even depressed if they needed pain relief or a Cesarean section, for example.

Pain is experienced differently for everyone and there is no right or wrong way to manage the pain of labor. Be sure you understand all your options for pain management, and be open-minded about what the best option is for you in that moment. Pain is subjective—no one else can feel your pain; if it is too much for you, then ask for help. Your options (see pp.402–407) will be explained to you by the doctor.

Childbirth is hard work, but the experience should not be so painful that it scars you. Being pain-free may mean that you have a more enjoyable, even empowering, labor experience. If you do decide you want pain relief, an epidural is the most common option—more than half of women having a baby in a hospital receive one.

> "Natural birth has many advocates, but the best birth is one that delivers your baby safely with minimum trauma for both of you."

ASK A PANEL

I want a natural birth, but everyone says I'll change my mind once I'm in labor. Are they right?

Mom: Nothing can prepare you for the pain of labor, and I found my carefully laid plans were unrealistic and impractical when the pain kicked in. No matter how well prepared you are, you may change your mind during labor, and it's worth being prepared for that. I did feel a bit disappointed that I couldn't manage without pain relief. It helps if you focus on what's important—delivering a healthy baby. If you achieve this aim, you've succeeded, no matter what happens along the way. I would say to stick it out for as long as you can, but you'll be doing yourself and your baby no favors if you both become exhausted and distressed.

Doctor: Many women are shocked by the intensity of the birth experience, and soon forget about their idealistic birth plan. It's better for all involved that you allow for contingency plans during labor, and keep an open mind. Pain relief (see pp.396–407) and interventions are designed to make the experience better for you and your baby, and will not be offered unless they're necessary, or you feel that you can't do without them.

A mom who has her pain who has her pain under control will find that the delivery is much quicker, and she'll have much more energy for her new arrival.

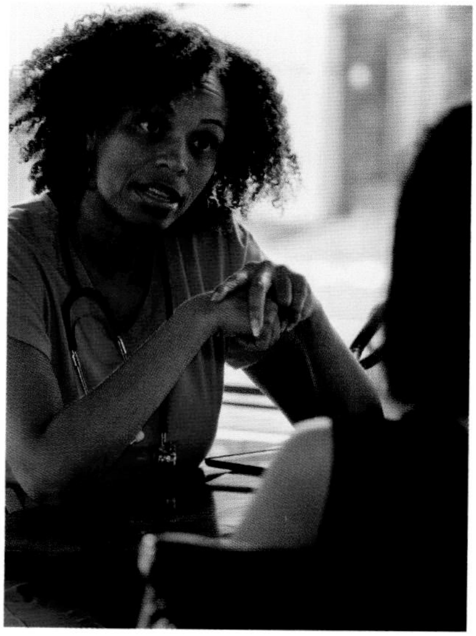

Twins

Just a few weeks to go. By now, you're probably quite large and, of course, excited at the imminent arrival of your twins, or more. However, you may also be concerned about how you will manage during and after the birth.

Getting ready for the birth

Although multiple pregnancies and births are more likely to have complications, they are now safer than ever as advances in prenatal and postpartum care have dramatically improved the outlook for premature babies—the main concern with multiples (see below).

You can prepare for the birth by getting plenty of rest. Putting your feet up, or even taking a nap during the day, helps improve the blood flow to the placenta, which in turn helps your babies grow. Practicing Kegel exercises (see p.69) is important with a multiple pregnancy since your pelvic floor muscles are under additional strain.

A shorter pregnancy Twins or more usually arrive earlier than singletons. Space in the uterus is one factor. As a result, the average length of pregnancy is shorter; for twins, 36–37 weeks is considered typical; for triplets, the average pregnancy is 33 weeks; and for quadruplets, pregnancy lasts about 30 weeks. The average birth weight for each twin is 5 lb 8 oz (2.5 kg) at full term.

You may deliver even earlier than this, since nearly 50 percent of twins are born prematurely. However, nowadays expert care for premature babies means that about 75 percent of babies weighing 3 lb 5 oz at birth, and 57 percent of babies weighing 2 lb 3 oz at birth, survive.

BONDING WITH TWINS

Often, expectant moms of twins or more worry about how they will bond with more than one baby. It's true that bonding can be harder with twins, and even more so with higher multiples. After all, it's hard to fall in love with more than one person at a time, especially when you're exhausted caring for two babies or more. Being aware of this and arranging extra help for after the birth may ease your anxiety. Also, accept additional offers of help that allow you to rest or spend time with one twin. If someone offers to take the twins out, you might consider one twin going and the other spending time with you.

Even if your twins are identical they're unique individuals, and relating to them as such will help their development and your relationship with them. Even in pregnancy, some expectant moms notice how different their babies are from their different movement patterns in the womb.

HOW YOUR BABIES LIE IN THE UTERUS

In the final weeks, your babies will take up their positions for the birth. The most common is both babies lying vertically. With 75 percent of twins, the first is head down (cephalic); the second twin may be head down or breech, or one twin may lie across the uterus (transverse). You may suspect their position from the kicks, but only a scan confirms this.

A cesarean will be recommended if you have triplets or more, or your first twin is breech or transverse (25 percent of cases). A vaginal delivery is most likely if both twins are head down. If the first is head down and the second is transverse or breech, discuss the options for delivery with your obstetrician.

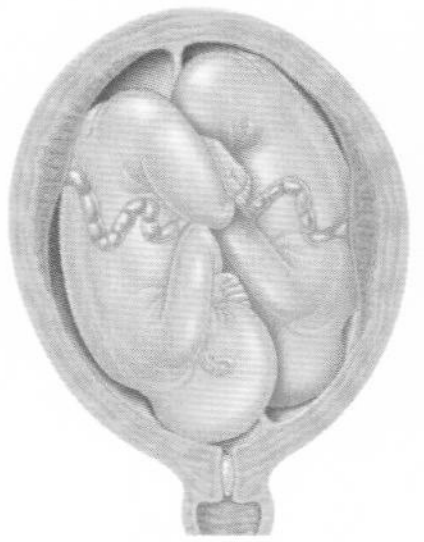

Both babies head down (cephalic)

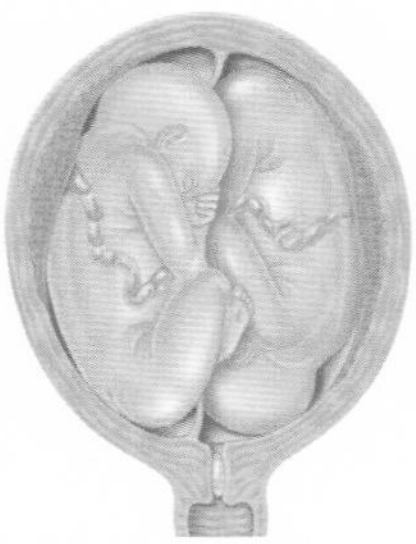

One baby head down, and one breech

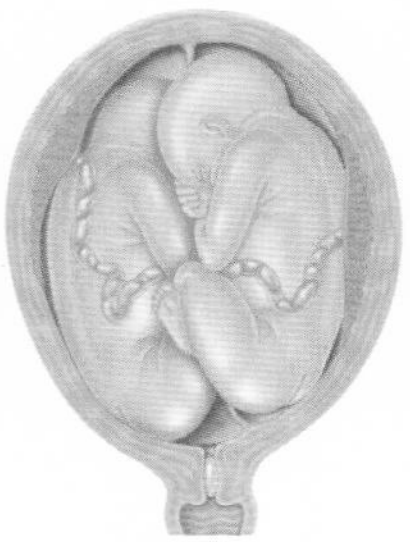

Both babies in a breech position

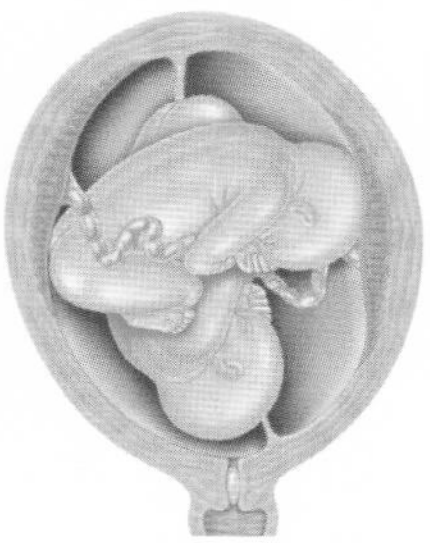

One baby head down and one transverse

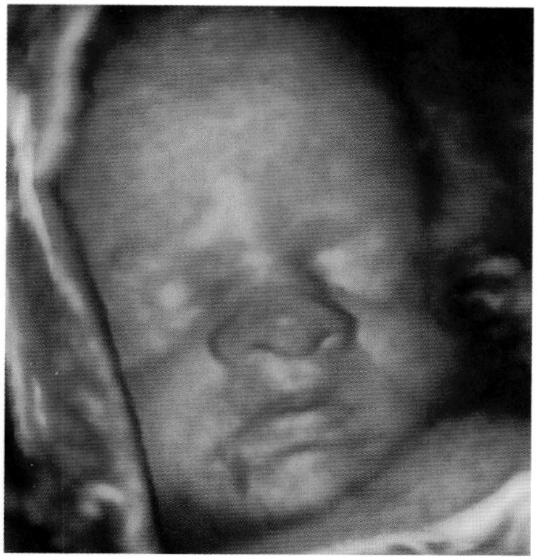

YOU ARE **30 WEEKS AND 4 DAYS**

66 days to go

YOUR BABY TODAY

In this 3-D scan, the baby's arm is held up next to the face. This type of scan shows external features but also looks inside the baby in 3-D so you may see some parts of your baby "through" an arm or leg. Here, the baby's ear can be seen through the arm.

> " In the uterus and in the first months of their life, your baby relies on your immunity to various infections. "

If your immune system thought your baby was foreign, it would mount an attack on them. You and your baby are designed so that this does not happen. Your baby does not have the ability to produce antibodies (which would attack you) in the uterus; they rely completely on you to protect them from infection, not only in the uterus but also after birth. Protection after birth is possible because antibodies from your immune system cross over the placenta into your baby's bloodstream, while you're pregnant. If you have immunity to a disease such as measles, mumps, polio, and many other severe infections, your baby will carry your antibodies to these conditions. This so-called passive immunity is lost with time and it is for this reason that, from two months onward, your baby will require a program of immunizations to protect against these and other illnesses.

EXERCISE MYTHS

There have been numerous studies involving women exercising while they're pregnant. The bottom line is that exercise performed effectively and safely, at a moderate intensity and in healthy women, is beneficial to both mother and baby.

In addition to being good for your health and making you feel more energized, exercising will get you into great shape for labor and childbirth, which is, in effect, a workout! Here are the myths:

- **Exercising will harm my baby if I move too much.** Your baby is protected by amniotic fluid and nourished by the placenta. By keeping within safe exercising guidelines (see p.18), and not doing any high-impact sports or activities where you are at risk of falling or injuries, you are not putting your baby at risk.
- **Exercise will use up some of the nutrients my baby needs.** Your baby's growth will be monitored at your regular doctor appointments, so you and your doctor will be able to tell whether your baby is growing at a usual rate. If you are losing weight while exercising during the pregnancy, you may need to increase the number of calories you eat.
- **Doing abdominal exercises will harm the baby.** You can perform exercises to strengthen your core but try to avoid laying flat on your back in the second and third trimesters. The risk of lying on your back is that your uterus and the weight of the baby can put pressure on the vena cava (the large blood vessel that returns blood to your heart), cause your blood pressure to drop, and can compromise oxygen flow to the baby. If you feel dizzy, roll on to your left side, and symptoms should disappear. Always consult your doctor if you're concerned. See p.250 for safe abdominal exercises after the first trimester.

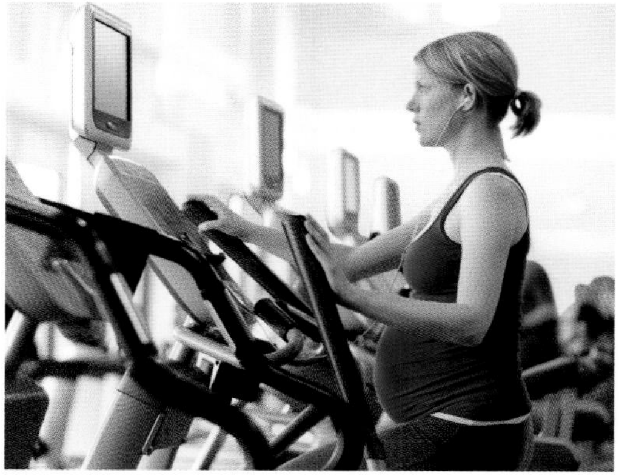

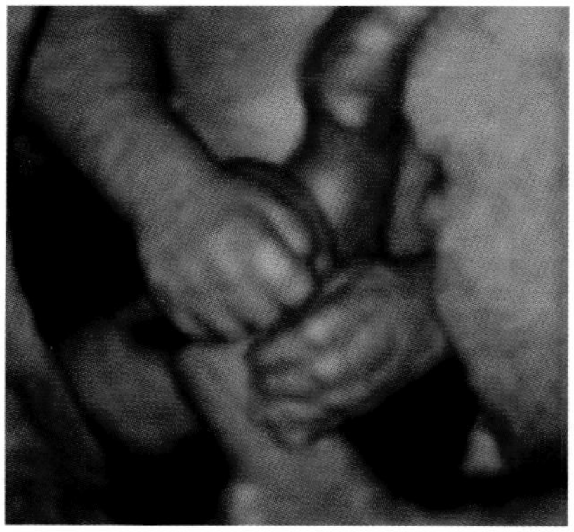

YOU ARE **30 WEEKS AND 5 DAYS**

65 days to go

YOUR BABY TODAY

Here the hands are holding the umbilical cord as it arises from what will become the belly button, or umbilicus. The umbilical coils and its covering of firm, clear jelly protect the cord from kinking and prying fingers.

> "If you want a home birth atmosphere with additional support, consider having your baby in a birthing center."

Birthing centers give moms-to-be a labor experience different than that of a hospital. The emphasis is on a natural birth. They can be attached to a hospital or on a separate site. Some hospitals have a birthing center facility in the maternity unit. Since the majority of women give birth without needing medical intervention, these centers provide a good alternative to a more medicalized hospital environment. The environment in a birthing center tends to be more relaxed and flexible than a hospital environment. You'll have continuous support from a combination of labor nurses and midwives. Your doctor may also be affiliated with a birthing center. Furthermore, the medical team in these centers is very experienced at handling a birth without medical intervention. All of these factors therefore increase your chances of having a straightforward birth. To be give birth in such a center, you need to have had an uncomplicated pregnancy and be unlikely to require specialized medical care or monitoring in labor and birth. If complications did occur, you would be transferred to the closest hospital, although this is rare.

HOME IS WHERE THE HEART IS

The prospect of sleeping in your own bed and being taken care of by people who love you are reason enough to opt for a home birth. It's natural to feel less inhibited at home, and you may be more inclined to move around more and for longer, be as vocal as you like, use gravity, and try different birthing positions, all of which can make labor and delivery shorter and easier. Your midwife will explain what's involved, so seek her advice. On the big day be flexible: you may want to head for the hospital.

ASK A DOCTOR

I'm having a home birth. Can my older children, four and six, be present at the birth? There is nothing more wonderful or miraculous than the birth of a baby, and it's natural to want your older children to be present and witness it for themselves. However, do consider this carefully before you give them the go-ahead. For one thing, even the easiest of labors are painful, and young children will be distressed to see mom in pain. What's more, they may be slightly daunted to see their new sibling emerging from your body, probably covered with various substances. Having said that, many kids handle the experience well if they know what to expect, so outline everything, and explain that any cries, shrieks, or swearing on your behalf are necessary to help get the baby out. You could also mention that you may cry or even vomit, just so they are prepared. Let them know to expect some blood, and that baby will be attached to a (rather gruesome!) cord. If they're squeamish, get them to position themselves by your head, or bring them in immediately after.

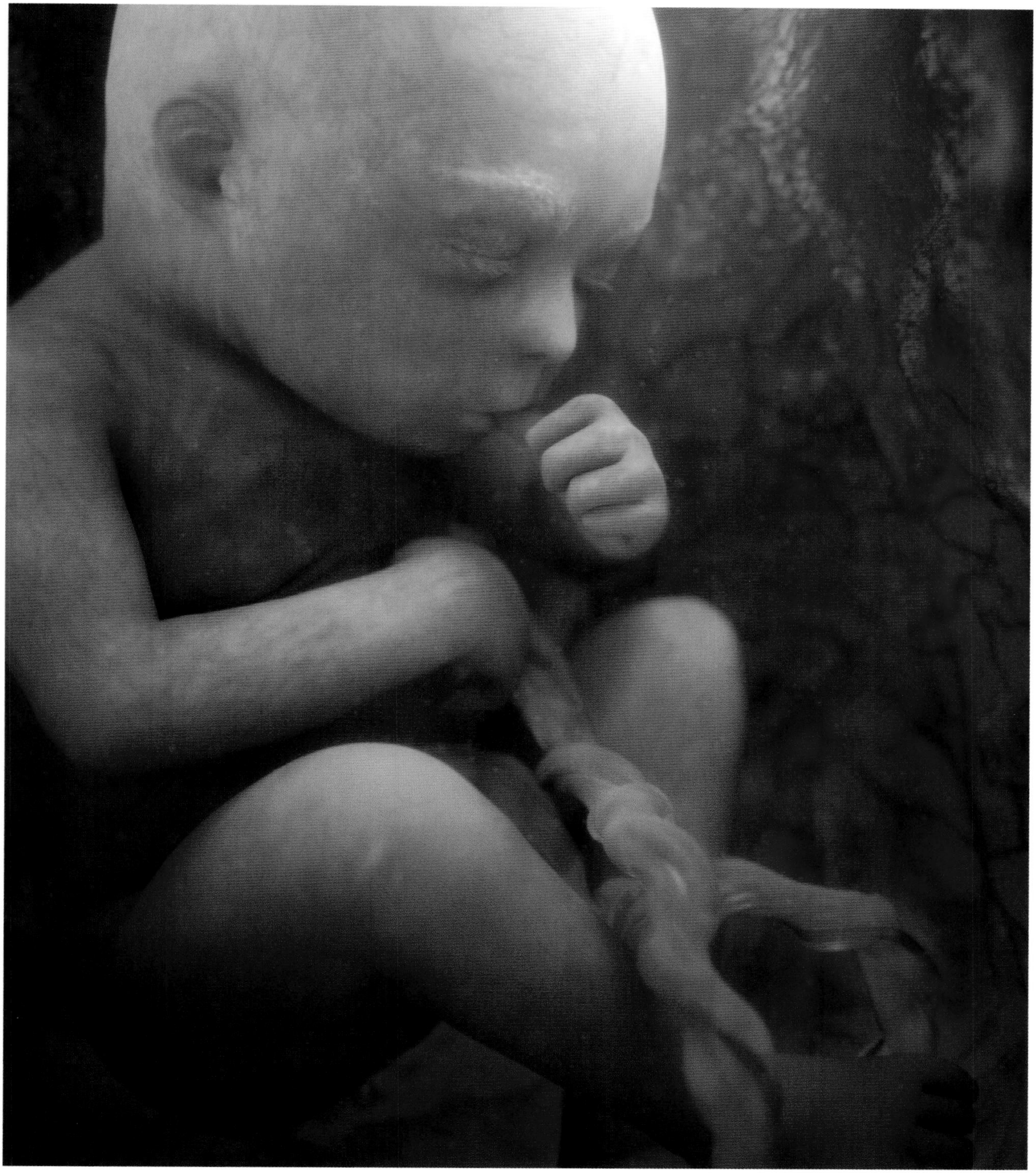

Your baby still has slender arms and legs and little fat under the skin. Their skin is covered with fine lanugo hair and waxy vernix and they now have eyebrows and eyelashes—their first mature hairs.

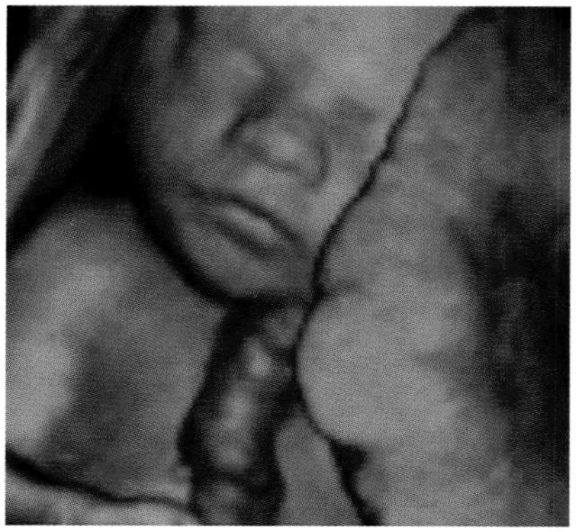

YOU ARE **30 WEEKS AND 6 DAYS**

64 days to go

YOUR BABY TODAY

Here the baby is resting on the placenta, seen at the right-hand side of the image, with the umbilical cord just below the baby's chin. The eyes are closed and this image was taken at a time when the baby was at their quietest, during deep sleep.

" Once your baby's production of red blood cells is in full swing, in theory your immune system could begin to harm your baby. "

At 30 weeks, your baby's red blood cell production switches from the liver to the bone marrow. Their blood type will be determined by your blood group and the baby's father's blood group. Small numbers of the baby's blood cells often leak across the placenta; your body may recognize them as foreign and may attack them.

Your blood group is not important because, although antibodies to blood groups A, B, AB, or O attack your baby's cells in your circulation, they are too large to cross the placenta and attack your baby. Therefore differences in ABO blood groups do not matter. However, everyone is also Rhesus positive (85 percent) or negative (15 percent). If you are Rhesus negative (see p.123) and the father is Rhesus positive, your baby may also be Rhesus positive.

Rhesus negative women produce antibodies to rhesus positive blood cells; these can cross the placenta. Once they do, large numbers of antibodies can attack your baby's blood cells, leading to anemia. First pregnancies are rarely affected. To prevent future pregnancies from being affected, a rhesus negative mother will be given anti-D during the pregnancy and after delivery, if it is confirmed that the baby is rhesus positive. Anti-D mops up fetal cells in the maternal bloodstream, preventing the mother from developing antibodies that could cross the placenta and destroy the baby's red cells, causing anemia.

A GOOD NIGHT'S SLEEP

Insomnia is a common problem during pregnancy and can lead to fatigue, feelings of stress and anxiety, and irritability. Whether it's brought on by your increased size, back pain, heartburn, getting up to empty your bladder, or something else, insomnia is not fun. Taking a warm bath or having a small snack before bed may help, as can relaxation techniques, such as deep breathing. A calming scent in a potpourri or fragrance on your pillow may aid relaxation. Make sure to exercise during the day. If you still can't sleep, get up and do something relaxing: read a book, watch TV, or listen to calming music until you feel sleepy. And try to make up for lost sleep with daytime naps.

AMNIOTIC FLUID

Your baby excretes and reabsorbs about 18 fl oz (0.5 liter) of urine daily, and the amniotic fluid reaches a peak volume of 35 fl oz (1 liter) at 35 weeks. After this time the volume starts to decline and can be as little as 3.5–7 fl oz (100–200 ml) in an overdue pregnancy (see p.393).

Low levels of amniotic fluid, known as oligohydramnios (see p.475), can be a sign of a growth-restricted baby or a baby with kidney problems. Excessive amniotic fluid, known as polyhydramnios (see p.475), may be seen in twin or triplet pregnancies, and is also associated with physical abnormalities in the baby or diabetes in the mother.

At 41 weeks, induction (see p.432) is usually recommended. If you do not want to be induced, you will have an ultrasound to check the amount of fluid around the baby. If the level is low, it is advisable to be induced.

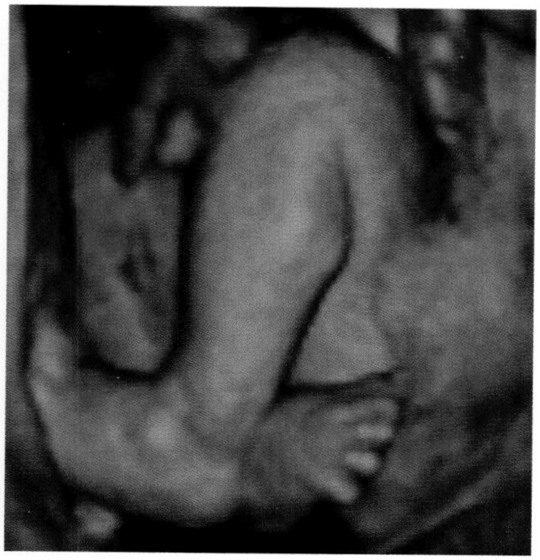

YOU ARE **31 WEEKS EXACTLY**

63 days to go

YOUR BABY TODAY

One leg is shown here crossed over the other. Your baby can still stretch the legs out fully and even curl up in such a way that the feet can rest on top of the head: just because you're kicked on one side doesn't mean that the head will be on the other.

“Epidural is a common form of pain-relief during labor and may be an option for you if you have a low pain threshold.”

Many women have decided that they want a pain-free delivery with an epidural (see pp.404–405) even before they go into labor. It's good to know, however, that labor has to be well established before you can have an epidural, so you'll still experience some painful contractions. Epidurals generally work well, but sometimes the block isn't complete or is more effective on one side than the other. Some women decide to have an epidural because they know they're unlikely to cope well with labor pain. Many women start off saying that they don't want an epidural and change their minds halfway through—if it's your first pregnancy, you can't possibly know how you'll feel.

A scheduled Cesarean (see pp.438–439) is one that is planned and generally performed for medical reasons—for example, because of a low-lying placenta (see p.212).

Some women will choose to give birth by Cesarean without having any medical reasons for surgery, but this is rare. It's important to discuss any concerns you have about your plan for delivery with your obstetrician.

TOCOPHOBIA

This condition is an intense fear or dread of childbirth. There are two types: primary tocophobia predates pregnancy and can start as early as adolescence; secondary tocophobia is associated with an earlier traumatic experience in childbirth. This fear can manifest itself as nightmares, intense anxiety, or panic attacks.

If you have tocophobia, your doctor will refer you to a consultant obstetrician who deals in mental health issues, or you may be referred directly to a psychologist to discuss your fears. Some experts believe that hypnotherapy can help to tackle any subconscious fears of childbirth. An elective cesarean (see pp.438–9) may be recommended if your fear of having a vaginal birth cannot be overcome.

HAVING SEX IN LATE PREGNANCY

You may need to experiment to find lovemaking positions that are comfortable. Most women find that the missionary position becomes increasingly uncomfortable as your partner presses on your belly. You may find being on top is enjoyable and does not put pressure on your belly. Lying in the spoons position, with your partner behind you, can also be pleasurable. Other positions that don't restrict your pleasure and are comfortable include sitting together, kneeling while your partner enters from behind, and lying side by side with your legs entwined.

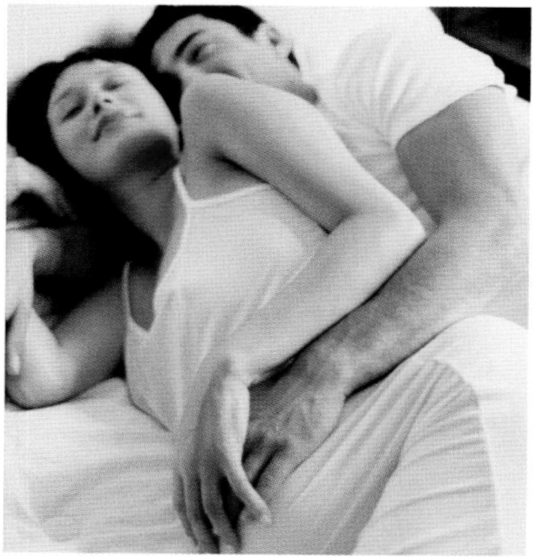

Your 32nd week

YOUR MIDWIFE WILL BE MONITORING YOUR BABY'S POSITION IN THE UTERUS. The baby has not settled into their final birth position just yet, but an assessment of how they're lying will be made at every routine checkup. There's still room in the uterus for your baby to exercise their limbs and they're getting much stronger and more active. You'll know all about it! As your belly gets bigger, it may become more difficult to be very active and to get comfortable when you're sitting or lying down.

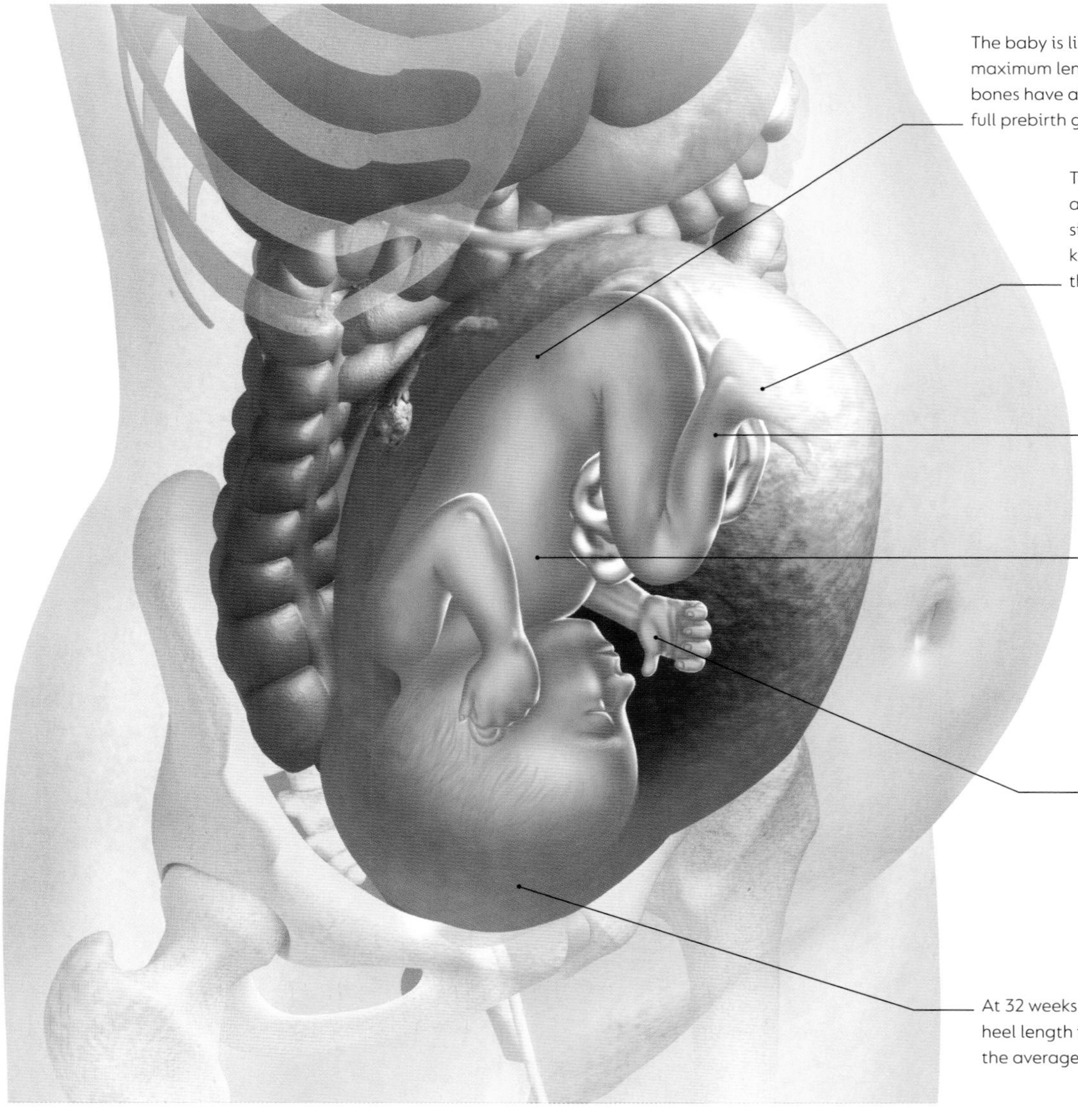

The baby is likely to be near their maximum length now, since their bones have almost reached their full prebirth growth.

The baby's movements are mainly from side to side, and you won't know where to expect the kicks to come from.

The skin starts to look pinker and less translucent.

Increasing layers of fat and muscle are rounding out the baby's body, and she looks a little less skinny.

Creases can be seen in the skin of the wrists and the palms of the hands.

At 32 weeks the average crown to heel length is 16.7 in (42.4 cm) and the average weight is 3.8 lb (1.7 kg).

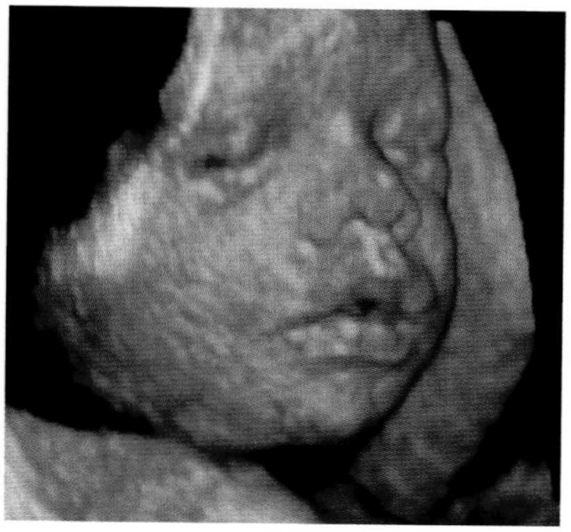

YOU ARE **31 WEEKS AND 1 DAY**

62 days to go

YOUR BABY TODAY

The amount of amniotic fluid reaches its maximum over the next two weeks but will then start to reduce gradually. Measurements of the four deepest pockets of amniotic fluid can add up to 6–8 in (15–20 cm), allowing space for your baby to move.

"If you listen to music while you're pregnant, your baby will be tuning in, too."

You might have noticed that your baby becomes more active when you're listening to music. It's been noted that unborn babies move and even breathe in time to music, and there have been claims that by exposing your baby to certain types of music, you can enhance brain development.

One study, relating to a "Baby Mozart" brain-enhancing product, claimed that the structure of, say, a particular Mozart arrangement, stimulated brain development to a greater extent than other genres, and even other classical composers. This theory has, however, been debunked.

Some research found that college-aged students who listened to classical music showed a brief and temporary improvement in spatial intelligence. However, the same research was not tested in children or babies.

The research has not been repeated and the results are open to several different interpretations.

Whether or not it enhances your baby's intelligence, listening to classical music can relax you, which is always a good thing during pregnancy. And if you gently sway to the music, your baby may enjoy being "rocked" to sleep.

PROTRUDING NAVEL

The pressure of your rapidly expanding uterus presses against your abdomen and can cause your belly button to pop out. A protruding navel is a normal consequence of pregnancy and will usually return to position a few months after the delivery. Like other areas of the body, however, it may not ever look exactly the same as it did before!

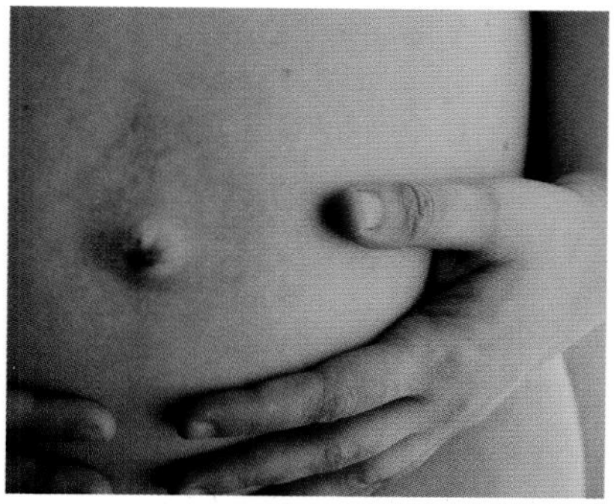

ASK A DOCTOR

What exactly is an "active birth"?
Having an "active birth"—staying mobile during the first stage of labor and remaining upright, squatting, kneeling, or on all-fours during the second stage—can make labor and delivery easier and less painful. Working with gravity helps your pelvis to open and encourages the baby's head to press on your cervix, helping it to dilate. To get active:

- **Practice squatting (see p.424):** it takes time to learn to do it, but it's an effective way to speed labor up. When squatting, make sure you have sufficient support—from your partner, or by using a wall or the back of a sturdy chair.
- **Relax by kneeling** and facing forward with a birth ball or beanbag.
- **Use a birthing pool** if you want to relax in water for a while.
- **If you need an IV,** because you've been induced (see p.432), ask for a mobile one so you can move around.
- **Choose a walking epidural,** which should enable you to stay active.
- **If lying down** makes your contractions stop, get up and start moving again.

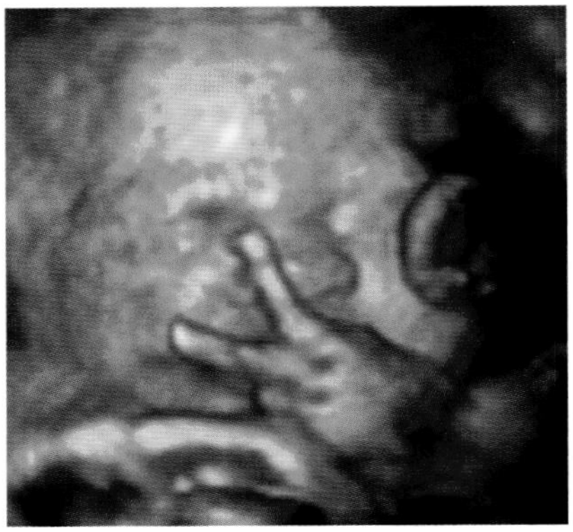

YOU ARE **31 WEEKS AND 2 DAYS**

61 days to go

YOUR BABY TODAY

Your baby's hand coordination continues to improve as their brain is better able to make sense of the feedback it receives. The eyes will often open but only for short periods at a time, reducing the chance of a stray finger coming too close.

" By this stage, your baby is the length they'll be at birth, but they're still very thin and need to gain fat and muscle. "

At this stage of pregnancy, your baby's muscle mass and fat are continuing to increase. Their skin is now thicker and less translucent, and begins to look pink rather than red as the underlying blood vessels are overlaid with more flesh. Growth hormone is being produced by your baby's pituitary gland but before they're actually born this does not influence their growth. Instead insulin and insulin-like growth factors are key. As your baby's skeleton is now close to its final size, their overall length is established. Your baby is still, however, very skinny.

A sonographer can make a good estimate of your baby's weight from an ultrasound scan, but this may vary to your baby's actual weight by plus or minus one pound. Your baby will continue to grow throughout the pregnancy, although in the last few weeks growth is mainly due to fat deposits rather than to muscle mass.

If you're trying to guess how heavy your baby will be at birth, the latest research indicates that the size of your baby has a lot to do with "imprinted" genes. These are genes that are marked as having come from the father, which promote the baby's growth, or the mother, which are growth limiting and attempt to preserve her resources.

FOCUS ON TWINS

Twins look adorable when they're dressed alike, so you may be buying—and certainly will be given—lots of sets of matching clothing. But it's much easier to tell identical twins apart when they're dressed differently. It also helps everyone relate to them as individuals, which is good for their development.

Also keep practicalities in mind: every time one of your twins gets dirty, are you going to change them both? You may find it pays to be flexible: if there are only two clean onesies, then that is what they'll have to wear, regardless of style or color match.

If you get into the habit of dressing them the same, all the time, they may grow conscious of this in toddler years and get distressed if they're dressed differently.

You could:

- **Dress your babies in matching outfits but different colors,** or the same colors but different styles.
- **Only dress them identically on certain occasions,** for instance, for a family photograph or when it's a special occasion.
- **Give any identical outfits you receive to one twin.** The next batch of identical outfits goes to the other twin.

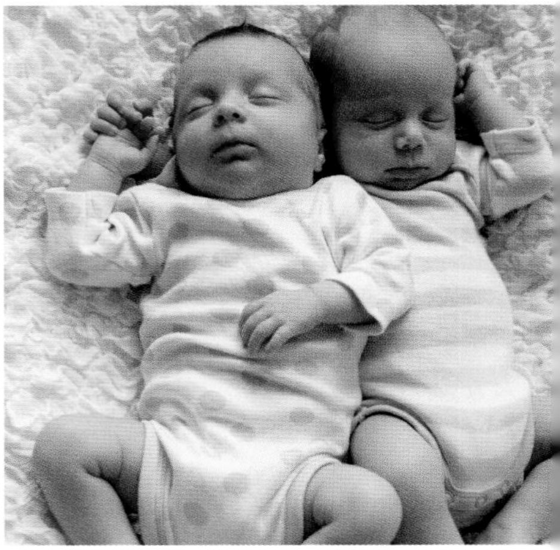

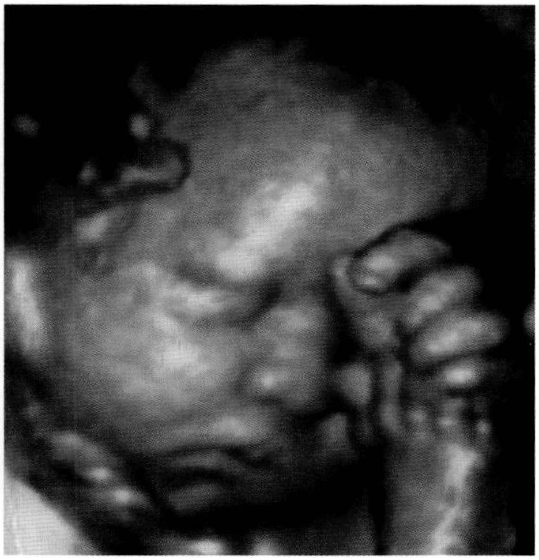

YOU ARE **31 WEEKS AND 3 DAYS**

60 days to go

YOUR BABY TODAY

Here the umbilical cord is seen lying over the baby's shoulder. This is very common; in fact at some time every baby will have the umbilical cord lying close, especially during these next few weeks while the baby frequently changes position.

> "Jolts and jostles are all part of being pregnant—and your baby probably won't even notice them."

Your belly is getting larger and larger. As you walk, you may notice that your belly also appears to move, swaying from side to side with each step. It can be difficult to remember that you're so much bigger than you used to be. You may find yourself trying to squeeze through tight spaces, or between tables and chairs in a restaurant that previously you would have fit through and now find yourself a bit stuck!

Even if you find that your belly is getting bumped around occasionally this really is nothing at all to worry about: your baby is safe, protected by the pool of amniotic fluid that acts as a cushion against the occasional jolt. Soon enough, though, you will be back to your normal shape, or nearly your normal shape, and it can be odd to think back to having to compensate for a belly.

HEART PALPITATIONS

Having a run of fast heartbeats, or missing a beat occasionally—or simply being acutely aware of your heartbeat—is defined as heart palpitations (see p.471). It's common to have these in late pregnancy. They are usually nothing to worry about and are simply the result of changes to your blood circulation, coupled with a large abdominal bulge, although unnecessary stresses and anxieties can play a part as well.

If, however, there is also chest pain or breathlessness, or if you think they are occurring more frequently, mention this to your doctor.

ASK A MOM

I'm finding it increasingly hard to focus at work. How can I best get through the next few weeks? As your baby—and you—get bigger, you may find that you have less energy and your concentration span decreases accordingly. This is normal, but it can pose problems if you have a job to do! First of all, take regular breaks, putting your feet up or closing your eyes for a few minutes to rest. Make sure you drink enough, since dehydration can affect your performance. Similarly, eating healthy snacks, little and often, can keep you from flagging. Iron-rich foods, such as dried fruit, are particularly important: low iron levels can make you tire easily.

Carry a small notebook with you, and jot down anything that you need to remember, no matter how trivial. This can help overcome lapses of memory, and keep you focused on what needs to be done. It may also help to start your day with a "to-do" list, and check your way down it in order of priority. Finally, try to get enough sleep, which will give you at least half a chance of feeling refreshed the next morning.

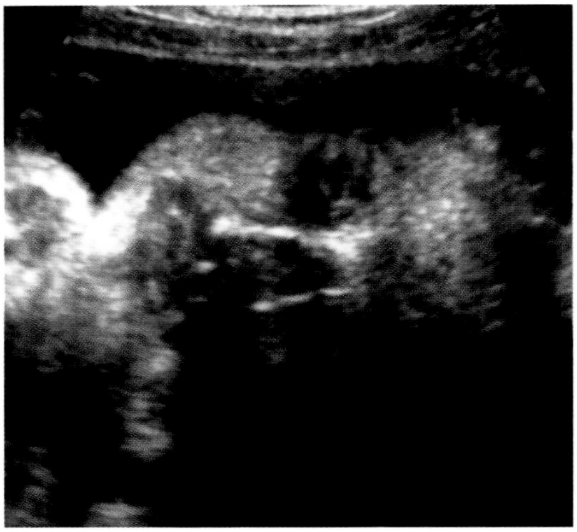

YOU ARE **31 WEEKS AND 4 DAYS**

59 days to go

YOUR BABY TODAY

Measurements around the head, abdomen, and thigh bones are used from the ultrasound image to estimate the weight of your baby. Interestingly, on average, boys are now starting to be slightly heavier than girls.

"As your baby puts on muscle and its tone improves, they begin to be capable of more complex and stronger movements."

Your baby's muscle tone takes some time to develop fully. By this week of your pregnancy, head control is improving and in the legs muscle tone now allows for smoother and more complex movements. For once, the arms and hands lag behind the legs and feet in development, taking another three weeks to achieve the same level of tone and movement.

In the last few weeks, the familiar "fetal position" is increasingly seen on scans: this is not only due to lack of space but also because your baby's flexor muscles (those that bend the elbows, hips, and knees) have a better tone than the extensor muscles (the muscles that extend the arms and legs) in each limb.

You will also be aware that your baby is moving more now than at any other time. You only feel the movements that hit the lining of your uterus, but there will be many more small movements of which you are completely unaware. Movements inside the uterus are important: they help your baby's coordination, strengthen their bones, and increase muscle mass. The number of muscle cells increases up until 38 weeks. From this point on, individual muscle cells lengthen and expand in response to exercise, further increasing muscle mass and strength.

REFRESHING DRINKS

Staying hydrated will continue to be an important part of maintaining your well-being through the end of pregnancy and through breastfeeding. Here are some ideas for nonalcoholic drinks:

- A milkshake made with nutritious fresh berries.
- Grapefruit juice/cranberry juice/ club soda or tonic water
- Sparkling apple juice/dash of angostura bitters/sugar to taste
- Orange juice/bitter lemon
- Lemon juice/pineapple juice/ orange juice/grenadine/club soda

Apple juice/pear juice/ginger ale If you have gestational diabetes, replace any normal full-sugar carbonated drinks with diet versions.

ASK A DOCTOR

Will having an orgasm cause me to go into labor? In a pregnancy without problems, an orgasm will not cause premature labor (see p.431), and at full term orgasm will only cause the onset of labor if it's going to happen anyway. If you have had any signs of premature labor, or vaginal bleeding, you'll be advised to avoid sexual intercourse. This is because the hormone oxytocin increases during sexual arousal, and oxytocin causes the muscles of the uterus to contract. Orgasm may increase Braxton Hicks contractions (see p.410). You should also avoid sexual intercourse if your water has broken, due to the risk of infection.

If you've gone past your due date and your body is ready to go into labor, sexual intercourse may help things start for two reasons: the prostaglandins in semen help the cervix soften at this stage of pregnancy, and the contractions stimulated by orgasm are more likely to develop into early labor contractions.

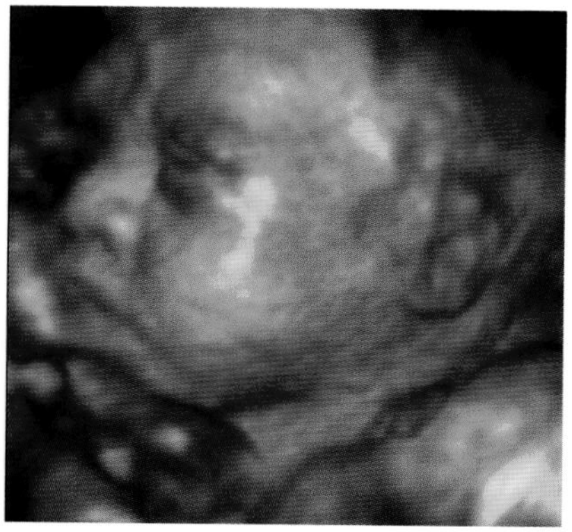

YOU ARE **31 WEEKS AND 5 DAYS**

58 days to go

YOUR BABY TODAY

This image shows a furrowed brow and an open-eyed expression. Just as the muscle tone in the limbs is strengthening, so the muscles of the face are being used and tested. This can produce some memorable facial expressions.

> “ How your baby is positioned can affect your delivery, but there is plenty of time at this stage for things to change. ”

As you get closer to your due date, your doctor may assess your baby's position during your prenatal appointment. Many babies are in the breech position earlier in the pregnancy, but most turn into the head down position by the end of the pregnancy. Still, breech births occur in about 3 or 4 percent full-term births. Between 32 and 37 weeks is the best time for your doctor to try to turn a breech baby. This is because there is plenty of room for the baby to turn around. After the 35th or 36th week, the baby is unlikely to change position since there is less room for large maneuvers. If your baby is breech, your doctor may try to turn the baby, a process called version and she may recommend an extra ultrasound scan at 37–38 weeks of pregnancy to check the baby's position. It may be difficult to be completely sure, on examination alone, whether the doctor is feeling the baby's bottom or head. If your baby is breech, your doctor may suggest a cesarean delivery.

FOCUS ON PARTNERS

Be prepared for the fact that in the last few weeks of pregnancy, your partner will not be able to maintain the same level of activity as she did before.

This reduced activity may range from doing less exercise to doing fewer household chores. She may find it challenging to muster the energy needed to care for other children, , especially a lively toddler.

It may be challenging for your partner to realize that she's not able to do things as easily as before and, to a certain extent, is less independent. So while you can be a great help to her in these final weeks of pregnancy, be aware that there's a fine line between being supportive and being overly protective. Deep down you may want to turn into "super hero" and do everything, but it might frustrate your partner if you become overly protective. Try to take the lead from her and give her help as and when she needs it, as well as space to do her own thing.

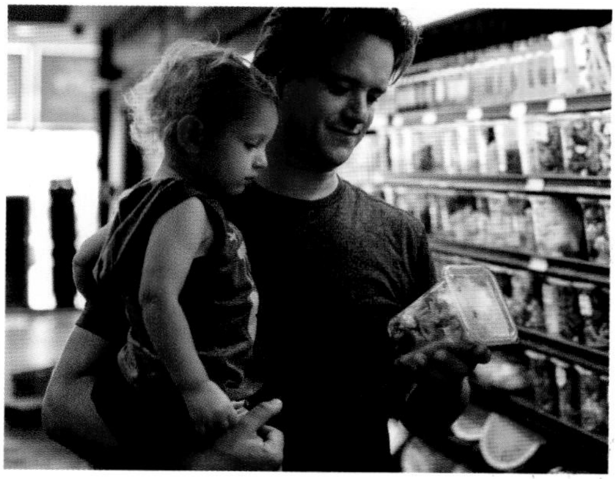

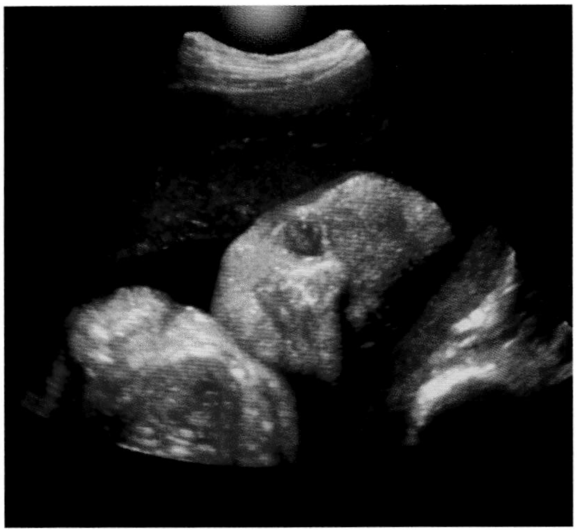

YOU ARE **31 WEEKS AND 6 DAYS**

57 days to go

YOUR BABY TODAY

This image shows the amount of amniotic fluid is around your baby at this time. Ultrasound displays the fluid as black on the screen. Sometimes there will be speckles within the fluid: these represent skin and hair cells that are shed as your baby grows.

> "If your third trimester coincides with the summer months, staying cool and comfortable can be a real challenge."

When the weather is hot, your baby makes it sweltering! Keep yourself hydrated by drinking lots of cool water. Consider carrying a spray bottle of water (keep it in the fridge overnight so that it's nice and cold the next day) to spritz you when you're too hot.

Opt for sleeveless clothing that is made of natural fabrics, such as linen and cotton, which will help keep the air circulating. If you want to keep some or all of your arms covered, wear short-sleeved jackets or cotton cardigans. Wear a sun hat and sunglasses, especially if you're in direct sunlight for any length of time.

Opt for flip-flops or low-heeled sandals to let your feet breathe—these can also be a good option if your feet are swollen (see pp.468–469).

LISTENING TO YOUR BABY'S HEARTBEAT

From the very earliest stages of pregnancy, your baby's heart will be beating, and there can be nothing more uplifting and reassuring than hearing this for yourself. Your doctor can use a variety of instruments to hear your baby's heartbeat, including a stethoscope and a Doppler monitor, which uses ultrasound technology (see right). A baby's heart beats between 120 and 160 times per minute (with slight variations)—quite a few more than your own heartbeat, which is normally under 100. The sole purpose of listening to the heartbeat is to ensure that it falls within a normal range, and to reassure moms-to-be that all is well. If there's an unusual rhythm or the heartbeat speeds or slows unexpectedly, your doctor can arrange for tests to confirm that all is well. Some women feel that hearing their baby's heartbeat helps the bonding process in advance of the birth.

FIRST HOURS AND DAYS

To help you prepare for what to expect in the first few days after your baby is born, here are a few interesting facts you might like to know:

- **You may shake all over** just after giving birth and don't be concerned if you vomit; this is quite normal and nothing to worry about.
- **Newborn babies don't always master breastfeeding** (see pp.450–451) immediately. Just like you, they need to practice.
- **After pains** (the cramping sensation in your uterus when your baby nurses) can hurt almost as much as contractions.
- **The first time you urinate** and defecate after giving birth can be uncomfortable.
- **You may feel very vulnerable,** and in need of your own mom, in the first few days of parenthood.
- **Lochia (after-birth bleeding)** can be a challenge at first, even if you're using larger-sized sanitary pads.
- **Bonding with a newborn doesn't always happen** immediately for all mothers, but it's worth the wait.

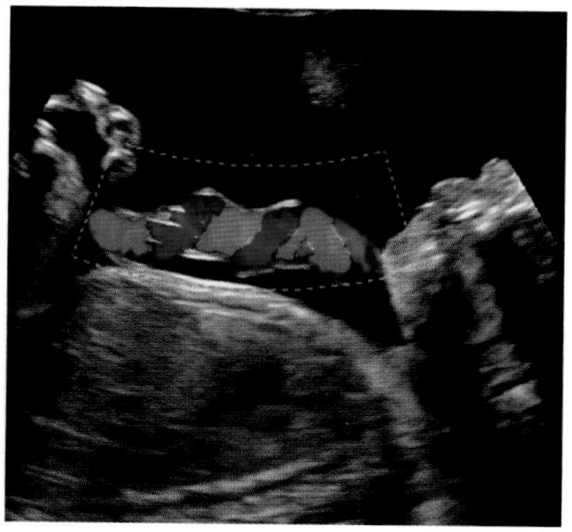

YOU ARE **32 WEEKS EXACTLY**

56 days to go

YOUR BABY TODAY

The blood flow in the umbilical cord is highlighted in this image. The colors show the direction of flow. The smaller umbilical arteries that carry blood toward the placenta are seen in blue as they wrap around the more central umbilical vein (in red).

You may be having difficulty sleeping, partly because your belly makes it uncomfortable to lie down in certain positions, but also because you have lots to think about. Try to take some time out with your partner relaxing and bonding together with your belly. Even 10 minutes doing nothing except focusing on yourself, your body, your partner, and you baby can be invigorating and rejuvenating.

At night, try to get yourself into a comfortable position, and then focus inward on your body, turning your mind away from all your external worries. First focus on slowing down your breathing. Then think about a place and a time when you felt relaxed and happy—for example, on vacation, walking on the beach. Next focus on clenching and then relaxing each set of muscles in turn, or imagine a ball of heat passing slowly through your limbs and body making them feel warm, heavy, and relaxed.

You might want to involve your partner, perhaps they could lie with you with their hands or head on your belly and try to adjust their breathing so it's in sync with yours. Just lying next to your partner can relax you and bring you close together.

> “ The best way to make sure you get enough sleep is to find ways to slow down mentally and relax. ”

DRESSING FOR EXERCISE

In this last trimester, dressing comfortably for exercise can make all the difference to you feel. Be sure you are wearing the correct size—trying to squeeze into clothes you outgrew three months ago will be uncomfortable and restricting and may make breathing difficult. There are exercise clothes designed specifically for pregnancy, but you can also just wear a large T-shirt and tracksuit bottoms or loose-fitting shorts.

Support belts may make cardiovascular exercise more comfortable. Most are made from elasticized fabric with Velcro fastenings that can be adjusted to suit your belly size. These belts, available at many maternity stores, are inexpensive and can help ease back pain, too.

Wearing a well-fitting sports bra is vital for any activity as the delicate breast tissue can weaken due to the increased pressure of your larger and heavier breasts. If your breasts are very large, and you feel they're unsupported by just wearing a sports bra, try wearing it on top of your usual bra.

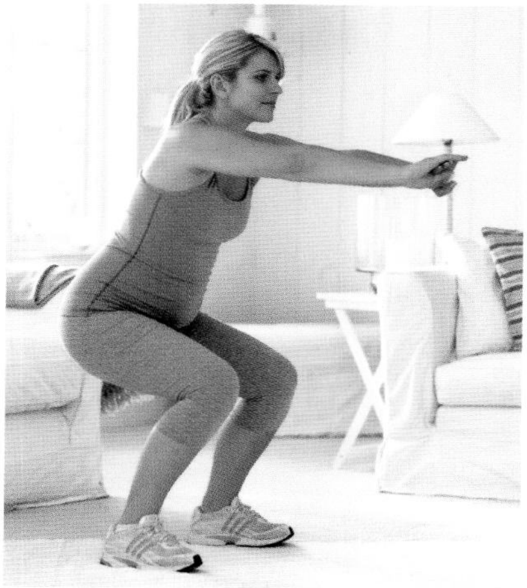

Your 33rd week

IT'S HARD TO IMAGINE HOW LIFE WILL BE WITH A NEW BABY. All prospective moms, and not just first-timers, find it difficult to envision the future after the arrival of the baby. The imaginings, dreams, and hopes of the last few months are about to become realities—which may be very different from what you expect. You may find that it helps to concentrate on practical matters, such as the birth celebrations and future child care. You could make plans for recovering your prepregnancy figure. The belly won't be with you forever, even if it feels like it!

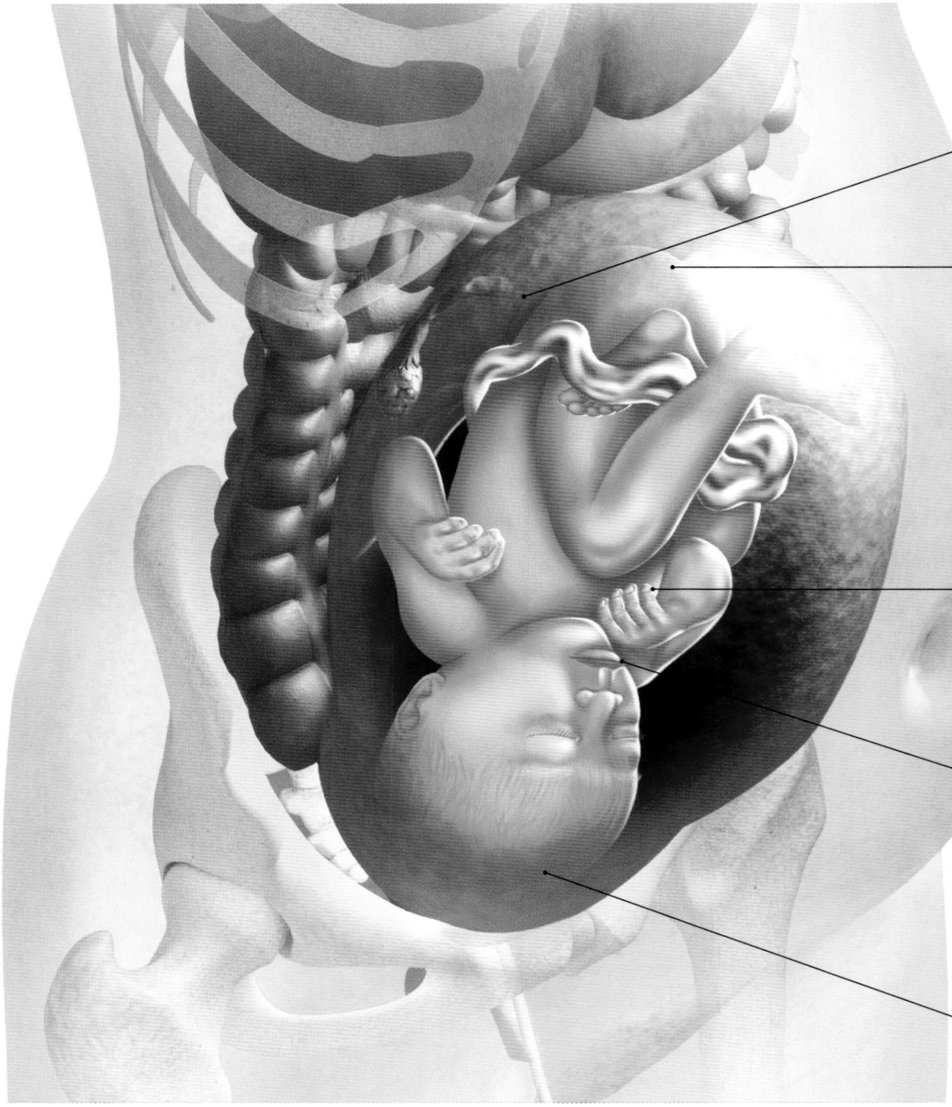
Calcium from your diet crosses the placenta and is used to help strengthen your baby's bones.
With bottom up, head down, and chin tucked into the chest, a baby is in an ideal position for the beginning of labor. Of course, not all babies are so obliging.
Fingernails have grown long enough to reach the tips of the fingers.
The amniotic fluid swallowed by the baby passes through the stomach and intestines in the same way that food travels through a mature digestive system. Waste is stored in the baby's colon to be excreted after birth.
At 33 weeks the average crown to heel length is 17.2 in (43.7 cm) and the average weight is 4.2 lb (1.9 kg).

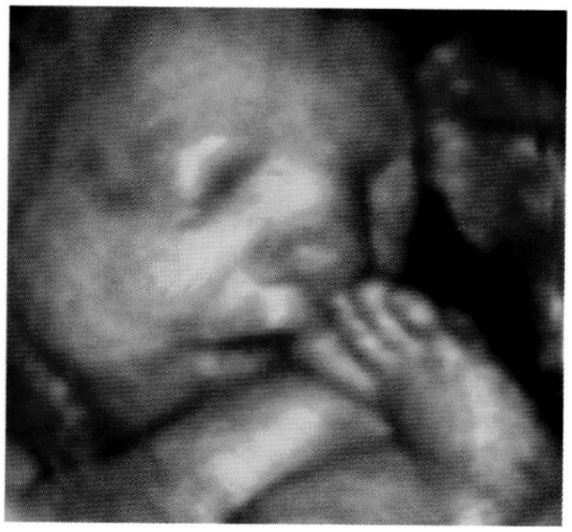

YOU ARE **32 WEEKS AND 1 DAY**

55 days to go

YOUR BABY TODAY

In this image, the hands are folded over beneath the chin and there's a foot up by the mouth and nose. It can look as if your baby is quite a contortionist but because they are still quite skinny, the joints allow for a great deal of flexibility.

" If you feel you have little control over your own body, it's natural to think your figure will never be normal again—but it will! "

At this stage, you'll still be gaining about 1–2.2 lb (0.5–1 kg) per week, but weight gain tends to slow down in the last few weeks. By now, your belly will have stretched and your belly button may have popped out—this can be quite protruding and may be seen through your clothes (see p.319). You may have developed a linea nigra in your second trimester, a dark line of pigmentation down the center of your abdomen (see p.170).

Like most women, you are probably happy and excited about having a baby but a little concerned about getting your figure back after the birth. Some women get quite upset at the thought that their abdomens may not return to their previous shape after the birth, and this is completely normal. Rest assured that with gentle exercise and the continuation of your healthy diet, your figure can return to its prepregnancy state and your belly button should pop back to its normal shape of its own accord. The key is to remember it will take a bit of time—it did, after all, take nine months to gain the weight.

NUTRITIOUS FIBER

Eating fiber is the most natural way to keep your bowel movements regular, so it will help prevent or relieve constipation—a common problem in the third trimester. The recommended 25g of fiber per day can be difficult to achieve, but if you base all your meals around fiber-rich whole grains and include legumes such as lentils, beans, and peas, and eat a minimum of five portions of vegetables and fruit a day, you'll be well on your way. Eating fiber will help you feel more full, which can help prevent overeating and excess weight gain. If you eat a fiber-rich breakfast, for example, you're less likely to snack an hour later.

Fiber also contributes to the management of diabetes, lowers cholesterol, and decreases the risk of heart disease.

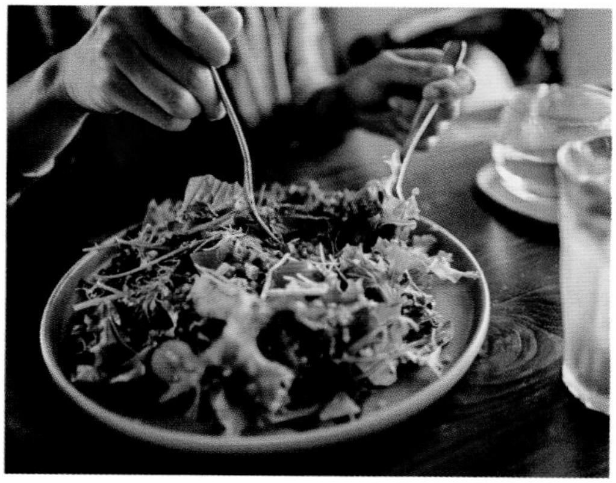

ASK A DOCTOR

I want to work right up to the birth—is that allowed? Yes. Many women do, so they don't waste any maternity leave before baby. Check with your doctor to make sure it's okay for you. Think carefully before making this decision. Late pregnancy can be extremely tiring and, if your job is mentally and/or physically taxing, it may be better to begin your leave before your due date. You will also need time to prepare for the arrival of your baby.

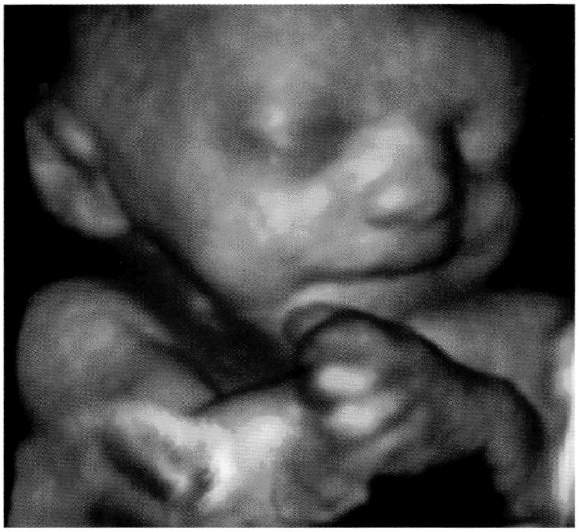

YOU ARE **32 WEEKS AND 2 DAYS**

54 days to go

YOUR BABY TODAY

During this week your baby's fingernails have become fully developed and now approach the tips of the fingers. Bathed in amniotic fluid, the nails are kept very soft: it's only after birth that your baby might tend to scratch and need to wear mittens.

> " Every 40 minutes, your baby swallows enough amniotic fluid to fill their stomach, before emptying it back into the amniotic sac. "

Your baby is swallowing and recycling almost half a liter (18 fl oz) of amniotic fluid each day. In addition to providing nutrients, especially proteins, this fluid is important for the healthy development of the gut. Your baby's sense of taste is thought to have developed to such an extent now that if you have eaten spiced food it can be distinguished in the amniotic fluid they drink.

Amniotic fluid does not enter the lungs but travels down the esophagus into the stomach where it is stored for a short time. At this stage, the stomach fills every 40 minutes, but, from 35 weeks, as the stomach enlarges, this rate slows down to every 80 minutes. Muscle contractions move the fluid in waves into the small and then large bowel. As it travels along the bowel, water is reabsorbed so that only waste material, or "meconium," enters the colon, the final section of the large bowel. This meconium accumulates in the large bowel, which is completely full by the time your baby is born. Babies don't usually pass meconium before the birth but do so soon after. Meconium consists mainly of skin cells, lanugo hairs, and vernix. It has a greenish color due to the presence of bilirubin, a breakdown product from red blood cells.

FALSE ALARMS

In the next few weeks, as you and your partner await your baby's arrival, you may experience one or two false alarms, especially if it's your first baby. A false alarm can come at any time of the day or night and it won't respect important meetings or deadlines.

It can help if you—as well as your partner—familiarize yourself with all the signs that indicate labor may be starting (see pp.409–411). If, however, you're ever in doubt, contact your doctor to ascertain that labor has not started, instead of assuming that this is the case. She will be very experienced in dealing with false alarms and won't mind you contacting her.

ITCHY SKIN

Having itchy skin on your belly is common. As the skin there stretches and thins, it can become dry. If, however, you have severe itching on your abdomen, or on the palms of your hands or soles of your feet, see your doctor. This itching can be a sign of obstetric cholestasis (see p.475), a rare pregnancy condition involving the liver, which causes bile salts to enter the bloodstream, making the skin (especially on the hands and feet) itchy, although there is no rash.

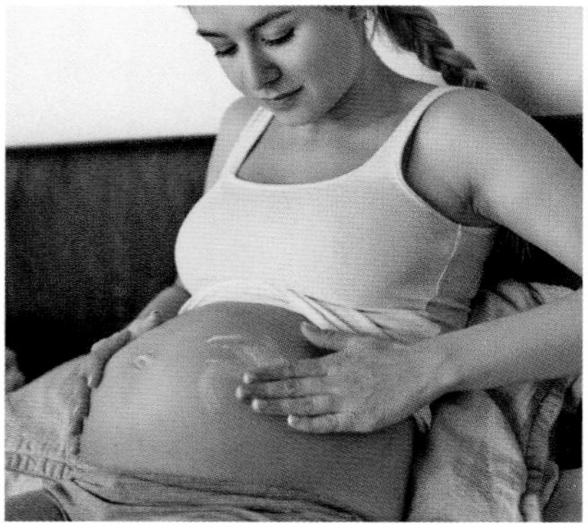

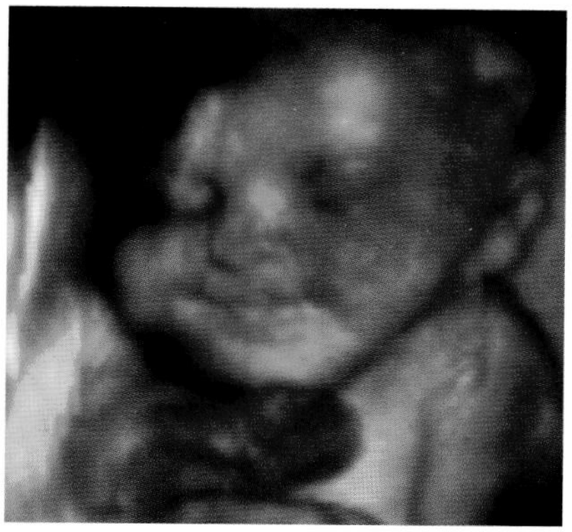

YOU ARE **32 WEEKS AND 3 DAYS**

53 days to go

YOUR BABY TODAY

Your baby's position in the uterus is influenced by your own posture. Gravity has some effect on your baby, so whether you are standing or sitting, and which side you lie down on, affects the way your baby's back is turned and which side he rolls onto.

"As your belly grows, it's normal to feel you want to support it when you're walking around."

You've probably had to change the way that you exercise by now due to your growing abdomen. You may well have had to replace jogging on the treadmill, for example, with going for long, brisk (or not so brisk!) walks. If you find that even walking makes your belly and pelvis sore or uncomfortable, you may find you naturally hold up your belly with your hands to try to give it some extra support and to give your pelvis and back a break. Some women say it feels as if the baby "might fall out."

You might want to invest in a pregnancy support band (see p.179); made of stretchy fabric, this useful item supports the belly and can help prevent lower back pain.

BUYING A BABY MONITOR

There are hundreds of baby monitors on the market, so choosing one that's right for you can be daunting. And although monitors vary, they have the same basic components—a minimum of two units: one to transmit your baby's sounds, and one that stays with you so that you can hear if your baby is crying or fussing

Video monitors that allow you to see, as well as hear, your baby are increasingly popular.

Features tend to include a moving lights-sound display, the option to plug it in or use batteries, a talk-back function, and a temperature sensor. Your choice depends on your personal preferences and your budget.

REPOSITIONING YOUR BABY

Your movements during late pregnancy can affect the position of your baby. Ideally, he'll lie head down, facing your back, with his chin tucked into his chest. You can encourage this optimum fetal position by:

- **Spending a couple of minutes on all fours,** gently wiggling your hips from side to side, without straining your lower back.
- **Sitting with your knees lower than your pelvis,** and your body tilted slightly forward.
- **Kneeling on the floor,** leaning over a beanbag, cushions, or birth ball.
- **Sitting on a birth ball,** with your legs positioned slightly apart and knees lower than your hips, then rocking your pelvis.
- **Assuming the tailor pose:** sit on the floor with your back straight and the soles of your feet together. Let your knees fall to the side and rest your elbows on your inner thighs.
- **Swimming:** breaststroke helps to open the pelvis.

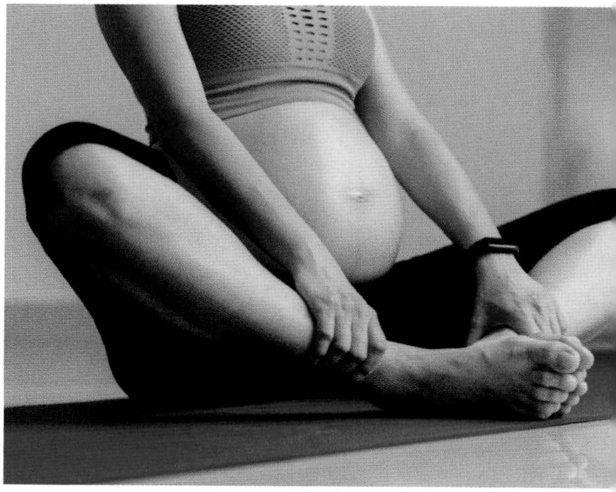

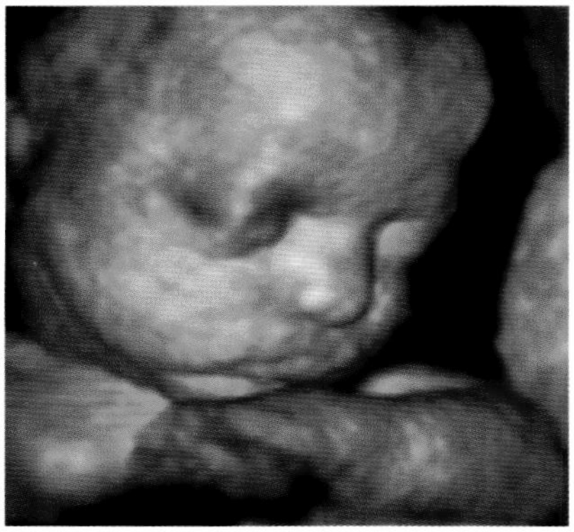

YOU ARE **32 WEEKS AND 4 DAYS**

52 days to go

YOUR BABY TODAY

The bridge of your baby's nose is now more fully formed. The face is taking on a more rounded shape and some babies may look quite chubby from now on. Shadows around the top and sides of the head will increasingly give the illusion of hair.

> " By this stage of pregnancy, your baby's fingernails have grown and reached the tips of their fingers "

Your baby's fingernails first appeared at 23 weeks, and because the development of the arms is consistently ahead of the legs, the toenails started to develop four weeks later.

The future nail begins at the tip of each finger or toe, where a nail fold is formed. At the base of this nail fold, the cells start to harden into nail, in a process known as keratinization. The nails grow from new cells formed in the soft nail bed. It takes nine weeks for the nails to reach the fingertips, and it will be another four weeks before the toenails reach the tips of the toes.

The nail is actually all the same color, but the white part of the nail appears white because it does not have the nail bed, with its rich blood supply, beneath it to give the illusion of color. Since the nails already reach the fingertips, it probably won't be long after the birth before your baby's nails need trimming. A newborn baby's nails are very fine and soft and you may find it easier to trim them by filing them away rather than trying to cut them. Or cut them with baby nail scissors while your baby is asleep and not wiggling around.

STRETCHING EXERCISES

The stretches shown below are great for opening up the pelvis and strengthening the legs. Practicing these exercises while pregnant will allow you to be able to use them more effectively and confidently during labor. When you're practicing squatting, it may help if your partner supports you from behind. Many women do pregnancy yoga; it may be a cornerstone of your birth preparations if you choose to take active birth classes (see p.333).

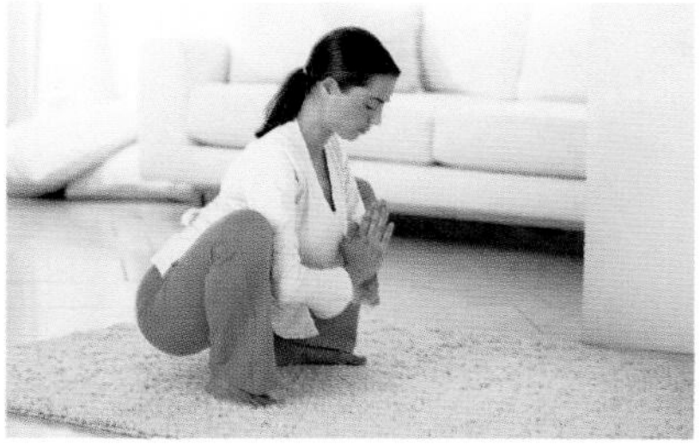

Get into a squatting position. Squat only if you find it easy to hold this position with your heels on the floor and your back straight.

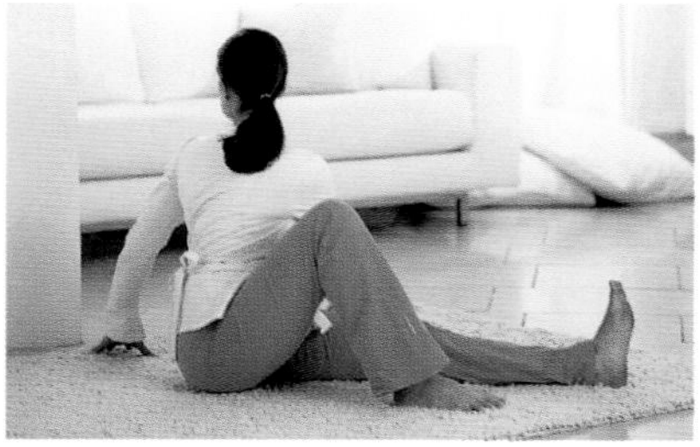

Sit with your left leg stretched out in front of you and right leg bent. Gently twist your body, placing your hands on the floor for additional support.

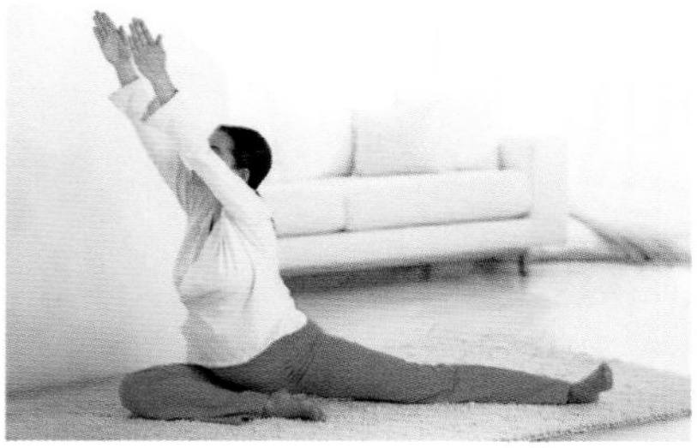

Sit with one leg stretched out behind you, and the other tucked beneath your belly. Stretch upward, breathing deeply throughout.

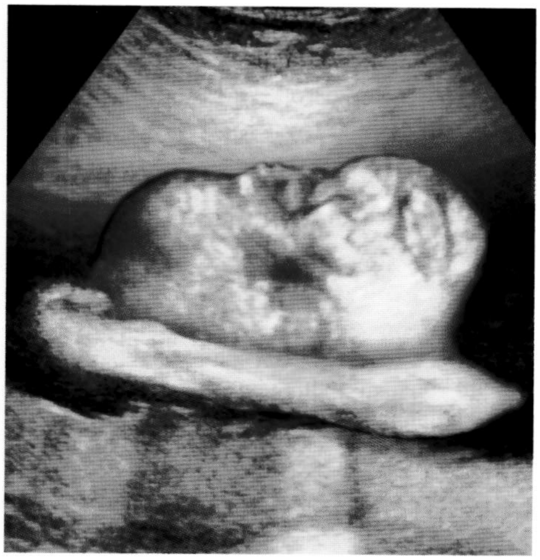

YOU ARE **32 WEEKS AND 5 DAYS**

51 days to go

YOUR BABY TODAY

In this image of the baby lying on their side, the arm is positioned beneath the head and is partly outside of the 3-D view, allowing structures within the arm to be seen. Part of the bones in the elbow and forearm show here as bright reflections.

Friends and family might now begin talking about what will happen after the birth and what it will be like for you to have a baby.

If this is your first baby, it may be hard for you to imaging what life will be like with your newborn, and even if you have had a baby before, you've never had a second or third and so you don't know what it will be like to have another one. Of course, you know that life will continue, but it can be difficult to see past the labor to the realities of life with a newborn. As ever, keep talking to those close to you about how you feel, be it excited or scared and unprepared (usually all three in rapid succession). Talk about what you think or hope it will be like after the baby is born, for example when are grandparents and other key people going to visit, and whether you would like a christening or naming party—or perhaps neither of these. This may help you get used to the idea that not only are you pregnant but there is a baby coming.

“ To get used to the fact that your newborn will arrive very soon, start focusing on life after the birth ”

ASK A DOCTOR

How will I benefit from going to prenatal classes? You'll get the opportunity to share information, ideas, fears, and concerns about childbirth in a comfortable environment, and to discuss and decide upon issues that will affect the way you choose to give birth. You'll also meet other parents-to-be. Often friendships formed at classes continue after the birth as you support each other in your new parenting role. In most classes, you'll be given advice about:

- **Tried-and-true labor techniques,** such as breathing through the pain, massage, suitable sustenance, and some positive visualization exercises.
- **Pain-relief options** and a range of natural alternatives (see pp.396–407).
- **How to present** (and preserve) your birth plan (see p.303).
- **The practical and emotional support** a birth partner can offer.
- **The items required** for a hospital or home birth (see pp. 341 and 358).

You'll be advised on how to prepare yourself for the birth, what to expect in the first few days postpartum, and how to encourage healing afterward. You will also be given information on caring for a newborn, including diaper changing, bathing, and establishing breastfeeding.

FIRST-TIME LABOR

In your first pregnancy, the cervix dilates (see p.415) by about 0.5 cm every hour, compared to 1.5 cm an hour for subsequent babies. You will probably push, on average, for more than one hour with your first baby. With your second baby, this may be less than 30 minutes.

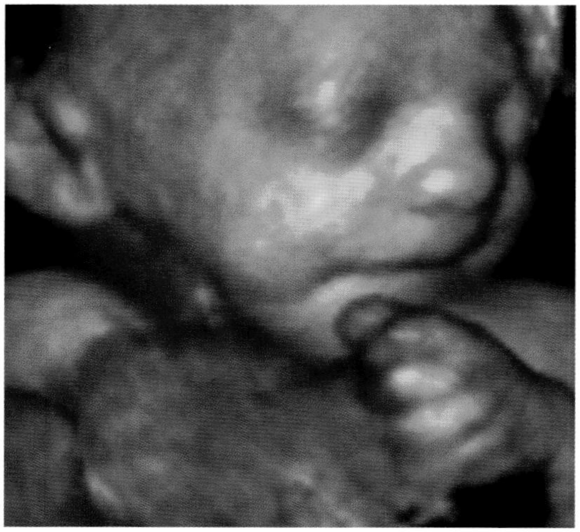

YOU ARE **32 WEEKS AND 6 DAYS**

50 days to go

YOUR BABY TODAY

This image may show the start of a smile. Your baby will often be smiling inside, sticking their tongue out, and making all sorts of faces. They may also still be experiencing hiccups that may be something that you are now becoming aware of.

> " The days and nights fly by with a newborn, so it's a good idea to start thinking about child care well before you need it. "

It may seem impossible to believe that you should be considering child care before your baby is even born, but it can be useful to think through the options while you have the time. There are two main types of child care: in and out of your home. In the first case, you can have a live-in or live-out nanny or mother's helper, an au pair (which may be acceptable if you work from home, for example, and can supervise), or perhaps a family member or friend who is prepared to come to your house to take care of your baby. If you choose outside child care, there are a number of options including day-care centers, relatives or babysitters in their homes, or on-the-job day care. Before you set your heart on one particular type of care, it's a good idea to investigate the costs and the availability in your area. You may want to pay a visit to some of the nurseries or other facilities close to you, just to get a feel for what's available, and establish now what you do and don't want. Secondly, remember that good-quality child-care facilities and babysitters are usually in demand, and, even if you aren't entirely sure when you will be going back to work, it's probably a good idea to put your baby's name (or last name, at least!) down for a few, to give you options when the time comes.

CALCIUM INTAKE

Calcium transferred across the placenta to your baby is essential for the healthy development of their skeleton and teeth, as well as for their blood.

Your body adapts to optimize the amount of calcium your baby receives. If your diet is, or has been, low in calcium, it will be mobilized from your bones to go to your baby—so your baby won't have a calcium deficiency, but you might.

Vitamin D is needed to help your body metabolize calcium, so take a 600–800 IU daily supplement. Also make sure you eat plenty of calcium-rich foods, especially dairy foods, since these are particularly good for helping to prevent loss of bone mass. Just one glass of milk provides 300 mg of the 800 mg calcium you need each day. See also p.114 for good sources of calcium.

FOCUS ON PARTNERS

Many partners are anxious about being there during labor and birth because they know they will be witnessing their partner experience one of the most intense things a woman can ever do and they may be unsure of how to help.

There are plenty of ways in which you can support your partner during labor; these include being aware of her wishes, speaking for her if she is unable to, and repeating what doctors have said if she didn't hear clearly; passing her a drink; rubbing her back; holding a warm cloth to her face; switching music on or off; being encouraging and reassuring her.

You can learn effective ways to support your partner physically and emotionally during labor by attending prenatal classes (see p.331).

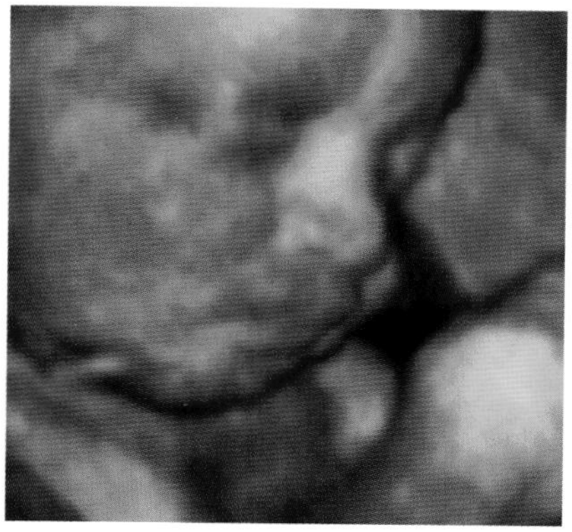

YOU ARE **33 WEEKS EXACTLY**

49 days to go

YOUR BABY TODAY

Soon your baby's lungs will be able to fully support them after birth. At 33 weeks, though, most babies would still need some help with breathing if born this early. Your baby will be regularly practicing breathing movements inside.

You can choose whoever you like to be your support partner at the hospital. During public health emergencies, your hospital may limit the number of support persons allowed. If you are allowed more than one person, you may consider whether you'd like to ask your mom, sister, or close friend to be present at delivery, or hire a doula. It's also good to have a backup plan in case your partner is unable to make it, whether planned or due to unexpected circumstances.

There may be many other people in your life who would like to be present with you and are unable—you can stay connected and share these special memories with them by taking pictures or even video calls. Not all hospitals allow you to record the birth, so be sure to ask in advance before you start filming.

"Choosing who will be present at the birth with you is a big decision, so start thinking about it in good time."

ACTIVE BIRTH CLASSES

The goal of active birth classes is to make women feel good about their bodies and give them the confidence that they have the mental and physical reserves to have a successful birth experience. Classes are generally appropriate regardless of fitness level, flexibility, and your stage of pregnancy.

- **Active birth classes** promote the benefits of yoga and exercise as both physical and mental preparation for childbirth.
- **Yoga strengthens the body,** improves posture and circulation, and teaches how to use relaxation and breathing techniques to relieve stress.
- **Like prenatal classes,** active birth classes allow you to meet other parents-to-be and share their pregnancy experiences.
- **The downside** is that these classes aren't widely available, so they get booked quickly and can be expensive. Ask your doctor about local classes. If you can't find a class in your area, read an active birth book or consider taking a prenatal yoga class.

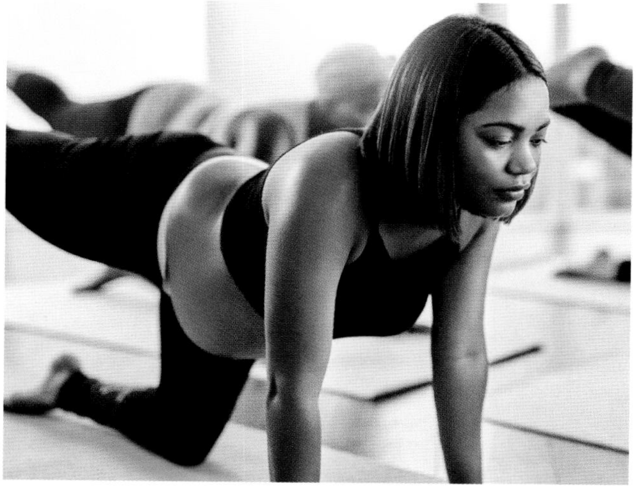

Your 34th week

YOUR BABY IS ALMOST FULLY EQUIPPED FOR THE OUTSIDE WORLD. If your baby was born this week, they'd still need some help with breathing and feeding. But it's reassuring to know that basically they're in pretty good shape for survival. However, you are unlikely to go into labor this early. Now is your chance to start practicing the relaxation and pain-relieving exercises that you've been learning at your prenatal classes. The more familiar you are with the techniques, the more they will help you during labor.

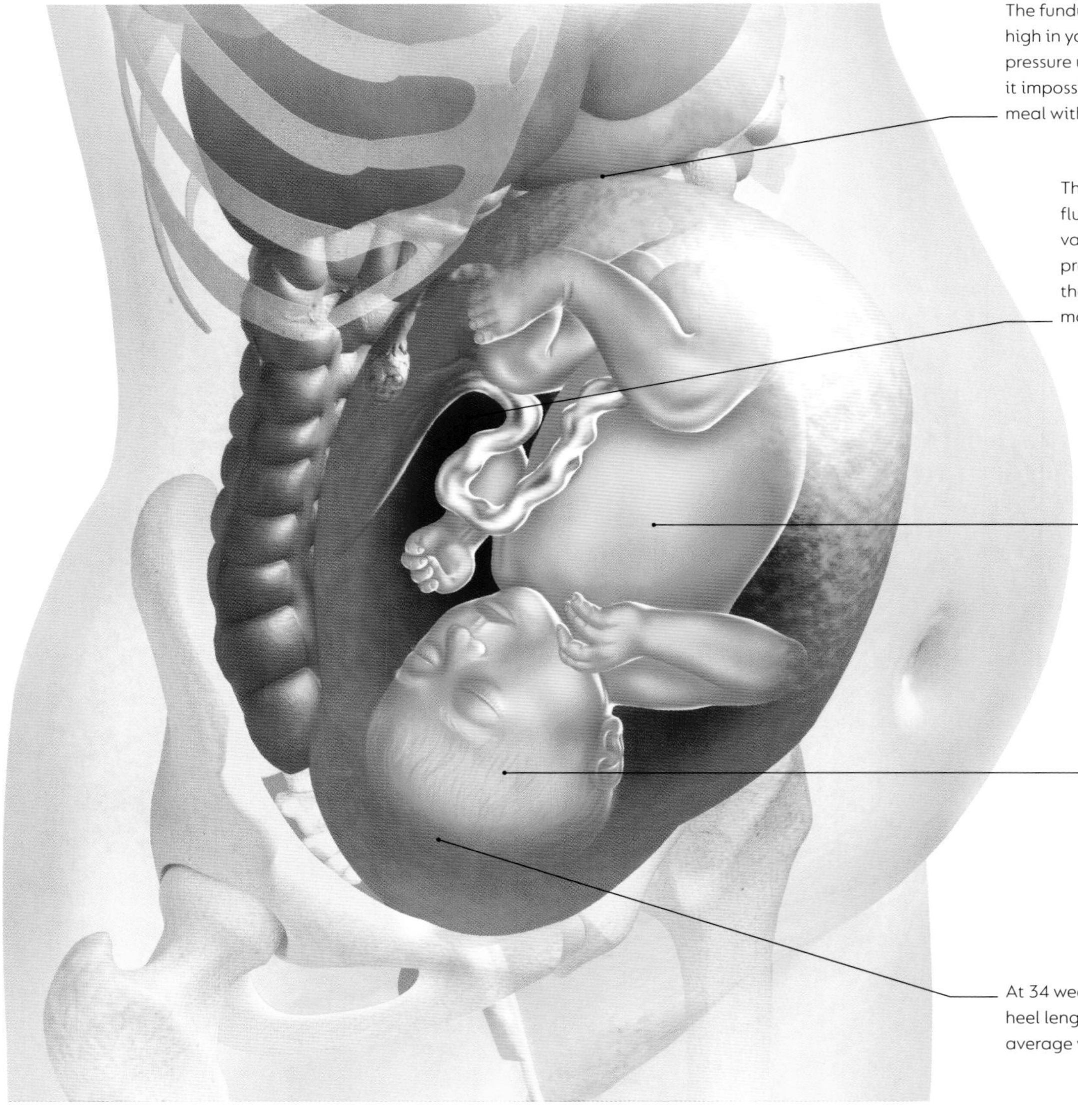

The fundus, or top of the uterus, is high in your abdomen and the pressure under your ribs may make it impossible for you to enjoy a full meal without discomfort.

The amount of amniotic fluid surrounding the baby varies in individual pregnancies. At this stage, the fluid has reached its maximum level.

Your baby's gut would be able to process food if they were to be born this week. All the digestive enzymes are now active.

The position of the baby is unlikely to change between now and the birth if this is your first pregnancy.

At 34 weeks the average crown to heel length is 17.7 in (45 cm) and the average weight is 4.7 lb (2.1 kg).

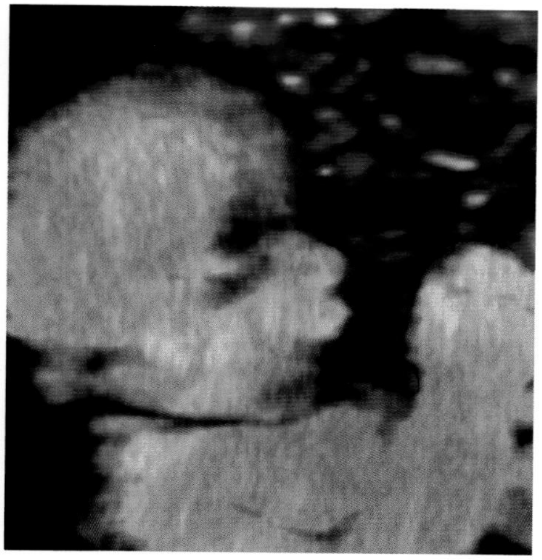

YOU ARE **33 WEEKS AND 1 DAY**

48 days to go

YOUR BABY TODAY

Your baby may well be head down by this stage. The head is the heaviest part and gravity plus the shape of your uterus favors a head-down position. Ask your doctor at the next visit whether they can determine the position for you.

“Premature labor is highly likely in a twin pregnancy, so your doctor will be on alert and monitoring you closely.”

If you're expecting twins they may arrive any time now. Most singleton pregnancies are 38 to 42 weeks, but if you're carrying twins, 37 to 39 weeks is optimal. But over half of twins are born before 37 weeks. Women expecting twins are at higher risk of high blood pressure, preeclampsia, placental insufficiency, gestational diabetes, and may need to be induced early. That said, many women do go on to deliver twins vaginally.

Depending on the type of twins you are having, your doctor may recommend delivering as early as 32 weeks, or up to 39 weeks, as well as anytime in between.

If the babies are in any position other than “head down,” or the placenta is in an awkward position, such as near the neck of the uterus, a Cesarean may be recommended. Some doctors prefer to deliver twins by Cesarean because the second twin may run into difficulties during the delivery, particularly if they are not head down.

Premature babies are more at risk of complications than those who go to full-term. A Cesarean ensures the babies are delivered quickly without having to go through hours of potentially stressful labor.

BIRTHWEIGHT OF TWINS

The average birth weight of twins is 5 lb 8 oz (2.5 kg). This is compared to 7 lb 8 oz (3.5 kg) for singleton babies. It's not unusual for there to be a difference in birth weight between the babies. In fact, one twin may weigh 2 to 3 lb more than the other.

ASK A MIDWIFE

I'm having my twins in a couple of weeks. Can they sleep in the same crib? Having shared the same tight space in the uterus for many months, it seems natural to allow twin newborns to sleep together and, in fact, research indicates that it may have some benefits. Not only has it been found to be safe for twins of roughly the same size to sleep together until three months of age, but one study found that putting newborn twins in the same crib helped regulate their body temperature and their sleep cycles. They can be placed side by side, or head to head. To be safe, don't overdress them or use blankets, bumpers, or pillows. Make sure the mattress is firm with a fitted sheet over it. Like singletons, twins should be put to sleep in the safe sleeping position, on their backs.

A double crib will last until your twins are old enough to move to a bed, but many experts believe twins should be given their own sleeping space from three months, so they can be given individual attention and the opportunity to develop their own sleep patterns.

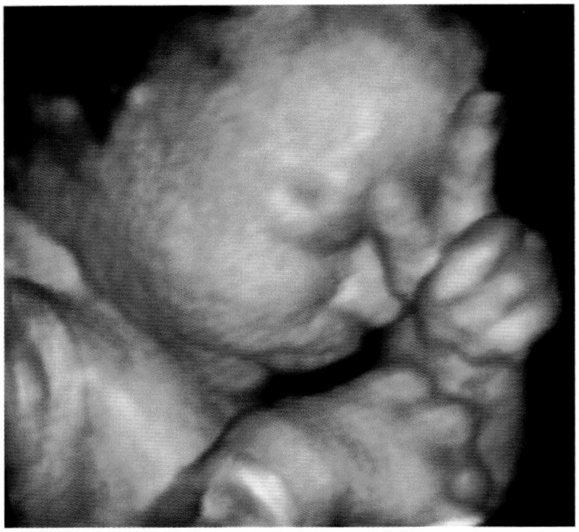

YOU ARE **33 WEEKS AND 2 DAYS**

47 days to go

YOUR BABY TODAY

Shadows give the impression of hair on the eyebrows and eyelashes on this 3-D image. Because this baby was lying head down, the view of the top part of the head is lost in the shadows caused by the mother's pelvis.

> "With well-developed hearing, your baby may not be getting as much peace and quiet as they would like in the uterus."

It is not quite as peaceful for your baby in the uterus as you might think. There will be a constant background noise produced by your heart beating, your breathing, and your stomach rumbling. While the uterus and amniotic fluid will prevent many quieter sounds from reaching your baby, voices do penetrate quite easily. Your baby has already learned to adapt to repetitive sounds but is now acquiring a memory for familiar noises. The most familiar sounds. Your baby will startle and turn toward loud or unfamiliar noises and these will also cause their heart rate to increase.

LIE AND PRESENTATION

Your baby's lie and presentation will be assessed by your doctor at every prenatal appointment. The "lie" refers to the position of the baby's spine in relation to the maternal spine. This can be longitudinal (vertical), transverse (horizontal), or oblique.. The "presentation" refers to which part of the baby is closest to the pelvis and would come out first during a vaginal delivery.

The most common presentation is head down, bottom up, called the cephalic presentation. Breech presentation (see far right) is when the baby is bottom or feet down with the head upward. A footling breech means that the baby is head up or both feet are below the bottom. In an anterior position (see below), your baby's head is down and faces your back. In a posterior position, their head faces your belly, which can prolong labor and may increase the chances of an assisted birth.

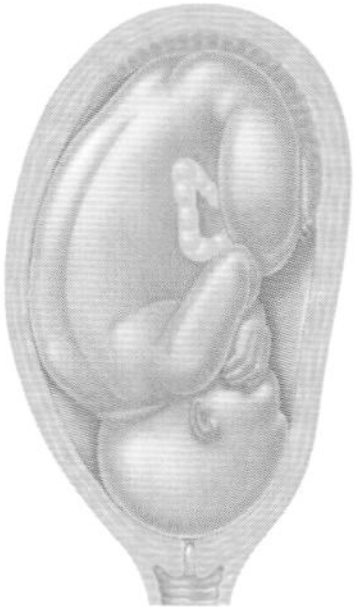

Cephalic presentation

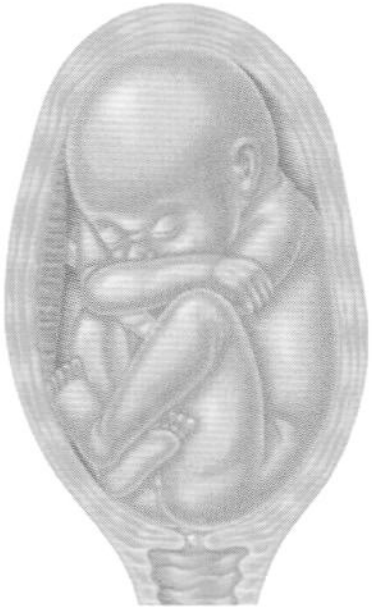

Breech presentation

ASK A DOCTOR

What is perineal massage and how do I do it? Spending just five minutes a day massaging your perineum (the area between the vagina and anus) with oil could reduce your risk of tearing or having an episiotomy (see p.427) during the birth. It also means you're less likely to experience pain in that sensitive spot after the birth—even after having an episiotomy. Follow these steps to perform a perineal massage:

- Wash your hands. Apply a mild lubricant, like K-Y jelly, to your thumbs, then slide them an inch inside the vagina. Gently stretch the vagina until you feel a slight stinging sensation.
- When you feel that sensation, hold the pressure steady until you no longer feel the stinging. Then gently massage the lower half of the vagina with your thumbs. With your thumbs hooked in the vagina, pull forward to stretch the skin as you massage.
- Not sure you're doing the first part properly? Insert your fingers into the corners of your mouth and pull your mouth open to the sides for a similar "burning" sensation.

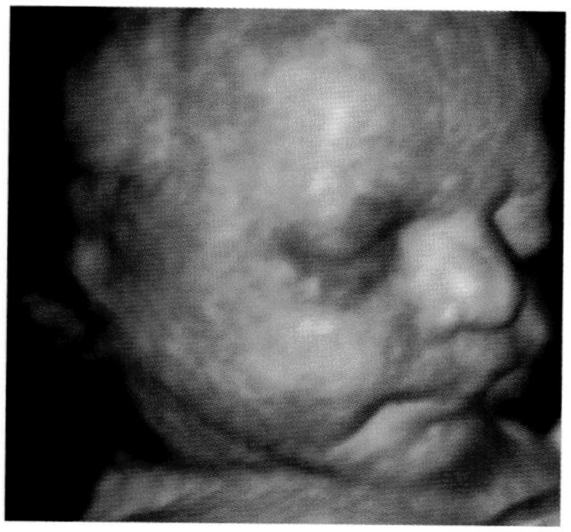

YOU ARE **33 WEEKS AND 3 DAYS**

46 days to go

YOUR BABY TODAY

At this stage, it is simply no longer possible to see the whole baby on a scan. The ultrasound scan cannot not step far enough back to include the whole baby in a single view. Instead it is necessary to move the probe around, to examine one area at a time.

> "Most women want to wait as long as possible to start maternity leave, but you must make the decision that is right for you."

You may decide to work right up until you deliver, and it is generally safe to do so, but by this week, you are likely to find yourself increasingly tired. If you want to start your leave sooner, speak to your employer. Hopefully, they will be understanding, but realize that if you start your maternity leave early, you may have to come back to work sooner (see pp.348–349). But if you are struggling to cope with the discomforts of late pregnancy, the decision to take leave of absence during the last four weeks, work flex-time, or work from home may be the right move for you. Talk to your doctor and your employer as soon as you make this decision.

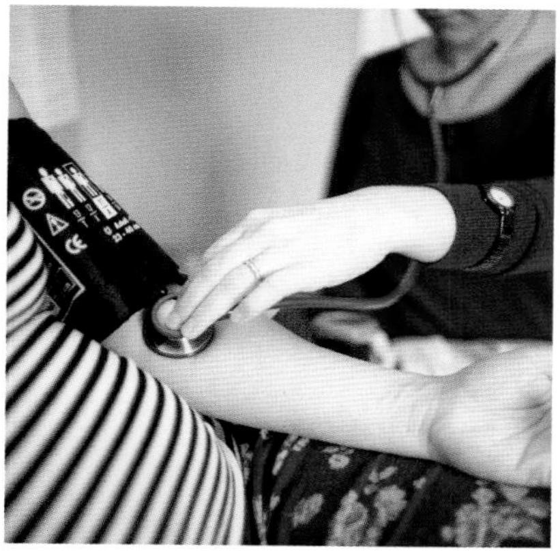

Your blood pressure will be monitored regularly at this stage because a high reading can be a sign of preeclampsia.

ESSENTIAL CHECKS

Some of the regular tests you will have in the third trimester are designed to check for preeclampsia (see p.474). A combination of high (or rising) blood pressure and protein in your urine can be an indication of preeclampsia; another sign of this condition is extreme swelling, particularly of the face and/or ankles.

ASK A DOCTOR

Will I have to give back my maternity pay if I decide not to return to work? This is a little bit complicated, and it's a good idea to get some legal advice. In a nutshell, if you do not return to work after your maternity leave, you must resign.

Bear in mind that every situation and every company is different. You should let your company know of your decision as soon as possible. Make an appointment with your human resources representative to discuss your company's policies so you have plenty of time to think about your options. Also keep in mind that if your company lets you take vacation or sick days that you haven't yet accrued as part of your leave, they may ask you to reimburse them for those days if you're not returning to work.

This happens quite often, and your boss may not be surprised to hear that you're not returning to work. If you're not 100 percent certain about not returning to work, it may be a good idea to ask your employer about coming back to work on a part-time basis or working from home.

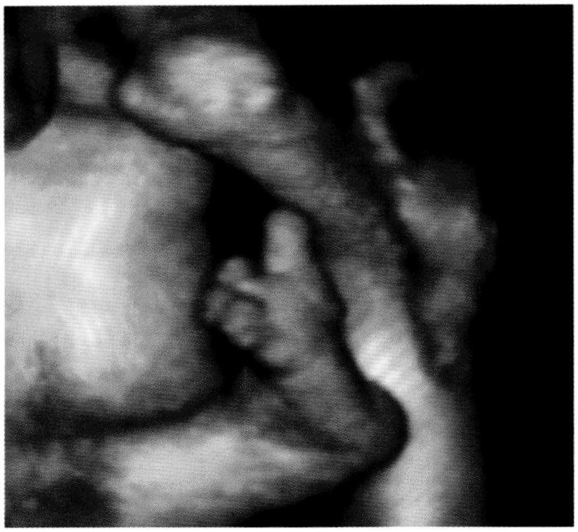

YOU ARE **33 WEEKS AND 4 DAYS**

45 days to go

YOUR BABY TODAY

A foot is shown here with the toes spread out. Not all of the movements that you feel will be due to kicks; some movements will be shrugs or punches and some from the bottom or head as it touches the sides of the uterus.

> “The size of your belly will increasingly be due to the baby alone as the amniotic fluid now reduces slightly each week.”

The amount of amniotic fluid that surrounds and protects your baby is now at its maximum and the placenta has almost completed its growth.

Amniotic fluid is essential for your baby's lung development, gut maturation, protein requirements, and temperature control. Adequate fluid also allows your baby to move easily since they are in an almost weightless state. There is about 1 liter (35 fl oz) of fluid around your baby. The range, however, is quite wide and "normal" can be anywhere between 300 ml to 2 liters (11–70 fl oz). Sometimes there is too little fluid (oligohydramnios; see p.475), or too much fluid (polyhydramnios; see p.475). In this situation you would be closely monitored and premature delivery might be necessary.

It's not surprising that the size of your uterus may not reflect the size of your baby since there can be so much variation in the quantity of fluid.

As the amount of amniotic fluid reduces in late pregnancy, your baby is not as well cushioned and her movements may become more obvious. If you are not feeling your baby move like normal, or having decreased fetal movement, it is important to notify your prenatal provider immediately..

WATERS BREAKING IN PUBLIC

One of the most common concerns for women in late pregnancy is that their water will break in public.

The reality is that the amniotic fluid is unlikely to gush out. It is much more likely to trickle out because in a head-down position, the baby will press down on the cervix and prevent the liquid from escaping. If it does happen in public, don't worry—you won't be short of people offering help.

FOCUS ON PARTNERS

Once your partner's labor begins, your attention will need to be focused on helping her both practically and emotionally. So in addition to helping your partner prepare her maternity bag (see p.358) in advance, it's a good idea to prepare a bag of your own.

You should plan to be at the hospital for several days, as you may be asked to stay and support your partner until they are discharged from the hospital.

Consider packing the following:

- Snacks
- Drinks
- A pillow
- Something to read or play
- Some money to buy tea and coffee or other snacks (including change for vending machines)
- A list of phone numbers, or enter them into your cell phone now
- A camera.

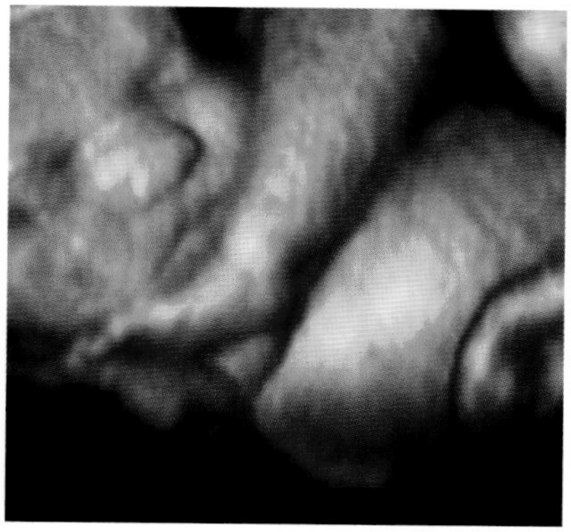

YOU ARE **33 WEEKS AND 5 DAYS**

44 days to go

YOUR BABY TODAY

At this stage your baby may lie transversely (see p.336) across your uterus as here, but such a position becomes increasingly less likely as the pregnancy advances. The more babies you have had the more likely it is that the shape of your uterus allows this lie.

When you are tense and frightened, pain can feel much worse, so teaching yourself to relax and stay calm can help. With around six weeks to go, you still have plenty of time to try out some of the breathing and relaxation techniques that will help you during labor. It's true that practice makes perfect, and it can take some time to train your mind to relax at will, especially if you are in pain.

Spend a short period of time as often as you can, every day if possible, practicing your breathing—close your eyes and slow your breathing down, breathing in through your nose and out through your mouth. As you breathe in, imagine your breath entering your body and relaxing you, and as you exhale you breathe out any pain or tension. You might want to involve your partner by asking them to breathe with you or count your breathing, a slow count to three or five for every inhale and exhale.

Some women like to practice using the techniques while pinching their arm temporarily to simulate a contraction—although of course it won't mimic the pain exactly! Practicing these techniques in a calm, relaxed manner in late pregnancy will help you to use them effectively on the big day.

“ You may be learning breathing and relaxation techniques at prenatal classes, but practice them at home, too. ”

FUEL FOR FITNESS

Demand for nutrients is higher when you're exercising and even higher when you're pregnant. This is not the time to reach for low-nutrient, high-calorie snacks; ensure you make careful choices when it comes to the nutrients you put into your body.

You should be eating a snack before you exercise, consisting of a complex carbohydrate and a protein. You should also eat frequent small meals and snacks if you are feeling hungry. It's fine to snack throughout the day.

Some healthy snack ideas are as follows:

- Half a bagel spread with two teaspoons of peanut butter
- An apple or banana and a handful of raw almonds
- A pear with two slices of Cheddar cheese
- Carrot, celery, and cucumber sticks and/or breadsticks dipped into two tablespoons of hummus
- Cottage cheese or cream cheese spread on two large crackers or whole wheat toast.

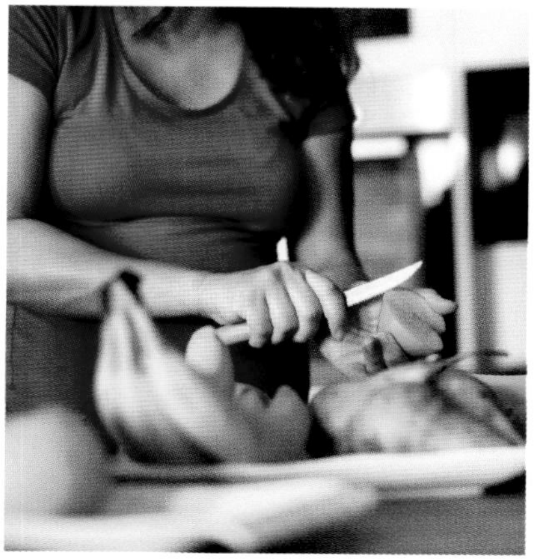

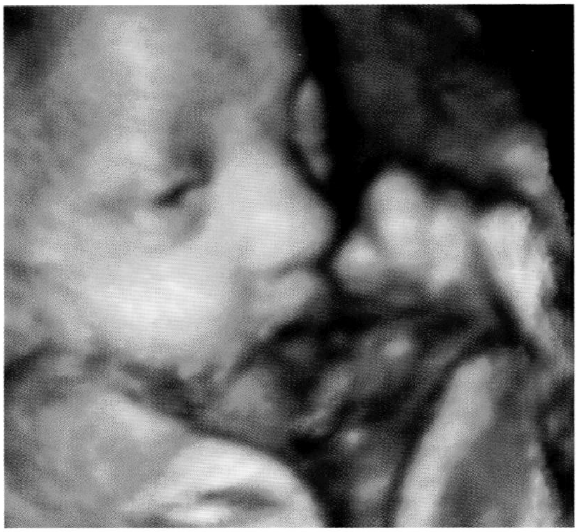

YOU ARE **33 WEEKS AND 6 DAYS**

43 days to go...

YOUR BABY TODAY

Your baby is now capable of producing all of the enzymes that will process food within the digestive tract. If born early, your baby could now feed normally, although some will still require help since they need to fine-tune the coordination of their suckling reflexes.

> "Your baby is naturally nourished inside the uterus and her own digestive tract is now functioning well."

Although the placenta grows most rapidly in the first three months, it becomes increasingly important in transferring nutrients and energy to your baby in the last trimester.

The carbohydrates you eat are broken down into glucose and the placenta transfers glucose to your baby for her own energy needs. This includes converting some glucose into protective fat reserves. These reserves are important because if your baby is born too early, she won't have had time to accumulate enough fat to keep herself warm.

The protein you eat is broken down into its constituent amino acids. The placenta keeps about 30 percent more amino acids circulating in your baby's blood than in yours. Eating protein is vital to build new cells and your unborn baby's vital organs.

Fats from your diet are essential this trimester. They are split up and cross the placenta to your baby as omega-3 fatty acids. These are used to make essential tissues, such as those that help develop the nervous system, and those that help the brain and eyes develop properly.

GETTING UP FROM LYING DOWN

After you've exercised on the floor, or have been resting in bed, you may find it a struggle to get up from lying down. This simple maneuver can put a strain on your abdominal muscles, which are stretched, and it isn't helped by your altered center of gravity.

The technique shown below was originally devised by yoga teachers. As with any strenuous maneuvers at this stage of pregnancy, always take your time and remember to breathe slowly and deeply throughout.

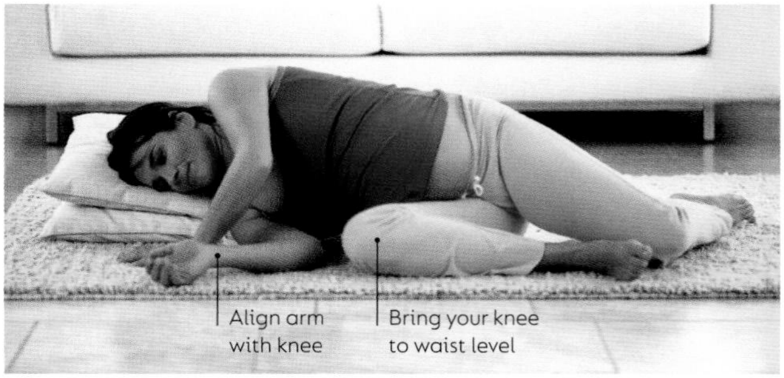
Align arm with knee
Bring your knee to waist level

With your knees bent, roll on to your right side bringing your knee to waist level. Keep your right hand aligned with your bent knee.

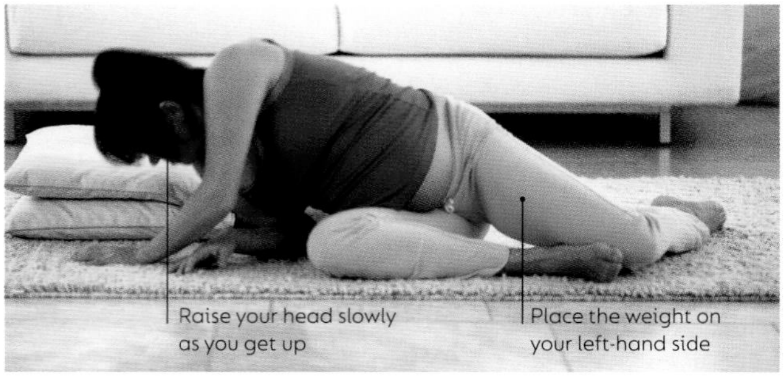
Raise your head slowly as you get up
Place the weight on your left-hand side

Shift your weight on to your left hand and knee. Position your right hand under your shoulder and come up slowly on all fours.

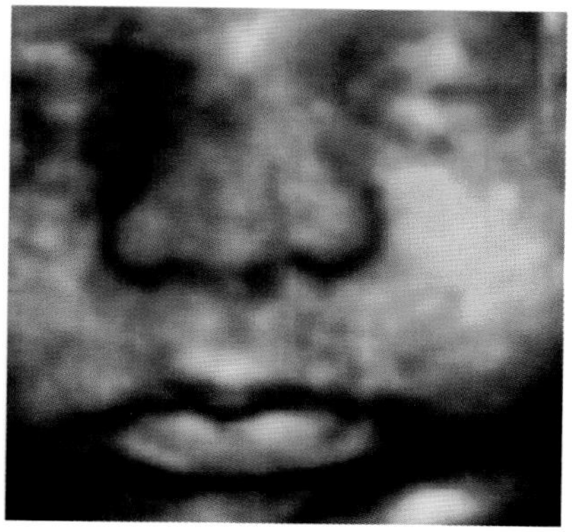

YOU ARE **34 WEEKS EXACTLY**

42 days to go...

YOUR BABY TODAY

A close-up of the baby's face clearly showing the lip shape and slightly separated eyelids. The slight shadowing seen to the left of the image is from the wall of the uterus, which at this stage of the pregnancy will always be very close to your baby.

Women had their babies at home for generations; it was only in the 20th century that women began to have hospital births. If you're considering a home birth, remember that the majority of pregnancies and births are normal and do not need any medical intervention.

Be reassured that if you have decided to have a home birth and then change your mind, for example you decide you want an epidural, or your midwife advises you that the baby needs help, you will be transferred to a hospital.

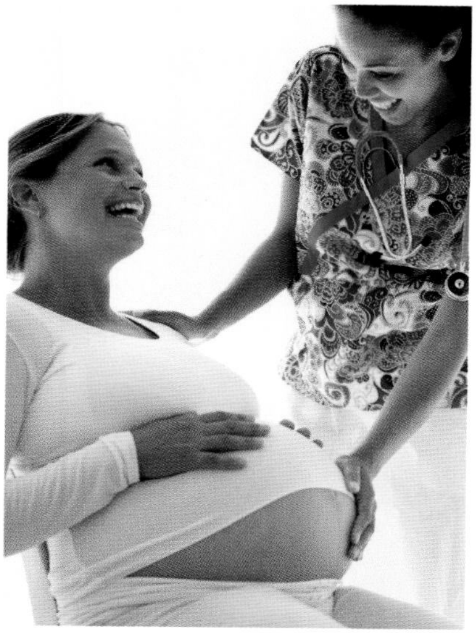

Your relationship with your midwife is even more important if you're giving birth at home as she will be your sole medical support.

> " If you've made the decision to have a home birth, you'll need to ensure you're fully prepared in good time. "

ASK A MIDWIFE

What additional things do I need to think about if I'm having a home birth? Have all the items you need for labor and birth gathered in the place you intend to deliver, and organize your items separately from the baby's items.

As well as practical items, such as clothing, toiletries, and sanitary pads, you may also want to have on hand music, phone numbers, and a camera. It's a good idea to have a well-stocked fridge, so make a list of nutritious foods to stock up on before your due date. This will help you during labor and in the first week of parenthood. Your baby will need diapers, cotton cloths, onesies, clothing, sheets, blankets, and a hat.

If you have other children, you may need to make arrangements for them to be taken care of.

Even though you're planning to have your baby at home, there are circumstances in which you may need to be transferred to the hospital. You should have an emergency bag packed (see p.358) just in case.

GROUP B STREP TEST

Ten to 30 percent of pregnant women carry the strep B bacteria in the vagina or rectal area. Known as group B streptococcus (GBS), it is usually harmless in adults, but can cause a rare and serious infection in newborn babies if untreated.

- Many women are now routinely screened for GBS, at 35–37 weeks of pregnancy. If the result is positive, antibiotic treatment can be given during labor that will reduce the risk of the baby becoming infected. Some hospitals don't screen but if the bacteria is detected in a urine test or a swab is taken for another reason and is positive, antibiotic treatment may given in labor.
- The test involves taking a swab of the area around your vagina and rectum.
- If treatment is given as soon as labour starts, there is little risk to the baby.
- It is possible to be infected with GBS in a second pregnancy, even if you didn't have it first time around.

Your 35th week

TRY TO STAY ACTIVE, EVEN THOUGH YOU MAY BE SLOWING DOWN BY NOW. Getting exercise is probably the last thing on your mind, but it's worth the effort. The more you move, the more energy you will gain. Gentle exercise will also help relieve some of the aches and pains of pregnancy at this stage. The baby's movements may also change as they have less room to move around. Instead of kicks, they may be shuffling around. They're busy, though, practicing for the outside world, learning to suckle and focus vision.

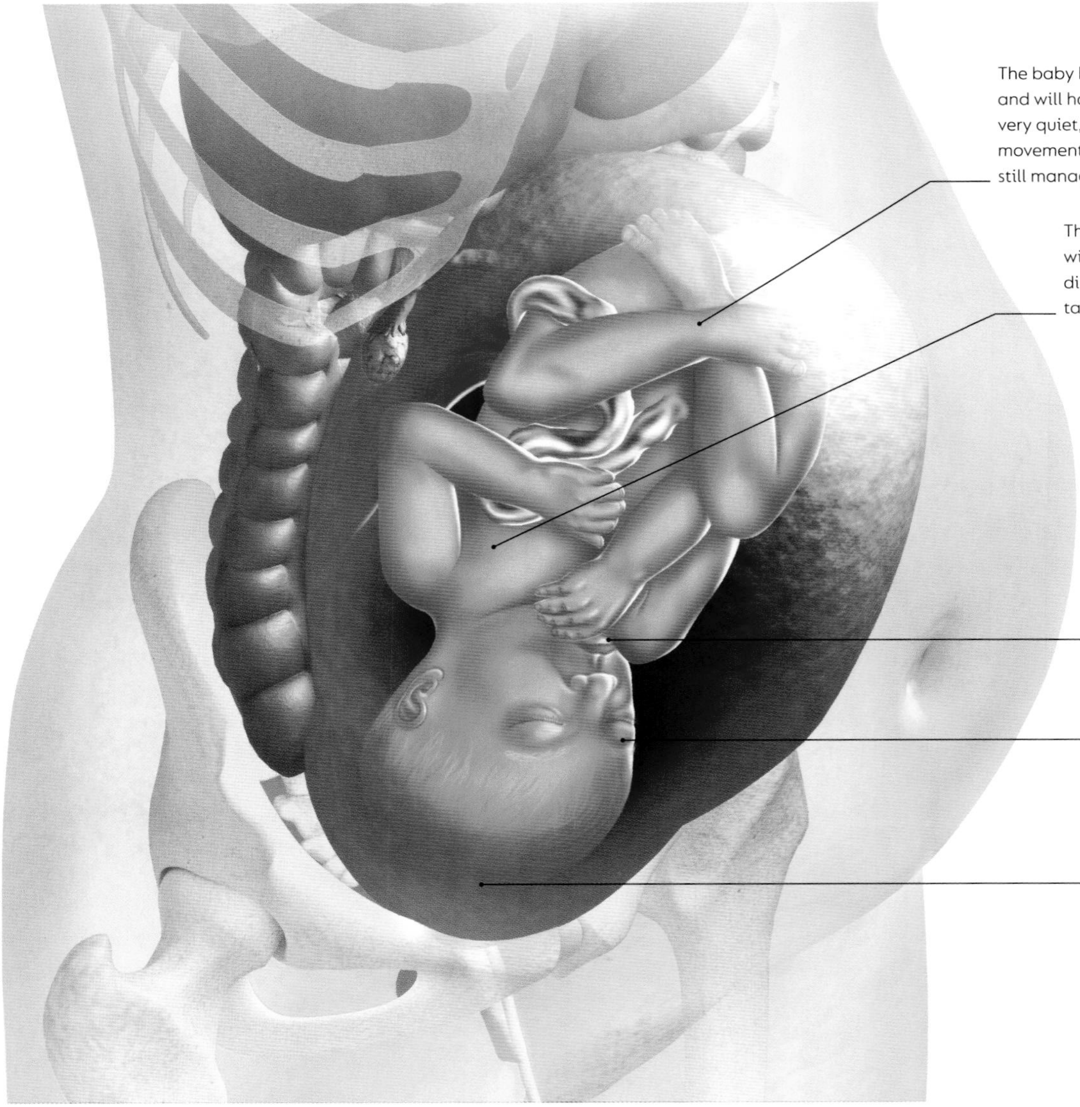

The baby has less room to maneuver and will have periods when he is very quiet, but you will feel some movements every day, and he can still manage some strong kicks.

The lungs are filled with fluid, which will disappear when the baby takes his first breath.

By practicing suckling movements, the baby is teaching himself how to feed when he is born.

The pupils of the eyes now dilate in response to light filtering into the uterus.

At 35 weeks the average crown to heel length is 18.2 in (46.2 cm) and the average weight is 5.3 lb (2.4 kg).

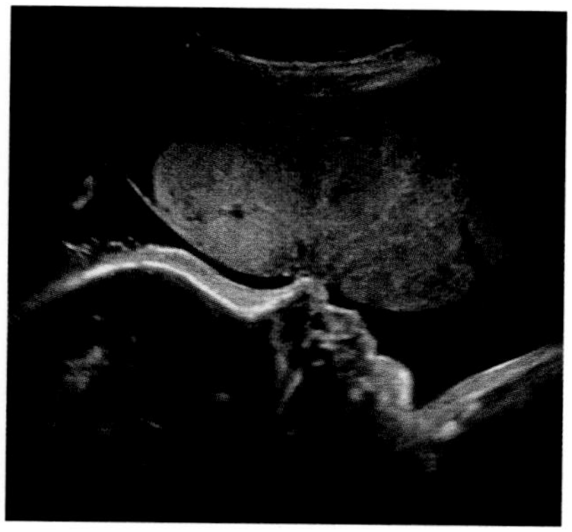

YOU ARE **34 WEEKS AND 1 DAY**

41 days to go

YOUR BABY TODAY

This profile of the baby shows the tip of the nose touching the placenta. Your placenta will not be growing any more and now thins slightly. Within, the placenta continues to mature and it remains a highly efficient means of supplying your baby's energy needs.

" As your size begins to have an impact on your daily activities, you'll find that a few practical adjustments are necessary. "

Your posture will change throughout pregnancy as your belly continues to grow. To compensate for the heavy weight you're carrying, you might find that you lean back slightly, especially when you're walking downhill. You might also waddle when you walk as you shift your weight from side to side. In a few weeks' time, when the baby begins to engage into the pelvis (see p.361), you may find that you waddle even more.

It's normal at this late stage of pregnancy to move more slowly than normal. You may find yourself struggling to get out of bed or out of a chair, and picking something up off the floor can be more difficult than usual. Tasks such as tying your shoelaces or painting your toenails can seem impossible. You can overcome tasks such as these—for example, by putting your feet on a stool to tie your shoelaces so you don't have to bend down so far. If you need help, there's no shame in asking. It can be difficult to be reliant on others, but remember it's only temporary.

ASK A DOCTOR

Can I have a water birth in the hospital? This depends on the maternity unit: some have birthing pools; others have facilities for you to rent a pool. More hospitals and birthing centers are offering this birthing option, so ask about renting a pool and bringing it in, but realize that just might not be an option.

Most hospitals will support you laboring in a pool or tub, however there are increased risks to your baby with a water birth and is usually not recommended.

A DIABETIC PREGNANCY

Whether you develop diabetes in pregnancy (known as gestational diabetes—see p.475), or have preexisting diabetes, you'll require special care from your doctor. They will figure out a plan for you, since diabetes poses risk in pregnancy.

In the mother, these risks include having high blood pressure, blood clots, preeclampsia (see p.476), polyhydramnios (see p.475), as well as an increased chance of having a Cesarean delivery. For the unborn baby, there is an increased risk of congenital abnormalities, and growth may be too fast or too slow.

Controlling blood-sugar levels reduces the risk of birth defects and stillbirth, or of you having a larger-than-expected baby, which can lead to problems during the birth. The key to a healthy pregnancy and baby when you have diabetes is blood-sugar control, often achieved through dietary changes. You will need special help to adapt your diet to include more carbohydrates and fiber and reduce your intake of fats and sugar.

Some women also require oral medication or, occasionally, insulin injections.

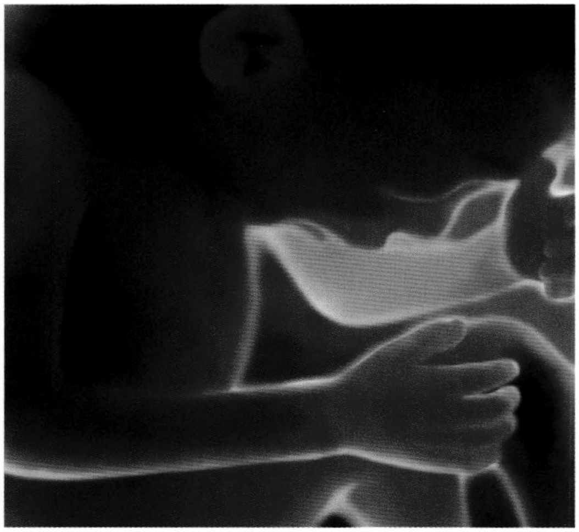

YOU ARE **34 WEEKS AND 2 DAYS**

40 days to go

YOUR BABY TODAY

At the back of your baby's eye, nerve cells that identify either black and white or color are maturing. The cells that respond to color signals are the last to develop, but will eventually process more than half of the information that the eyes receive.

" Your baby is blinking and learning to focus, and their pupils will dilate in response to light filtering through the uterus. "

Your baby's eyes first began to develop two weeks after conception, and then all of the major eye structures are formed over the following four weeks. The eye, however, keeps growing during the pregnancy and the optic nerve continues to develop after birth.

The eyes have been opening since 26 weeks of pregnancy but, until now, eye movements have been poorly coordinated. Eye movements are first seen at 18 weeks, but they are random and infrequent. Movements become more frequent from 26 weeks and now, in the final few weeks, movements settle into a cycle of rest alternating with rapid eye movements (REM).

Some light does get through into the uterus and your baby is now much more responsive to strong lights.

ASK A MOM

I'm concerned my maternity leave substitute will do a better job than me. Are these fears normal? Yes, completely normal. I remember being worried that the man filling in for me would outshine me. The amazing thing was that once my baby was born, anything work related was eclipsed by my new role. Far from losing skills, I became an efficient multi-tasker and when I returned to work, found the job easier than taking care of a baby.

Feeling this way is normal, but try not to worry. Not only do you have legal rights regarding the safety of your job (see pp.348–349), but you will have your chance to shine once again when your baby has settled into childcare. In the meantime, enjoy your leave. It goes quickly, but also presents you with an opportunity to hone some important life skills.

GETTING OUT AND ABOUT

In most cases, it's perfectly safe to drive in the months leading up to the end of your pregnancy. However, if you feel that you're not able to concentrate at the wheel, or driving makes you uncomfortable, then give it a pass. When driving, it's very important that you position your lap belt directly under your belly (see p.253), to ensure that there is no danger to your baby if you are involved in an accident.

Traveling by public transportation is fine, too, but for your safety, be sure to request a seat, even if they are all occupied. Being jolted around on a train or bus won't hurt your baby, but you are more likely to fall because of the shift in your center of gravity and could injure your abdomen. Long periods of standing can also cause your ankles and feet to swell.

If you're feeling uncomfortable or dizzy, get off the train or bus and sit down in a cooler environment, preferably with your feet up, for about 20 minutes. Always carry water with you when you're out.

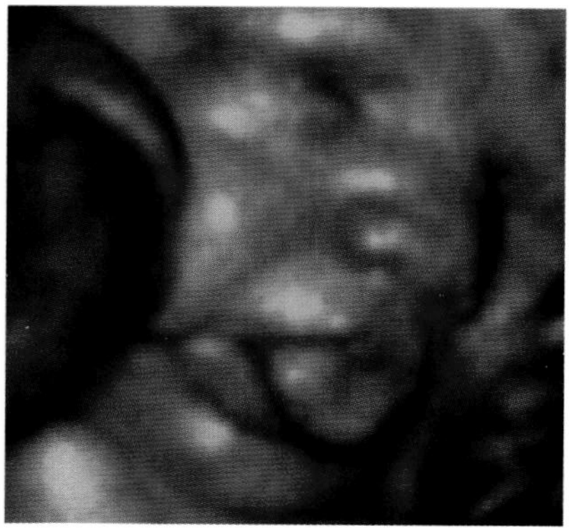

YOU ARE **34 WEEKS AND 3 DAYS**

39 days to go

YOUR BABY TODAY

Your baby will often stick their tongue out, as part of the development of the reflexes needed to feed. The rooting reflex enables your baby to find the nipple, then the strong suckling reflexes take over to coordinate breathing, feeding, and swallowing.

Dressing your newborn baby doesn't have to be expensive. Don't be shy about asking friends and family members for hand-me-downs, and consider getting together with your prenatal group, and arrange a clothing swap. While the idea of your baby wearing "used" clothing may feel strange at first, it's actually ideal for the environment and your budget as most babies grow out of clothes very quickly.

Look on the internet for end-of-season sales, and even on some of the auction sites, where you can often pick up designer goodies for a fraction of the original price. Visit yard sales or garage sales. Shop around; you don't have to pay a lot for items such as sleep sacks and will find inexpensive prices in the superstores. Make a purchase with your weekly grocery shopping and you won't notice the cost as much.

Remember, too, that you will probably receive numerous gifts of clothing from friends and family when your baby is born. If you know exactly what you'd like, you may like to create a gift registry from a favorite store or ask people for gift certificates for that store. When looking for more expensive items of clothing, head for the three- to six-month-old rack, so that your baby will get plenty of use out of them. It can be disappointing if your newborn only gets a couple of weeks' wear out of an outfit you like.

" When it comes to buying baby clothes on a budget, there are many creative ways to save money. "

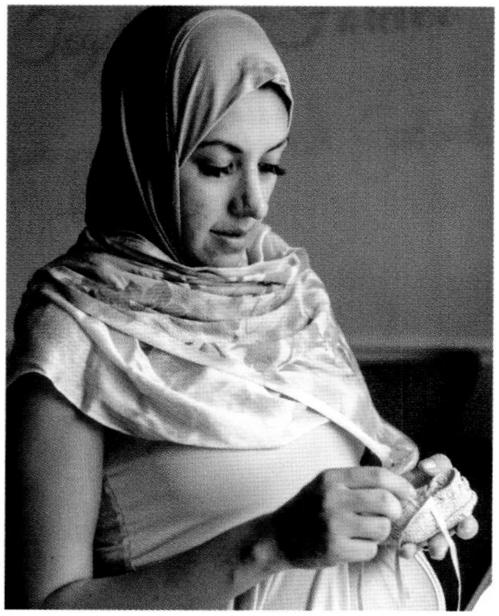

FOCUS ON PARTNERS

It's quite normal to feel concerned about getting through labor on the day, and focusing on your partner and attending to her needs may help keep you distracted and reduce your anxiety. If possible, try to develop a good relationship in the coming weeks with your partner's caregivers. This way you'll feel more able to express any worries you're having, and hopefully get the reassurance and information you need.

If you find yourself feeling woozy on the day, try to leave the room since the nurses and doctor will be focused on caring for your partner. If you don't have time to leave the room to seek help when you feel faint, sit down immediately, with your head lower than your hips, or lie down with your feet raised. Try to stop yourself from panicking by taking slow, deep breaths. You'll find that the feeling passes quickly.

A good tip is to make sure that you are not too hot and to eat and drink regularly to prevent you from feeling faint due to low blood sugar.

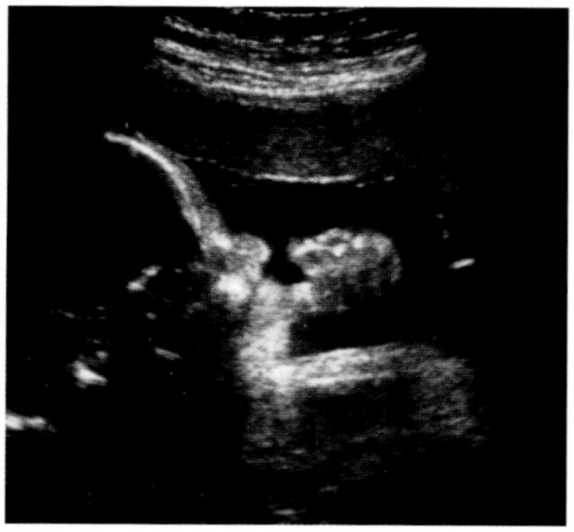

YOU ARE **34 WEEKS AND 4 DAYS**

38 days to go

YOUR BABY TODAY

This 2-D ultrasound has captured the moment that the baby is sucking their thumb. Your baby is gradually learning to coordinate this complex activity with breathing movements even though they are surrounded not by air but by the amniotic fluid.

“Inside the uterus your baby is already practicing the suckling reflex, which will enable them to feed when they’re born.”

The suckling reflex is present earlier in pregnancy but it is known from assessing premature babies that it’s usually not until around this time that the baby is strong and coordinated enough to suckle with ease. Your baby regularly practices suckling and this, in combination with the rooting reflex, will enable your baby to feed.

After birth you will see the rooting reflex as your baby turns toward anything that strokes his cheek. The head will turn, and your baby will move his mouth in a series of gradually diminishing circles until the object is found. Once feeding is well established, at about four months, the rooting reflex disappears. From this point on, your baby has much more control over the process, able to turn and directly latch on (see pp.450–1) to the nipple.

While in the uterus, there is no chance of your baby accidentally swallowing amniotic fluid into the lungs. The lungs are already filled with fluid and the high pressure of this, together with your baby’s larynx, keeps out amniotic fluid. After birth, babies have a series of reflexes designed to keep breathing and drinking separate. To help with feeding, babies always breathe through their nose.

ASK A DOCTOR

My mom has offered to stay with us after the birth. Is this a good idea? Some couples prefer to get to know their baby on their own, taking the first few days to settle in and get used to the idea of being new parents. It’s also good to try to do things your own way when it comes to caring for your newborn. Having said that, you’ll find an extra pair of hands invaluable.

It really depends on your relationship with your mom: if it’s good and you feel she’ll be supportive, then it’s more likely to help than hinder. However, gently establish some guidelines—namely that while you welcome her help, you’d like to do things your way and have space to bond with your baby. Encourage your mom toward helping around the house, rather than just with the baby, not least so that your partner doesn’t feel excluded at this important time.

ARE YOU READY FOR THE BABY?

You may find that you soon become too tired to go out shopping and carry lots of bags. Buy a few items at a time and shop online when you can.

There are certain things that are worthwhile purchasing by around 37 weeks, just in case you go into labor before your due date. First, buy the small baby-care items you’ll need right after the birth (see p.269) plus a car seat and a bassinet or crib. If going out shopping becomes difficult in late pregnancy, consider buying some items online.

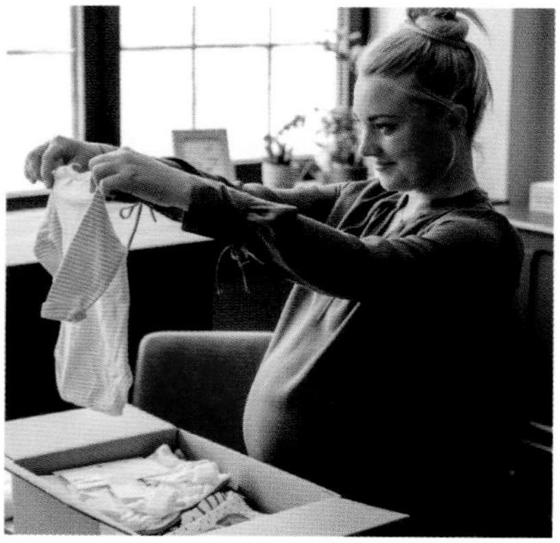

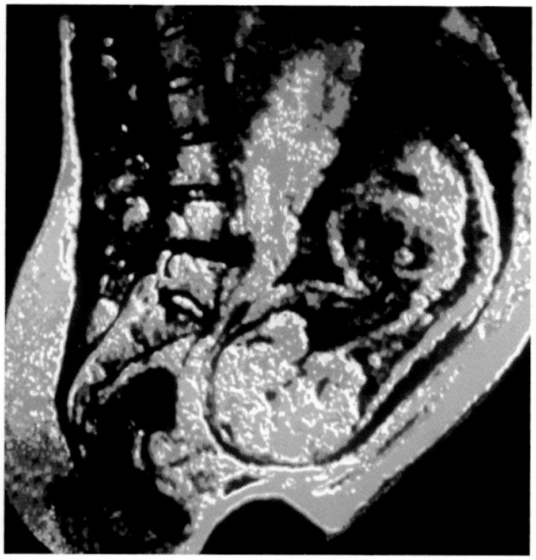

YOU ARE **34 WEEKS AND 5 DAYS**

37 days to go

YOUR BABY TODAY

This is an MRI image showing a cross section of the entire pregnancy. The mother's spine is on the left of the image, and the baby is lying head down within the pelvis. An MRI is rarely needed during pregnancy, but if recommended, it is entirely safe.

> "You'll probably find yourself analyzing every ache and pain in these final weeks of your pregnancy."

By this stage of pregnancy every time you get a twinge you may worry that it's the onset of labor. This is a normal concern, but try to remember that, even though you're heavily pregnant, most aches and pains are still likely to be due to constipation, or stretching ligaments, rather than labor.

You may begin to have Braxton Hicks contractions; these practice contractions occur as the uterus tightens as a warm-up for labor. They also help direct more blood to the placenta in the final weeks of pregnancy. Some women are unaware of them, while for others they can be quite uncomfortable. Relaxing the uterine muscles by changing your position, walking around, or taking a warm bath can help.

If you're unsure whether the pains you're having are Braxton Hicks, always consult your doctor.

ASK A MOM

What will I need if I'm planning to breastfeed? I found all the following items really useful:

- **Nursing bras** that can be unclipped at the front or have zip-open cups. Get properly fitted (bearing in mind that your breasts will be bigger once your milk comes in). You'll need several nursing bras.
- Nipple **cream:** this is soothing if you have cracked nipples.
- **Breast pads** (disposable or washable). Slip them inside your bra to absorb any leaks between feedings. Alternatively, breast shells slot inside your bra to catch any excess milk.
- **Breastfeeding pillow:** a V-shaped pillow isn't essential, but it will help you and your baby get comfortable.
- **Burp cloths** to catch dribbles.
- **Breast pump** and bottles or bags for storing expressed milk.

PREPARING FOR BREASTFEEDING

If you've decided to breastfeed (see pp.450–451), know that it doesn't always come naturally, so make it easier by being prepared:

- **Read all about it.** If you're expecting some of the discomforts, they won't come as such a shock and you may be able to take measures to prevent them. It can help, for example, to know how to latch on your baby correctly (see p.450).
- **Address any concerns** before your baby is born: ask your doctor, or friends who've breastfed.
- **See how it's done** by visiting a breastfeeding group (ask your doctor to recommend one). You may have been concerned about breastfeeding in public, so it can help to see how discreetly it can be done. You could also ask a friend to let you watch her position and breastfeed her baby.
- **Look for a lactation consultant**—available from your doctor, or maybe a friend can recommend one, or contact the La Leche League (see p.482) for a list of counselors.

Your rights and benefits

Having a baby is a huge life change, and many new parents find time and money are in short supply. Maternity and parental leave and pay can help ease the transition, so it's worth finding out what you're entitled to.

Your rights

When you have a baby, you can take up to 12 weeks off work during a 12-month period and retain your right to return to the same, or an equivalent, position, including equivalent pay and benefits, if you are eligible to be covered by the Family and Medical Leave Act (FMLA). Employees eligible for FMLA have worked for their employers for at least 12 months, including at least 1,250 hours during the previous 12 months. Additionally, the employee must work within 75 miles of where 50 or more employees work. FMLA leave is guaranteed unpaid, but employers or employees can opt to use paid vacation or sick time, when this is allowed by an employer. Both men and women are eligible for FMLA leave, which applies to private employees, all state and local government employees, and some federal employees.

Your employer is required to continue your health insurance coverage during your FMLA leave. If you've been paying a portion of your health insurance premiums, you'll have to continue doing so during your FMLA leave. If you don't want to take all 12 weeks of FMLA leave in a row, you may be able to break it down into shorter blocks of time, or even a shorter work week or work day. When possible, employees who are planning to use FMLA leave are required to tell their employers 30 days before the leave would begin. But if you have pregnancy complications that require you to stop working before the baby is born, the 12 weeks of FMLA leave would begin then.

Maternity pay

According to 2015 data from the US Department of Labor's Bureau of Labor Statistics, just 12 percent of all workers were eligible for paid family leave. According to the Institute for Women's Policy Research, which analyzed 2006 rankings for America's 100 most family-friendly employers, 93 percent of those best-ranked companies provide at least one week of paid maternity leave, but 52 percent of the companies pay for six weeks or less. Every company has its own policies for maternity leave. If an employer does provide compensation, the amount you'll receive may depend on what you earn and how long you've been working for the company. The best way to find out what you may be eligible for is to meet with a human resources representative or read the employee handbook. You may be allowed to use paid sick time, vacation days, or the company's short-term disability coverage, in addition to paid leave.

Partners at home

Far fewer employers offer paid leave to partners than paid maternity leave

PAID LEAVE: THE FACTS

Some states have passed laws that offer new parents paid maternity leave and, in many cases, paternity leave. California was the first state to pass such legislation. Through its Paid Family Leave Program, employees who participate in the State Disability Insurance Program can receive up to six weeks of partial pay for time off within the first year of their baby's birth. Two other states, Washington and New Jersey, have passed similar legislation, and other states may follow suit. Find out about the laws in your state.

BETTER BREAKS FOR PARENTS ABROAD

A recent report from researchers at Harvard University and McGill University found the US lags behind most other countries when it comes to paid maternity and paternity leave. Out of 173 countries studied, 168 offered working women guaranteed paid maternity leave. The US was one of only five countries that did not, along with Lesotho, Liberia, Papua New Guinea, and Swaziland. Sixty-six countries offered men paid paternity leave; the US did not.

to new moms. According to the Institute for Women's Policy Research, only 50 percent of 2006's 100 most family-friendly companies offered paid parental leave. Of them 35 percent paid for one to two weeks leave, and no companies paid for more than six weeks of parental leave. Partners who want to be home for a newborn's earliest days may be able to use paid vacation or sick leave, or they can take FMLA leave.

QUESTIONS AND ANSWERS

If I have to take a pregnancy-related absence, will my employer hold my job for me or will I be left without my job when I'm ready to return to work? According to the Pregnancy Discrimination Act, employers must hold open a job for a pregnancy-related absence for the same length of time that jobs are held open for employees on sick leave or on disability leave.

What happens to my eligibility for a bonus if I go on FMLA leave? You'll still be eligible. The Family and Medical Leave Act requires an employee to be given her same, or an equivalent, position, and that would include eligibility for bonuses, including perfect attendance bonuses. If you don't miss days before or after your FMLA leave, you will still be eligible for that bonus.

I've just been offered my dream job, but I'm eight weeks' pregnant. Should I keep mum or should I say something to my new employer? The Pregnancy Discrimination Act states that employers cannot refuse to hire a woman because of her pregnancy or a because of a pregnancy-related condition.

Going back to work

Before returning to work, consider:
• Will life as a working mom be easier if you switch to a flexible working arrangement, such as a job share or part-time work? Give your employer ample time to consider any request.
• If you're breastfeeding, will your employer provide a private, clean, and safe room for you to express and store breast milk?
• You're entitled to time off (it may be unpaid) for family emergencies.
• You may be eligible for working and child tax credits, which can help with child-care costs..

Breastfeeding

Most states (47 of them) have laws that protect a mother's basic right to breastfeed her child. But women still experience negative reactions when they nurse in public. Nearly half of the states (21 of them) have laws that protect women's rights related to lactation and employment. Being able to pump at work prolongs the amount of time that you can breastfeed your baby, so these protections are important to breastfeeding moms. According to La Leche league, during an 8-hour workday, many moms find time to pump three times a day: during morning, lunch, and afternoon breaks. Since time is a premium at work, many moms get by with double-pumping with electric pumps, which should supply enough milk for the following day. La Leche League recommends that working moms should breastfeed their babies when they are at home mornings, evenings, and weekends.

Child care

If you will be returning to work, you will likely need child care for your baby. It is wise to look into your child care options while you are still pregnant, because it may take time to make a decision, and some programs may have long waiting lists. Contact a local child-care resource and referral center for recommendations. Some employers offer flexible spending accounts to employees that reduce salary by a set amount to pay for tax-preferred expenditures like day care. You won't pay taxes on the set-aside funds. Check with your human resources department to see if a flexible spending account is available to you. .

BABY AND CHILD BENEFITS

Your baby will need health insurance coverage just like you do. When your baby is born, you'll need to add them to your health insurance plan so they can get the coverage they will need. Most health insurance companies make the process easy. Typically you'll just need to call your health plan and tell them your baby's name and the date of your baby's birth, and your baby will automatically be added to your plan. For most insurance plans, you will have 30 days to give notice of the birth. From then, your baby will be covered for doctor appointments in the same way that you are.

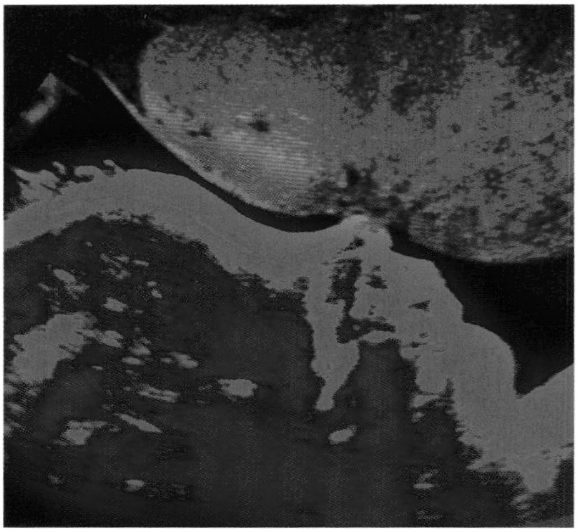

YOU ARE **34 WEEKS AND 6 DAYS**

36 days to go

YOUR BABY TODAY

The placenta, shown in red above the baby's green profile, is now receiving 18 fl oz (0.5 liter) of blood each minute from your circulation. In order to accommodate this increase, your blood volume expanded dramatically in the first few months of the pregnancy.

"It's never too late to improve your fitness, and whatever you do now will serve you well in labor."

ASK A DOCTOR

Why are some babies born prematurely? There are certain factors that can increase your risk of going into preterm labor, but the truth is the exact cause of preterm birth is not known. Some lifestyle factors, such as cigarette smoking, are strongly associated with preterm delivery. Twin pregnancy or a prenatal infection can also increase the risk of preterm labor. Some people may need to deliver early due to complications such as preeclampsia or diabetes, or if the baby is not growing well enough due to poor placental function. Having a previous baby who was born preterm also increases the likelihood of having another baby born prematurely.

You might be in the final few weeks, but you will want to stay active. Exercising regularly and consistently will enable you to reap the rewards of your efforts: increased fitness, higher self-esteem, and much more energy.

Find activities that you enjoy: swimming and walking are often favored by pregnant women in this late stage. As well as helping to improve fitness, both of these activities will help you to relax and unwind.

Always listen to your body and stop if you feel that you are over-exerting yourself.

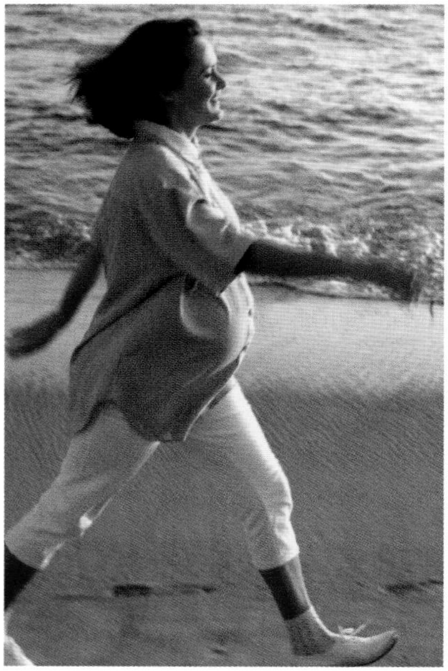

If you go for a daily walk you will feel energized and it will be good preparation for all those strolls you'll be doing with your baby.

KANGAROO CARE

If your premature baby goes into a Neonatal Intensive Care Unit (NICU) (see pp.454–455) you may be able to take care of him using a method called kangaroo care. You will be asked to hold your baby on your chest between your breasts with his head turned so that his ear is next to your heart.

Developed in Bogota, Columbia, in response to a lack of incubators, kangaroo care is shown to have many benefits for NICU babies—mainly that their heart and breathing rates regularize quite quickly, allowing them to sleep for much longer periods. The baby's temperature is regulated by the temperature fluctuations in your breasts, meaning he doesn't have to expend energy keeping himself warm.

This, in addition to the extra sleep, preserves his energy for other vital functions, such as brain development and weight gain. Breast-feeding is also more successful and some kangarooed babies lose none of their birth weight.

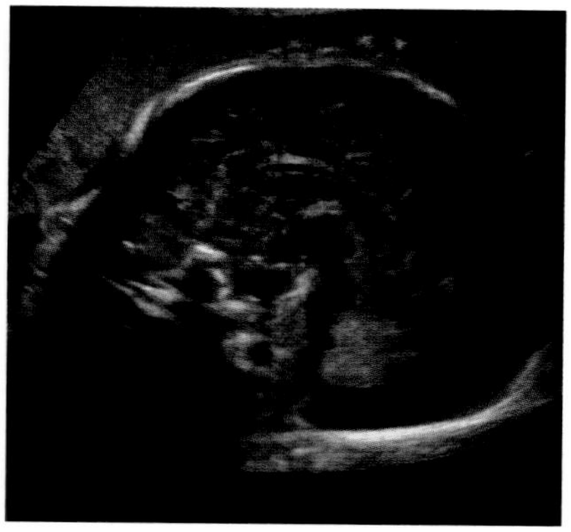

YOU ARE **35 WEEKS EXACTLY**

35 days to go

YOUR BABY TODAY

Your baby's brain continues to mature. This image shows that the folding pattern overlying the cerebral hemispheres has now developed, giving rise to the familiar folds and grooves on the brain's surface. The bright reflections are from the bony skull.

Before the birth, it can be difficult to imagine having a relationship with your baby, even though you may feel a close bond during pregnancy.

Fortunately, bonding is a chemical process in your brain when you give birth. Other people's babies may leave you feeling cold, but it's highly likely that your own baby will spark all kinds of feelings that you never even knew you could experience.

It's normal to worry about being a mother—coping with the responsibility, taking care of a helpless baby, being "good enough," and making lifestyle changes. However, when your baby is born, your priorities will become abundantly clear, as will your affections—although bonding may not always be instant.

In some cases, postpartum depression (see p.477), or even the short-term baby blues (see p.452), can interrupt the natural progression of feelings a mother has for her newborn baby.

> "The reality of being a mother will begin to hit you in these final weeks, and you have everything to look forward to."

PAMPER YOURSELF

You may not feel particularly lovely, but that's all the more reason to pamper yourself. There's unlikely to be time for beauty rituals once the baby is born.

- **Treat yourself to a manicure,** but don't have nail extensions for when your baby is born—sharp implements and babies don't mix.
- **Indulge in a facial:** it will make you feel good and help you relax.
- **Have your hair cut** since it may be some time before you get to the hairdresser again. It's a good idea to opt for a style that will be easy to manage once your baby arrives.
- **If you have aches and pains,** book a massage with someone who specializes in pregnancy.
- **Have a pedicure** a week or two before the birth. You'll be thrilled once your belly is gone and you're able to see your feet again.

ASK A DOCTOR

Will I be able to breastfeed my twins?
Yes, but if possible, arrange for a lactation consultant with experience in feeding twins to be available after birth. If you get the positions correct and know how to latch on your babies (see p.450) at the outset, you'll feel much more confident continuing on your own.

Many moms of twins find that feeding them simultaneously, using a specially designed breastfeeding pillow, is the easiest way to manage. This is something you may want to buy now. There are a variety of effective breastfeeding positions for twins that the consultant or a midwife can show you.

Your 36th week

GET TOGETHER WITH YOUR PARTNER AND TALK THROUGH YOUR BIRTH PLANS. Don't leave crucial arrangements until the last minute. Have an action plan ready for when you go into labor—it might be sooner than you think. Babies can arrive ahead of schedule, so make sure you and your partner feel confident about managing. Figure out practicalities, such as arranging care for other children, or even the cat. Rope in your parents or friends to help if need be, pack your hospital bag, and relax.

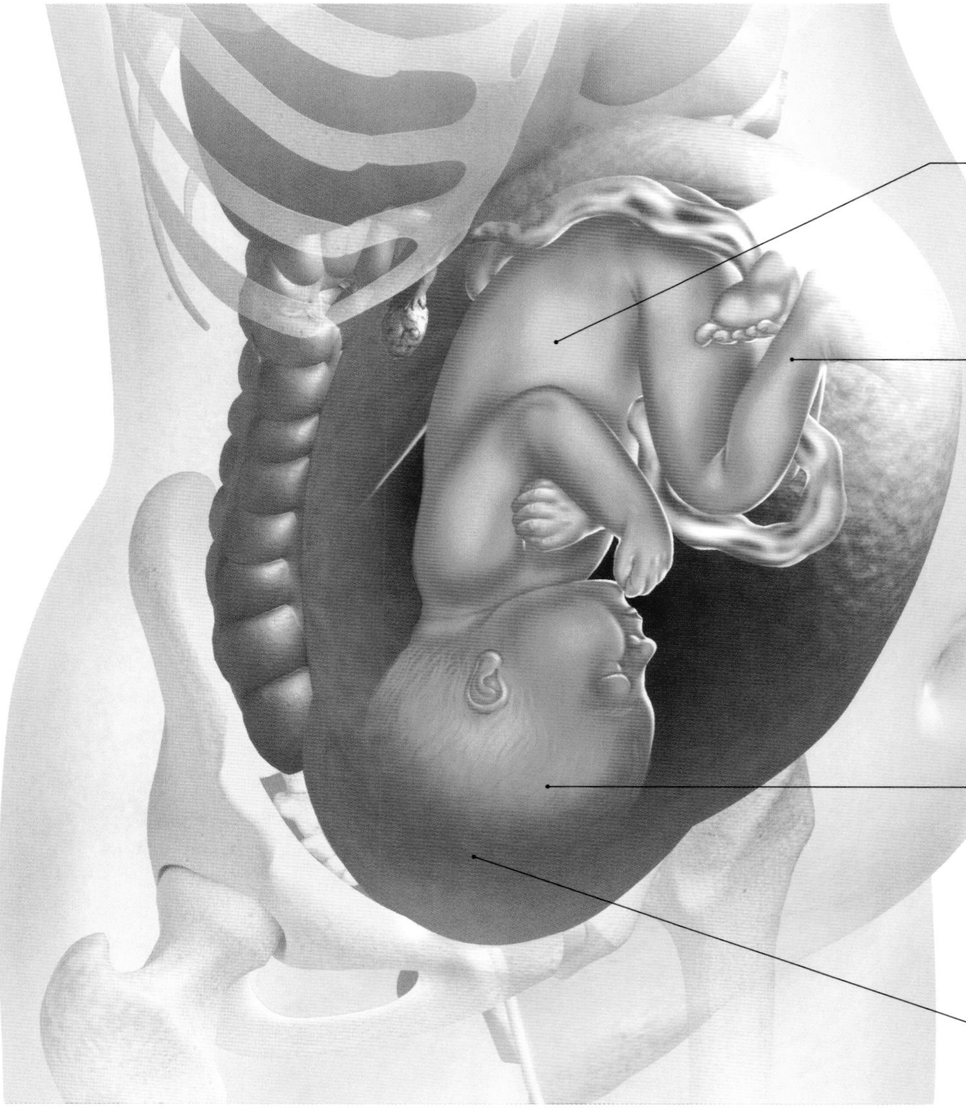
The lungs are structurally complete and the air sacs, or alveoli, are producing a lubricant called surfactant, which will help keep the sacs open when the baby takes her first lungful of air.
The uterus has very little remaining space, so most babies lie curled up, with their limbs folded closely against their bodies.
The head may be starting to engage, dropping down lower in the pelvis toward the birth canal in readiness for the start of labor. Your doctor will be keeping a close eye on the baby's position.
At 36 weeks the average crown to heel length is 18.7 in (47.4 cm) and the average weight is 5.8 lb (2.6 kg).

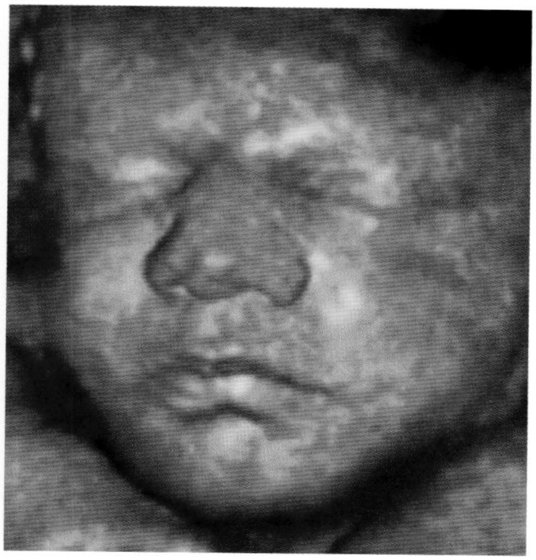

YOU ARE **35 WEEKS AND 1 DAY**

34 days to go

YOUR BABY TODAY

Your baby's hair and eye color are both determined genetically and set before birth. Unfortunately, however detailed an ultrasound image is, it can only show the shape of structures and will never be able to show true color information.

"You may be surprised to find that your social life is already changing, and the baby hasn't even arrived yet!"

If you've become a homebody recently, be reassured it's quite normal. Wanting to stay at home is common in the final stages of pregnancy. You may be reluctant to plan social engagements for the next few weeks, just in case. For example, you don't want to spend money on a theater ticket that might not get used. Do, however, pencil in dates with friends because they will understand if you cancel at the last minute. You'll also find that on some days, you're glad to get out of the house in the evenings.

Take the opportunity to go out with your partner in these last few weeks of your pregnancy as dinner dates may not be on the agenda once the baby arrives.

ASK A DOCTOR

My feet are swollen and tight; can I do anything about it? Swollen feet and ankles, known as edema, is due to excessive fluid seeping into the tissues because of the increased volume of blood (see pp.468–469). By late pregnancy, as blood volume continues to rise, this is a common problem. The swelling is usually worse later in the day and when the weather is warmer.

Steps you can take to help reduce the swelling include elevating your legs when sitting, rotating your feet, and lying on the floor with your feet up the wall. Wearing support stockings or hose (see p.225) also improves circulation. Make sure you drink plenty, particularly water, since this improves kidney function and reduces water retention. Don't take diuretics—studies have found that these can adversely affect an unborn baby.

A SOOTHING SWIM

Although you may feel too big to be exercising, swimming is a great activity for late pregnancy. The water supports the weight of your belly, so you may feel much lighter than you do normally. Try to do some gentle swimming as well as just relaxing in the water. Also consider going to prenatal water aerobics classes, which have exercises tailored for pregnant women.

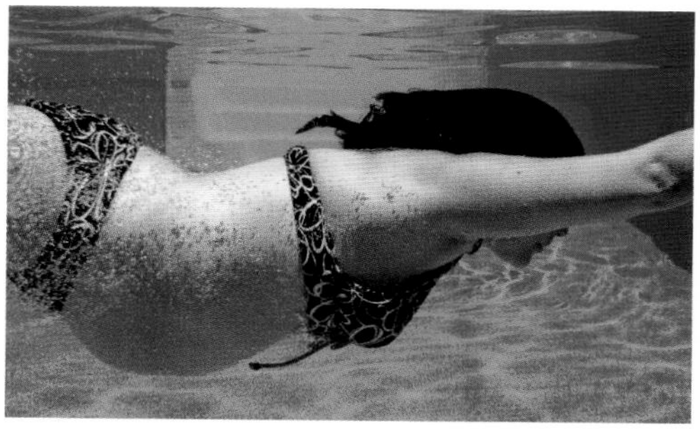

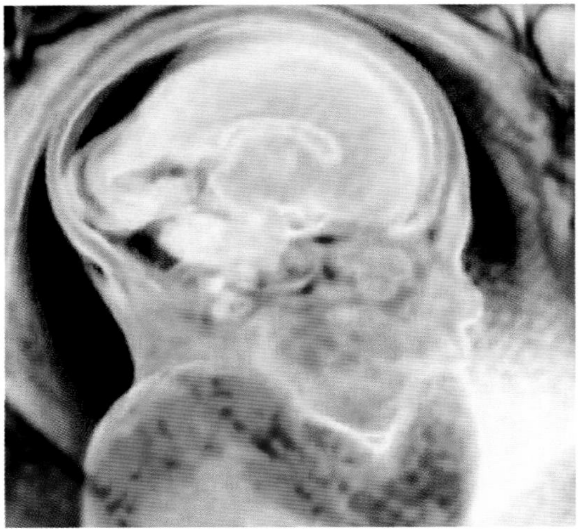

YOU ARE **35 WEEKS AND 2 DAYS**

33 days to go

YOUR BABY TODAY

This MRI scan shows detail of the baby's brain. MRI is particularly good at showing structures within the central nervous system. Obtaining and interpreting these images remains difficult and time-consuming, however, so they are not part of routine testing.

“ Although the color is developing in your baby's eyes, the final color will not be known for some time. ”

What color will your baby's eyes be? The iris controls the amount of light that enters the eye and gives the eyes their color. Eye color is determined by the amount of melanin within the iris; this is the substance in the skin that gives different skin tones.

It certainly doesn't follow that your baby will have an identical eye color to that of you or your partner. Most fair-skinned babies will be born with only a small amount of melanin in the eye and the iris will appear gray or blue. If dark-skinned, there is a great deal of melanin and the color is usually dark gray or brown. The color continues to change after birth as melanin is produced in response to light. Your baby will be a year old before the final color of her eyes is fully developed.

PRACTICING VISUALIZATION

Visualization is an effective and positive way to help prepare for labor. Try practicing it in these final weeks of your pregnancy, beginning with this basic relaxation exercise.

Start at the top of your head and gently flex and relax every muscle down to your toes, concentrating on each muscle, and your breathing, as you do so.

Now imagine the birth, with every step given a positive connotation. For example, your baby is floating in water, and is gently rocked as the contractions begin; the tightening you feel is the strong walls of your uterus, guiding your baby into the world; the contractions are waves on which you and your baby are riding, as your baby is washed out—you are both swimming together with the tide.

CESAREAN BIRTH

If you know you're going to have your baby by Cesarean, it's good to be aware of what to expect following the birth. Although you should remain mobile after Cesarean surgery, it's also important to get plenty of rest. Keep in mind that a Cesarean section is major surgery, so you will need to avoid lifting and carrying heavy loads for the first few weeks. Since this may be difficult if you have other small children or you are at home alone, you should try to recruit as much help as possible after the surgery. You should avoid doing any shopping since this usually involves carrying heavy bags. Order online if you can.

The advice is not to drive for six weeks. If you feel up to it before this time, check with your doctor that it is okay and make sure you're comfortable wearing a seatbelt and doing maneuvers, including stopping short.

It is generally thought to take up to six weeks to fully recover from a Cesarean delivery.

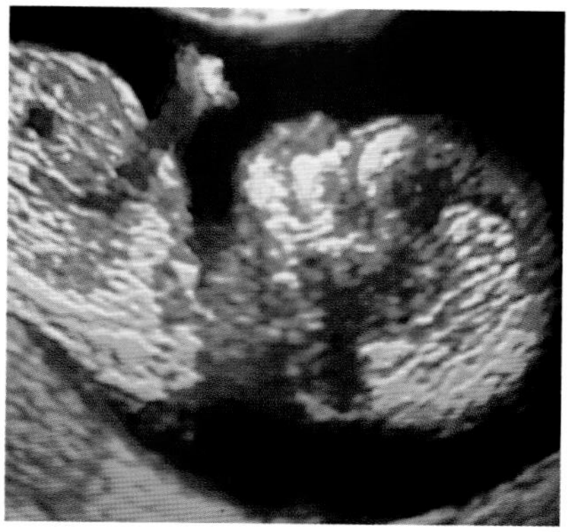

YOU ARE **35 WEEKS AND 3 DAYS**

32 days to go

YOUR BABY TODAY

In this week, the lungs become almost fully functional and able to support the baby if delivered early. However, the baby at this time is still preterm, and will not be mature enough until 37 weeks to be considered full term.

"Don't forget this is a life-changing time for your partner, too, so find positive ways to involve them in the time preceding the birth."

There is, understandably, a lot of focus on the mother in the lead-up to childbirth, but it's important not to neglect your partner, who may be getting anxious about the birth itself, about how to cope being in the delivery room or just concerned about you being in pain. Some partners feel guilty that they cannot take their share of the pain and help more during labor.

Aside from thinking about the birth, your partner may be anxious about the fact that they will be sharing the responsibility for a newborn baby in just a few weeks!

Talk to your partner if they appear anxious and involve them as much as possible—from helping you cope with pregnancy discomforts to preparing for the birth. If you've written a birth plan (see pp.181 and 303), go back over it now and discuss what might happen and how your partner could help on the day.

You could practice positions and breathing techniques for labor so that they feel more confident about helping you manage. If possible, your partner could go to your final prenatal appointments with you, where they can discuss any concerns with the doctor.

ASK A DOCTOR

Will I be able to love my newborn twins equally? Yes, but it may happen that one baby needs more attention than the other, and it is natural for your time to be diverted to the baby whose needs are not yet met. It is possible that the strain of having two babies may increase the likelihood of delayed bonding, although this can also happen if the birth has been traumatic; if the parents are exhausted; or if one baby has taken time to establish feeding, or is more irritable than the other.

When a parent has two children born at different times, that parent may love one child differently than the other, but this does not mean that the love a parent has for one child is to the detriment of the other. If once your babies are born you still have concerns, speak to your doctor.

FOCUS ON PARTNERS

Have you done everything on the to-do list? This may include:

- **Buying a car** seat and making sure you know how to install it safely in the car. You can't leave the hospital with your newborn without one.
- **Assembling the crib** if you're going to use one in the early weeks.
- **Making sure there is storage** space for the baby's clothes, bedding, diapers, and other bits and pieces.

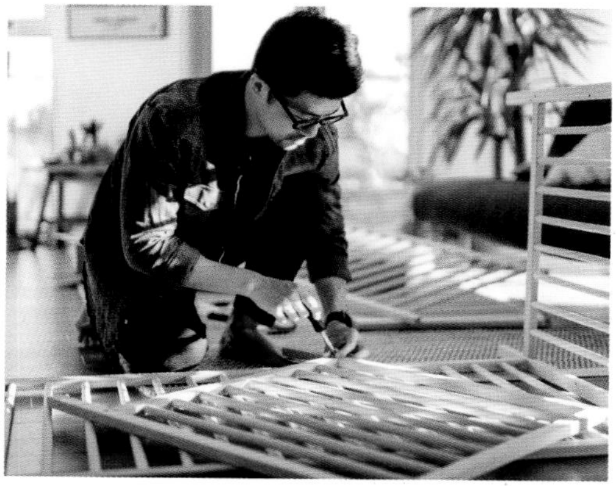

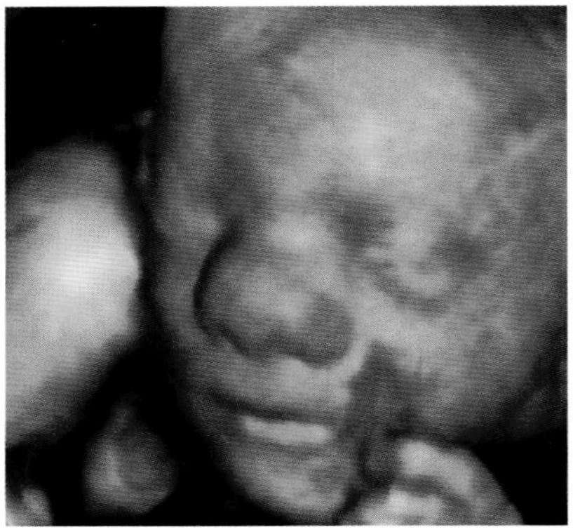

YOU ARE **35 WEEKS AND 4 DAYS**

31 days to go

YOUR BABY TODAY

Your baby's heart will beat quite fast, at between 110 and 160 beats every minute. Even after birth, your baby's heart will continue to beat at this speed. It will be several years before the heart rate is 70 or so beats per minute, the same as an adult.

> "The lungs don't become fully functional until these final weeks, but important development is taking place now."

If you imagine the lung as a tree, then the windpipe or "trachea" is the trunk of the tree. This then forms several branches or "bronchi," which divide several times, like twigs, to then produce the most delicate structures: the alveoli or leaves of the tree. It is within the alveoli that gas exchange will take place.

The alveoli began to develop at 24 weeks but they continue to increase in number throughout the pregnancy. The alveoli contain surfactant-producing cells to keep them open and these now become fully functional.

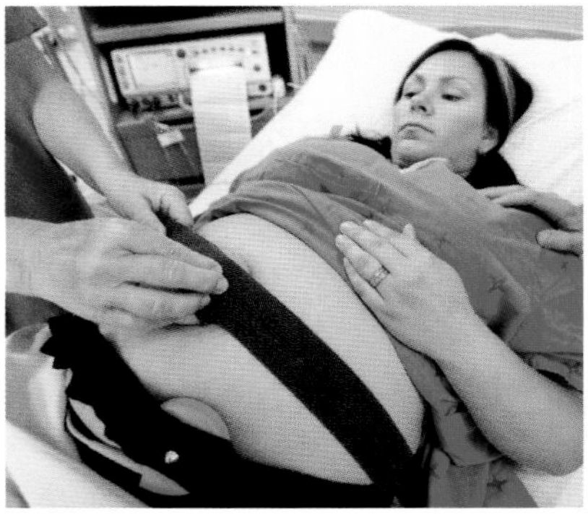

You may be closely monitored in the hospital toward the end of your pregnancy if there is any concern about your health or that of your baby. A fetal monitoring machine will be used to check your baby's heartbeat.

PRESCRIBED BEDREST

Toward the end of pregnancy, there are some circumstances when you may need to be admitted to the hospital for observation.

- **If you have developed preeclampsia** (see p.476), so that measures can be taken to reduce your blood pressure.
- **If you have any vaginal bleeding** that may be due to a low-lying placenta (see pp.212) or a placental abruption (see p.475).

GETTING STRONG

Maintaining muscular strength, stretching, and doing gentle exercise right up until you give birth will help your posture—minimizing backaches, reducing stress on your skeleton, and making you feel more energized and relaxed. As long as you feel good and adhere to the guidelines outlined on page 18, you can continue with your activities.

Most importantly, at this time you should use common sense and listen to your body. If you're in pain, feel fatigued, or have dizzy spells, see your doctor immediately and stop exercising. You'll be feeling tired carrying around all that extra weight, so adjust your activities accordingly. This could mean that you lower the intensity of your exercise and exercise for a shorter time, but if you feel good don't stop exercising altogether.

Look at the routines on pages 90 and 250, but don't do any exercises at this stage that require you to lie on your back for extended periods of time.

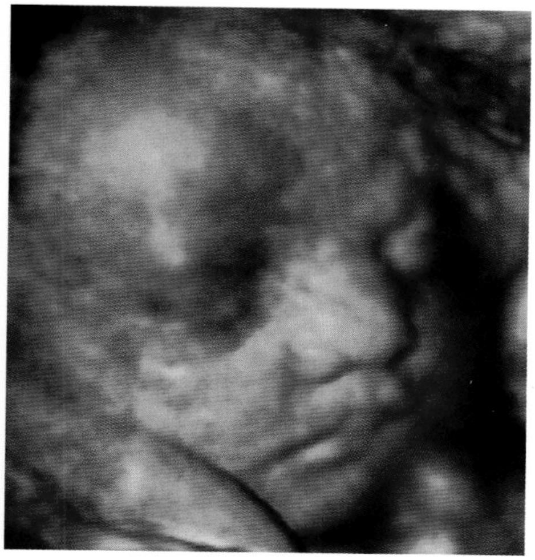

YOU ARE **35 WEEKS AND 5 DAYS**

30 days to go

YOUR BABY TODAY

Many babies will still have a good volume of amniotic fluid around them, but shadows from the placenta or side of the uterus, coupled with the curled-up fetal position, will make imaging the baby harder and harder.

> " It's a good idea to make practical arrangements now for what might happen if you go into labor. "

With only around four weeks to go, now is the time to make sure you have all your partner's contact details and know exactly how to get a hold of them in case you go into labour when they are at work. They might discuss with their employer being able to keep their cell phone nearby or minimizing any travel.

If you have other children or other dependents (pets, for example), then you should arrange what will happen to them when you go into the hospital. You may want to explain to any older children what is going to happen so that they are prepared for when they go to stay with Grandma, or whoever will be taking care of them. If you're having a Cesarean, you might need more help once you are home to care for your older children after you've had surgery.

Reassure your children that you will be coming back and that you're not sick, but that you have to go to the hospital when the baby comes. Depending on the age of your children, you could go with them to buy a present for the baby or you could give them a special job such as opening all the new gifts. Presents from the newborn to elder siblings is also a good gesture.

PAIN RELIEF DURING LABOR

In one study of women who anticipated that they would not need pain relief, 52 percent actually used it.

The best time to talk about pain-relieving options is during your prenatal visits. This will help you set an accurate expectation about pain in labor and how you may cope with it.

ASK A DOCTOR

If my baby is born prematurely and is in the neonatal intensive care unit, is it still helpful to express milk? Yes, definitely. Breast milk helps to ensure that the mother's natural immunity is passed on to her baby via her milk. Because premature babies are more prone to infection, expressing your breast milk is a great way to help your baby if she is in the intensive care unit. Breast milk is much easier for a baby to digest: this is important for premature babies since their digestive tract may be less developed than a full-term baby's.

This is also a great way for you to bond and develop a relationship with your baby. This situation could be a time of considerable stress for you and you may feel helpless, so knowing that you're doing such a great thing to help your baby could help.

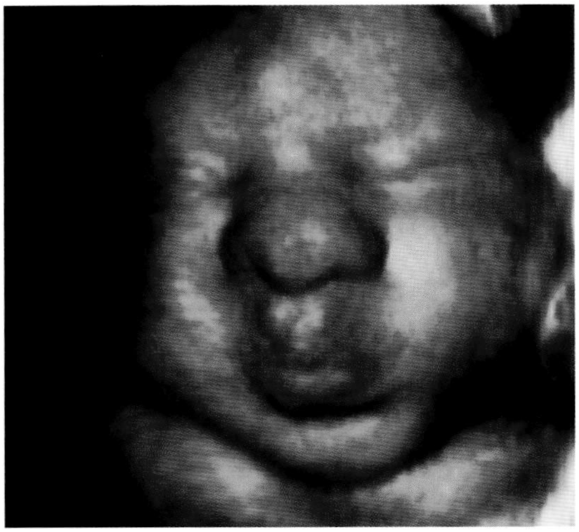

YOU ARE **35 WEEKS AND 6 DAYS**

29 days to go

YOUR BABY TODAY

Most babies will now be positioned longitudinally (lying straight up and down, with their head well in the pelvis). Even now, when space is limited in these final weeks, there is still time for the position to change to head down if your baby is bottom first (breech).

“ Complex developments are taking place in your baby’s lungs that will enable her to breathe unaided once she is born. ”

The blood flow to your baby’s lungs mirrors the development of the airways. Blood leaves the right side of the heart through a one-way valve into the main pulmonary vein. This then divides to give a pulmonary branch to each lung, and also a duct that allows blood to bypass the lungs and travel to the body directly. This will close soon after birth as the lungs expand and their resistance to blood flow falls.

Because your baby doesn’t use their lungs for gas exchange in the uterus, the blood supply to them is quite small—only 10 percent of the postbirth supply. At this stage of pregnancy, the lungs’ blood supply has completed its development, branching into finer and finer vessels as they come to lie closer to the alveoli.

When your baby is born, their chest is compressed in the birth canal. This helps push the fluid out of the lungs to prepare for that incredible first breath. If your baby is born by Cesarean, they will need to bring the fluid up themself. This is why planned Cesareans are done after 39 weeks. Babies born by Cesarean before this sometimes have a problem clearing the fluid and may need a little help breathing in the first few hours after the birth.

ITEMS FOR YOUR HOSPITAL BAG

Include items for yourself, as well as your baby. If you’re having a cesarean, pack for a few days

For yourself:
- Pajamas
- Underwear
- Nursing bras
- Slippers and robe
- Hairbrush
- Toothbrush
- Toiletries
- Maternity sanitary pads
- Breast pads and nipple cream
- Comfortable loungewear.

For your baby:
- Undershirts
- Footed onesies
- Blanket
- Diapers
- Diaper bags
- Cotton pads
- Diaper cream, such as Desitin
- Baby wipes if you intend to use them.
- Hat and cardigan for going home. Babies lose a lot of heat through their head, so it is a good idea for your baby to wear a hat.

Other useful items:
- A phone or camera for photos and videos
- Music for the delivery room
- Books and magazines
- Massage oil
- TENS machine (see p.399)
- Washcloths.

Your partner should also get a bag ready (see p.338) and make sure the car seat is installed properly..

Pack snacks and drinks close to the time, such as nuts, cereal bars, rice cakes, dried fruit, and bottled water.

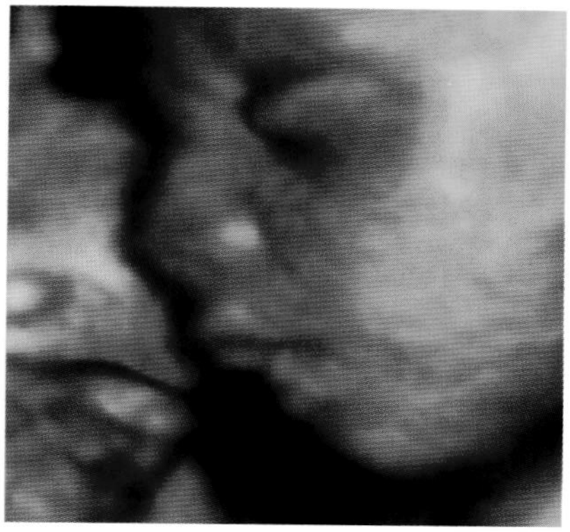

YOU ARE **36 WEEKS EXACTLY**

28 days to go

YOUR BABY TODAY

You may notice a change in the character of your baby's movements, reflecting the reduced amount of amniotic fluid and, consequently, space to move around in. Each movement is more likely to be felt, however, as they touch the side of your uterus.

> “All pregnant women need support in the final weeks, but if you're single, this can be even more important.”

Whether you're single by choice, or have unexpectedly found yourself in this position, you may be experiencing mixed feelings about the weeks to come. There is no doubt that going solo involves extra responsibilities and worries, but with a little help from your close friends and family, you can make these final few weeks of your pregnancy positive.

If you're concerned about going into labor alone, line up a close friend or family member who is on call at all times. They might want to get permission from their place of work to take leave to be with you should you go into labor. Keep yourself busy before your baby arrives, planning plenty of activities during your maternity leave.

Don't be afraid to ask people for help with shopping for last-minute baby buys or getting your home ready for your new arrival. Most people will be delighted with the honor of being asked to keep you company, and helping you get things ready.

Most importantly, take care of yourself: get organized by preparing meals you can freeze so you have plenty of healthy food in storage for the weeks after the birth.

BABY SHOWERS

Throwing a baby shower to celebrate the imminent arrival is a great opportunity to get together with friends.

Organize it yourself, or ask one of your best friends to do the honors. Note to best friend: surprise parties are great, but consider whether the mom-to-be will want to be the center of attention.

Think about:

- **A pampering theme:** the guests could give each other manicures and pedicures, or you could even hire a beautician for the afternoon.
- **Chipping in together to buy the mom-to-be something useful,** such as a car seat, or indulgent, such as a relaxing day out at a spa.
- **Games you could play,** such as inviting guests to guess the baby's sex, weight, and date they'll be born.
- **Refreshments:** Champagne, nonalcoholic drinks, nibbles, and a “birth” day cake.

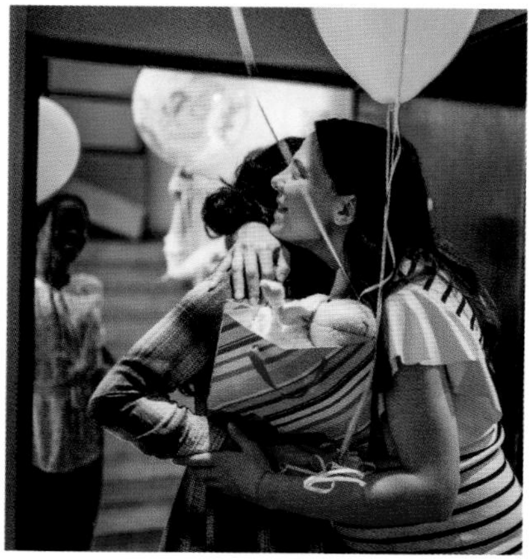

Your 37th week

YOUR BELLY MAY LOOK AS THOUGH IT'S STARTED TO SLIDE DOWNHILL. You're now about as big as you're going to get. Soon—maybe this week—the baby will drop down lower into your pelvis, ready for birth. Your belly may shift downward, too, giving you a different shape. This doesn't necessarily mean that labor is imminent, so don't worry about the baby "falling out." You're likely to still have some time to enjoy maternity leave and get organized.

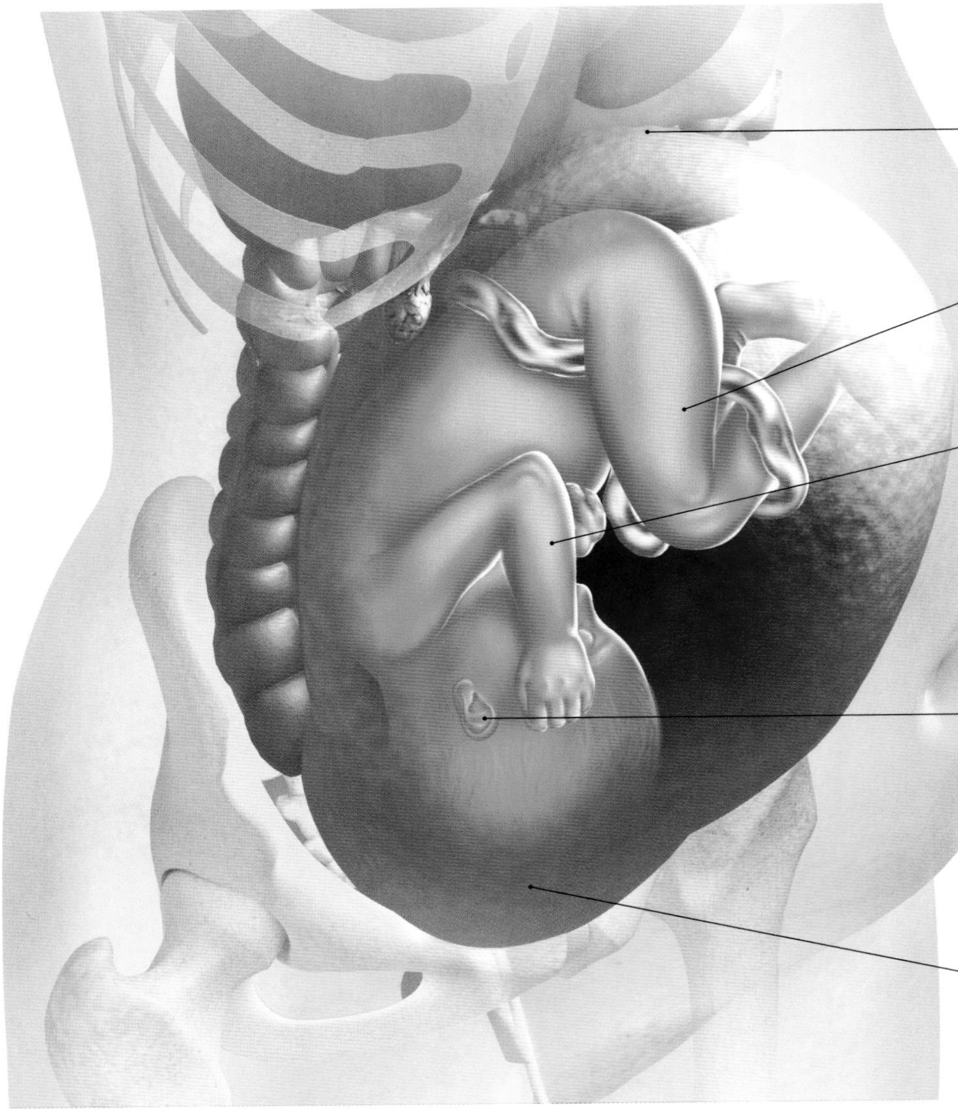
Some of the pressure under your rib cage may be easing off as the baby continues to descend into the pelvis.
The baby is still gaining weight as more fat covers his limbs and abdomen. As a newborn, he will look much the same as he does now.
Short, very fine hairs, called vellus hairs, are growing in place of lanugo hair on most parts of the baby's body.
Your baby turns toward a familiar sound and practices looking for its source: your voice is the most familiar sound to him.
At 37 weeks the average crown to heel length is 19.1 in (48.6 cm) and the average weight is 6.3 lb (2.9 kg).

YOU ARE **36 WEEKS AND 1 DAY**

27 days to go

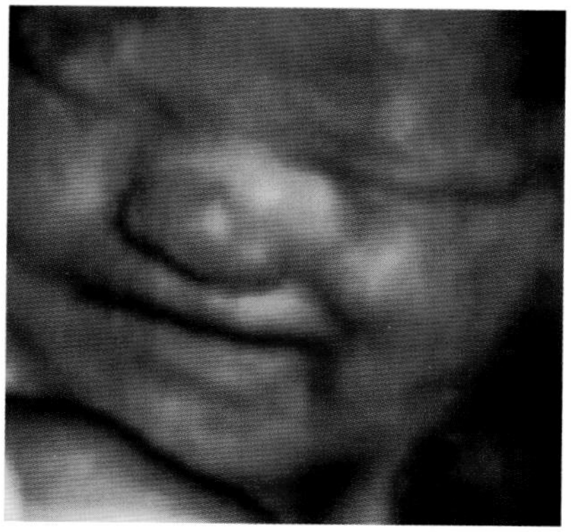

YOUR BABY TODAY

When scanned, this baby was lying with their back to their mother's. This "back to back" position is common at this stage but becomes less so as the pregnancy continues. Your doctor will be able to feel for the position of your baby's back from this point on.

If you're lucky enough to have the opportunity to start maternity leave at this point, take advantage of it. As you leave your working role, the reality of beginning your role as a mother may hit you—but hopefully you will have a few more weeks to get used to the idea!

It can be a welcome respite to take it easy and not have to rush around in the mornings, and you'll feel less tired by not having to travel to work. Although you need to take it easy, it's a good idea to plan some outings during the daytime, as not having a routine can take some getting used to. Although it's good to stay in touch with colleagues, try not to fall into the trap of logging on to work email or staying up-to-date with what's happening at work. You might be worrying about losing some of your identity while you're on maternity leave; this is a common feeling, but you'll find that before you know it, your leave is over and you're settled back into work again.

Try to enjoy this lead-up to the birth and make the most of the time (see p.366) to get organized and prepare for your new arrival.

> "You're in the home stretch now. This can be a relief but also a time of mixed emotions."

ASK A DOCTOR

Will I feel different when my baby drops? Breathing will be easier, as your lungs have room to expand. Your abdomen may seem smaller, with your belly shifting down and forward, as your baby's head enters the birth canal. You may have more pelvic pain and may need to urinate more.

WHEN YOUR BABY ENGAGES

Engagement is the process by which your baby's head moves through the pelvic brim and into the birth canal in preparation for birth, and this can occur any time in these final few weeks of pregnancy, until the start of your labor. In the last weeks of pregnancy, your doctor will check to see if the head has started to engage, or drop, sometimes called "lightening."

Your doctor will do an examination to see where the baby's head is. This is called the station, and it's measured from –5 (the baby's head is floating above the pelvis) to +5, the head is at the opening of the vagina. This last stage is called crowning.

When your baby drops, you may find it easier to breathe, since your lungs will have more room to expand, or the need to urinate more because of more pressure on your bladder.

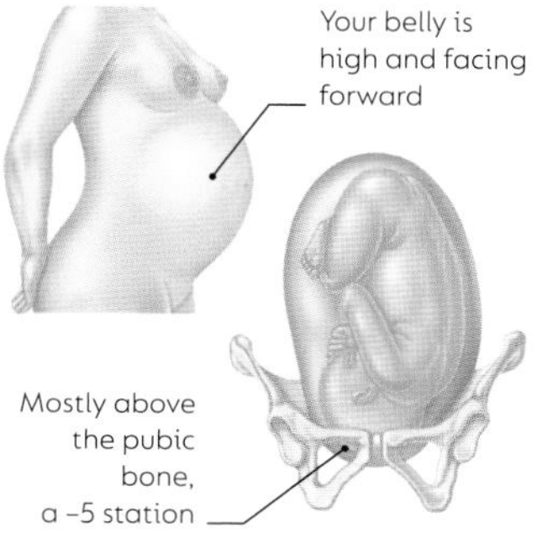

Your belly is high and facing forward
Mostly above the pubic bone, a –5 station

Not engaged: The baby's head has started to move into the pelvis, but more than three- or four-fifths can be felt above the pubic bone.

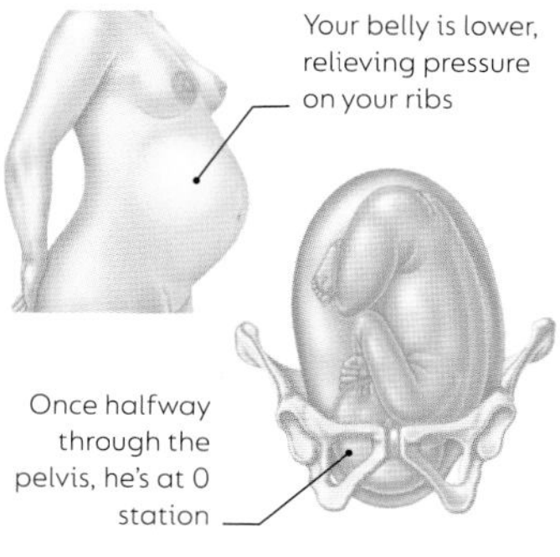

Your belly is lower, relieving pressure on your ribs
Once halfway through the pelvis, he's at 0 station

Engaged: The baby has dropped into the pelvis in preparation for birth. This causes your belly to change position and shape.

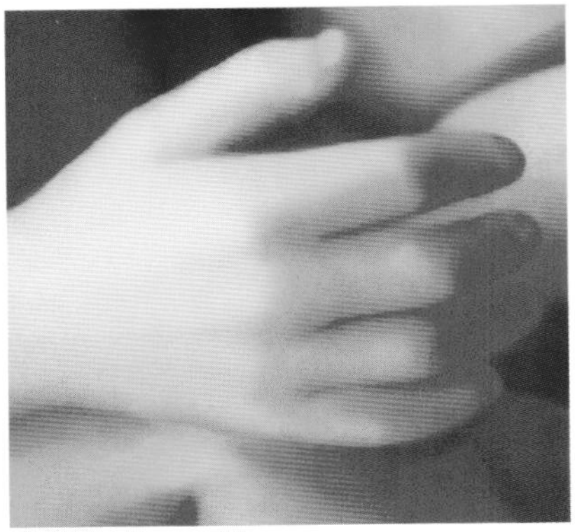

YOU ARE **36 WEEKS AND 2 DAYS**

26 days to go

YOUR BABY TODAY

Although almost invisible in the image, a very thin layer of vernix covers your baby. At first this helped to reduce the amount of water leaving your baby's skin, but now it helps to prevent direct contact with the skin and amniotic fluid.

> “Have you started nesting? The need to provide a safe, comfortable space for your new baby is a primitive desire.”

The nesting instinct usually begins in the final weeks of pregnancy, accompanied by a surge of energy and an uncontrollable urge to get your home in ship shape.

Give in to your inner domestic goddess: cook, clean, organize, and declutter, but take it easy. If you spend hours on your hands and knees scrubbing, you may find yourself in labor sooner than you expected.

Not feeling the urge to nest? Pay the professionals to do a spring cleaning. Or forget it: your baby won't care whether the cabinets are clean.

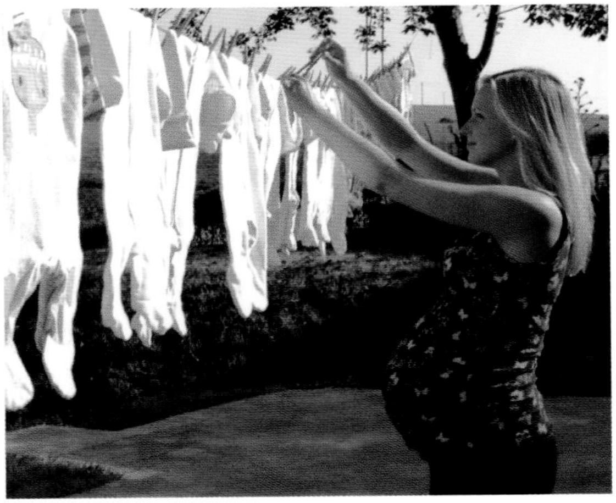

Washing your newborn baby's clothes ahead of the birth, may be one of the many nesting urges you have in late pregnancy.

PLASTER CASTS

Preserve your belly for posterity by making a plaster belly cast. You can either buy a kit or (far cheaper) purchase the plaster separately; it's all available online.

You will need:

- Plaster of Paris bandages, cut into strips
- Large tub of petroleum jelly
- Bucket of warm water
- One or two people to help you

Here's how to do it:

1. Strip down except for some old underwear (the smaller, the better)
2. Apply petroleum jelly liberally to your belly and breasts
3. Assume a comfortable pose
4. One by one, dip the plaster of Paris strips into the water, then apply, overlapping the layers until you have a thick coating.
5. Sit and wait for it to dry (rock hard).
6. Slip it off and paint it if you'd like.

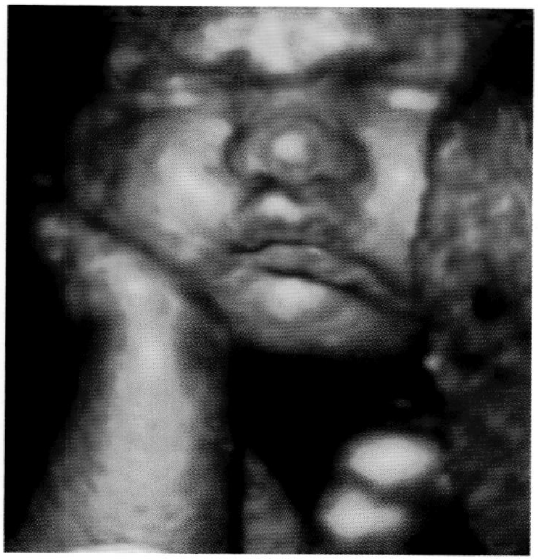

YOU ARE **36 WEEKS AND 3 DAYS**

25 days to go

YOUR BABY TODAY

A short portion of the umbilical cord is lying close to the mouth, which makes this baby appear to have a rather grumpy-looking expression. The placenta is seen to the right of the image, partially obscuring the view of the face.

“You’ll find that your beautiful belly is intruding on your life more and more, affecting your movements and eating patterns.”

You might be feeling frustrated by your size around now, which can make everyday activities more difficult. Simple maneuvers, such as fitting through doors or getting off the sofa, can be more difficult and you may find that everything takes a bit longer to achieve. All you can do is be patient and focus on getting through the next few weeks. .

During pregnancy, it’s common to eat more often than previously but to eat less at each meal. This is because your uterus has grown so much that all your other organs have moved around and are squashed into much less space. Your stomach simply has less room in it to fit the food, so you can’t eat as much before feeling full. When your stomach empties, you may find yourself hungry again. It’s fine to snack, but make sure you’re reaching for healthy foods whenever possible and not indulging in too many sweets.

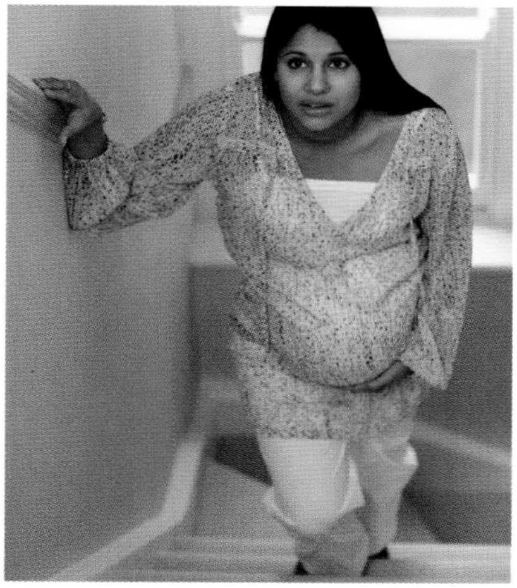

Everyday activities, such as climbing the stairs, are likely to take longer and be more tiring in the final weeks of pregnancy.

VBAC

Doctors used to think that if you had one baby by Cesarean, all future babies must also be born that way. But doctors now know that 90 percent of women who delivered by Cesarean are candidates for VBAC, or Vaginal Birth after Cesarean. Depending on the reason for your prior Cesarean, you may be able to deliver vaginally, especially if you have no major medical problems, the baby is healthy and in head-down position, of normal size, and any condition that necessitated your last Cesarean isn’t present. If you have diabetes, high blood pressure, or are pregnant with multiples, you are not a candidate for VBAC.

THINKING ABOUT BREASTFEEDING

You may have started thinking about whether to breastfeed. At this stage, try to remain open-minded. Some women who are adamant they will breastfeed find it harder than they expect, while others who don’t like the idea of breastfeeding take to it very easily. Whichever camp you fall in, know that it’s okay to change your mind and your method of feeding. Even if you don’t manage to breastfeed for as long as you’d like, try to start your baby off at the breast. Breast milk provides unique antibodies and protective substances to boost your baby’s immunity.

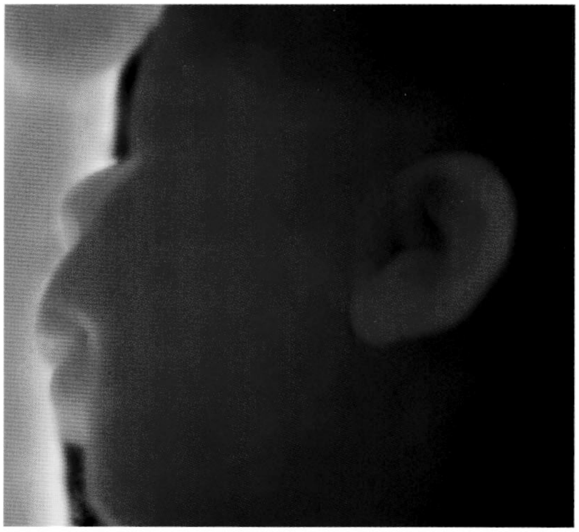

YOU ARE **36 WEEKS AND 4 DAYS**

24 days to go

YOUR BABY TODAY

Your baby is now more well equipped for the time after birth. Their ears are fully formed on the outside and inside and they are used to hearing the sound of your blood circulating and your heart beating, and they recognizes your voice.

> "Your baby is losing the downy hair that they've had for several weeks, but if they're born now there may still be some visible."

Lanugo is extremely fine hair that covers your baby's body and, unlike adult hairs on the body, it is not associated with sweat glands. Lanugo hairs begin to be shed now since they are lost into the amniotic fluid in the last few weeks before birth. Your baby then swallows these lanugo hairs in the amniotic fluid, but this is not a cause for concern: these hairs provide your baby with an important source of protein, essential to his development. It's been estimated that two-thirds of the protein in the fluid is swallowed and absorbed by the baby's gut each day, providing 15 percent of his protein needs.

The fine lanugo hairs are gradually replaced by vellus hairs, which are short, soft, nonpigmented hairs (often seen more on women and children). Terminal hair is the thicker, coarser, and longer hair that first grows on your baby's eyebrows, then his eyelashes, then his scalp. In adults, facial hair (beards), armpit, and pubic hair is terminal hair.

NEEDING THE BATHROOM

In the third trimester you'll be frequenting the bathroom regularly, as you did in the first trimester. At this stage, it's due to the increasingly heavy baby pushing down on your bladder from above. If you find that it hurts when you expel urine, you may have a urinary tract infection and should contact your doctor for a test.

ASK A DOCTOR

I've heard about doctors "turning" breech babies. How does this work? Some obstetricians may try to turn a baby in late pregnancy using external cephalic version (ECV), which has a success rate of around 65 percent. They'll try gently to guide the baby into a head-down position by pressing their hands on the mother's abdomen, using ultrasound as a guide. You may be given medication to relax the uterine muscles. You will be scanned first and if the baby is in an awkward position, the procedure may not continue. If your baby is large, this can affect the procedure, as can the amount of amniotic fluid (a low amount offers less protection to the baby).

If you're Rh negative, you may get an Rh immunoglobulin (RhIg) injection after the ECV due to the small risk of a bleed around the placenta. An ECV is not recommended if you have a multiple pregnancy, have had bleeding, your placenta is low-lying (see p.212), your membranes have ruptured, there is a known problem with the baby, or you should not have a vaginal delivery.

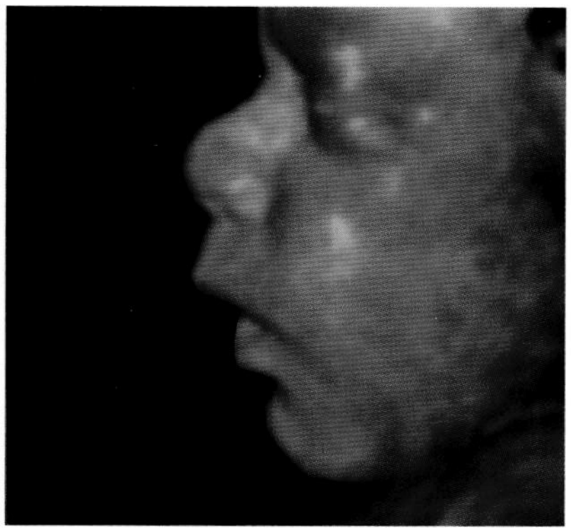

YOU ARE **36 WEEKS AND 5 DAYS**

23 days to go

YOUR BABY TODAY

3-D views at this stage of the pregnancy will be extremely clear. Every part of the face is fully developed and your baby will be very expressive. Your baby is only a few days away now from being full term.

> “Don't be concerned about embarrassing yourself in labor—your caregivers will have seen it all before.”

Many women worry about losing control during labor—for example, that they will urinate or defecate when they are pushing. You might well pass a bit of stool when you're pushing, but you probably won't notice; your doctor will put on a pair of gloves and use gauze to remove it.

The reality is that when you're in the throes of labor, you really won't care—you'll just want that baby out!

ASK A PANEL

What if I can't deal with the pain of labor?

Doctor: If you're concerned, take time to investigate the pain-relief options in advance of labor, so that you're aware of what's available, even if you don't plan to use it.

There's no shame in deviating from what you requested in your birth plan; the ultimate goal is to deliver a healthy baby, and to keep your energy levels and your spirits high. It's also important to ask for pain relief as soon as you feel that things are getting away from you.

Mom: When I was in labor, the pain literally took my breath away, and I really did feel that I would be unable to continue. Changing position, walking around, and using a birthing ball proved to be a good distraction, even if they passed the time rather than provided relief, and I chanted to myself, over and over, “You can do it!”

I dimly remembered that when the pain is at its worst you've hit “transition,” which signals the beginning of the delivery itself, and it did help to know I was near the end, even if it did seem a long time in coming. Focus on how much you want your baby in your arms, and view every contraction as one step closer to that moment.

Midwife: Moms who are prepared for the pain seem to find that it isn't as bad as they thought it might be, and are able to cope using breathing exercises and massage. The best advice is to know your limits. If you find the pain unbearable, then ask for some pain relief. Ask the doctor or nurse what pain options are available to take the edge off of the discomfort, and make the process more bearable.

No woman can anticipate how her labor and delivery will proceed, and sometimes babies make things difficult by presenting themselves in awkward positions, or simply enjoying life inside a little too much to arrive promptly. Take things one step at a time, and when you know you've had enough, conserve your energy by getting the help you need. Any woman who delivers a healthy baby has had a successful delivery, and that's what's most important.

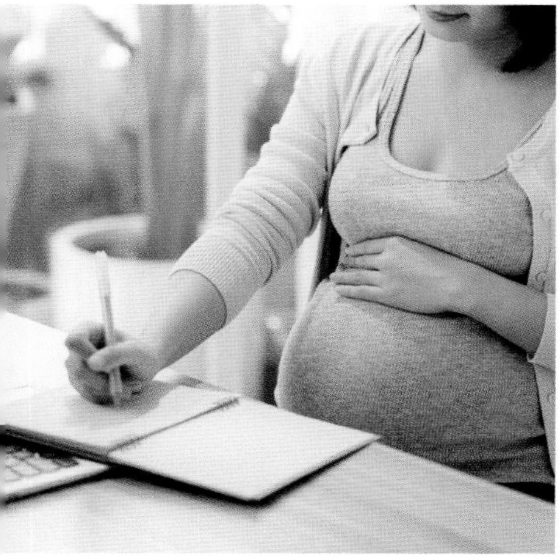

Do some research about pain relief to become as informed as you can and weigh the pros and cons of each option. Speak to your doctor if anything is unclear.

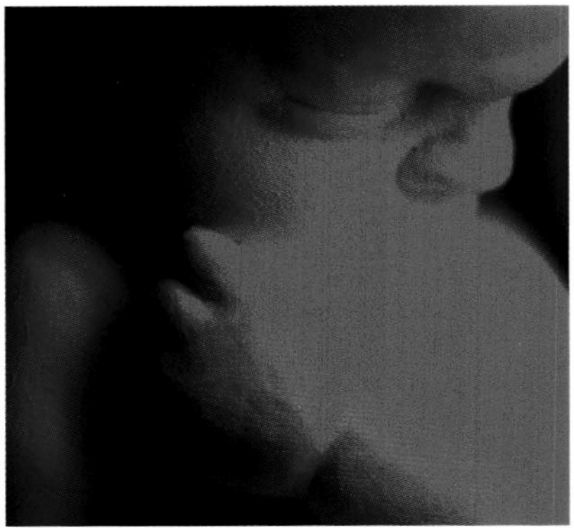

YOU ARE **36 WEEKS AND 6 DAYS**

22 days to go

YOUR BABY TODAY

Your baby will be able to recall and recognize the frequency and pattern of the most familiar sounds they hear within the uterus—your voice. Also, you might have noticed that loud noises may startle your baby during these final weeks.

> "If you're lacking in energy, rest when you can and make sure you continue to eat a well-balanced diet."

Like many women, you may find that in the third trimester you have a poor appetite and cannot manage to eat a full meal.

It is important to keep up your calorie intake to maintain good energy levels, so try to eat small meals little and often, and make sure you continue to balance your diet with plenty of carbohydrates, protein, fruits, and vegetables (see pp.14–17).

As well as eating small meals, you'll find you snack more—take healthy snacks with you when you go out.

Doing a little gentle exercise, such as a walk, every day will also help you to maintain good energy levels.

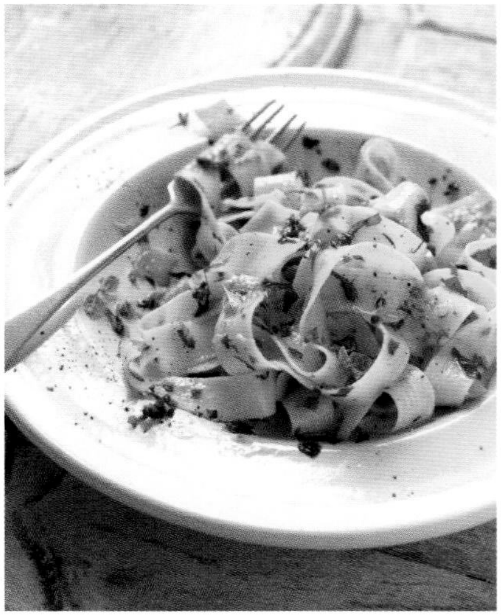

Eating pasta, or other carbs, such as a baked potato, is a great way to boost your energy in late pregnancy. Eat little and often if you can't manage big portions of food.

MAKING THE MOST OF MATERNITY LEAVE

Maternity leave offers a great opportunity to prepare yourself for the birth of your baby.

- **Take time to rest.** While it may seem like the optimum time to rush through a long "to-do" list, it's important to conserve your energy for the birth, and the weeks after.
- **Prepare your hospital bag** (see p.358), or anything you may need for a home birth (see p.341).
- **Make a list** of everyone you'd like contacted after the birth.
- **Put together some natural remedies** to help you through labor and its aftermath. Lavender oil can be sniffed during labor to relax and calm. You may need ice packs if you end up having an episiotomy (placing ice pads or chilled witch hazel pads on the area may soothe your pain). Ask your doctor about safe pain medications for after delivery, or, if you want to avoid medications, ask him or her for drug-free suggestions.
- **Prepare a few freezer meals.** There is nothing better than having an already prepared, meal on hand in those early weeks.
- **Sort your baby's new clothes** into sizes, so you don't find yourself searching through piles to find something that fits.
- **Get a manicure, pedicure, or massage.** Not only will time be tight after your baby arrives, but money may be, too!
- **Produce something creative**—paint your baby's nursery, cross-stitch a little pillow or picture, make a crib bumper, start a scrapbook, or simply write a letter to your baby to put in a keepsake box. These personal touches are satisfying, and will be treasured for years to come.
- **Catch up with friends and family for lunch.** It may be some time before you feel like going out again when you're getting used to being a parent and enjoying your new baby in the comfort of your home.

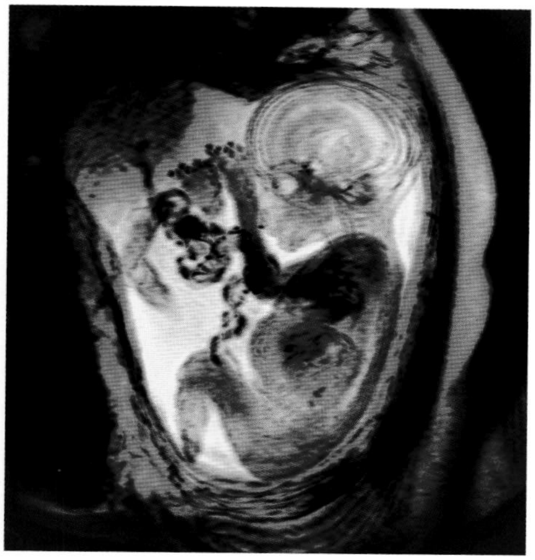

YOU ARE **37 WEEKS EXACTLY**

21 days to go

YOUR BABY TODAY

This baby is lying in the breech position, with the umbilical cord seen as it travels toward the placenta in the top-left side of the image. Approximately 3 in every 100 babies will be in a breech position after 37 weeks.

> "Your baby is now able to hear many sounds that will all be familiar to him once he's born."

In this late stage of pregnancy, sounds penetrate the uterus easily and there is no doubt that the baby can hear and respond to these before birth. Your baby will startle at loud sounds, but now also will turn toward familiar sounds, and practice looking for the source of the sound. Your baby is not only recognizing a wider range of sound frequencies but also discriminating between different sounds as well as learning and remembering familiar sounds, such as your voice and that of your partner.

Your baby breathes more quickly when they're concentrating on sounds and their heart rate increases. Although the baby can hear at birth, the ear drum continues to thin out, at the same time becoming more mobile and responsive to sounds. Your voice will be the most familiar sound to your baby at birth.

ASK A DOCTOR

What if I can't breastfeed? It's normal to have doubts, but be reassured that most women have enough milk, and with some help with positioning, the baby can breastfeed without any problems. By this stage, you may even be leaking colostrum (see p.295).

Try to keep an open mind and remember that the breast milk does not come in right after the birth (see p.450). Even if you have problems, try to persevere and don't feel pressured to give up just because it's convenient for the hospital staff or your partner, or because a friend or family member tells you it's not necessary.

Even if you don't end up breastfeeding, you can still get close to your baby by bottle-feeding.

FOCUS ON PARTNERS

You aren't alone if you're a partner who's feeling a bit bewildered and shell-shocked by the imminent arrival of your baby. To begin with, you can expect a lot of changes at home. Once your partner starts maternity leave, she may start a whirlwind of activity in preparation for the new arrival and will need your help to get everything ready.

While supporting your partner both practically and emotionally will be important in the coming weeks, take care of yourself, too. Take every opportunity to get some rest. Even if you've agreed that your partner will do the majority of the nighttime baby care, your sleep will still be disrupted in the weeks after the birth. Catch up with friends now, but not to the point where you tire yourself out, and keep up your exercise routine, if you have one.

It's normal to feel anxious about what's ahead—both being a birth partner and a parent—but be reassured that somehow everything will fall into place. Focus on the thought of holding your newborn baby.

Your 38th week

EVEN IF YOU HAVE ENJOYED YOUR PREGNANCY, YOU MAY BE LONGING FOR IT TO BE OVER. The baby is nearly ready, you are more than ready, so when is the birth going to happen? Probably not yet—especially if this is your first pregnancy. For another week or so, the uterus is still the best place for your baby while the finishing touches to their development take place. If you have other children, you can tell them that their new brother or sister won't keep everyone waiting much longer.

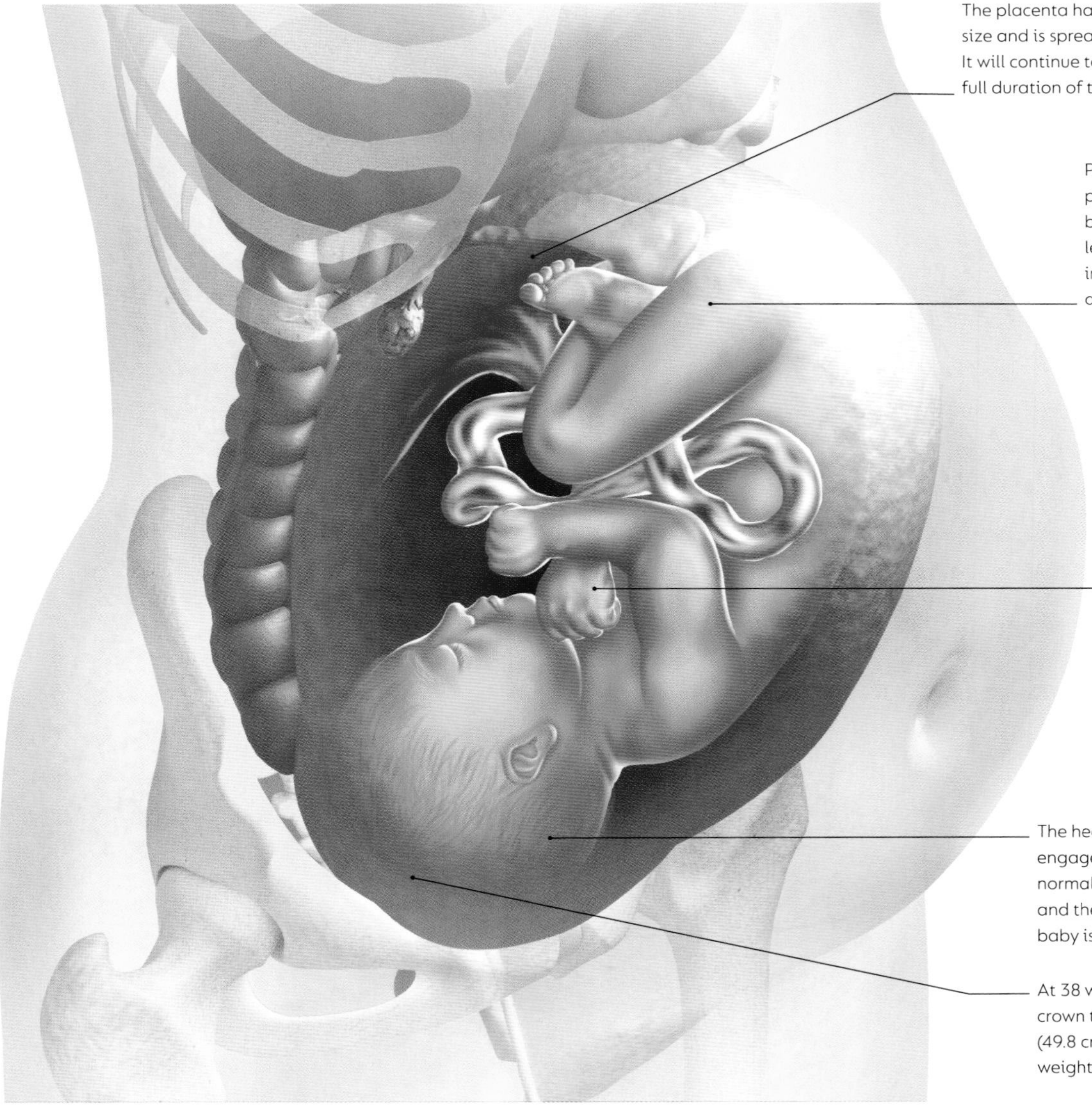

The placenta has reached its full size and is spread out like a plate. It will continue to function for the full duration of the pregnancy.

Parts of the skeleton, particularly the long bones of the arms and legs, have hardened, in a process known as ossification.

The hands may be curled into fists, grasping the umbilical cord, or free-floating with fingers outstretched. The grasp reflex is very strong.

The head may now be fully engaged. There are several normal variations in position and the direction in which the baby is facing.

At 38 weeks the average crown to heel length is 19.6 in (49.8 cm) and the average weight is 6.8 lb (3.1 kg).

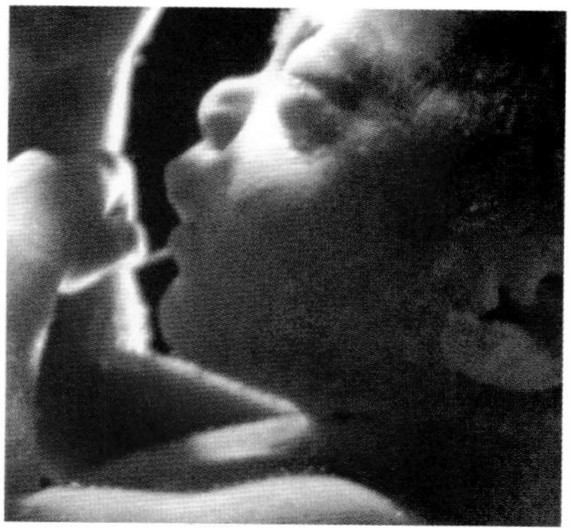

YOU ARE **37 WEEKS AND 1 DAY**

20 days to go

YOUR BABY TODAY

Full term has been reached and your baby's features are now very clearly formed. From now on, your baby is simply growing and gaining weight—factors that are necessary to provide energy after birth and help with temperature control.

" Start preparing for the birth now: by being practical and positive, you can make it memorable for all the right reasons. "

Probably the most effective way to remember as much as you can about your labor and the birth of your baby is to try to remain as healthy and rested as possible prior to the start of your labor; this will give you the best chance of staying strong and clear-headed throughout.

Feeling strong and having plenty of energy may also help you remain upright and active during the course of your labor, reducing the need for pain relief such as Demerol (see p.403), which can sometimes cause memory loss that makes it more difficult to remember the finer details of the birth. It's also helpful to have your birth partner with you throughout your labor so that they can help fill in any blanks later. Photographs and videos are also good prompts.

If you find that there are parts of labor and delivery that you can't remember, you can ask your doctor to review this with you. You might want to consider writing about your experience in a journal.

HYPNOSIS

Being hypnotized during pregnancy can make you more confident in the lead-up to labor. A study found that first-time pregnant women also experienced a shorter labor. The average amount of time they pushed in the second stage was one hour, compared with the usual two hours for a first baby.

FOCUS ON PARTNERS

When you get closer to the birth, and especially during labor, you will find that there is inevitably more contact with health professionals. These individuals are a source of reassurance and a font of knowledge, but as a partner, you may sometimes feel that you're being sidelined or that your opinion doesn't count.

This can be very frustrating if you want to be highly involved in the pregnancy and birth.

Bear in mind that the health professionals are trying to provide care for the person who needs it the most—namely your partner. If you want to be heard, it's a good idea to write down any questions that you may have before you meet with health professionals. Labor nurses will make every effort to help you feel involved and assist you in supporting your partner.

Try to keep in mind that the most important relationship your partner has is with you, and that a positive attitude on your part can make a substantial difference to your partner's pregnancy and birth. Do your best to be patient and persistent but not pushy.

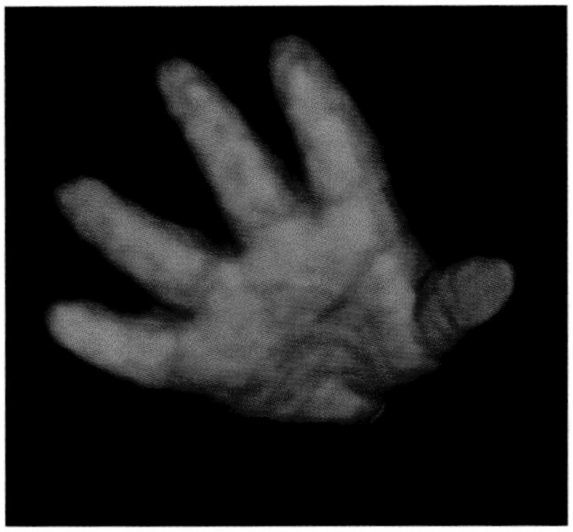

YOU ARE **37 WEEKS AND 2 DAYS**

19 days to go

YOUR BABY TODAY

A 3-D close-up of the hand shows the skin folds. Just as fingerprints are unique, so are the deeper skin folds seen on the hands and feet. The grasp reflex is strong and your baby will start to grasp anything that touches the palm of their hand.

" Your baby will benefit from extra time in the uterus, but their development is almost complete and they're now "full term." "

There is now less space for your baby to move and they will soon, if they hasn't already, settle down into a comfortable head-down position. The shape of the uterus encourages this head-down position and, once in it, turning would be a major effort for your baby. Plenty of amniotic fluid remains to cushion and protect your baby, who will still be attempting to be active in this more confined space.

Your baby's behavior is now exactly the same as a newborn: they'll turn toward light and yawn just as much as a newborn, and they'll continue to practice breathing the amniotic fluid in and out with regular rhythmical movements.

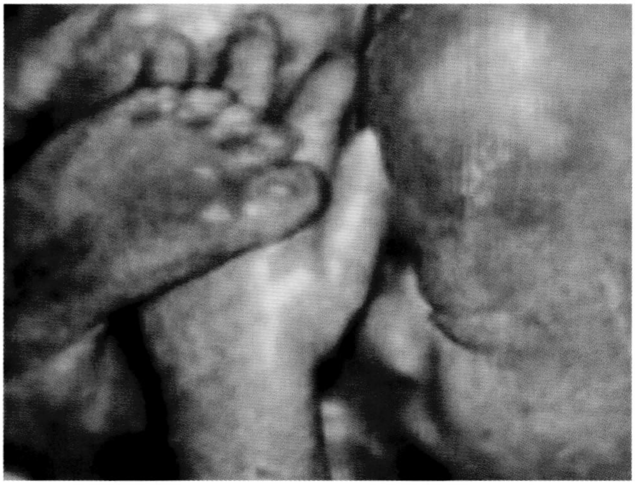

Your baby will be very cramped in the uterus. It won't be long, however, until she's positioned head down and begins to engage in the pelvis as she prepares to make her entry into the world.

HAIR REMOVAL FOR BIRTH

One dilemma that's rarely discussed— but much pondered—among moms-to-be is whether they should shave or trim their pubic hair before giving birth.

This is a personal choice and depends on your preferrence for grooming. There is no medical reason to remove your pubic hair, so don't feel pressured to wax or shave—aside from anything else, itchy regrowth will not be welcome in the days following the birth of your baby. If you prefer a more tidy appearance, you can consider trimming, plucking, or shaving any stragglers, though, in the interest of postpartum hygiene. Postpartum blood loss will cling to the hair.

If you're scheduled to have a Cesarean, your obstetrician may ask to shave the top part of your pubic hair if it is going to interfere with your surgical incision, although it's common to leave the hair as is.

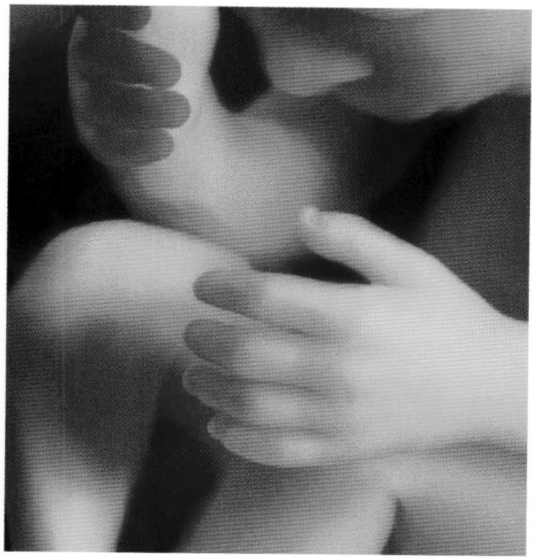

YOU ARE **37 WEEKS AND 3 DAYS**

18 days to go

YOUR BABY TODAY

As your due date approaches, you may experience Braxton-Hicks contractions, which help to soften the cervix and prepare for labor. The amniotic fluid that surrounds your baby ensures they'll hardly notice these mild tightenings.

> "It's a good idea to give some thought to life after the birth, and ensure you have adequate help and support lined up."

HEALTHY SNACKING

Large meals are likely to leave you feeling uncomfortably full, especially late in the third trimester. If you go long periods of time between meals, you may become lightheaded and feel weak from hypoglycemia—low blood sugar. This is because the baby is constantly drawing glucose from your bloodstream.

Healthy snacking is the key to eating well and comfortably:

- **Keep lots of fresh fruit** in the fridge or fruit bowl and snack on it to get your sugar fix, rather than chocolate.
- **Stock up and nibble** on dried fruits and nuts.
- **Keep hard-boiled eggs in the fridge** as a handy nutritious snack.
- **Buy or make some frozen juice pops** and keep them in the freezer. Some women also find it refreshing to suck on these during labor.

Even at this late stage of pregnancy, it may still be hard to imagine your baby being born and living in your home. You and your partner may settle into life with your newborn with ease, and manage without any help, but it's still a good idea to have backup support just in case.

What you may not be prepared for is the fact that you're likely to be exhausted after weeks of poor sleep during pregnancy, and the rigors of labor itself. Add to this interrupted nights' sleep and the adjustment to being a new parent, and you may well find you'll need to call on people to help practically and emotionally.

It can help enormously to have a good support network set up in advance of giving birth. Ideally, this will be close family and friends who you know you can rely on to drop in to help, but who will also know when you need to be left alone. Even an hour's help to prepare you a nutritious meal, or hold your baby while you get a much-needed rest or a shower, can give you some welcome respite.

Have the number on hand for your lactation consultant so you can ask for advice. Also get on the phone to moms-to-be whom you've met at prenatal classes; they, more than anyone, will be able to relate to how you're feeling.

Don't be too proud to accept help with housework and shopping. Knowing these tasks are taken care of will help you relax and focus on your baby.

Try to limit the number of guests you have in the early days, and make sure that they are warned that visits will be short. Although you will be desperate to show off your new baby, visits can be draining, so it's better to wait until some routines are more established.

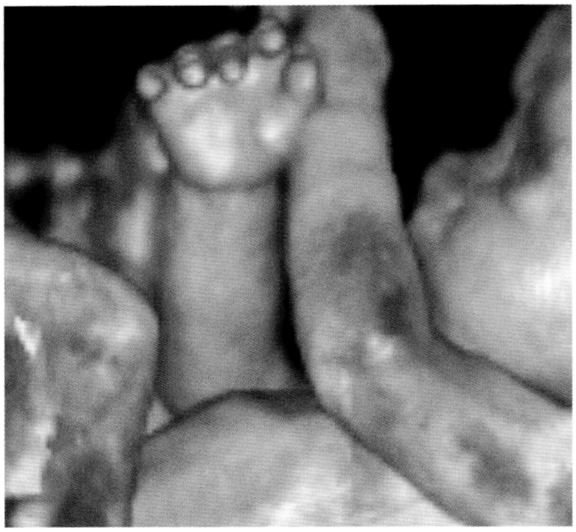

YOU ARE **37 WEEKS AND 4 DAYS**

17 days to go

YOUR BABY TODAY

What exactly triggers the start of labor is still a mystery. Does the signal come from your own body or does the baby play a part in the decision? Every labor is different, and the timing of your first labor can be quite different from your second.

> "Gradually, each of your baby's bones is becoming strengthened thanks to adequate amounts of calcium."

Your baby's bones are strengthened by the process of ossification in which hard bone is formed from calcium. To meet this increase in demand, you absorb calcium much more readily from your diet.

By this stage of pregnancy, the baby's humerus in the upper arm, femur in the upper leg, and tibia in the lower leg have undergone this process. As ossification occurs at specific weeks in your pregnancy, ultrasound scans can use these as markers to estimate the date of the pregnancy, if necessary.

The time at which this ossification occurs may be seen a few days earlier in girls than boys and, interestingly, the patella (knee bone), does not ossify until after birth.

ASK A DOCTOR

I've had a small amount of bleeding. Should I be concerned? Bleeding in late pregnancy is common and usually not harmful to your pregnancy. However, you should always let your doctor know if you are having any bleeding, and you will need to be seen by an obstetrician to confirm that there are no serious concerns. Serious causes of bleeding include placental abruption, when the placenta separates from the uterus wall. A low-lying placenta can also cause painless vaginal bleeding. A sticky mucousy discharge, which is often tinged with blood, is called "bloody show" and may indicate labor is starting (see pp. 391 and 411).

BACH FLOWER REMEDIES

Flower essence blends are designed to calm and center your energy, which some think can help you relax and encourage you to focus. Rescue Remedy and Emergency Essence, types of Bach Flower Remedy, are thought by some to be effective when used in labor, and in the weeks prior to and after the birth. The remedies are taken for a variety of symptoms, including anxiety, shock, worry, stress, or simply for a boost during a long or painful labor.

A few drops may be taken on your tongue as required or mixed in water. Both of these blends also come in cream form, to apply topically, or as a spray, to spritz yourself and your environment.

Ask your doctor before you try these or other natural remedies, since they haven't been thoroughly studied.

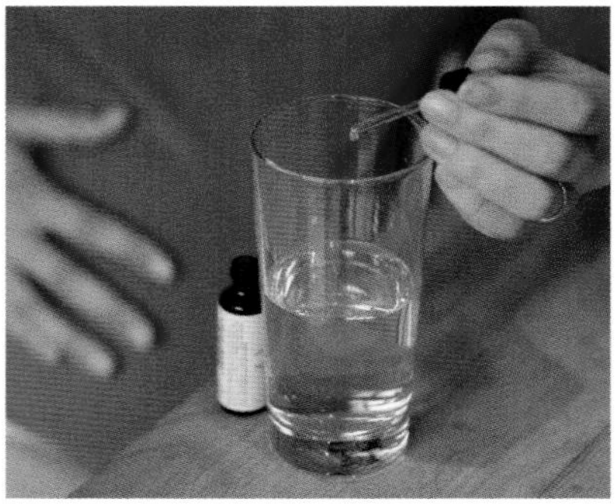

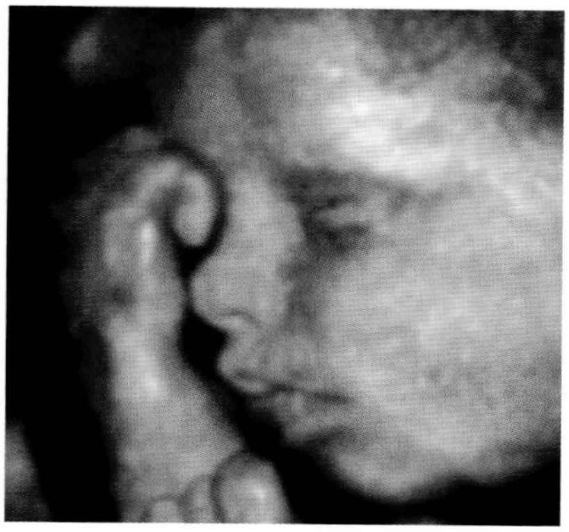

YOU ARE **37 WEEKS AND 5 DAYS**

16 days to go

YOUR BABY TODAY

The size of your uterus may have reduced slightly as your baby's head becomes more deeply engaged within your pelvis, allowing their body to move down. This can take some of the pressure away from your ribs, which is a welcome relief at this stage.

> "When there's going to be a new arrival on the scene, it's important to prepare the little members of your household."

ASK A DOCTOR

My mom had a difficult delivery with me. Am I likely to have the same experience as her? Like many women, you're aware of the details of your own birth.

Some say you'll have the same sort of delivery your mom had with you—for example, your baby will be early or late or you'll have a very quick labor or a slow, assisted one. This isn't necessarily true.

Remember, depending on how old your mom is, there have probably been significant developments in obstetrics since your mom's days and, even if you face the same hurdles during your labor, they might be managed differently.

Also, you might be healthier and stronger than your mom was, so don't assume you're in for a difficult labor just because she had one.

How you handle introducing the new baby to your children will depend on their age. A toddler might be totally indifferent and unfazed, being more interested in your new baby's toys than the fact that they have a new brother or sister. An older child might be shocked and jealous by the arrival of a new baby, who appears to steal their limelight, and divert their parents' attention.

It's a good idea to prepare your little one several weeks in advance, explaining that the new baby will need a lot of time and attention, will need to be fed and changed regularly, and probably not be much fun for a few months. Focus on how your child can be a great helper, and show them what the new baby will need when they are born. Check some books out from the library that explain how families change when a new baby is born, and ask your child to talk about how they're feeling, and how they think things will be different when the baby arrives.

Encourage your child to choose a gift to give to the baby, and find something your child really wants as a gift from their new sibling. Ask grandparents or close friends to arrange a few treats or outings for your child both now and after the birth so that they're occupied and getting extra attention.

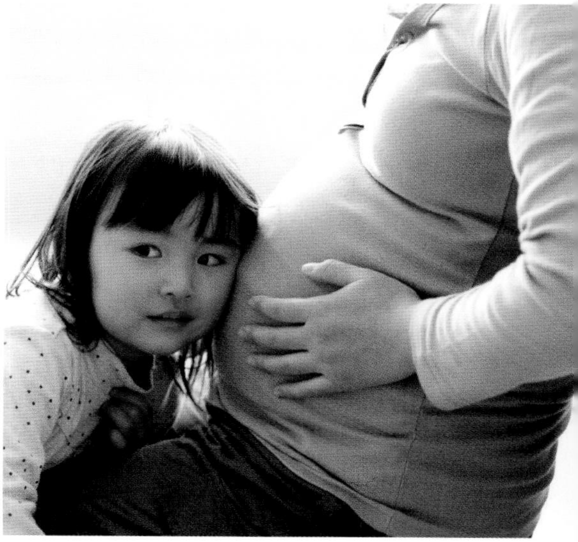

Try to encourage a bond between your older child and your baby. They might want to listen in or gently feel your bump for movements. Ask them to imagine what the baby might be getting up to inside there.

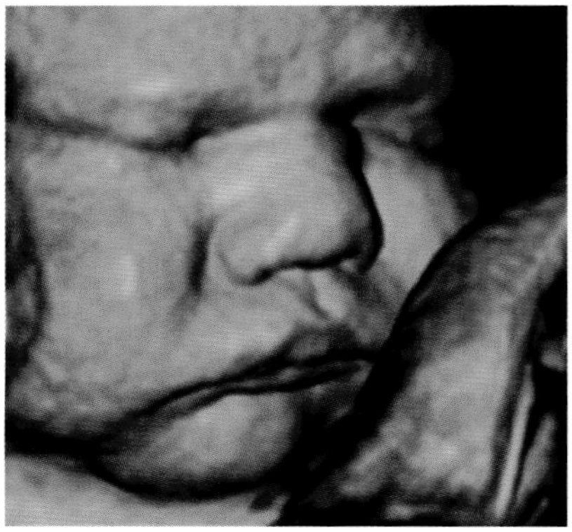

YOU ARE **37 WEEKS AND 6 DAYS**

15 days to go

YOUR BABY TODAY

Estimating your baby's size by measuring from the top of the uterus to the front of your pelvic bone is less accurate now. Your baby may not yet have moved down into the pelvis and the amount of fluid around your baby is variable.

" Newborn babies can tightly hold someone's finger because of the grasp reflex, and this is already functioning in the uterus. "

Inside the uterus, your baby has developed a strong grasp reflex. The grip is so strong after birth that it could support your baby's weight. This grasp reflex persists until your baby is about six months old; they will then have more choice over whether to grasp an object or not.

Interestingly, your baby also has a similar reflex in the foot. This is the "plantar reflex" and it causes the toes to attempt to curl around your finger if the sole of the foot is stroked. The plantar reflex takes slightly longer to disappear after birth, typically persisting until 12 months of age. Another reflex action causes the toes to spread out if the side of the foot is stroked. These reflexes and others seem to be quite primitive in nature and although they are thought to protect the baby, the precise function of each reflex is not fully understood.

SECOND LABORS

Second labors are usually shorter in duration than first labors.This usually means an easier labor, but a second baby could be bigger than a first, or positioned differently. There are many factors to consider.

ASK A DOCTOR

Is it true that natural or water births are best for the baby? Most childbirth experts would agree that a straightforward vaginal birth is the safest form of birth for both mother and baby. It is also generally considered safe to use water as a method of relieving the pain in uncomplicated labors.

However, it is sometimes not possible to achieve a straightforward vaginal delivery due to certain situations that can arise during labor and birth. If a problem with either the mother or baby occurs, the medical team will advise you on the safest way of delivering the baby.

It's important to think about the type of birth you would prefer, but be prepared to be flexible and to see how labor unfolds. Ask your doctor if there's a birthing pool you can use at your hospital.

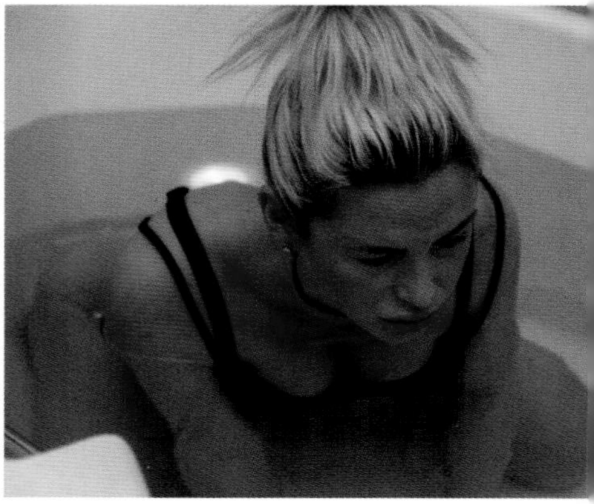

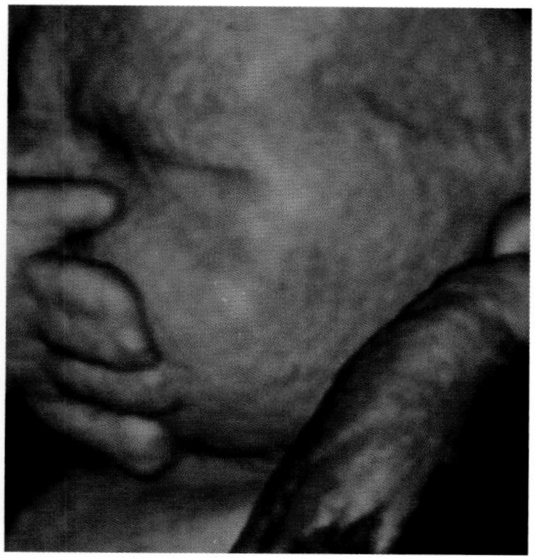

YOU ARE **38 WEEKS EXACTLY**

14 days to go

YOUR BABY TODAY

The back of the hand is held up against the mouth in this image. Your baby will be practicing suckling at every opportunity, but this will be with parts of the hands, thumbs, or fingers, since it's no longer easy to reach the toes.

> "If you haven't found out the sex of your baby, the excitement will be building; if you have, you can decide on a name, at least."

Knowing the sex of your baby can be useful. In addition to choosing a name, you may want to buy items that you feel are more suitable for a boy or a girl. Remember, however, there's a chance that the scan (see pp.214–215) gave you misleading information. The only way to be absolutely certain of the baby's gender is if you found out following a diagnostic test, such as amniocentesis or chorionic villus sampling (see pp.152–153).

If you know the sex, you won't have the same incentive of a surprise at the end of your labor, but you may feel you can bond more closely with your baby during pregnancy and picture what they will be like as a newborn.

If you don't know the sex yet, then you will have a well-earned surprise after your hard work in labor. Some women who don't know the sex of their babies say that they have a strong instinct that the baby is a particular sex but may be quite surprised when they have a baby of the opposite sex.

It may help to know that, overall 105 male babies are born for every 100 female babies worldwide.

If you're really curious and want to guess the sex of your baby, you might want to bear in mind these old wives' tales:

If your hands are soft, it's said you're having a girl; if they're rough, you're having a boy.

If the mother picks up her coffee cup with two hands, it's a girl; if she picks it up by the handle, it's a boy.

If you have a sensitive belly button, it's a girl; if you have cold feet, it's almost certainly a boy!

TRUST YOUR BODY

Be reassured that your body is designed to handle the pain of labor! Nobody likes pain, but your body's endorphin levels will increase during labor to help you cope with it. So it's reassuring to know that as the intensity of the contractions builds, so does your ability to handle them.

ASK A DOCTOR

My baby is in a posterior position. How will this affect my labor? In the posterior position, the baby faces your belly instead of your spine (see p.336). This position may prolong your labor, and cause more of a backache.

Most of the time, the baby turns into an anterior position, with the help of contractions as the head descends down the birth canal. If the baby doesn't turn on their own, your obstetrician may be able to gently turn their head, or use forceps or a ventouse (see pp.436–437); occasionally a Cesarean birth may be needed.

Your 39th week

TIME MAY FEEL AS THOUGH IT'S STANDING STILL AND EVERY SMALL TWINGE HAS YOU ON THE ALERT. Know the signs that mean labor is really about to start. You may have some false alarms, so don't hesitate to call your doctor for advice and reassurance. Excitement will be competing with nerves—and that goes for your partner as well. No one can predict how labor is going to turn out, but before the big day it's helpful to agree on what your partner's role should ideally be.

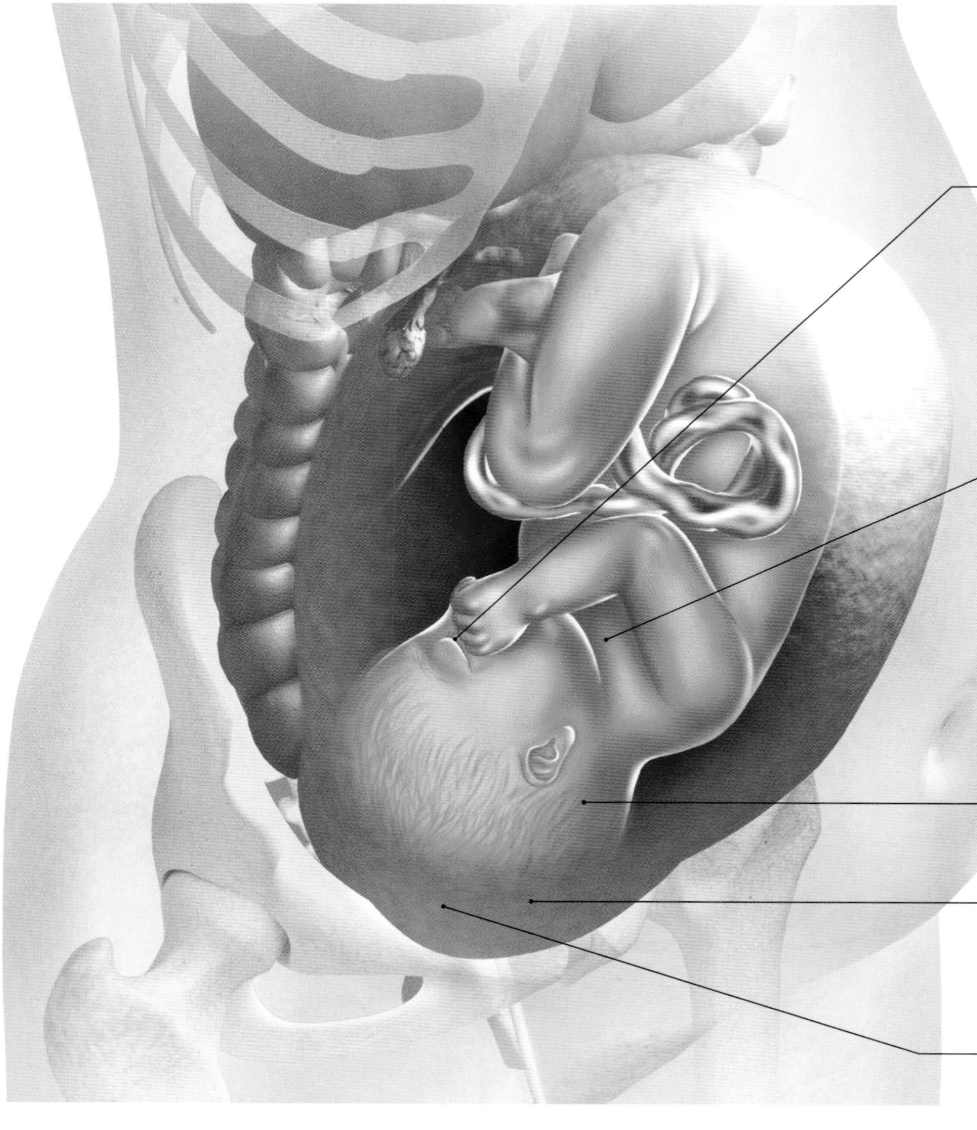

The eyes are large and well formed, although the neural networks are not yet sophisticated enough for the baby to focus. Vision in newborns remains poor for a few weeks after birth while the eyes continue to develop.
Breathing is now rhythmical, with your baby making around 40 breathing movements every minute.
The head may be covered with hair, a few wispy strands—or no hair at all.
The baby is so low down in your pelvis that you have probably exchanged discomfort in your upper abdominal area for pressure on your bladder.
At 39 weeks the average crown to heel length is 20 in (50.7 cm) and the average weight is 7.3 lb (3.3 kg).

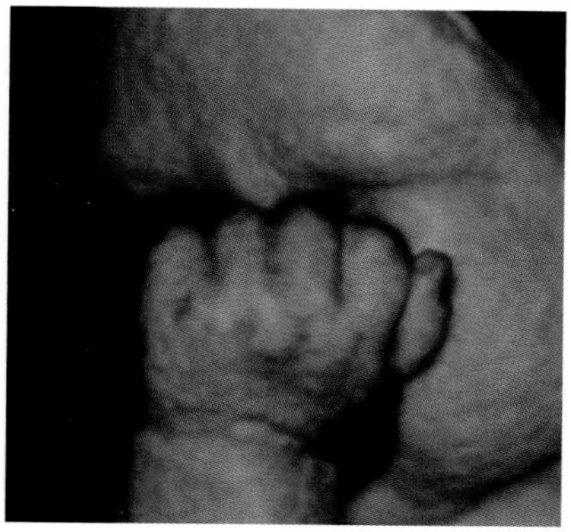

YOU ARE **38 WEEKS AND 1 DAY**

13 days to go

YOUR BABY TODAY

This baby's hand is in the same position as in the image opposite, with the fist held tightly in front of the face. All of your baby's movements help build muscle strength and aid coordination, whether it's a kick or simply curling and uncurling the fingers.

" With labor imminent, you'll be playing the waiting game. Staying active will help the time pass much more quickly. "

Try to rest a lot in the next two weeks. As your figure expands and you become more tired, it's natural to want to sit out the remainder of your pregnancy at home with your feet up, and turn on your voice mail to field all the "Has it arrived?" inquiries!

It's fine to do this, but it's good to remember that the very best way to stimulate labor is to keep active. What's more, the hormones produced by even gentle walking will lift your mood and help you feel more positive when your labor begins.

Try to do something nice each day—perhaps meeting a friend for lunch, going for a very gentle swim, or purchasing some last-minute items for baby—being careful to stop and put your feet up when you feel tired. Be sensible about the type of activities you undertake, and avoid anything that could be exhausting or potentially dangerous; for example, bear in mind that your center of gravity is way off balance at the moment, and that wallpapering the nursery or carrying heavy groceries should definitely not be on your to-do list.

It may feel as though your life is on hold at the moment, so that's why it's good to fill your time as best you can. Don't forget, however, that in just a couple of weeks you'll have your newborn occupying all your time.

THE POWER OF MUSIC

Research has shown that women who listen to music during labor tend to feel less stressed and are less likely to need pain relief. There's also some evidence to suggest that babies born to the accompaniment of music are calmer.

One study compared different beats and found that classical, instrumental sounds were the most relaxing. Familiar tunes and rhythms could distract you from the pain and—if you choose the right track—help you focus on your breathing. Create your playlist well in advance of labor.

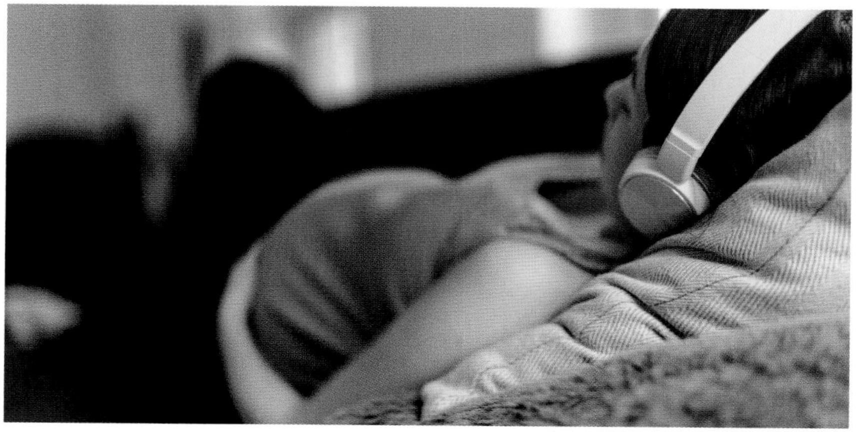

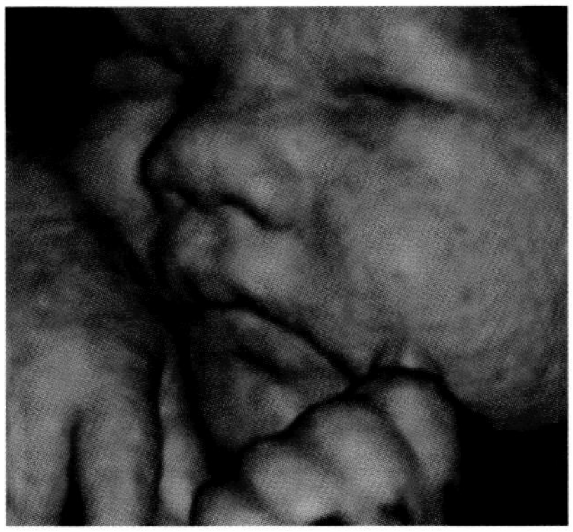

YOU ARE **38 WEEKS AND 2 DAYS**

12 days to go

YOUR BABY TODAY

Your baby's head, deep within your pelvis, remains rounded in shape. It is not until labor starts that the bones of the skull move closer to each other, elongating the shape of the head, and allowing your baby to pass more easily along the birth canal.

" Although your baby will be born with beautifully big eyes, it will be some time before they will see clearly at a distance. "

Your baby's eyes are almost their adult size at birth. Although the eyes continue to grow very slightly until adolescence, and the lens within the eye grows throughout life, the eye is three-quarters of its adult size at birth. Both color (cones) and black and white visual cells (rods) are present in the retina, but vision is still rather poor—equivalent to being able to just see the top letter of the optician's chart. This is referred to as 20/400 vision. This means than if the baby could read, then they could read a letter at 20 ft (6 m) that a person with perfect vision could read when 400 ft (122 m) away. Because of this, your newborn may not seem to pay much attention at first; they'll have some difficulty focusing and their eye muscles will be quite weak. They will, however, be able to see objects 12 in (30 cm) away (roughly the distance between your breast and face), so they can see your face as they feed. They'll be six to eight weeks old before fixing onto and following an object, four months before they can judge distances, and two years of age before their vision has perfected to 20/20.

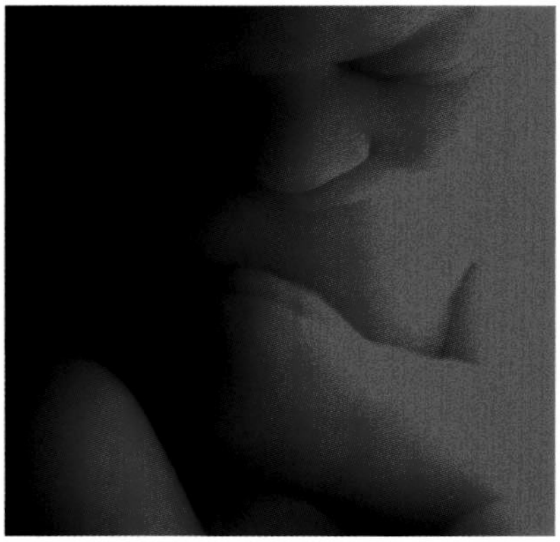

Your baby will have gained weight steadily during these final weeks, with fat being laid down under the skin. If born now, they would have a plump, rounded appearance.

ASK A MIDWIFE

I don't often swear but is it true that I'm likely to subject my partner to verbal abuse during labor? Possibly, but no one will blame you if you do! Giving birth can be incredibly painful, and you may feel emotional, irritable, shaky, and even nauseated. Don't worry too much about what you say and do: try to stay focused on the birth and ask for pain relief if you need it. Most birth partners will be forgiving and are unlikely to take the abuse personally. They will realize that you might not quite be yourself during childbirth—and if they've been by your side throughout labor will be fully understanding of what you're going through. You may also be irritable with your caregivers, but they will be used to this!

THE DUE DATE

95 percent of babies don't arrive on their due date—of these, 25 percent come early and 70 percent late.

There's a 5-week window (37–42 weeks) of pregnancy that's regarded as normal and safe for a baby to be born. Due to recent evidence, however, elective delivery before 39 weeks is not recommended.

Five weeks is a long time to wait, so put a message on your voice mail along the lines of "We'll be in touch as soon as the baby's here." Keep busy: have your hair done, catch up with friends, and, most importantly, get some sleep!

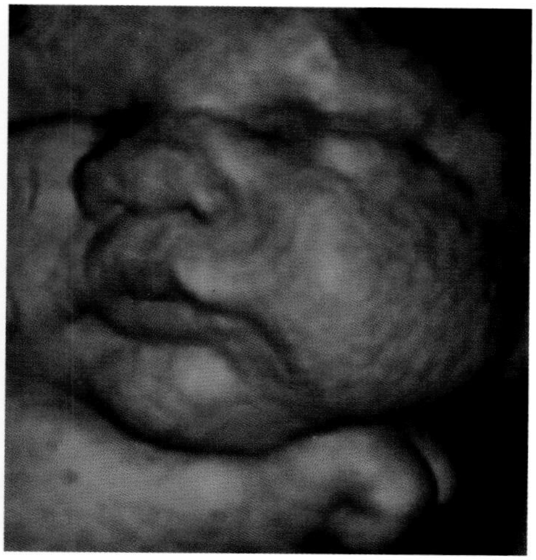

YOU ARE **38 WEEKS AND 3 DAYS**

11 days to go

YOUR BABY TODAY

This image demonstrates how your baby has laid down fat reserves, nicely rounding out the cheeks. In these final weeks, your baby will continue to grow in the uterus, although at a slower rate than previously.

> “If you’re having a home birth, you can make the midwife’s task as easy as possible by being well organized.”

If you’re having your baby at home, spend this week ensuring that everything is in order and that the room in which you plan to give birth is clean, comfortable, and adequately heated.

Your midwife may bring around a pack about now, which contains all the items they will need. To make their task easier, make sure the bed on which you’re going to deliver (if you plan to use a bed) is easily accessible from all sides. You might also want to ensure you have plenty of extra pillows on hand as well as several changes of bed sheets.

Even if you plan to labor in dim lighting, remember that there needs to be a good source of light for the midwife, especially after the birth when you may need to have stitches.

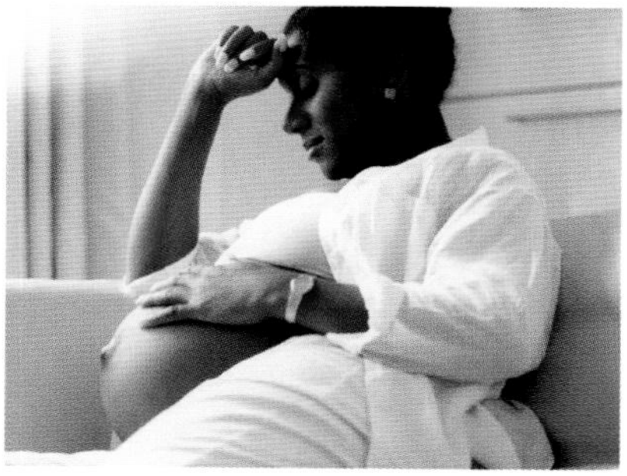

Learn to catnap for 10–20 minutes. This will help you rest and revive you, and it’s a good technique to use once the baby is born.

ON PUSHING

You will feel a strong urge to push during labor, but because it’s painful you might resist doing so. Medications such as an epidural (see pp.404–405) will reduce the sensation of wanting to push. Your labor nurse will help you throughout and guide you as to when it’s safe and most effective to push.

ASK A DOCTOR

I’m so tired already. How will I ever get through labor? First of all, take every opportunity you can to rest—even if this means napping several times during the day. Every bit of sleep you get will make a difference to your energy levels, especially if you’re having broken sleep at night.

When you are feeling good, try to do some gentle exercise as this encourages healthy, restful sleep. Swimming can be a great way to expend energy and take your mind off things, and it puts little or no pressure on your belly or your aching muscles and joints.

Try eating food containing tryptophan (see p.177) before you go to bed, which can encourage sleep, and make sure that you get plenty of high-energy carbohydrates (see p.92) during the day, to keep your blood-sugar levels stable and prevent energy slumps.

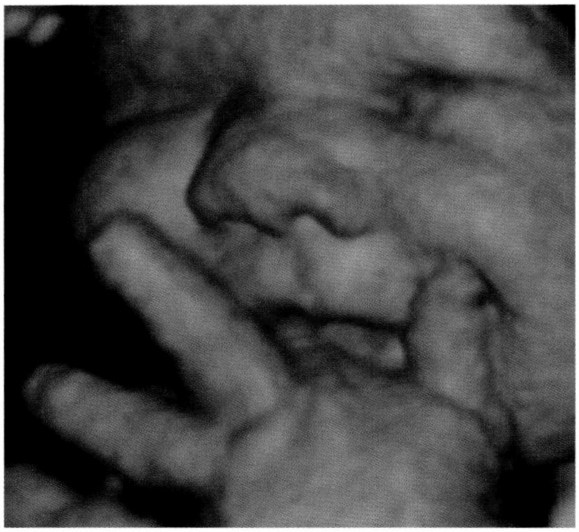

YOU ARE **38 WEEKS AND 4 DAYS**

10 days to go...

YOUR BABY TODAY

Your baby's neck muscles have strengthened, so the head can be held well away from the chest wall. Once delivered, though, the buoyancy provided by the amniotic fluid will be lost and you will need to support the head at all times while holding your baby.

> "Could your baby be dreaming already? A lot of their movements are occurring when they're fast asleep."

Your baby has been practicing breathing since week 10, but now the pattern has changed from short practice bursts lasting 10 seconds or so, to a regular rhythmic breathing pattern of approximately 40 breaths per minute, just as the baby will breathe after birth.

Eye movements have also matured with periods of rapid eye movement (REM) lasting for just over 25 minutes at a time and rest periods lasting just under 25 minutes. REM sleep is closely coupled with periods of increased activity and a faster heart rate. So just because your baby is moving it doesn't always mean that they're awake.

Although your baby cannot stretch out as freely now, movements at least 10 times a day should continue in the same familiar pattern.

FUEL FOR LABOR

Labor is definitely tiring and thirsty work! Thankfully, it is now accepted that unless a woman is known to need anesthesia, she can eat and drink in the early stages of labor. Having said that, many women find that they don't have much of an appetite as labor progresses.

Try isotonic sports drinks, as well as drinking water, since they provide some energy to counter the fatigue of labor. It is better to sip drinks during labor instead of drinking large amounts at a time. Pack healthy snacks and drinks in your hospital bag (see p.358).

ASK A DOCTOR

What is "stripping the membranes" and could I have this instead of being induced if I end up being overdue?
Depending on your health and the baby's condition, and many other factors (for example, you're more than 42 weeks along, you have high blood pressure, you have an infection), your doctor may induce labor. There are many ways to do this, including stripping the membranes. With a gloved finger, your doctor checks your cervix and sweeps her finger over the membranes that connect the amniotic sac and the uterine wall. The goal of this is to stimulate the release of hormones that may start labor contractions. Although this procedure may feel uncomfortable and can cause a little bleeding, it should not cause you actual pain. Following the sweep, you may have a mucousy "bloody show" (see p.411), which is quite normal.

The procedure can be done at your doctor's office or in the hospital (see p.432). Your doctor will advise you of your due date.

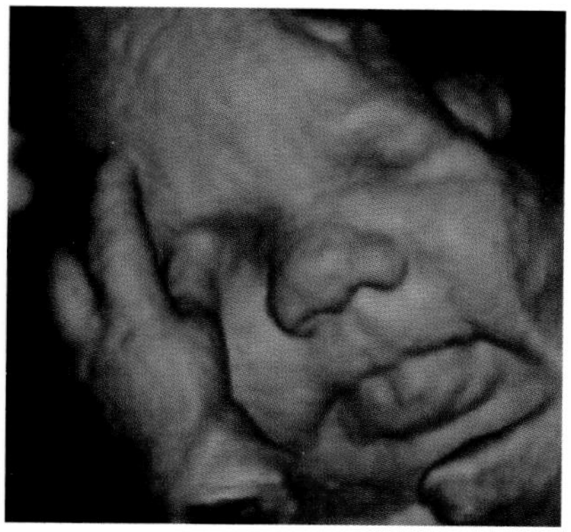

YOU ARE **38 WEEKS AND 5 DAYS**

9 days to go...

YOUR BABY TODAY

It can be hard to accurately predict the size of a newborn baby. An ultrasound can estimate the weight, but as with all other measurements at this time, it has a fairly wide margin of error.

“ Don’t just wait for contractions—it’s worth familiarizing yourself now with the signs that may mean labor is imminent. ”

If it’s your first pregnancy, it can be difficult to recognize the signs that the baby is on their way. Some women get lower back pain that is minor before becoming painful. You might notice a bloody show (see p.411), which can happen well before true labor actually starts. Your water may break as the sac containing the amniotic fluid bursts open. Even if your water breaking is not accompanied by contractions, you should still inform your doctor of what is happening.

Finally, the most obvious sign is contractions: these painful tightenings of your uterus will increase in intensity and become more regular as labor progresses. Contractions are associated with the dilation and shortening of your cervix, so your doctor will examine you to see how far you’ve progressed (see pp.414–415).

If you think that you are in labor, stay calm and call your doctor or prental provider. Inform them of your symptoms and, especially, describe your contractions and whether your baby is moving. If you’re having contractions every 5 minutes that last for a minute (time them), and they’re so uncomfortable that you’re forced to stop what you’re doing, you should think about going to the hospital.

FETAL MONITORING

If there are no complications or reasons for concern, your baby’s heartbeat will usually be monitored using a handheld device much like the one used during your prenatal appointments. You may be hooked up throughout the entire labor and birth, or your nurse may listen to your baby’s heartbeat every 15 to 30 minutes, which means that you can move around as much as you like in between these checks.

If you’ve had complications in pregnancy, or problems develop during labor, the doctor may monitor the heartbeat using a CTG (see p.418) and transfer you to a labor ward.

ASK A DOCTOR

How long am I likely to stay in hospital after the birth? After a vaginal delivery, you will usually stay 1–2 days after in the hospital. If you had a Cesarean delivery, you will typically stay 2–3 days postpartum.

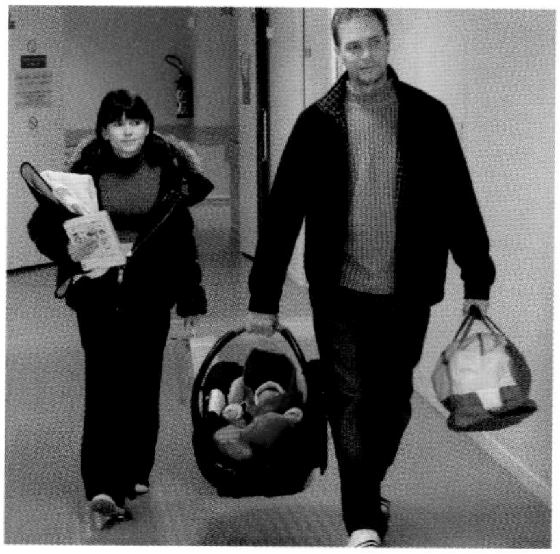

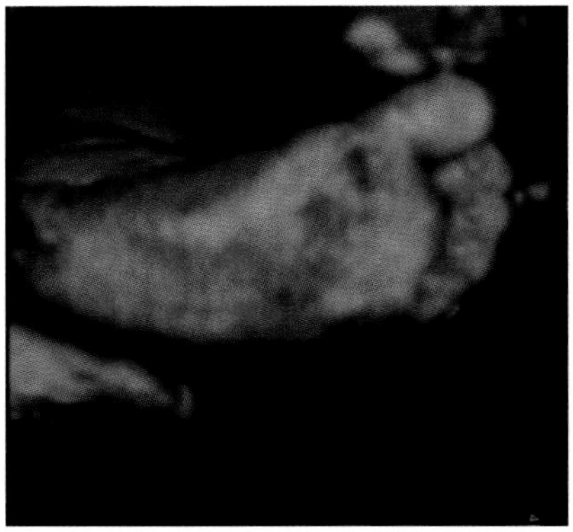

YOU ARE **38 WEEKS AND 6 DAYS**

8 days to go...

YOUR BABY TODAY

The movements that you feel will usually be concentrated in a few areas since your baby cannot readily change position. Although the character of these movements will have changed, you should still experience many movements each day.

> "Because you're heading into the final week, you're bound to feel a little anxious, but hopefully excited, too."

It's normal to feel a little anxious about your impending labor, especially if it's your first baby. Try not to keep your feelings bottled up: share anxieties with your partner, since you might find that they are in need of reassurance, too. Do confide in friends and family, but remember not to get drawn into stories of their birth experiences, or someone else they know, as these can often add to feelings of anxiety!

If you have specific concerns, call your midwife. She'll be used to handling these worries and will be able to put your mind at rest.

Plan your time to keep busy and active, but always be aware of your limitations at this stage of pregnancy and invite people to visit you at home, rather than you visiting them. An ideal outing in this final couple of weeks might be a gentle stroll in your local park with a friend or relative.

ASK A DOCTOR

What are the signs that it's too late to go to the hospital? If you're having an uncontrollable urge to push, then that's the point where it may be too late to reach the hospital before your delivery.

If you do find yourself in this situation, call your doctor who will advise you. They may arrange to send paramedics to you for the delivery of the baby. Or you can contact the emergency ambulance services yourself and follow their advice while you wait for their arrival.

FOCUS ON PARTNERS

As your partner's primary support, you have the difficult job of trying to take charge, exude calm, and give emotional and practical support. Don't hesitate to call the doctor—a short discussion may help you to gauge how far your partner has progressed. You must allow plenty of time to get to the hospital and you should be familiar with the route.

There may be periods when your partner is not lucid, but you will know what she wants better than anyone else. It's therefore your role to advocate for her and to engage with the medical staff when she can't do it herself. You'll also know how to reassure and encourage her.

The time taken to complete the first stage of labor (see pp.408–421) is varied. In a first pregnancy, the prelabor or latent phase can last for over 24 hours. With a second baby, this phase is very short and labor is usually much quicker.

In the second stage of labor, your partner may change position frequently and you will need to help and support her and provide lots of encouragement.

In the third stage (see pp.428–429), once the baby is born, you may cut the cord. Watching the birth of your baby is likely to be a very emotional experience. Do not worry if you are moved to tears—this happens frequently.

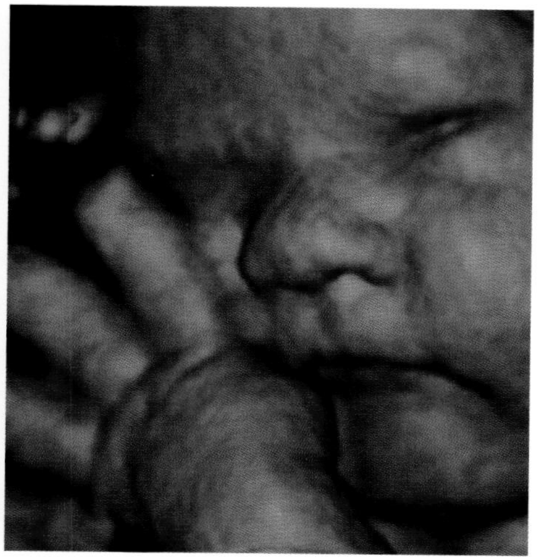

YOU ARE **39 WEEKS EXACTLY**

7 days to go...

YOUR BABY TODAY

This baby can easily be seen at this late stage in the pregnancy because there is ample amniotic fluid present. The amount of amniotic fluid at this point is still extremely variable, but it is usually in the region of 18 fl oz (0.5 liter).

> “Use this time in the run-up to labor to get your partner fully up to speed on how they can help you on the big day.”

FINAL PREPARATIONS

It's amazing that even after 40 weeks of pregnancy, when labor begins, there is still a scramble before heading off to the hospital. So to avoid last-minute panic:

- **Make sure your bag is packed** (see p.358). You may also want have a list handy of any extras you'll need at the last minute.
- **Decide who will do what:** For example, perhaps your partner could prepare snacks.
- **Do a trial run** of the trip to the hospital—anticipating areas where there is likely to be traffic, seeking out shortcuts, and figuring out where you are most likely to find a parking space. It can also help to time the run at various points in the day, so you can avoid school-zone hot spots or commuter traffic. Also find out how to get into the maternity unit at night.
- **Above all, don't panic.** The majority of parents-to-be do get to the hospital in plenty of time.

It's a good idea to prepare your partner in advance, and figure out what may help the proceedings once labor does begin. If you're planning on listening to music during labor, laboring in a tub, or walking around, inform your partner ahead of time what you think you'll expect from him.

Ask your partner to practice some massage strokes, and teach him how to do them (see p.163). Some women can't bear to be touched during labor, but others find it helpful to have their back, or even just their hands and feet, massaged. You won't really know what works for you until you're in labor but practicing massage now won't hurt.

If your partner has been going to prenatal classes with you, they will be familiar with the breathing and relaxation techniques so practice these together and, if necessary, get advice from your doctor about techniques.

It may be helpful for your partner to speak to friends or relatives who have recently had a baby. Hearing the experiences of others and learning some do's and don'ts of being a birth partner might be useful.

THE BABY'S LENGTH

Whatever their weight, most babies at 40 weeks are approximately the same length— 95 percent are between 17.7 in (45 cm) and 21.6 in (55 cm) long. The length of newborn babies is remarkably consistent and relates to skeletal growth, whereas birth weight may vary considerably.

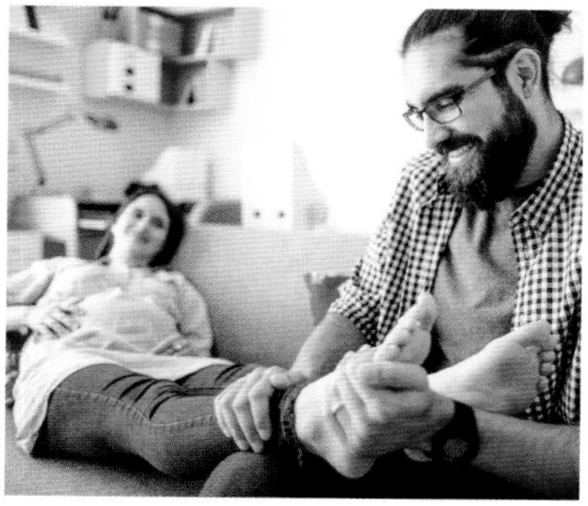

You may find it relaxing to have your feet massaged in the early stages of labor, even if you don't want your back or shoulders touched. A massage helps to relieve tension.

Your 40th week

ALL THE MILESTONES ARE SAFELY PASSED AND YOU WILL MEET YOUR BABY ANY DAY NOW. Like many moms, you may have to linger in suspense beyond the "last" day of pregnancy. Without a doubt, the big event is about to happen very soon and it will be worth the waiting, wondering, and worrying. Once you see and hold your baby, you won't spend much time looking back over the past 40 weeks, but you'll certainly marvel at the miracle of it all.

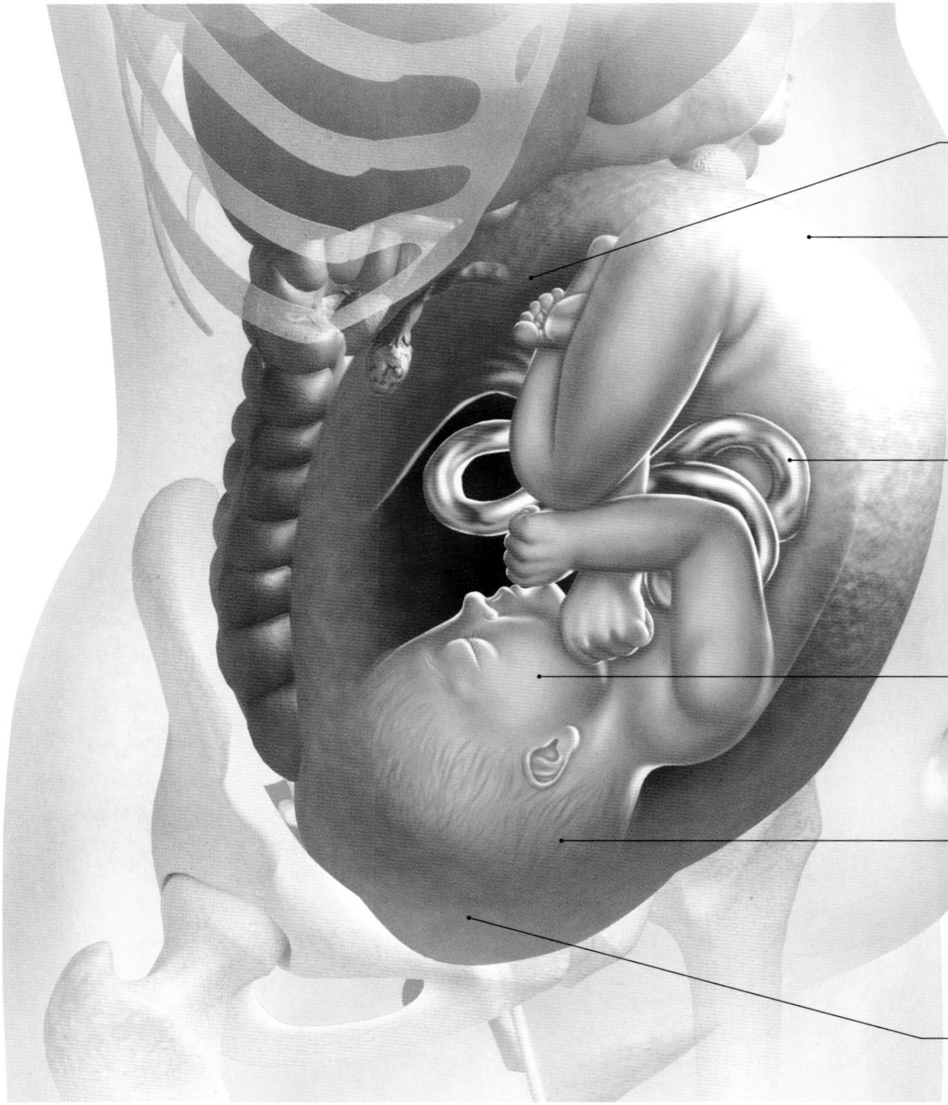

Shortly after the baby is born, further contractions will separate the placenta from the wall of the uterus. The doctor may gently deliver it by pulling on the umbilical cord.

The membranes of the amniotic sac will rupture once labor starts, and the fluid that has cushioned the baby for months will drain away.

The umbilical cord is about the same length as your baby.

At full term the baby has the rounded chubby cheeks typical of new babies.

The skull bones are separated by membranes that allow for movement between bones and an easier passage of the head through the birth canal.

At 40 weeks the average crown to heel length is 20.2 in (51.2 cm) and the average weight is 7.7 lb (3.5 kg).

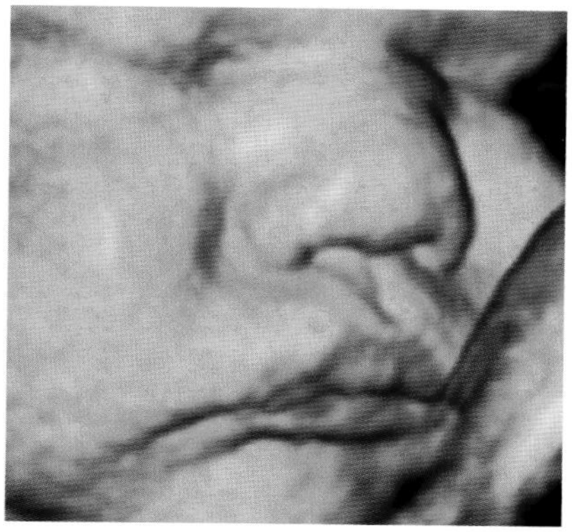

YOU ARE **39 WEEKS AND 1 DAY**

6 days to go...

YOUR BABY TODAY

If you are having a planned Cesarean delivery, this is usually offered now—in order to balance the chance of labor starting unexpectedly with that of delivering your baby too soon. It is best for babies to be delivered as close to the due date as possible.

" It's good to revisit your birth plan at this late stage since you may feel differently now about some of the requests you made. "

A birth plan is usually filled in earlier in pregnancy, and reviewed at 36 weeks (see pp.181 and 303). Now that the birth is imminent, look over it with your partner to consider things like your preferred method of pain relief, how you would like to be directed in pushing, and any other interventions that might be needed during labor. Adapt your birth plan as needed and discuss any changes or new concerns with your doctor.

Since your partner will be your advocate in labor, putting your requests forward to your labor nurses and doctor if you're unable to express them, it's important that they understand your wishes and they're fresh in mind.

Remember, though, that you won't really know how you'll feel or what you want until you're in labor, so keep an open mind and be prepared to adapt your plans on the day if it's in the best interests of your baby's well-being.

Discuss with your partner how you think they can best help you, whether it be giving you a massage or holding your hand. Talk to them about your concerns, hopes, and expectations.

STAYING CLOSE

It can be difficult to think of anything but the birth this close to the end of pregnancy. Try to focus on other things:

- **Spend time with your partner:** Enjoy quality time together while it is still just the two of you.
- **Have sex:** you might feel you are too big, or too tired, but it is good to remind yourselves of your sexual relationship. And, you never know, having sex could just get your labor started (see p.393).

ASK A DOCTOR

Can I refuse to be induced? You have a right to say no to any intervention, but generally, induction is recommended when there is a risk in continuing the pregnancy. Make sure you understand why an induction is being recommended. Your doctor will review the process with you. Discuss any concerns you have and why you don't want an induction. If you decide against an induction, you may need additional monitoring for the remainder of the pregnancy.

Many doctors induce labor by 41 or 42 weeks. If your pregnancy goes beyond 42 weeks and you don't want to be induced, your doctor may offer monitoring with scans to measure the baby's pulse and volume of fluid around the baby; or you may have an NST (see p.418) once or twice a week until labor to pick up any signs that the placenta is failing. If a problem is found, you'll be advised to have a Cesarean or an induction of labor.

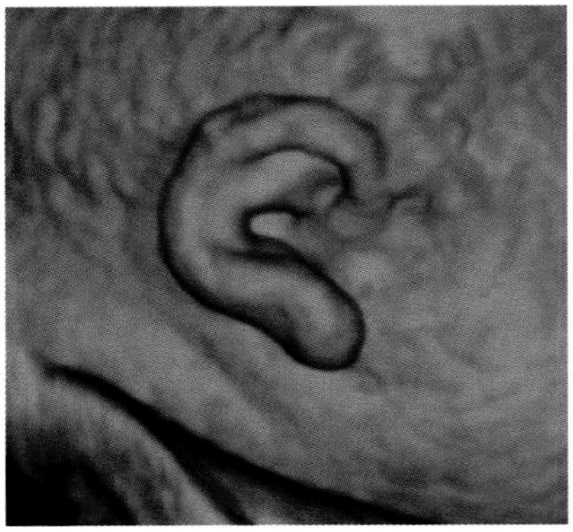

YOU ARE **39 WEEKS AND 2 DAYS**

5 days to go

YOUR BABY TODAY

This close-up 3-D ultrasound view shows that this baby's earlobe is particularly prominent. The dark flecks around the ear look like hair but are in fact shadows (although many babies have hair at this stage).

“Your baby's bones have hardened to a certain degree, but this process will continue right up to the teenage years!”

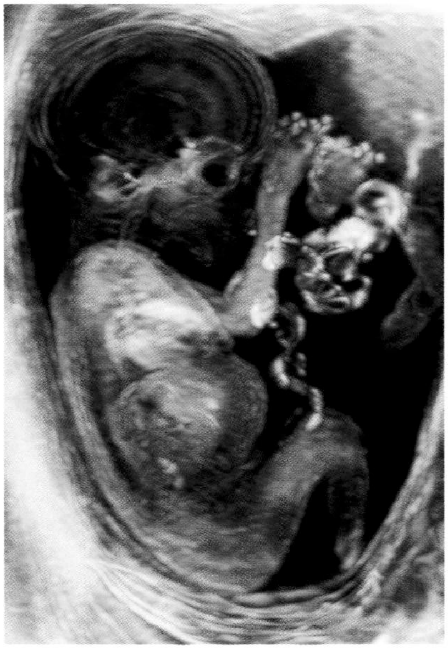

This magnetic resonance imaging scan (MRI) shows a fetus approaching full-term. The baby's brain, spinal column, heart, liver, and lungs are visible, and the umbilical cord can be seen to the right of the image.

Your baby's skeleton has gradually transformed, from soft cartilage to bone, a process called ossification (see p.372). This process starts in the center of each bone spreading outward. By the end of pregnancy, ossification is complete along the length of each bone, but the ends of the long bones and the tips of the bones in the fingers and toes remain as cartilage. This is necessary to allow later bone growth as the child develops.

The bones in the upper part of the skull are slightly different, developing from membranous structures rather than cartilage. These do not fully fuse until several years after birth and remain separated from each other by connective tissue. This connective tissue forms areas called sutures, and where more than two bones meet, wider spaces called fontanelles. Their function is to allow space for movement or “molding” between the skull bones making it easier for the head to descend into the pelvis during labor. It is also these suture lines and fontanelles that help your doctor determine the position of the baby's head during labor.

After delivery, you will notice that your baby's head shape is often elongated, but this soon changes as the bones realign back into their usual positions.

PLACENTA ON TOAST?

The thought of eating the placenta may turn your stomach, but some women choose to do exactly that. The organ is revered for its spiritual properties, and devotees of placentophagia believe the nutrients it contains, including vitamin B6, will help prevent them from developing postpartum depression. However, the evidence in favor of the health benefits of consuming a placenta is purely anecdotal.

An alternative and less controversial custom involves dressing the placenta with herbs, then burying it at a party to celebrate the baby's birth; this is thought to be an important bonding ritual for the extended family.

Art is another option: press the placenta against a piece of paper and you'll get a tree-shaped print.

Some cultures use the dried organ to make medicinal herbs.

Not sure how to cook placenta? Well just look online and you'll find plenty of placenta recipes, from pâté to lasagne, but, understandably, these might not be to everyone's taste.

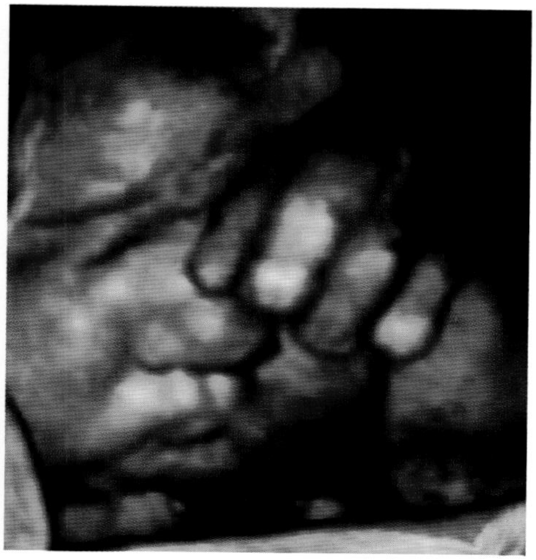

YOU ARE **39 WEEKS AND 3 DAYS**

4 days to go

YOUR BABY TODAY

Once labor starts, your baby will no longer have room to place their hands on top of their head or by their face, although, interestingly, they're still moving around—you probably won't notice these movements since you'll have other things on your mind.

> "The inquiries may begin flooding in this week and it will feel as though the whole world is awaiting news of your baby's arrival."

In this final week of your pregnancy, the weight of expectation can be immense. It can feel as though everyone is waiting for you to pop, especially if it's your first baby.

You'll no doubt cope with it this week—and you may even enjoy getting all the attention—but if you happen to go overdue, you might get frustrated by the constant calls and by having to repeat yourself. Try to be patient and remember people are simply excited for you and are just as frustrated with waiting as you are. Matters aren't helped by the due date. Everyone will have this estimated date in mind, but unfortunately not many babies stick to a schedule and they enter the world exactly when they are ready (see p.378).

By 42 weeks and beyond, fewer than 1 percent of women will still go into spontaneous labor.

FALSE LABOR

You may experience deep and painful twinges, and practice contractions, known as Braxton-Hicks, particularly toward the end of pregnancy. It's easy to mistake these for the real thing, and you may find yourself rushing to hospital, even though you are not yet in labor. You may also experience regular contractions for a period, which then stop. All of this is normal.

One sign that labor may be imminent is that you lose your mucus plug (see p.411); another is your water breaking. In some cases, however, neither of these events takes place until labor is established, so don't panic if they don't happen to you.

You'll definitely know that you're in labor when your contractions are occurring regularly, approximately every 15 minutes—time the gap between them. True contractions will get longer, stronger, and closer together as time goes on and won't go away when you walk around or change position.

ASK A DOCTOR

How much should my baby be moving? Good fetal movements are the most important reassurance that your baby is doing well. You will notice a pattern to the movements; if this changes or you have concerns that the movements are different, contact your obstetrician and go for an immediate check. Your doctor will ask what has changed, monitor the baby's heartbeat, and may offer a cervical exam. If you've had two or more episodes of reduced movements in the last three weeks, they may perform an ultrasound to check the baby's amniotic fluid levels or recommend an induction; reduced movements may indicate a problem.

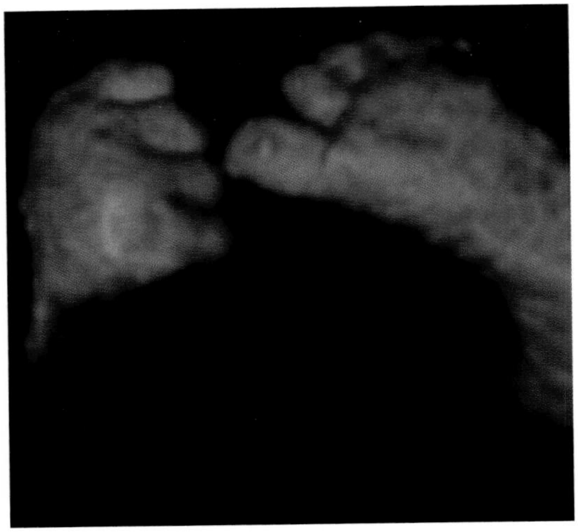

YOU ARE **39 WEEKS AND 4 DAYS**

3 days to go

YOUR BABY TODAY

This image shows that even at this time your baby will be able to reach down and touch their toes (see the foot on the right and the hand on the left). Because there is less space your baby will no longer be able to place their feet on top of their head.

> “Don’t be too concerned if your baby hasn’t engaged yet since this won’t have any bearing on the final delivery date.”

There are many reasons why your baby may not have engaged yet: the shape of your pelvis may mean that you need the pressure of the contractions to get the baby’s head to engage. Second and subsequent babies tend to engage later because the abdominal muscles are very loose, so the baby may move freely without feeling any need to get her head down.

There is also a small possibility that the baby’s head has not engaged because the head is too big to enter the birth canal. This can only be confirmed once labor has started.

HOW YOUR BABY IS POSITIONED

Once the baby is head down and moves into the pelvis there are several positions she may adopt: six of the most common are shown below. The position is determined by where her back and occiput (the back of her head) are lying. The most usual position is LOT. If the baby is breech (see p.433), the position is determined by how the bottom is lying.

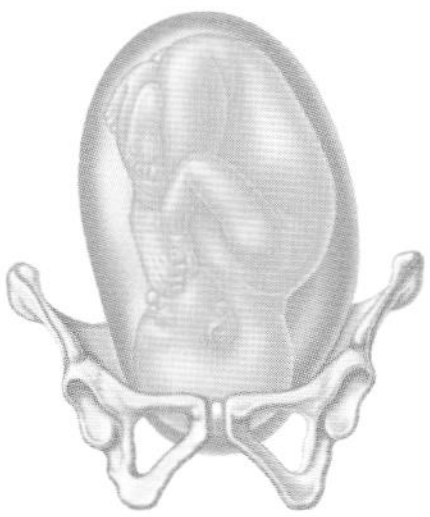

LOT: left occiput-transverse

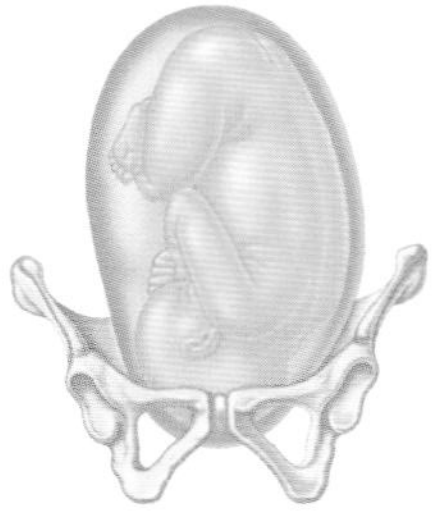

LOA: left occiput-anterior

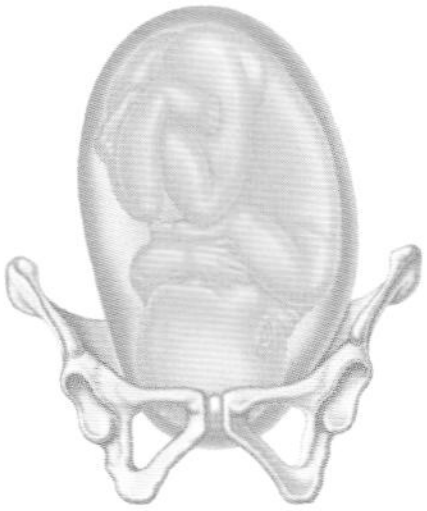

LOP: left occiput-posterior

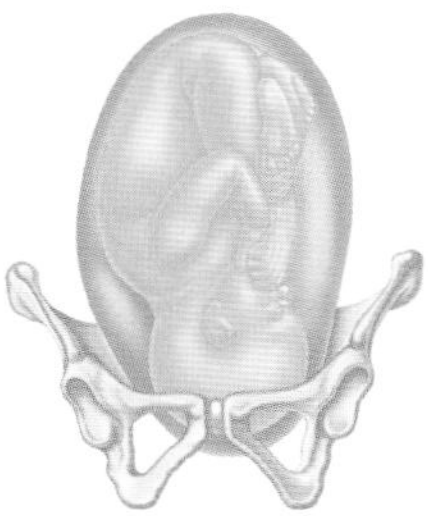

ROT: right occiput-transverse

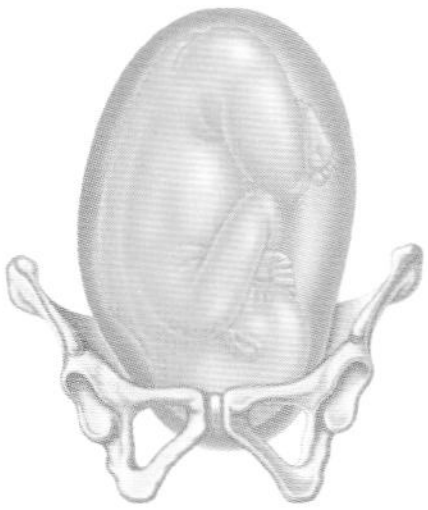

ROA: right occiput-anterior

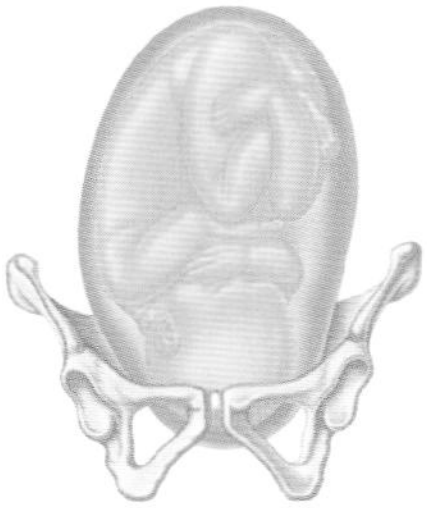

ROP: right occiput-posterior

LOT (left occiput-transverse): the back and occiput are positioned on the left-hand side of the uterus at right angles to the spine.

LOA (left occiput-anterior): the back and occiput are positioned closer to the front of the uterus on the left-hand side.

LOP (left occiput-posterior): the back and occiput are toward the spine on the left-hand side of the uterus.

ROT (right occiput-transverse): the back and occiput are at right angles to the spine on the right-hand side of the uterus.

ROA (right occiput-anterior): the back and occiput are toward the front of the uterus on the right-hand side.

ROP (right occiput-posterior): the back and occiput are toward the spine on the right-hand side of the uterus.

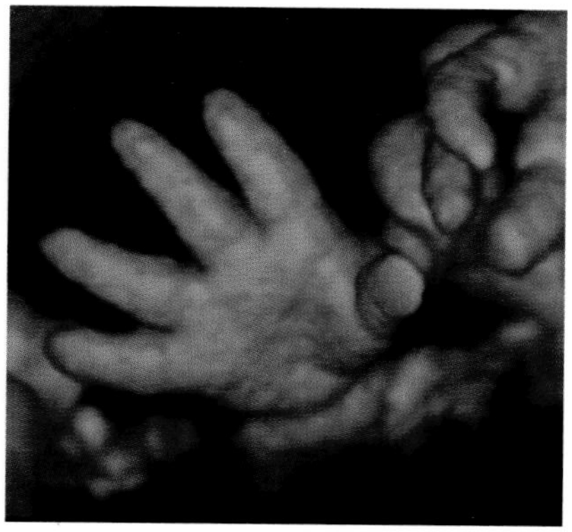

YOU ARE **39 WEEKS AND 5 DAYS**

2 days to go

YOUR BABY TODAY

This great image of the hands even shows the fine folds that have formed in the palms. Every baby has a unique pattern of folds on the palms and on the soles of the feet that you'll see when your baby finally arrives.

> " You'll be in labor very soon and it's normal to be anxious about what you need to go through to meet your baby. "

You're bound to have mixed emotions about going into labor. While you'll want your baby to be born, you may be apprehensive about going through childbirth. Most women are understandably concerned about the pain and may worry about their health and that of the baby. Remember that the majority of deliveries are normal and without complications and the majority of babies are fit and healthy.

Even though you've spent the past nine months preparing for the birth, you may still feel that you're not ready for the baby and that you won't be able to manage. Some of this will be the fear of the unknown—you have not yet met your baby and it's impossible to predict what the labor—and the weeks that follow it—will be like.

Although you may not feel fully prepared, be confident that you'll know how to take care of your newborn. In fact, you'll have probably already started the process of becoming a mother, wanting to nurture and protect your baby, even before they're born, and this natural instinct will continue.

MRSA: IS IT A RISK?

MRSA is a bacteria that can live harmlessly on the skin of healthy people but can lead to infection in vulnerable individuals. Good hygiene, particularly in the form of precautions such as hand washing, is an effective method in the prevention of MRSA and your chances of acquiring the infection in the hospital are low. Health-care workers use antiseptic solutions, and hospitals also have alcohol gels for hand cleaning in all units.

In addition to general hygiene measures, hospitals prevent the spread of MRSA by treating those infected with antibiotics and by detecting cases early so that they can isolate affected patients. Infected patients are moved to a single room or to a room with others who have MRSA.

Many hospitals now screen women before admission for MRSA, particularly if they are having a Cesarean, with the goal of treating those who carry MRSA before they are admitted for surgery.

ASK A DOCTOR

What's the difference between an emergency and elective Cesarean? An elective Cesarean is when a planned decision is made during pregnancy to deliver the baby by Cesarean section before the onset of labor. This is usually decided upon for medical reasons, although some women may decide to have an elective Cesarean for practical reasons or to avoid having to go through labor.

An emergency Cesarean is when a situation arises, usually in labor, that means the safest route for delivery is by Cesarean section.

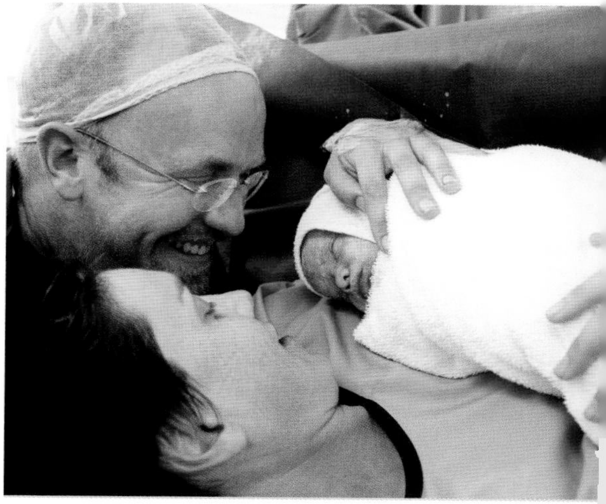

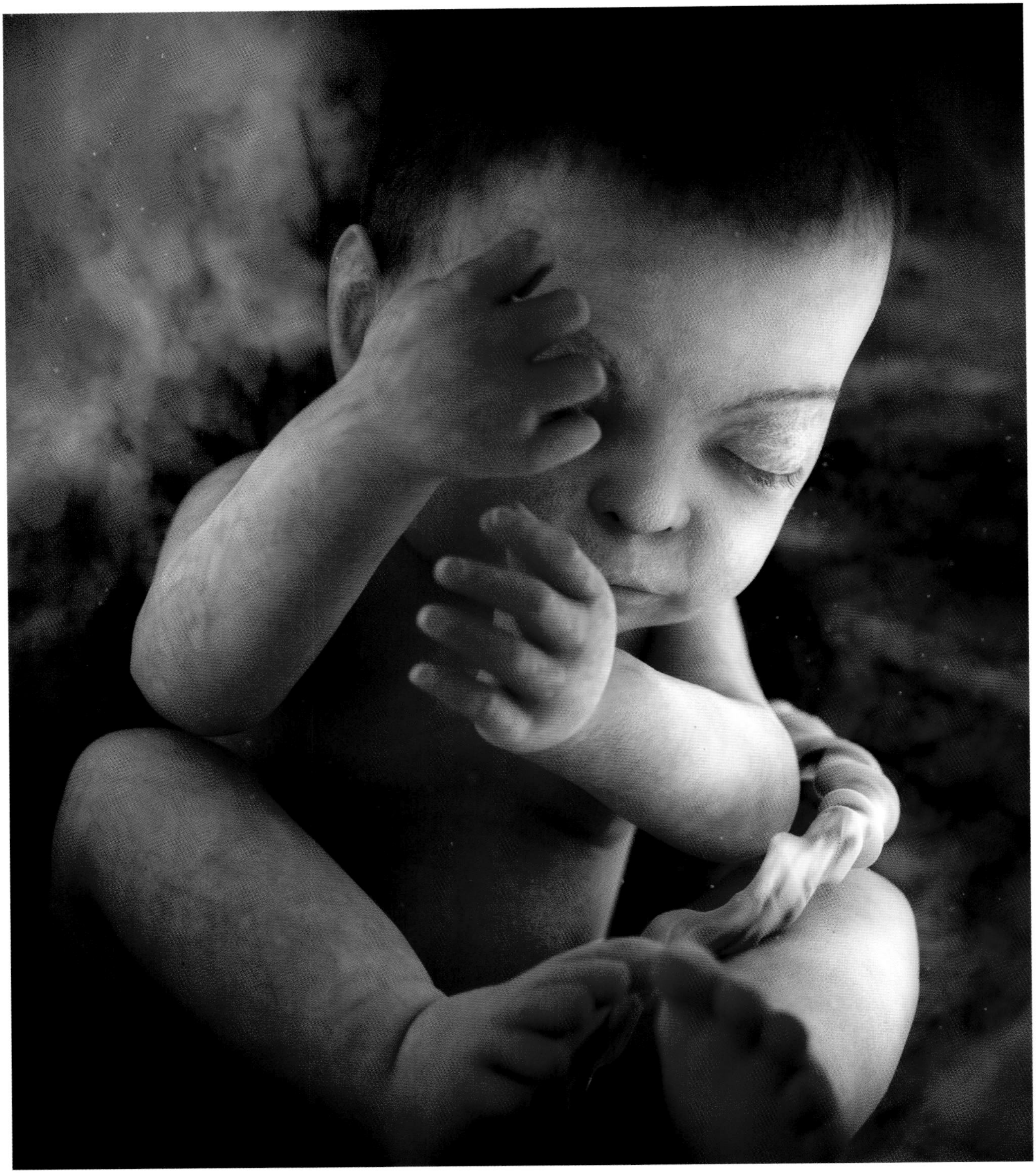

The final details of your baby's appearance—including eyebrows, eyelashes, and nails—are now in place and all their internal organs are sufficiently developed for life outside the uterus.

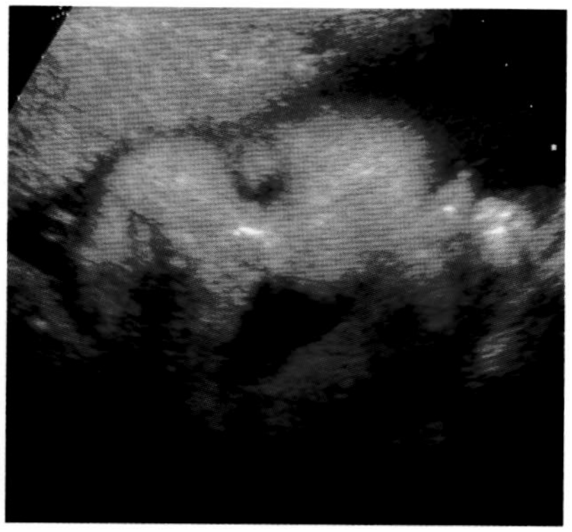

YOU ARE **39 WEEKS AND 6 DAYS**

1 day to go

YOUR BABY TODAY

It's been wonderful to see your baby's progress and facial features as each day of the pregnancy has passed by. 2-D and 3-D ultrasound images, as well as MRI, have all played a part in giving us a glimpse into the fascinating and complex world of life before birth.

" For most women, it is safe to go past your due date, but you should speak with your doctor about your options. "

If you are deemed to be at a higher risk of complications, you may be offered an induction of labor at or after 39 weeks.

High-risk factors include being 40 or over, having a big or small baby, and a previous birth complicated by shoulder dystocia (see p.476). The option of have a Cesarean delivery will also be discussed, depending on the severity of the problem.

At this stage, some women begin to try natural ways to trigger labor, with varying degrees of effectiveness, one of which is drink raspberry leaf tea.

Not to be confused with raspberry tea, it has been used for many years to stimulate labor. Some small studies have demonstrated that pregnant women experience a shorter second stage of labor after drinking raspberry leaf tea. Drinking this tea after 37 weeks is not likely to be harmful.

Some added benefits to raspberry leaf tea include nutrition as it contains vitamins A, C, E, and B, and the minerals calcium, magnesium, and iron, all of which are required for a healthy pregnancy.

Drunk after the birth, raspberry leaf tea can help the uterus to contract to its prepregnancy size, and also encourage the flow of breast milk.

ASK A DOCTOR

What exactly is a "show"? During pregnancy, a plug of jellylike mucus seals the lower end of your cervix and this prevents infection from getting into your uterus (see p.411). This "plug" comes away toward the end of pregnancy—known as a "bloody show"—and although this can mean that labor is going to start soon, it can also dislodge up to six weeks before your labor actually starts.

TAKE A "BABYMOON"

Consider now whether you might want to take a "babymoon" once the baby is born. Getting to know your newborn can be difficult if there's a constant stream of visitors. A "babymoon" allows you to shut out the world and spend a few days home alone. Your newborn baby will sleep a lot, so take the opportunity to do the same. There will be plenty of time for people to meet the new member of your family.

Your hormones will be all over the place, so expect to experience lows as well as highs, especially when your milk comes in (see pp.450–451).

Your partner also needs time to bond with the baby, nurture you both, and figure out diaper changing.

So stick a message on the front door, put your phone on silent, and snuggle up with your new family.

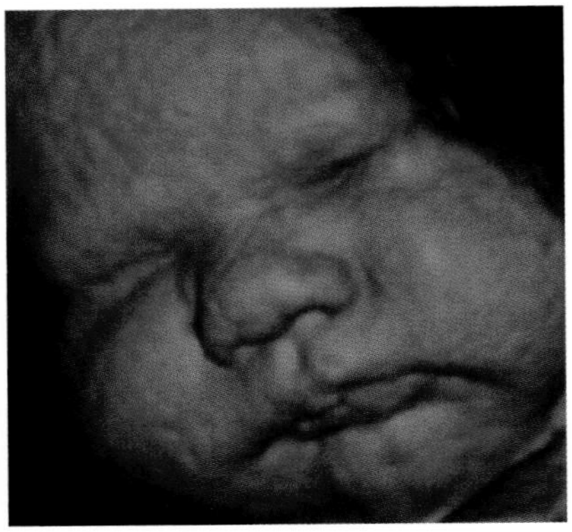

YOU ARE **40 WEEKS EXACTLY**

0 days to go

YOUR BABY TODAY

Your baby is now ready for the outside world. Sudden changes will take place with that first breath after delivery, as they immediately adapt from their time within the fluid-filled environment of the uterus to life in the air outside.

> “You’ve reached 40 weeks exactly! It may have seemed like a long wait, but it will be worth it once you’re holding your baby.”

Congratulations! If you don’t yet have your newborn baby in your arms, you soon will, and your life will be changed forever. Even the longest pregnancy seems unaccountably short when your labor begins, and the reality begins to hit that you’ll soon be holding your newborn.

You’ll get through the labor; and you’ll forget about the discomfort after a few good sessions detailing it to family and close friends. In fact, everything that precedes that moment when you hold your newborn baby for the first time becomes inconsequential when you realize that you have created the most wondrous thing of all: a new life. So good luck and well done! This is only just the beginning of the most amazing years of your life.

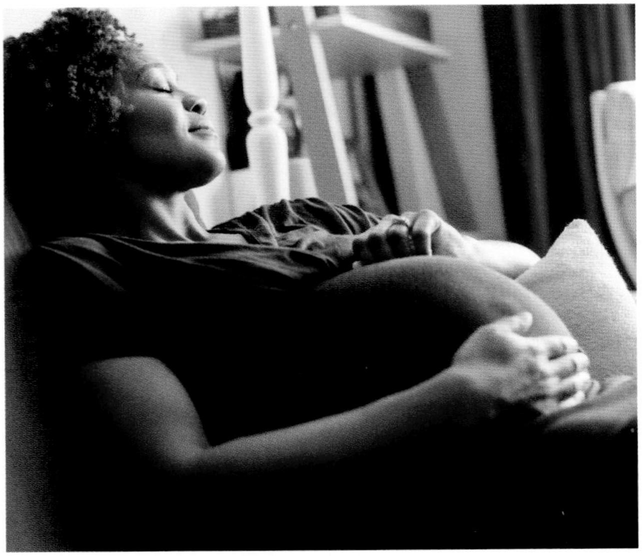

Your pregnancy is coming to an end, so instead of nurturing your belly, you’ll soon be nurturing your amazing newborn baby.

WHAT’S IN A NAME?

In one survey, 58 percent of parents questioned believed that the name they gave their baby would contribute to their success in life. More found it easier to name a boy than a girl, and just 3 percent said they would change the name they’d given their baby if they could.

Induction of labor

Your baby is described as being overdue if you have not gone into labor by the time you are 40 weeks pregnant. This is not unusual since most women do not go into labor at exactly 40 weeks, and anything between 37 and 41 weeks is considered to be normal.

As the exact mechanism that initiates labor is unknown, it's not clear why some women don't go into labor on their own and go past their due date.

What will be done

After 41 weeks, there is an increased risk of stillbirth, and even more so after 42 weeks. Most doctors recommend inducing labor by 41 weeks to avoid the risks of late pregnancy. This involves softening, shortening, and dilating the cervix by either inserting a balloon into the cervix or a prostaglandin pessary into the vagina. This first part of the process can take up to 24 hours. Once the cervix has opened slightly, the next part involves breaking the waters and using an oxytocin drip to start contractions. On average, it will be another 12 hours before baby is born.

Being induced increases the chance of having an epidural and an assisted birth. While it may sound long and complicated, induction is a gradual and safe process and important to consider if there is a risk to the health of the baby.

Stripping the membranes After 40 weeks, your doctor may do an internal examination. They'll insert a gloved finger into the cervix and pull the membranes in a circular pattern. This can soften the cervix and increase the chance of you going into labor by 30 percent in the next 48 hours. It's safe for you and your baby but can cause cramps and slight bleeding.

Assessments after 42 weeks Many doctors induce labor by 41 or 42 weeks. If your pregnancy goes beyond 42 weeks and you don't want to be induced, your doctor may offer monitoring with scans to measure the baby's pulse and volume of fluid around the baby and you may have an NST (see p.418) once or twice a week until labor to pick up any signs that the placenta is failing. If a problem is found, you'll be advised to have a Cesarean or an induction of labor.

If you decide to go past 42 weeks, it is very important to immediately seek help if your baby's pattern of movements change.

How you're feeling

Although it can be stressful, going past your due date does not significantly increase your health risks. You may be worried, that your baby will grow too large, but they'll unlikely put on enough weight in the last week or so to make a big difference, and most overdue babies have a normal birth weight.

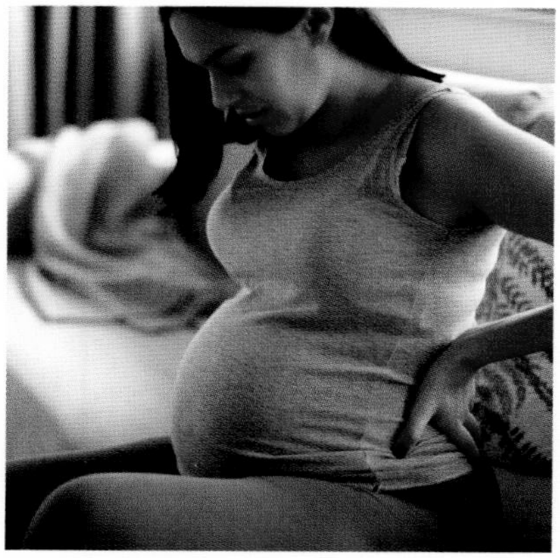

Going over your due date can be stressful, but it may help to remind yourself that it's also extremely common and quite normal.

BRINGING ON LABOR

Although no "home" or alternative remedy has been proven to bring on labor, there are several harmless techniques that are thought to assist the body's natural processes in the countdown to labor.

- **Probably the most enjoyable way to try to bring on labor is to make love** with your partner. Sperm contains prostaglandins that may act as a natural uterine stimulant, although the evidence that this works is inconclusive. Making love is not dangerous to your baby, unless your doctor has specifically told you to refrain from intercourse for a medical reason, such as fetal growth restriction or placental bleeding.
- **Nipple stimulation during sex** or by itself can cause the release of oxytocin from your pituitary gland, which is linked to contractions and cervical ripening.
- **Walking and exercise** may cause a mild increase in uterine contractions by helping the baby move down the pelvis, putting pressure on the cervix.

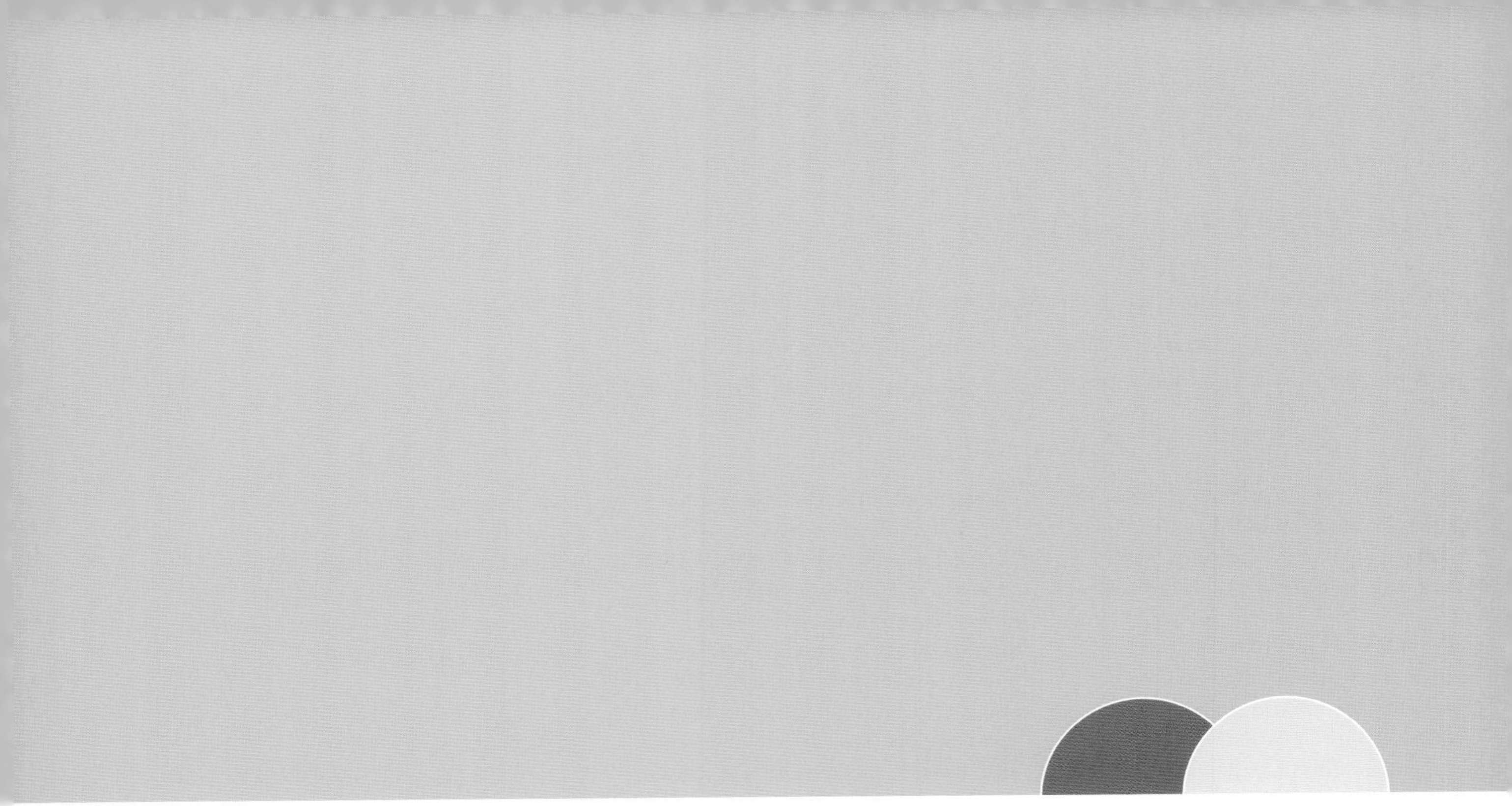

LABOR AND BIRTH

As the moment you have so eagerly anticipated approaches, you may be thinking about what lies in store for you during labor and wonder how you can best prepare for the physical and mental demands during this crucial time. Being as informed as possible about the progress of labor and your options for pain relief are both important first steps in enabling you to face labor and birth with a positive mindset.

Pain relief options

A PRIOR KNOWLEDGE OF PAIN RELIEF WILL HELP YOU MAKE INFORMED CHOICES IN LABOR. Once in labor, in addition to needing emotional and physical support, which your doctor, nurse, or midwife and birth partner will provide, you may also need some form of pain relief to help you cope. They will help you work with your labor pain by employing natural methods such as breathing techniques. If you need stronger pain relief, they'll advise you on medical methods, such as analgesics or an epidural (see pp.402–407).

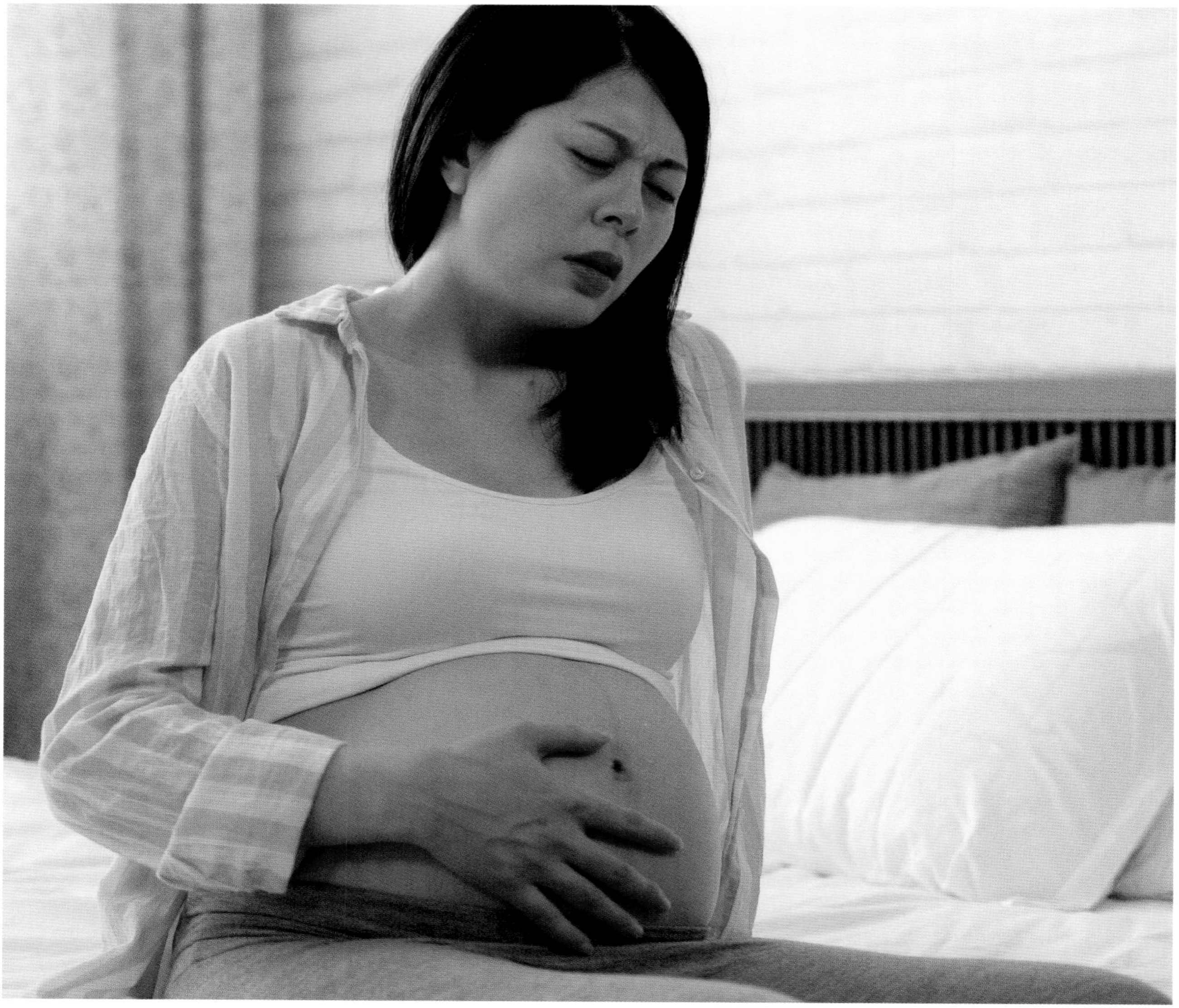

Coping with pain

To help you cope with labor and birth, it's important to have an understanding of the progress of pain during labor.

Labor pain is unique and quite different from everyday chronic and acute pain. Generally, pain is a warning sign that something is wrong, but labor pain acts as an "alert" that the birth process is underway and that you need a safe environment in which to give birth. Some women prefer a homelike environment, which has been shown to have many benefits, including reducing the need for medical forms of pain relief. For this reason, many labor rooms in maternity units and especially birth centers have homey decoration and furnishings to make them feel less medicalized. Other women need the reassurance provided by hospitals that stronger forms of pain relief and medical backup are available.

How women react to pain

The pain associated with labor can vary enormously between women. Some have relatively painless labors, while some describe the pain as moderate, and others experience severe pain. One thing that seems clear is that anxiety and fear increase the levels of adrenaline, which in turn can increase the intensity of the pain experienced. The strength of labor pain can also be affected by factors such as your emotional state and anticipation of labor; your previous experiences, if any; cultural beliefs; and, in particular for first-time mothers, the fear of the unknown. Thorough preparation prior to labor and sensitive and caring support throughout labor and birth can help reduce anxiety and fear considerably.

Thinking ahead

The sensation of pain is different during the different stages of labor, and as labor progresses, the intensity and duration of the pain increases. The most effective methods of dealing with pain will also change as your labor progresses (see box, left).

The more familiar you are with the methods of dealing with pain and with the several natural and drug-induced methods of pain relief available (see following pages), the easier it will be for you to manage during labor and birth. To make decisions about pain relief, you will also need to understand the changes that take place in your body during the three different stages of labor (see pp.408–429).

PAIN RELIEF THROUGHOUT LABOR

Your pain-relief requirements may change during labor, so it helps to be aware of when different types of pain relief can help.

Early first stage In this phase, the cervix begins to dilate. Contractions are mild, and you may find that natural methods, such as massage and breathing, are helpful. If you need stronger pain relief, you may be given analgesics, such as Demerol, which dull pain but allow you to remain active.

Active first stage The cervix now starts to dilate more quickly and contractions are stronger and closer together. Some women are happy to continue with natural or analgesic pain relief; others may need stronger relief and an epidural may be given at this point (see pp.404–5).

Transition Contractions are intense and frequent as the cervix dilates fully. Systemic (IV) analgesics aren't usually given this close to the birth since they could affect the baby. If you have an epidural already in place, this can be topped off.

Second and third stages Stage two lasts from full dilation of the cervix until birth; contractions are strong and longer lasting, but easier to manage since you start pushing. Analgesics may be used. In the third stage, delivery of the placenta, contractions are mild and you shouldn't need pain relief.

Natural pain relief

Many women opt for natural pain relief in labor, or choose to complement medical pain relief with natural methods.

During your labor, encephalins and endorphins (feel-good hormones) are released to provide you with some naturally induced pain relief. Many women now are also more aware of natural techniques, such as staying active, and of the availability of complementary therapies that they can use in addition to, or instead of, medical pain relief during pregnancy, childbirth, and following the birth. Some of these therapies are self administered and some are practitioner administered. A knowledge of the benefits of different therapies and how to use them is important if you are considering using them to deal with pain in labor.

Staying active

Being active in labor has been shown to help women to deal with pain and reduce the length of labor. Historically, women have been active in labor for centuries, but a medicalization of childbirth in the West led to an acceptance that women lie in bed, and a common image of a laboring woman is one lying in bed. Although during labor you may want to rest on a bed between contractions, many women find that when they feel supported, they will instinctively move around and do not cope well lying down, which can increase pain and hamper the progress of labor as your baby pushes against gravity. You may find it helpful to take a walk, roll on a birthing ball, rock in a rocking chair or change positions when you get too uncomfortable. There are certain interventions, such as the use of electronic fetal monitoring (see p.418), IVs, and some types of analgesia, that will limit your mobility.

RELAXATION TECHNIQUES

There are various techniques you can use to help you relax during labor; if you're relaxed, it will be easier to stay calm and in tune with your body. These techniques include focusing on your breathing (see below); listening to music (perhaps humming to the beat of a favorite tune during a contraction); and listening to a meditation.

Learning how to breathe slowly and steadily in labor helps you focus and stay calm. Usually, your breathing responds to how you're feeling and may increase slightly during a contraction, or you may hold your breath, which can make you feel lightheaded. If this happens, you need to focus and steady your breathing. Your nurse will remind you to breathe slowly and steadily. Breathing in for five and out for seven slows your breathing down, helps you relax, and stops you from panicking.

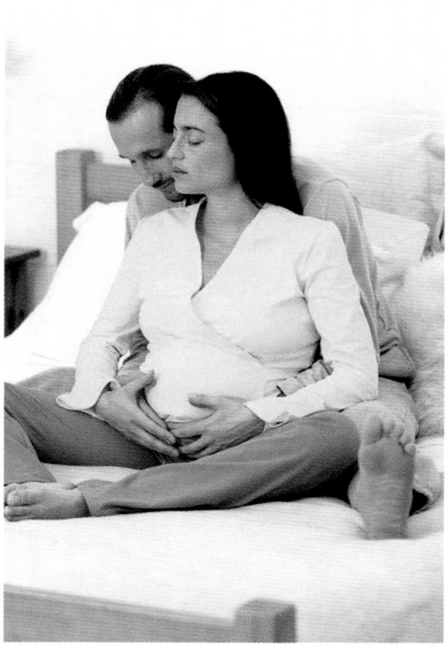

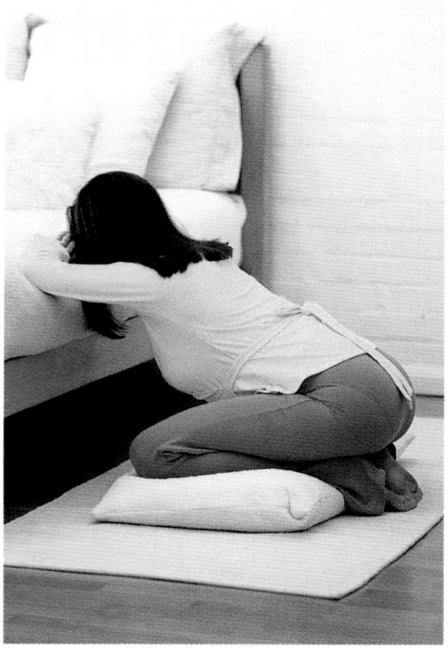

Concentrating on your breathing in labor is calming and helps you focus (above left). **Leaning forward while breathing** steadily can be comforting during contractions (above right).

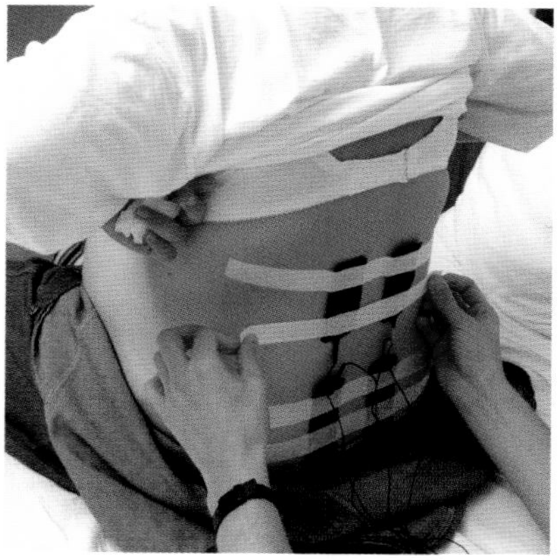

Once the electrodes for TENS are positioned on your back, you will be free to move around and find comfortable positions.

TENS

TENS stands for Transcutaneous Electrical Nerve Stimulation, and is a small electrical device that reduces pain signals sent to the brain. In addition to being used in labor, the device can also be used at the end of pregnancy (after 36 weeks) if you have a backache or uncomfortable Braxton Hicks contractions (see p.410).

The battery-operated TENS machine has thin wires that are connected to four electrodes, or sticky pads, which are taped to the lower back. The machine is thought to work by sending electrical impulses from the machine along nerve roots to the pain pathways in the brain, thereby blocking pain impulses. It's also thought to stimulate the brain to produce "feel-good" encephalins and endorphins, which can modulate the pain.

TENS is most effective in early labor, particularly for lower back pain, and it is therefore important to have the device available at the beginning of labor. It's therefore worth finding out if your hospital has TENS machines or whether you need to rent one in advance. You can hold the device or have it near you in labor and can increase the strength of the electrical impulse with a button as your contractions get stronger.

There are several advantages to TENS. It has few side effects; it allows you to remain active; and it can be used in combination with other types of pain relief. The disadvantages are that there hasn't been much research done about its safety for the baby, so a theoretical risk exists, and it is generally effective with just mild to moderate pain; the sticky pads mean that a back massage is not possible; and it isn't possible to labor in water or have an epidural inserted while using the device.

Water

Many women find being in warm water during labor very soothing and a helpful way to cope with labor pain. In addition to taking some pressure off your pelvis, water also relaxes your muscles, and eases tension and stress. The warmth of the water soothes your muscles and promotes relaxation. Being in water aids buoyancy, which can help relieve the pressure on your pelvis. Over the last decade or so, this natural method has become more available for women, and many hospitals and birth centers provide bathtubs. Due to increased risks of infection, however, it is recommended that you do not deliver in the water.

Hypnosis

Self-hypnosis, using visualization and breathing techniques to induce a state of deep relaxation and banish fear, is an increasingly popular means of dealing with labor, and is referred to as "HypnoBirthing." This is based on the "fear-tension-pain" syndrome of childbirth first described by the British obstetrician Grantly Dick-Read, who believed that fear prevents the release of the "feel-good hormones," endorphins and encephalins. He maintained that when fear is eliminated, most women can give birth naturally. With HypnoBirthing, you are fully aware of what is happening around you, but may feel as though you're daydreaming or drifting off to sleep. You and your birth partner can 111attend HypnoBirthing classes anytime during pregnancy to learn

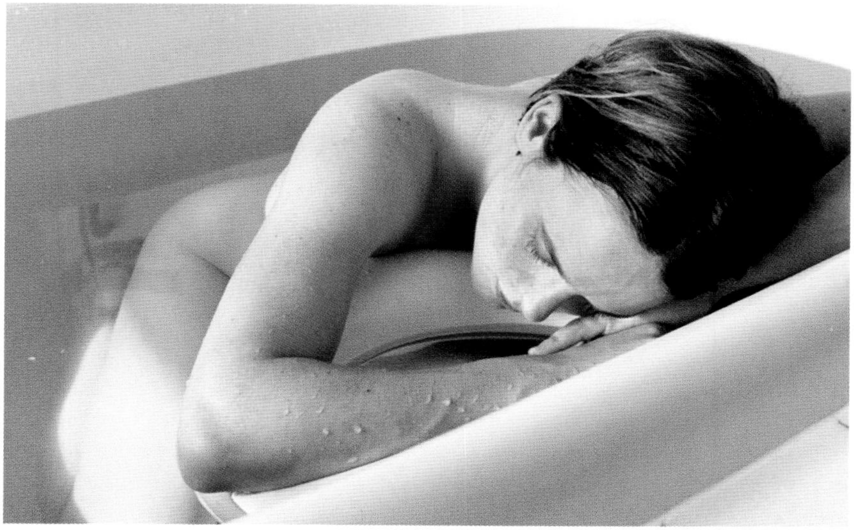

Laboring in warm water can be deeply soothing. In addition to helping take the pressure off your pelvis, water also relaxes muscles, in turn easing tension and stress.

QUESTIONS AND ANSWERS

Will I be able to stay active in labor? Most women are able to remain active through labor and are encouraged to do so, perhaps using props such as a chair, beanbag, or birthing ball. Staying active can help since this can speed up labor, and changing your position can help you deal with labor pain. When you arrive at the hospital or birth center, discuss your birth plan with the doctor and inform her that you want to be as active as possible.

Will I lose control if I use hypnosis during my labor? No, you will simply feel deeply relaxed, but will still be in control and know what you are doing. Don't worry—self-hypnosis will help you be less anxious and frightened during your labor, which will help you to deal with labour pain.

I've had a previous Cesarean. Does this mean that I won't be able to labor in water this time? It depends on the procedures that your health-care provider follows for women who have already had a Cesarean. After a Cesarean, the doctors will want to monitor you and the baby either continuously or frequently during labor, because there is a very small chance that your uterus may rupture, which is often only detected through a change in the baby's heartbeat. But waterproof monitoring systems are widely available and many practices perform WBAC—water birth after Cesarean

At what point can I get into the birthing pool? This is up to you. Relaxing in warm water is often suggested in the early stages of labor, as long as your contractions are progressing. You can sit in the warm water for 1½ to 2 hours for pain management, but then get out. Changing your environment helps keep your labor active.

the techniques before labor. To find a class in your area, visit hypnobirthing.com/findapract.htm.

Acupuncture

This uses fine needles placed at specific points on the body to reduce pain by stimulating the production of endorphins. Acupuncture is a traditional form of Chinese medicine that believes there are channels within the body through which energy, or "chi" runs. Blockages can occur in these channels, and so by inserting needles at certain points, energy is unblocked, relieving pain and restoring balance to the body. Many women find acupuncture helpful to treat mild pregnancy symptoms, and some women use this therapy during labor. Acupuncture has no harmful side effects for the mother or baby and in labor, needles will usually be inserted in points that do not restrict your movement, for example in the ear. If you want to have acupuncture during labor, you will need to look for an acupuncturist who specializes in this area and arrange to have him or her with you during labor.

Homeopathy

This is based on the principle of treating like with like. Talk to your doctor before using any homeopathic products during pregnancy or labor, since homeopathy is an area of complementary and alternative medicine that's associated with

MASSAGE AND TOUCH

Many women find massage helpful in labor to induce relaxation, bring about a sense of well-being, and alleviate pain. Your birth partner may find it relaxing and therapeutic too. Ideally, they will have had a chance to see massage techniques demonstrated in prenatal classes and to practice before labor. Massaging the lower back helps relieve pain in this area; head, neck, and shoulder massage is beneficial for relieving tension and fatigue.

The touch therapies shiatsu and acupressure can also help relieve pain and tension. They involve application of pressure to specific points to increase endorphin levels. You or your partner will need to learn the techniques from a trained practitioner. Ask your doctor whether they can put you in touch with a practitioner.

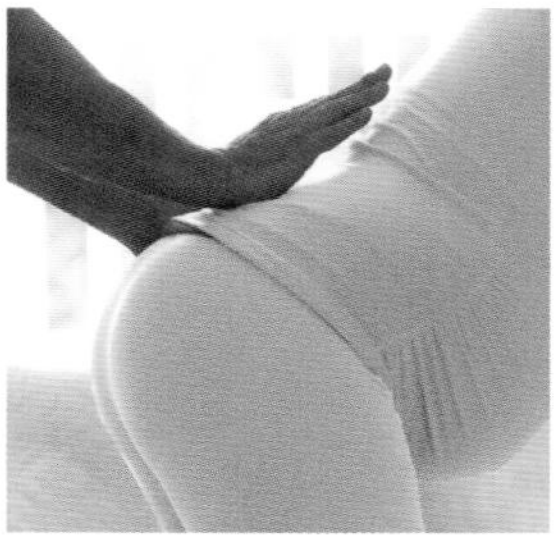

Your partner can use the heel of their hand to apply firm pressure to your sacrum. The hands can be alternated to stroke around the lower back.

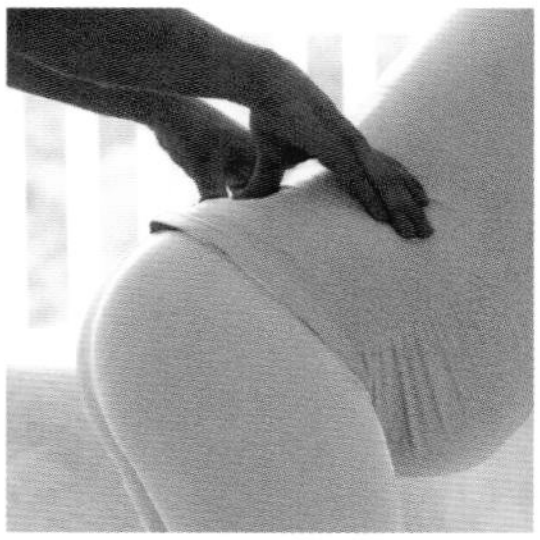

Using the thumbs to massage the lower back in a circular motion, working from the base of the spine down to the buttocks, can release tense muscles.

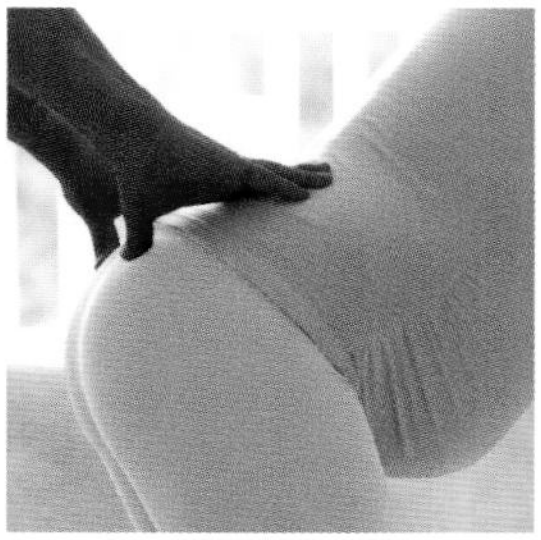

Applying deep pressure to the buttocks and lower back with the thumbs can help you focus and release held-in tension during contractions.

much debate and scientific controversy. If your doctor gives you the okay, a certified homeopath can prescribe remedies based on your individual needs. There is a lack of scientific evidence on the effectiveness of homeopathy, although many women find the remedies helpful.

Aromatherapy

Aromatherapy (essential) oils are derived from plants and used for their therapeutic properties. The use of these oils in childbirth can stimulate, refresh, and soothe you and your partner. Some evidence shows that oils, such as lavender, reduce anxiety in labor, which helps you cope with pain. Hot and cold compresses with essential oils added can be soothing, and massaging diluted essential oils (in a carrier oil) into the skin is therapeutic. Many experts recommend against aromatherapy during pregnancy and labor because some scents may be hazardous to pregnant women. The effects of most plant oils on pregnant women is unknown.

Reflexology

Reflexology involves massaging reflex zones on your feet that correspond with different parts of your body to improve your blood circulation and relax any tension you may be feeling. Reflexology is gaining some popularity as a coping technique in the early stages of labor. However, because many women naturally want to be active and move around during their labor, this may be more helpful in between early contractions.

BIRTH STORY: A NATURAL HOME BIRTH

Jenna is a 31-year-old mom and this is her second labor. She had a straightforward birth with her daughter, now three. This pregnancy was uneventful, so she decided to have a home birth this time.

Jenna's story: When I was eight days overdue, my midwife did a "stretch and strip" (see p.393) of my cervix to encourage labor. After that, I had a couple of bloody shows (see p.411) and irregular contractions. In the night, I woke with contractions 20 minutes apart. I couldn't get back to sleep, so I had a warm bath, took a couple of acetaminophens, and went back to bed. My little girl woke at 6:45 a.m. My contractions were every 10 minutes and getting stronger, so my husband stayed home.

By 8:00 a.m., my contractions were every 5 minutes, stronger, and lasting 50–60 seconds. My husband called the midwife. She said she was on her way and advised me to stay active. I started to use the TENS machine (see p.399) on a low setting, which helped me focus. I found standing and rocking my pelvis back and forth and from side to side helpful and I used a birthing ball. My husband was supportive, massaging my shoulders and under my abdomen where it hurt most; I found the heat from his hands soothing. My daughter held my hand.

At 8:40 a.m., the midwife arrived. She checked my blood pressure, pulse, and temperature, felt my belly, listened to the baby's heart, and took a urine sample, which relieved some pressure in my pubic area. She confirmed that I was in established labor since my cervix was 5 cm dilated. My cervix was thinning, the head was pressing down, and my membranes were intact. I stayed active, using TENS, and leaning forward. My partner put on relaxing music.

At 9:50 a.m., my contractions were every two minutes, very strong, and lasting 60 seconds. I tried walking and marching on the spot. My mom arrived and took my daughter to the park. I felt hot and so I had a cool drink and my midwife dabbed my face with a cool, wet cloth. I found kneeling on all fours, rocking and arching my back, helpful.

By 10:30 a.m., my contractions were very painful. My midwife listened to the heartbeat intermittently.

By 11:00 a.m., I felt an urge to push. My water broke and my contractions were very strong and each minute. I felt panicky, but my midwife encouraged me, saying she thought the baby would be born soon; my husband helped me focus by breathing slowly. My midwife confirmed that I was fully dilated and ready to push. I somehow found the energy to bear down and felt the head emerge. I took a breath, concentrated, and pushed my baby out.

My baby boy was born at 11:14 a.m., 8 lb 2 oz, and my husband cut the cord once it had stopped pulsating. I delivered my placenta without drugs (see p.429). My midwife advised me to put my baby to my breast to stimulate the hormone oxytocin, which causes contractions and helps the placenta to come away. My placenta was delivered at 11:40 a.m.

The midwife's comments: Jenna and her husband prepared well and worked as a team. Jenna was active for most of labor and stayed focused. Her feelings of panic in the transition period were normal, but her husband and I gave her extra support. By working with her instincts, she found inner strength and had a normal birth. Her labor was nine hours, about average for a second-time mom.

Drugs for pain relief

Various types of medication are available for pain relief during labor; many can be used alongside natural forms of pain relief.

For some, natural pain relief may not be sufficient to enable them to deal with the increasing intensity of contractions, and they may choose to use medication in combination with natural techniques. In some situations, for example if labor is induced (see p.432) or augmented (see p.415), contractions may start strongly rather than build up gradually and a stronger type of pain relief may be needed.

There are several types of medical pain relief available, which fall into two groups. Analgesic drugs dull the perception of pain, while anesthesia, which may be regional or general, numbs pain totally. In regional anesthesia, also known as a nerve block, local anesthetic drugs are injected around nerves that supply a particular area. There are several types of regional nerve block: epidurals and spinal blocks numb sensation in the abdomen and are used to reduce the pain of contractions; a pudendal block numbs sensation in the vagina and perineum and may be used in a forceps delivery. Rarely, a general anesthetic is given during a cesarean.

Since all labors are different, it's not possible to have a "one size fits all" approach to pain relief. Being flexible and informed will help you feel in control. Read any literature from your doctor, go to childbirth classes, and ask questions. Try to eliminate any worries by increasing your knowledge, for example by asking if it's possible to attend a childbirth education class at the hospital that discusses the pros and cons of each type of pain relief. Keep in mind that some childbirth classes, like Lamaze and the Bradley method, can teach you breathing and relaxation techniques that may help reduce your need for pain medication during labor.

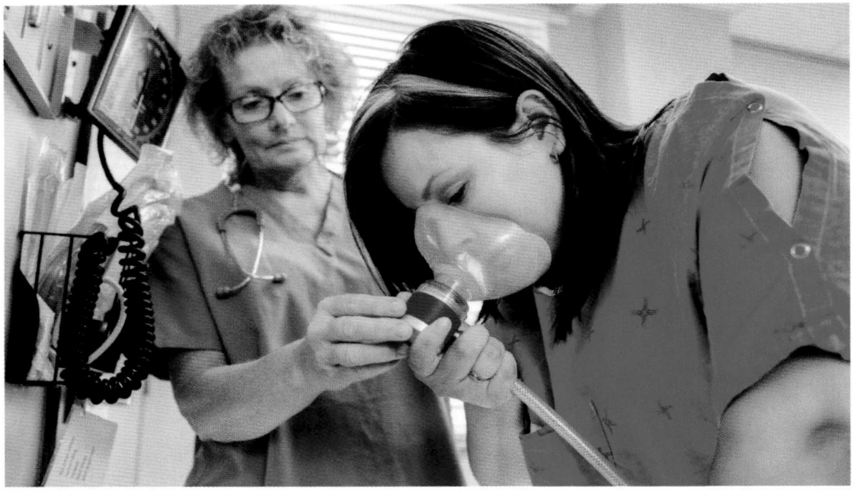

Nitrous oxide is a common way to manage the pain of contractions. Your midwife will guide you so that you know when to inhale for the most effective pain relief.

Pain relief plan

Having a birth plan ahead of time that outlines the circumstances during which you would resort to using medication for pain relief may be helpful for some women. For example, you may want to try to remain medication-free unless the pain is so intense, it interferes with your ability to hold a normal conversation, or it doubles you over in pain. Perhaps you'll seek relief if your labor drags on hours longer than you expected and you need some respite to sleep for a while to regain your strength for the upcoming pushing that you'll be doing. Whatever the case, you may feel more in control if you know

A HISTORY OF PAIN RELIEF

The history of modern obstetric pain relief began in the mid-19th century with the discovery of chloroform. Nitrous oxide and opioids followed; at the start of the 20th century, enthusiasm for pain-relieving drugs was so great that they were overused, with women in labor in a state of near-unconsciousness. The natural childbirth movement in the 1960s and 1970s was a reaction to such overuse of drugs. In the 1970s another revolution was at hand as epidurals became available.

ahead of time what your limits are and when you want to say yes to pain medication, rather than being overwhelmed by the situation, if you don't give it much thought beforehand.

Opioids

These belong to a group of drugs called narcotics and are sleep-inducing. They are similar to morphine and include drugs such as Demerol. They attach themselves to receptors in the brain or nerves and block the transmission of pain.

Tranquilizers

These drugs don't relieve pain, but they can help to relieve anxiety and help a woman relax for several hours during early labor. Some women who are very anxious about the impending pain or of labor and childbirth may seek this sort of medication. Tranquilizers may be given orally, intravenously, or injected into a large muscle. Oral dosage takes the longest to take effect. Some women dislike what tranquilizers do to them, since they may feel drowsy and out of control. If the dose is very high, women may nod off between contractions. It may be hard for a woman to fully remember her labor experience if she's taken tranquilizers. The drugs also affect the baby, decreasing his activity and muscle tone during and after birth. For these reasons, tranquilizers are not for everyone, but in certain circumstances, they can help a woman feel less anxious about labor.

Epidurals

An epidural is a regional anesthetic that can be given at any stage of labor to numb the abdomen and therefore block the pain of contractions, but it's typically given when the woman is at least 4 cm dilated. In some cases, if a woman's labor progresses very quickly and she doesn't request one right away, she may not be able to get one before delivery. Epidurals are the most popular form of pain relief during labor in the US, with more than half of pregnant women delivering in hospitals choosing this treatment.

ASPIRIN: NOT FOR LABOR PAIN

When you start to experience the pain of labor contractions at home, no matter how tempting it may be, do not reach for an aspirin to relieve your pain. Aspirin can be extremely dangerous during pregnancy, particularly in the third trimester and leading up to labor and delivery. The drug interferes with your blood-clotting ability, which means that your risk of a hemorrhage during delivery increases if you take aspirin in the weeks leading up to your baby's birth. Taking too much aspirin in the last trimester may actually prolong labor. Bleeding problems may even develop in your newborn. Taking aspirin regularly toward the end of your pregnancy can also affect your baby's heart or blood flow, so it's best to avoid aspirin, unless your doctor recommends you take it. Your best bet for dealing with labor pain at home is to keep active until it's time to head to the hospital. While you wait, do something to distract yourself from the pain, whether it's counting the length of time between contractions, packing your bag for the hospital, or anything else that feels right. Ask your partner for a massage or try a warm shower. No matter what you do, refrain from drug use. This way, if you need pain relief when you get to the hospital—many women do—you won't have any medication in your system.

OPIOIDS (PETHIDINE AND DIAMORPHINE)

Advantages

• Opioids help you to relax during labor, which can help you to conserve your energy between contractions.

• Opioids can produce a feeling of well-being, which many women find beneficial during labor.

Disadvantages

• Many women report feeling nauseated with opioids, which can be an unexpected and unpleasant side effect on top of your pain and contractions.

• Opioids can cause dizziness, and this can be disorienting during labor.

• Some women have reported feeling out of control with some opioid medications and therefore out of touch with how their labor is progressing.

• Opioids cross the placenta easily and pass into the baby's bloodstream. This can have the affect of sedating the baby and can affect the baby's breathing after the delivery. The administration of opioid medications therefore needs to be carefully timed during labor so that they are not given too close to the time of the delivery of the baby.

• Opioids can depress the mother's breathing during labor. However, this side effect is more common when the mother has a preexisting respiratory illness, such as asthma or emphysema.

• Opioids cause a delay in emptying the bowels and therefore increase the overall risk to the mother should general anesthesia be needed later on (see p.406).

How epidurals work A hollow needle is inserted between two vertebrae in the lower back. A tiny plastic tube is then passed through the needle and into the epidural space surrounding the spinal cord. A local anesthetic is injected into the needle and flows through the tube into the epidural space so that the nerve roots carrying the pain stimulus to the brain are coated with anesthetic and pain is reduced or completely blocked.

This will affect sensation in your legs so that you need to remain in bed and your baby will be closely monitored. A stronger epidural also affects sensation in your bladder, so you will need to have a catheter. Used late in labor, a stronger epidural may mean that you need help to push the baby out, since the pelvic floor muscles will be heavy and ineffective. In this case, your doctor will put a hand on your abdomen to feel when a contraction starts and will tell you when to push. In some cases, an assisted delivery (see pp.436–437) becomes necessary.

When are epidurals used? Epidurals can be used throughout labor, but they're typically given during active labor when a woman is 4–5 cm dilated. Since everyone has varying pain thresholds, the time when one is requested varies. There are factors to bear in mind should you opt for an epidural late in labor. To minimize the risks, you must remain completely still during the placement of the epidural tube. If your labor has progressed too far to enable you to do this, the anesthesiologist may be unable to proceed with an epidural for your own interest. Also, if you choose to have an epidural late in labor, it may be necessary to give a high dose so that it takes effect in time, which has disadvantages (see below).

If you're considering using an epidural, inform your doctor early in labor so that she can consult the anesthesiologist. The anesthesiologist may then discuss this with you and take a brief medical history to ensure that it's safe for you to have an epidural. She will discuss any risks, and answer any questions that you or your partner has, all of which can save time later on if you decide to go ahead.

There are occasions when an epidural is not advised. These include cases where a woman has had spinal surgery or is taking blood-thinning medication. Rarely, a woman may have an infection that could be exacerbated by an epidural.

Side effects There are a number of minor side effects. The medication can cause blood pressure to fall, so this will be monitored (see opposite page). If it does fall, you'll be given fluids and medication, and subsequent doses may be reduced.

It's common to experience itching with epidurals, caused by the release of histamine from the opioid component of a mobile epidural. Histamine is a substance released by the body during an allergic reaction that can cause itching. The itch can be treated, but in most cases it gets better on its own. If you develop an itch, a greater concentration of local anesthetic alone will be used.

It's not unusual to shiver with an epidural, although this is a more common side effect if a concentrated local anesthetic is used, as is the case for a cesarean delivery.

Epidural pain relief can cause a rise in temperature. If this occurs, you'll have a blood test to eliminate an infection since this can also cause your temperature to rise. You will be

THE PROS AND CONS OF AN EPIDURAL

Pros

- An epidural provides absolute pain relief in 90 percent of cases; 10 percent of women have some degree of residual pain but still have a marked improvement in their overall discomfort.
- Epidurals do not pose a risk to the baby.
- The presence of an effective epidural means that if intervention is needed at any time, the epidural can be topped up with an anesthetic for either an assisted delivery (see pp.436–437), or a Cesarean delivery (see pp.438–441). This also reduces the likelihood that a general anesthetic will be needed.

Cons

- Around 1 in 10 women do not experience absolute pain relief with an epidural.
- Some women develop a headache that persists after an epidural (see p.406).
- A rare complication is patches of heaviness in the legs or feet.

There are some very rare risks:

- As with all invasive procedures, inserting an epidural can result in infection. Meningitis occurs in around 1 in 100,000 women and an epidural abscess occurs in about 1 in 50,000 women.
- There is a 1 in 170,000 risk of developing a blood clot in the epidural space (epidural hematoma).
- There is a 1 in 100,000 risk of the epidural tube moving into the fluid around the spine and resulting in unconsciousness, and there is a 1 in 250,000 chance of the epidural causing some form of paralysis.

HOW AN EPIDURAL IS DONE

If you opt for an epidural, the doctor should explain the procedure to you, and you should have the opportunity to ask the anesthesiologist any questions.

Getting ready for an epidural Before starting the epidural, a plastic tube will be placed in a vein in the back of your hand or in your arm, to which an IV containing fluid will be connected. You are given fluids during an epidural to stop your blood pressure from dropping. The doctor will then help you into the correct position to receive the epidural, which will either be sitting up with your legs over the side of the bed leaning forward, or curled up on your side on the edge of the bed. The position may depend on the preference of the anesthesiologist.

Your lower back will be cleaned with antiseptic and a drape placed over the rest of your back to reduce the risk of infection. Before the epidural needle is inserted, a local anesthetic will be given into the skin and surrounding tissues. This creates a numb patch to ensure that the insertion of the large epidural needle is not painful. When the local anesthetic is injected, you may feel a scratching sensation and experience a very short-lived sting in the area between the vertebrae bones.

The procedure Since it's important for you to remain still during the procedure, the anesthesiologist will insert the epidural between your contractions. If this is difficult, you should try to concentrate on your breathing and remain as still as possible. You will feel a pushing sensation in your back while the anesthesiologist is trying to find the very small epidural space with the hollow needle. When the space is located, a tiny plastic tube will be fed into it through the needle. The epidural needle is then removed and the tube, which is secured onto your back with sticky tape, remains in the epidural space. The tube remains in place until your baby is delivered and, because it is very thin, soft, and pliable, it is perfectly safe to lie on the tube and to move around.

Managing the epidural Once the epidural tube is successfully in place, the anesthesiologist will give the first dose of medication. Once they are satisfied that the epidural is in the correct position and is working effectively, all subsequent doses, or "top offs," can be given without another injection. Your blood pressure will be taken once the epidural is in place and will be monitored for the next half an hour or so, and then regularly thereafter, including after each top off. Each dose of medication takes around 10–20 minutes to take its full effect and can last between one and two hours. The epidural will be topped off as required, usually around every three to four hours, to keep you comfortable throughout your labor. An anesthesiologist should be available 24 hours a day to manage any concerns or problems that may arise with the epidural.

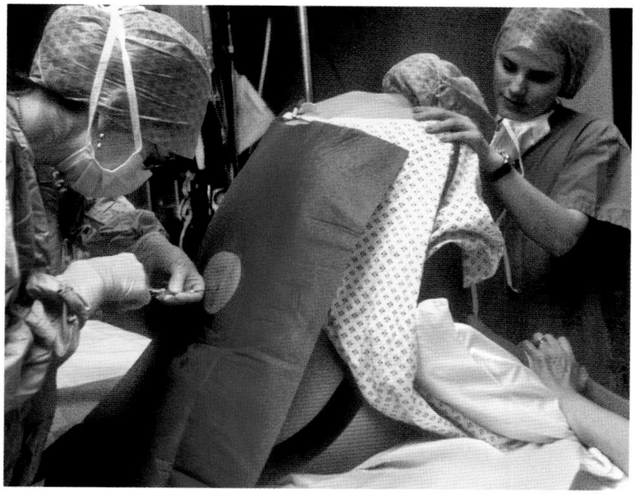

Before the epidural is given, your back will be covered with a sterile sheet and then a local anesthetic will be given to numb the area so that you don't experience pain when the larger epidural needle is inserted.

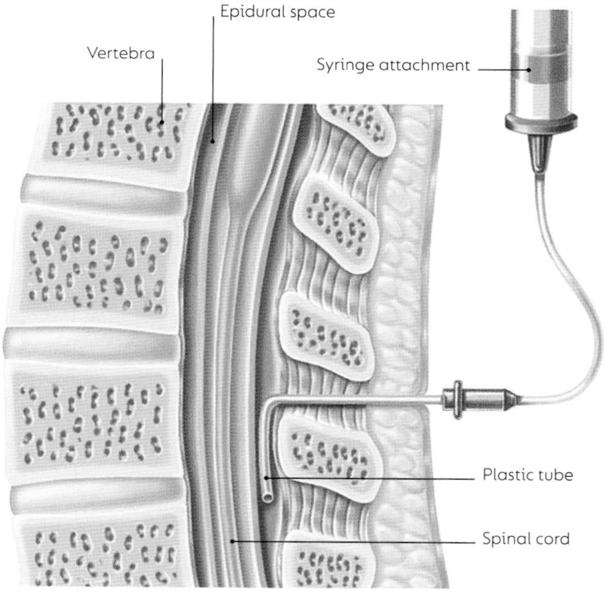
Epidural space
Vertebra
Syringe attachment
Plastic tube
Spinal cord

The anesthetic is given through a tube that is inserted into the epidural space, avoiding the spinal cord and its covering.

given preventative antibiotics while waiting for the blood test results, and acetaminophen to bring your temperature back to normal.

Problems with epidurals In addition to side effects, there can occasionally be problems with the effectiveness of an epidural. The anesthetic may not spread evenly in the epidural space, which may be caused by the epidural tube sitting on one side of the epidural space. This can mean that pain relief only occurs on one side of the body. If this occurs, the anesthesiologist will try to reposition the tube and give another dose of anesthetic. If this doesn't work, the only other solution is to redo the entire epidural.

Sometimes, one spot can remain painful, usually in the groin area or low down in the front of the abdomen, which is referred to as a "missed segment." This results from a single nerve root not being coated with the local anesthetic. Again, the anesthesiologist may reposition the tube. Sometimes, a stronger local anesthetic or an opioid is used to numb the area. If a persistent missed segment is too uncomfortable, the anesthesiologist may do a combined spinal epidural block, known as a CSE (see right).

It's thought that epidural pain relief may prolong the second stage of labor. It also increases your chances of having an assisted delivery, especially if a high dose of anesthetic is given toward the end of labor, which affects your ability to push. However, an epidural doesn't increase the chance of a cesarean and doesn't, despite common misconceptions, cause long-term backache after the birth.

Spinal block

This is similar to an epidural in that a needle is put in your back and pain relief is achieved by blocking nerve fibers that supply the pelvic organs. However, in a spinal block, the needle is passed through the epidural space to pierce the membrane covering the spinal cord (the dura) so that anesthetic can be injected into the fluid around the spinal cord; no tubes are left in place. The needle used for a spinal block is smaller than that used for an epidural, which means it's less painful to insert. There is still a risk of a headache as with an epidural (see left) and the side effects should be treated the same way.

A smaller dose of anesthetic is needed and it works very quickly: pain relief is almost immediate, whereas an epidural takes 10–20 minutes. However, the use of a spinal block is limited because only a single dose of medication can be administered. As a result, spinal blocks are usually reserved for use during a cesarean, or for an assisted delivery when an epidural isn't in place.

Combined spinal epidural (CSE) or "walking epidural"

This involves both a spinal injection and putting an epidural in place. It's sometimes done when problems are encountered with an epidural (see left) and for a Cesarean. A CSE gives pain relief for about two hours, but additional medication can be put into the epidural so that it lasts as long as necessary. However, it's a specialized technique and isn't offered in all units.

Pudendal blocks

This type of regional anesthesia involves injecting a local anesthetic into the vagina where the pudendal nerves are located to reduce pain in the vagina and perineum. The pudendal needle is quite long and thick, so before the injection is given, a cold anesthetic spray is applied to the area. The anesthetic has no effect on the

AN EPIDURAL "HEADACHE"

Some women report a headache after an epidural, which can develop more than 24 hours after the delivery and tends to be at the front of the head. It is made worse by sitting up and moving around and is much improved by lying down. This occurs in around 1 in 100 women and is caused by the epidural needle moving too far forward and cutting the dura sheath, the membrane maintaining the fluid around the spinal cord and brain. This small hole results in a loss of fluid from the sheath, which causes a headache. The risk is hugely reduced by remaining still during the placement of the epidural. In around 70 percent of women, the hole heals on its own. You will be advised to drink plenty of fluids and to take simple painkillers, such as acetaminophen and ibuprofen and you will be reviewed at regular intervals by an anesthesiologist. If the headache persists, a procedure called a "blood patch" will be done. This is done in the sterile environment of an operating room by two anesthesiologists. One places an epidural needle in your back, while the other takes around 20 ml of blood from a vein in your arm. The blood is then passed down the needle into the epidural space. This forms a clot that seals the hole and prevents further leakage of fluid from around your spine, therefore relieving the headache.

baby and can be used with other medications. It takes effect very quickly and is sometimes used just before birth to aid an assisted forceps delivery.

General anesthesia

Most cesareans are conducted using regional anesthesia. However, in some cases general anesthesia, where the mother is put to sleep, is necessary. This may be because of a failure of regional anesthesia, blood-clotting problems in the mother, an infection in the mother's bloodstream, or persistent fetal distress.

The procedure Precautions are taken to minimize the risks to you and your baby. You'll be given an antacid to reduce stomach acid. A urinary catheter will be inserted into the bladder and antiseptic applied to the abdomen before you're put to sleep to minimize the baby's exposure to the anesthetic.

As the mother is put to sleep, a face mask is held tightly over her nose and mouth. Because a major risk during general anesthesia is undigested food or liquids in the stomach reentering the mouth and going into the lungs (which can cause damage), you'll likely be told not to eat or drink anything once labor begins (because labor usually slows digestion), in case you need general anesthesia. You may be able to have ice chips, though. Once asleep, an anesthesiologist inserts a tube through your mouth and down your throat so that oxygen can easily reach your lungs. You may therefore have a sore throat when you wake up.

During the surgery the anesthesiologist cares for the mother, giving painkillers and anti-nausea medicine when needed. If you need general anesthesia for your Cesarean, your partner will not be able to be present in the operative room due to how rapidly everyone is working to help deliver your baby in a safe manner. However, your partner may be invited in after delivery to be present with your baby as the remainder of your surgery is finished.

After the surgery The procedure takes about an hour. The mother is woken shortly after the surgery is completed. The baby will typically stay with your partner until you have recovered enough from anesthesia to safely hold them. Since general anesthesia doesn't give localized pain relief, it's normal to need pain relief afterward. Morphine-based medication may be given for a day or two.

BIRTH STORY: EPIDURAL PAIN RELIEF

Alice was having her first baby. Her pregnancy had been uncomplicated and she had written a birth plan outlining her desire for a natural childbirth by keeping active and using TENS and then warm water to deal with contractions. She wished to avoid an epidural if possible.

Alice's birth story: My husband and I arrived at the delivery suite in early labor. I started to use a TENS machine for pain relief. However, as my labor progressed, I became very distressed since I hadn't anticipated that the contractions would be so painful. When I was around 3 cm dilated, I decided to remove the TENS machine and get into the bath. My husband gave me a back massage and provided emotional support. However, I think he struggled to understand my discomfort and he needed support from the nurse. After 15 minutes, I decided to get out of the bath since it was providing little pain relief. I used a birth ball to stay active and my husband gave me more massage and acupressure. I coped well for the next hour, but then became increasingly exhausted and upset. When I was examined, I was only 5 cm dilated. We both felt despondent because we had hoped I was further along.

My nurse then suggested that I talk to the anesthesiologist about my options for further pain relief, and as a result of my conversation with the anesthesiologist, I decided to have an epidural. I told the anesthesiologist that I'd had an epidural a few years ago for knee surgery and how it had provided excellent pain relief, but that I had itched for hours afterward. The anesthesiologist surmised that the itch was caused by one of the painkilling medications (fentanyl) in the epidural top-off and agreed that this medicine wouldn't be used. The anesthesiologist agreed to do a low dose combined spinal epidural that gave absolute pain relief within five minutes. My legs were a little heavy at first, but they felt fine within an hour. I felt that we were both able to take time out after the epidural and that I was able to refocus on my labor. I felt pleased that I'd managed a large part of my labor without pain relief, and was happy with the decision to have an epidural when I did. I had an unassisted delivery later that evening.

The anesthesiologist comments: Alice kept an open mind regarding pain relief and understood that different methods of pain relief could be used at different times during labor. After the epidural, she no longer felt that her labor was an endurance test and was able to focus again on her labor and on delivering a healthy baby.

1st stage of labor

WAITING FOR YOUR LABOR TO START CAN BE BOTH FRUSTRATING AND TERRIBLY EXCITING. You may be anxious to get your delivery over with, or feel that you aren't ready for labor. This can be an emotional time, so try to stay calm. This section helps you identify the symptoms and signs of labor and takes you through the changes that occur as your body gets ready to give birth.

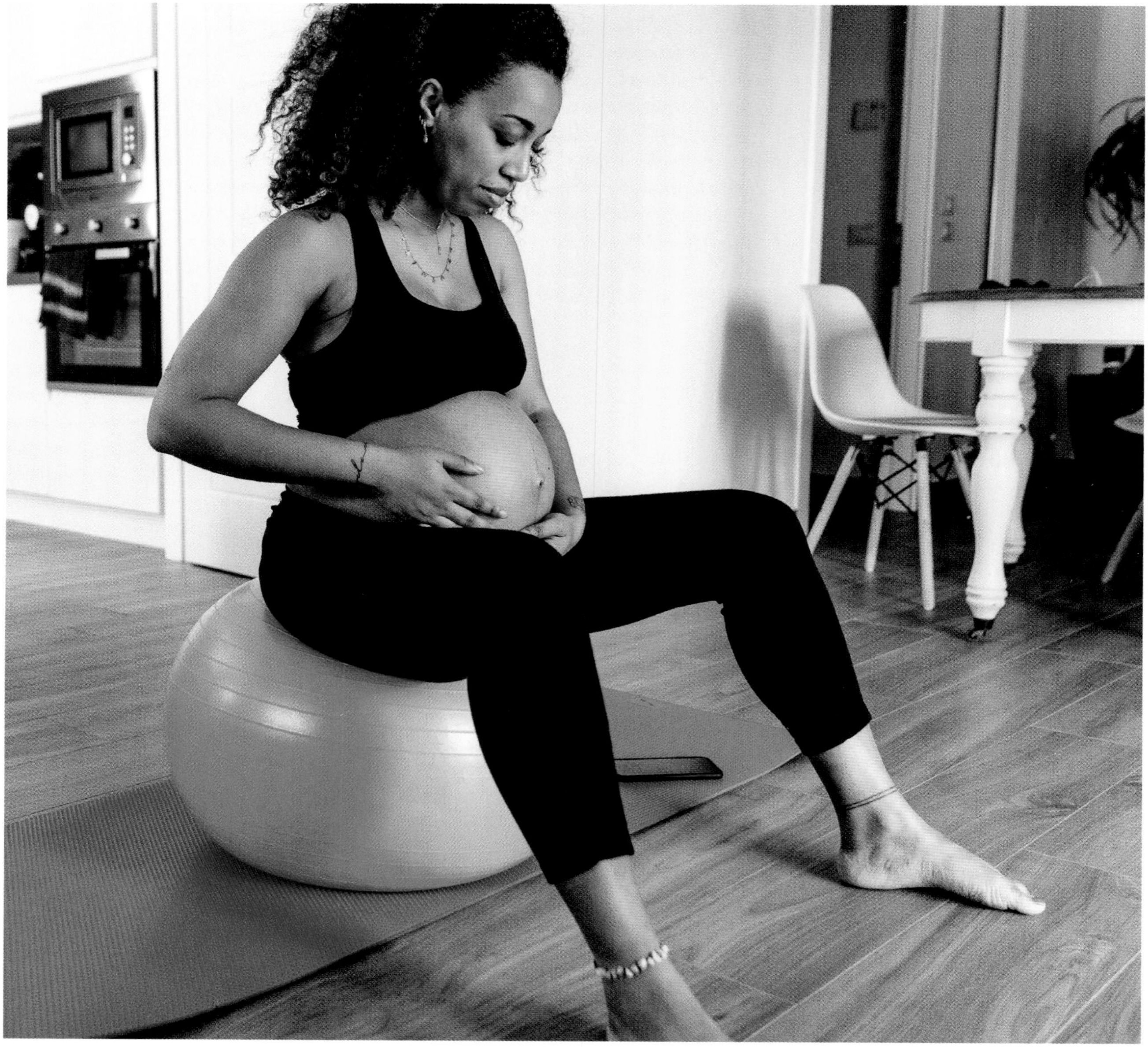

Approaching labor

As your pregnancy comes to an end, your cervix starts to soften as your body prepares for the forthcoming labor and birth.

As labor approaches, your body starts to prepare itself for the task ahead and you may notice various physical symptoms and signs that labor is about to start. Not every woman experiences labor in the same way, and certain signs can occur either before labor starts or during labor.

Common physical symptoms

Toward the end of your pregnancy, you may experience a sensation of building pressure or cramping in your pelvic or rectal area. This pelvic cramping can feel very similar to monthly menstrual cramps. A dull pain in your lower back that comes and goes is common too. You may also notice an increase in heartburn (acid reflux) and gassiness. Unless you have a high-risk pregnancy, there is no need to go to the hospital or call your doctor if you experience any of these symptoms in the later stages of your pregnancy.

Your emotional state

This is a time of waiting and many women busy themselves with household tasks. These bursts of activity are often thought to be instinctual, as the mother prepares the home for the new arrival, referred to as "nesting." The anticipation of what will happen during labor can give rise to a mixture of emotions, from fear and anxiety to excitement and impatience. Women may feel fearful about how much pain they will feel or how uncomfortable they will be with bodily functions. Nothing can prepare you fully for how you will feel in labor, but the more you understand about pain relief options (see pp.397–401) beforehand, the more confident you will feel about your ability to manage. It's also thought that by being informed and prepared, you are likely to reduce your anxiety during labor, which in itself can enable you to cope better with the pain of contractions.

Journaling can be a good way to process and record emotions as you approach the end of your pregnancy. It is normal to experience a range of feelings, from fear and anxiety to excitement and curiosity.

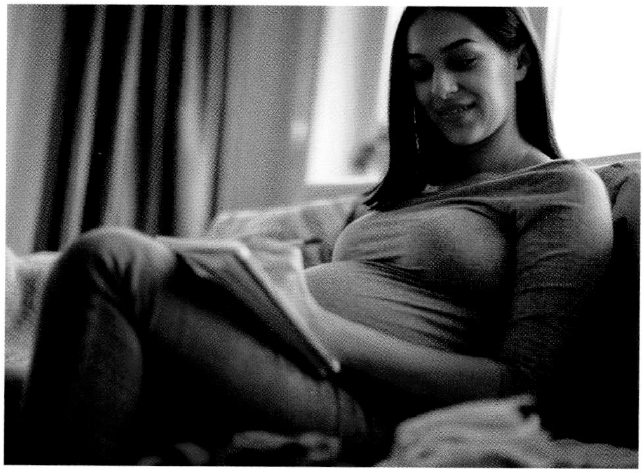

PREPARING FOR LABOR

The period before labor starts can last for hours or even days, particularly with a first labor. So that you can manage when you go into labor, you need to take care of yourself during this prelabor stage.

- **Stay well rested** so that you aren't completely exhausted when you go into labor. If you're having trouble resting due to anxiety, try practicing some relaxation techniques.

- **Trouble sleeping is usually due to physical discomfort,** such as being too hot, not being able to get into a comfortable position, or having trouble breathing from congestion. Measures that can help include using body pillows, a dehumidifier, and fans or air conditioning in the summer.

- **Continue eating to keep your energy levels up** and provide fuel for the days ahead. You may not feel like eating a large meal; instead, eat little and often.

- **If you're suffering with back pain, try showering in warm water or taking a warm bath.** However, be careful when showering, since pregnancy increases your chances of feeling dizzy, and avoid a prolonged bath in very hot water since this may not be good for your baby.

- **A lower back massage is comforting** and a good way to relax and ease discomfort—ask your partner to give you a soothing massage.

Braxton Hicks contractions

One of the most common symptoms of approaching labor is an increase in the strength and frequency of Braxton Hicks, or practice, contractions (see p.387), which may be occurring up to four times an hour. The purpose of these practice contractions is to prepare your uterus to deal with real labor contractions so that labor progresses smoothly. Some women find Braxton Hicks relatively painless, while others find these practice contractions fairly uncomfortable, especially if the baby is quite low and contractions cause increased pelvic pressure.

Apart from the level of pain, one of the main ways to distinguish Braxton Hicks from real contractions is that Braxton Hicks are irregular and they fade away, whereas labor pains occur at regular intervals and gradually become stronger, more intense, and closer together. The other main difference between Braxton Hicks contractions and real ones is that, unlike Braxton Hicks, real contractions cause your cervix to dilate, which indicates that labor is beginning.

Engagement of the head

With a first baby, dropping down of the baby's head into your pelvis, known as engagement, usually means that labor is likely to start soon. In second and subsequent pregnancies, engagement may not occur until the start of labor.

You can usually tell that your baby's position has changed in two ways. First, you may notice that you have less discomfort in your upper abdomen or around your ribs because the downward movement releases some pressure. Second, you may notice increased pressure or pain in your pelvic or vaginal area as the baby's head moves into position. Your walking may become more of a waddle and you may have to use the bathroom more frequently than before. In some cases, your baby's head may pinch some of the nerves that run through your pelvis and you may

A NATURAL OCCURRENCE

No one is sure exactly what triggers labor, but it seems the process varies with each species. In sheep, a drop in progesterone signals the start of labor. In mice, babies release proteins to signal their maturity. In humans, little is known about the signals that start labor, although there are many theories. Studies suggest that the production of hormones such as corticotrophin-releasing hormone (CRH) by the uterus and placenta may play a role. It's also thought that an increase in pro-inflammatory substances known as cytokines may be involved. Whatever the trigger, it's likely that the onset of labor involves a biological communication between your baby and your body.

SIGNS OF APPROACHING LABOR

Although each woman's experience of labor differs and there are no hard and fast rules as to what will happen when, there are signs that indicate that labor is likely to start either imminently or within a matter of days. One of the classic signs that labor isn't far away is a "bloody show" (see opposite), when you lose the plug of mucus that has protected your baby during pregnancy. The other indisputable sign that labor will be shortly underway is that your cervix begins to dilate, although of course this will only be visible during an internal examination.

One other sign that labor may be about to start is if your water breaks (see opposite). However, for the majority of women this happens later on during established labor.

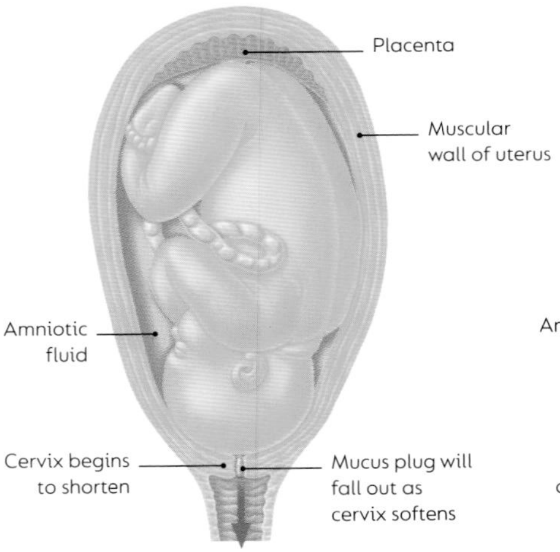
Placenta
Muscular wall of uterus
Amniotic fluid
Cervix begins to shorten
Mucus plug will fall out as cervix softens

As the cervix starts to soften and shorten, the thick plug of mucus that protected your baby from infection during pregnancy comes away and falls out of the vagina, an event referred to as a "bloody show." When this happens, you may notice a yellowish discharge.

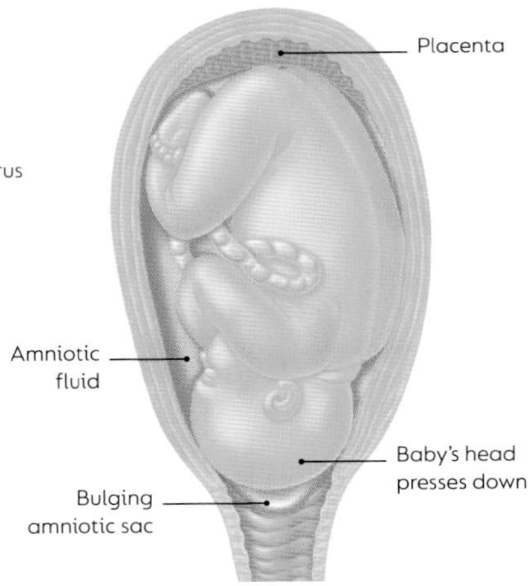
Placenta
Amniotic fluid
Baby's head presses down
Bulging amniotic sac

The amniotic membrane bulges through the cervix as the baby's head presses down. When the membranes break (water breaking), labor is imminent, or may have already started. The amniotic fluid may pass out as a gush of fluid or a trickle.

experience sciatica, a sharp electric pain that runs down the outside of your leg to your outside toes (see p.472).

The "bloody show"

In pregnancy, a plug of mucus forms at the end of the cervix to prevent infection from entering the uterus. At the end of pregnancy, as the cervix softens and widens, this plug is dislodged and comes out through the vagina. When this occurs, you may see a discharge known as the "bloody show"; although some women don't notice anything. The discharge may appear as a thick, clear or yellow clump that looks like mucus from your nose. It's common for small amounts of blood to be present.

Many women think that losing the plug means that labor is imminent, but this is not necessarily the case. In fact, it may be many days before labor starts. However, if loss of the plug is accompanied by other symptoms, such as painful, frequent contractions, heavy bleeding, or leaking fluid (indicating your water has broken), you should call your doctor or hospital immediately.

Water breaking

Rupture of the amniotic membranes, called the water breaking, usually occurs once labor has started but can happen earlier, and often means that labor is imminent. For some, a big gush of fluid is a clear sign that their water has broken, while for others there may be a trickle and it can be hard to determine if the amniotic fluid is leaking. Also, since many women have trouble controlling their bladder in pregnancy, telling the difference between urine and amniotic fluid can be hard. One way to tell is to wear a sanitary pad. If the pad quickly becomes soaked, your water has probably broken. Amniotic fluid also has an odor that is different than urine, even to nonprofessional noses.

Monitoring after the water breaks

If you think your water has broken but contractions haven't started, contact your doctor or the hospital for advice. If you're due, there are no complications, and your baby's head is engaged, you may be advised either to stay at home for a while to see if labor starts, or will be asked to be seen at the hospital. This is because, once your water has broken, your baby has lost the protective membrane surrounding them, which means there is an increased risk of an infection reaching your baby. The doctor should check your file to see if you're Group B Strep (GBS)-positive, and if you are, you'll be admitted and started on IV antibiotics. They may also monitor your baby's heartbeat (see p.418) to check that your baby is isn't distressed. If you're GBS-negative and all is well, you may be able to return home, or stay at home, for a set amount of time and an appointment will be made to see how you're progressing. If labor doesn't start within 24 hours (the timeframe may be shorter in some hospitals), the hospital may suggest an induction (see p.432).

Early contractions

As your body prepares to go into labor, you will start to experience mild and irregular contractions. These differ from Braxton Hicks since they build gradually and will soften and dilate the cervix.

WHEN TO SEEK HELP

Make your way to the hospital or seek advice if any of the following occurs:

- You have vaginal bleeding that is like a period or heavier.
- You're leaking amniotic fluid or leaking greenish fluid that could indicate the baby is distressed.
- The baby isn't moving as expected (ask your doctor for advice).

WHEN AM I IN LABOR?

A common concern of many women is how they will know when they are in labor. The following are indications that labor is truly underway.

- **You are having contractions that are becoming stronger** and more intense, lasting longer, and the interval between the contractions is getting shorter.
- **Changing your position or** walking around doesn't ease the intensity of the contraction.
- **The contractions start high in your abdomen and** move down through the uterus and lower back, instead of occurring only in the lower abdomen.
- **Your water breaks** (see above) while you're having contractions.

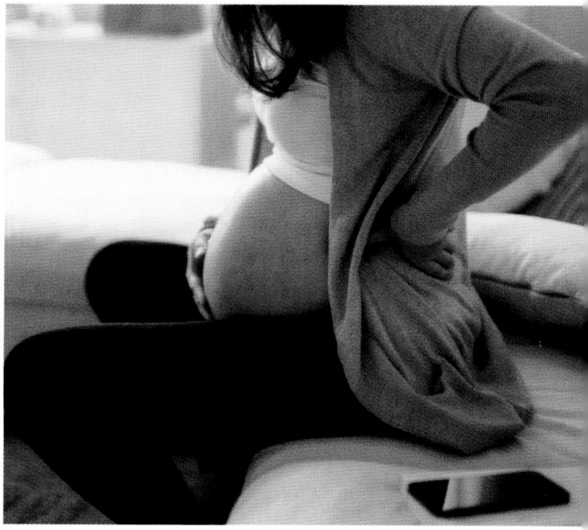

How labor progresses

Stronger and more regular contractions continue to stretch your cervix until, at around 10 cm, it is fully dilated.

Since every woman's experience of labor is different, it's hard to say exactly what your experience will be like. However, the stages of labor are common for all women. The first stage, when labor becomes established, starts when contractions start to open, or dilate, the cervix (see box, p.415). For some women, especially those who don't want strong pain relief, this is the hardest part of labor. Waiting for the cervix to dilate can be a long process with your first baby, and there isn't much you can do to hurry the process. The first stage of labor can be broken down into different phases, referred to as the early, or latent, phase, and the active phase (see below). After these phases comes transition, when your cervix becomes fully dilated and before you start to push your baby out (see p.416).

The early (latent) phase During the early phase, which can last for over a day or so in a first labor, your contractions gradually become more uncomfortable, but are still relatively mild, and occur more frequently, although they may be irregular. During this phase, your cervix gradually shortens, a process known as effacement (see box, p.414) and begins to dilate. When the cervix is approximately 3–4 cm dilated and you're having regular, strong contractions, the active phase has begun (see right). The changes to your cervix during the early phase can be slow or fast and are hard to predict.

SUDDEN BIRTH

Although uncommon, labor and birth can occur unexpectedly fast, resulting in an unplanned home birth or a birth on the way to the hospital. Sudden birth is more likely to happen in second and subsequent labors or if you've had a previous sudden birth.

If you're at home. If your contractions start coming very rapidly and you begin to feel some pressure in your bottom, try to stay calm and call 911 for an ambulance. Also ask them to contact your doctor. Try to contact a friend, relative, or neighbor who can help.

Wash your hands and gather newspapers, clean towels, or clean clothing, or if you have an assistant ask him or her to prepare in this way. If there is time, the floor or bed should be covered with a plastic sheet or newspapers; have a plastic bowl on hand for the placenta.

If you have an urge to push, breathe slowly; panting and blowing can help. Sit or kneel on the floor or your bed on top of a clean towel so that your baby doesn't fall onto a hard surface. Your water may break and an assistant can watch for a sudden bulging of the perineum and for your baby's head to appear, at which point you can push.

Once the head is delivered, you will feel another contraction and can push the body out. You may be able do this alone, or an assistant can put his or her hands on either side of the head and apply gentle pressure. If your baby is born in the amniotic sac, this can be punctured with fingers; the baby's face will need wiping so that the airway is clear. Try to record the time of birth.

Give your baby immediate skin-to-skin contact to keep him warm; then dry him and wrap him in a towel or blanket. Putting him to your breast stimulates contractions to deliver the placenta. An assistant can watch for a gush of blood or lengthening of the cord, a sign that the placenta has come away. Put the placenta in a towel in a bowl to be checked. Clamp the cord with string or a shoelace; the doctor or paramedic will cut it when he or she arrives.

If you're in a car. If you feel an urge to push, your partner should pull over and put the hazard lights on. If your baby is born in the car, your partner can put him on your belly for warmth. If you have towels, dry your baby, wrap him in a clean towel, and call an ambulance.

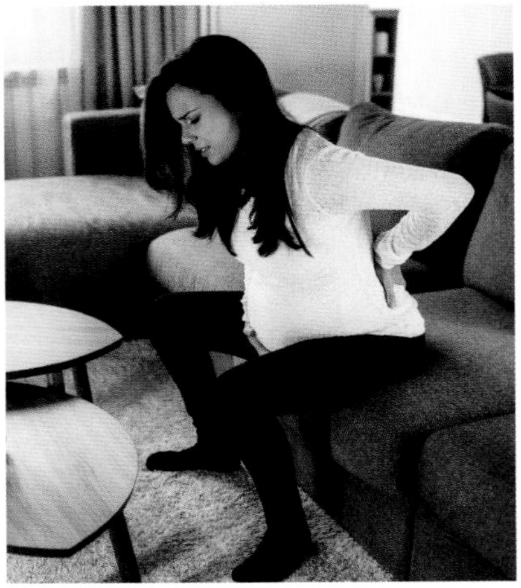

WHEN IT'S TIME TO GO TO HOSPITAL

Many couples feel unsure about when to go to the hospital. If your pregnancy is low risk, you will almost certainly be more comfortable at home at the start of labor and should wait until you're in active labor, when your contractions are regular, occurring every 5–10 minutes, and painful, before going to the hospital. At this stage, the hospital will want to assess how your baby is responding to strong contractions, and you may want some medication for pain. This needs to be administered in a setting where you can be monitored and, in the case of an epidural (see p.404), can only be given in the hospital.

If your pregnancy is high risk, you have had a prior cesarean, have a breech baby, or carry the streptococcus B bacterium, call the maternity ward to discuss when to go to the hospital.

Once you're in active labor, a final reason to go to the hospital is to make sure your baby is born there. An unplanned home (or car) birth is not best for you or your baby. This is unusual in a first pregnancy, but with subsequent births women are more likely to arrive at the hospital quite dilated or to have an unintended home birth.

Getting to the hospital Arrange for someone to drive you to the hospital, either your partner, or a friend or relative; don't consider driving yourself. Map the route ahead of time, consider a dry run before the big day, and have a bag packed with everything you will need for you and your baby (see p.358).

Admission procedure When you get to the hospital, you'll be checked in and will be put into a labor room if you look like you're in active labor, or into an assessment bed if this isn't clear. Usually you will be asked for a urine specimen, and a nurse will check your temperature, pulse, and blood pressure, check your cervix, and review your pregnancy history. If you're in early labor, you may be sent home. This doesn't mean you were unwise to come in; it's good to ensure all is well.

Once you've been admitted, you and your baby will be assessed by a doctor or nurse. Sometimes an intravenous (IV) line will be placed and blood tests may be done. You can make your room comfortable with items from home.

AS LABOR BEGINS

If you're having a home birth, your midwife will have talked to you in advance about how to contact her once you're in labor. This may be via her cell phone or via the birth center. Since she will be traveling to you, bear in mind local traffic conditions. If the streets might be busy, it's worth phoning her in early labor. She may ask you to phone again when your contractions are closer together.

While waiting for the midwife, you may want to move around, or relax in a warm bath. If you've purchased or rented a birthing pool, ensure that this is ready to use. Ask your partner to lay down old sheets or plastic sheeting over the floor. Eating small, nourishing snacks and drinking water will provide energy for the hours ahead.

Home births are not for everyone. They're only an option for you if you're having a healthy, low-risk pregnancy, and you may need to be transferred to a hospital before delivery if complications arise. The American College of Obstetricians and Gynecologists opposes home births because of the potential for complications, even in low-risk pregnancies, as does the American Medical Association. Only 6 out of every 1,000 U.S. births are home births.

The active phase The active phase of the first stage is the individual point for each woman where cervical change happens more quickly and predictably. However, exactly when you enter active labor can be hard to establish, even for a doctor. For most women, active labor occurs at around 4 cm dilation. Your contractions are regular and may be every 5 minutes or so and getting closer together until they're 2 to 4 minutes apart and lasting from 45 seconds to one minute or more. From the start of active labor to the birth can last for around 10 to 12 hours, although this may be considerably shorter when it is a second labor.

In active labor, the nature of your contractions changes, with pain becoming less concentrated in the lower abdomen, instead starting higher in the abdomen and moving down toward the pelvis and lower back as your baby is pushed down. Contractions are caused by a painful tightening of the muscles that may start off feeling like a severe period pain and increase in intensity as they reach their peak. Your doctor will assess if you're in active labor by observing your pain levels, the frequency and strength of contractions, and by using a tool called a labor curve, which plots cervical change and the position of your baby's head in relation to your pelvis over time (see labor graphs, p.419).

It's important for your doctor to determine when you enter active labor so she can assess how labor is progressing. For first labors, 90 percent of women have a cervical dilation of about 1 cm per hour, whereas labor moves faster in subsequent births. If you've had an epidural (see p.404), labor may be slower. Once it's established that you're in active labor, the doctor can predict when you may deliver. However, since women vary widely in how long it takes them to have a baby, bear in mind that this is only an estimate.

During active labor, you may want to have medical pain relief if you haven't so far, such as analgesics or an epidural (see pp.402–406).

Abdominal and vaginal examinations

You will have several internal vaginal examinations and your abdomen palpated to assess the baby's position. If your doctor is assessing whether amniotic fluid is leaking, they may do a speculum examination. Usually, the doctor uses their fingers to assess the baby and the progress of labor. They will try to check you often enough to make sure that your labor is progressing, but not so often that it causes you extra discomfort or increases your risk of infection. The following are assessed during a vaginal examination.

The station The doctor will check to see how far the head has descended into the pelvis (see box, below).

Cervical effacement The doctor will assess that the cervix is shortening and getting ready for dilation (see box, below).

Cervical dilation The doctor will assess how dilated, or open, your cervix is (see box, opposite). Active labor is established at 3 to 4 cm dilation and full dilation occurs at around 10 cm. You can't push your baby out until you're fully dilated.

Fetal position Fetal presentation refers to the part of your baby that is coming out first. Babies can be born head first or bottom first (breech; see p.433). Your doctor will also assess which way your baby is facing in the birth canal.

The easiest way for a baby to be born is head down with the back of the baby's head (occiput) and spine facing toward the front (anterior) of

CHANGES TO THE CERVIX

The cervix is comprised of firm muscle that forms a strong base at the bottom of the uterus. For your baby to be born, the cervix needs to shorten and soften so that it can open, or dilate, and your baby can pass out of the uterus and into the vagina.

Toward the end of pregnancy, substances in your blood called prostaglandins start to soften the cervix so that it becomes more malleable. While you are pregnant, your cervix is usually around 2 to 3 cm long. In late pregnancy or early labor, contractions start to shorten the cervix, a process known as effacement. Most women have a cervix that has shortened to 1 cm during the very early stages of labor. This is also referred to as 50 percent effaced. As the cervix continues to shorten, the cervix is gradually drawn up by the uterus, and by the time it is 100 percent effaced, the cervix will have started to open. Eventually the cervix becomes fully dilated (see box, opposite), and the baby can be pushed out.

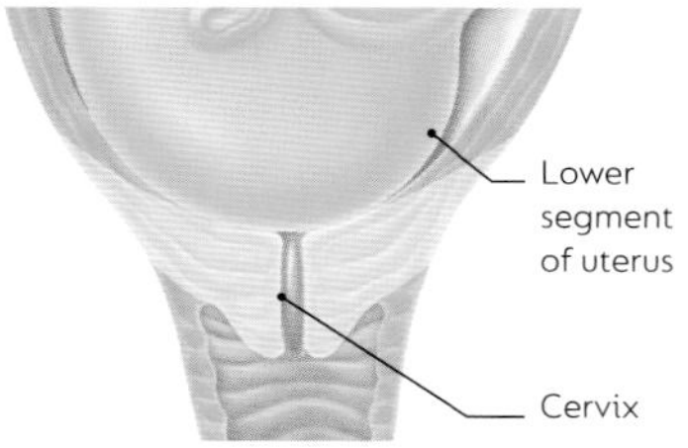

As labor approaches, the cervix starts to lose its firmness and starts to soften in response to the presence of prostaglandins in the blood and contractions.

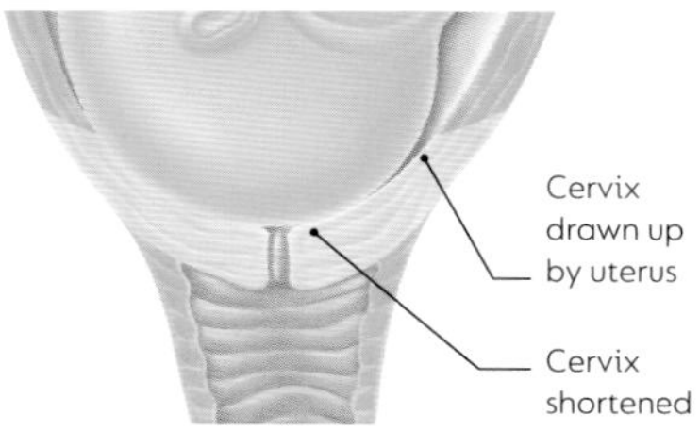

Once the cervix has softened, it starts to shorten. This process is referred to as effacement and needs to occur before the cervix can begin to dilate.

THE "STATION"

The "station" refers to the position of your baby's head in relation to your pelvis. This is recorded as a number between –5 and +5. Zero station means the head is "engaged" and has entered the vaginal canal within the pelvic bones. A negative number (–5 to 0) means that the head isn't engaged in the pelvis. A positive number (0 to +4) means that your baby's head is moving down the pelvis and +5 means your baby is crowning (being born). Ideally, you should not push until the head is engaged in the pelvis, even if you're fully dilated.

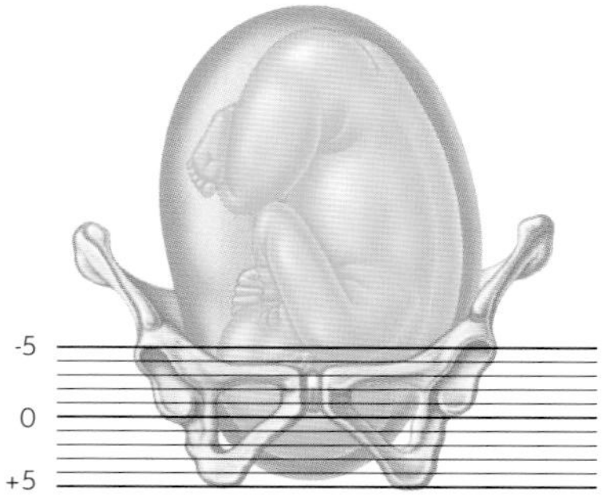

The position of the head in relation to the pelvis is marked on a scale of –5 to +5.

DILATION

Once your cervix is stretched and softened (see box, opposite), it begins to open, or dilate, so that your baby can pass through into the vagina to be born. Regular contractions cause the cervix to dilate, and in first labors the cervix dilates at an average of 0.5 cm per hour; this rate is often faster for subsequent labors. You cannot push your baby out until you are fully dilated, which occurs at 10 cm.

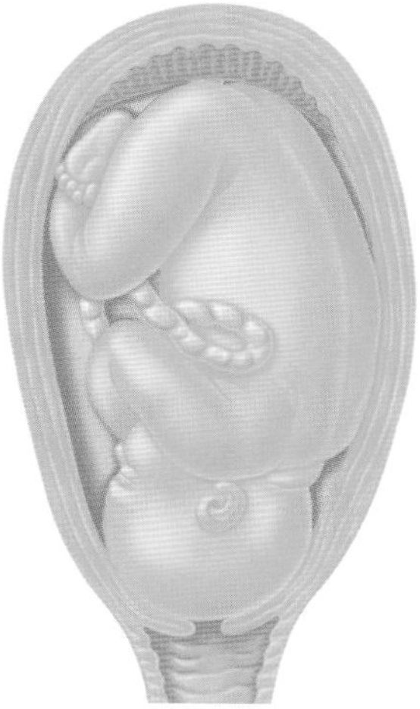

At 2 cm dilation, the cervix has shortened and is beginning to open. Contractions may still be irregular at this stage of your labor.

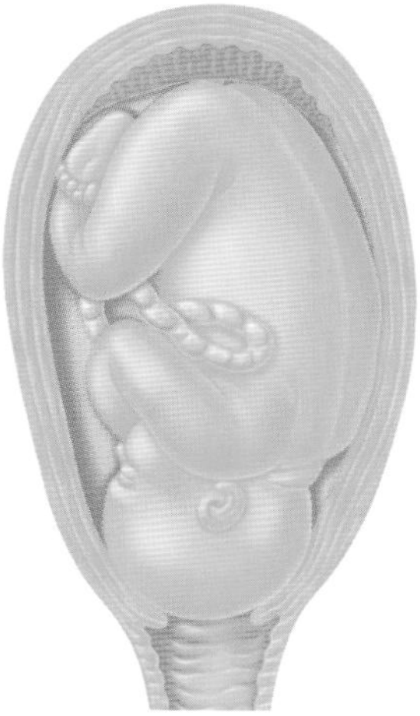

At 6 cm dilation, you are in active labor. Your contractions will be more frequent, regular, and stronger.

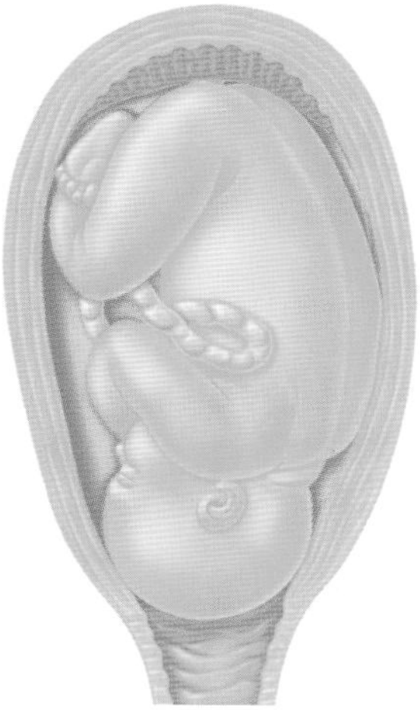

At 10 cm dilation, you are fully dilated. Contractions may be very frequent and you are nearly ready to start pushing your baby out.

your uterus, known as an occiput anterior position (OA).

Your baby can also be born vaginally from an occiput posterior position (OP; back of baby's head and spine face toward the back of your uterus), but this can take longer and be more painful. Vaginal tears are more common when babies are born in the occiput posterior position.

A final position is when your baby faces your side, known as occiput transverse. Full-term babies can't be born in the transverse position since the head is too big to fit this way. However it's usual for babies to rotate around during labor, although this would need to happen before you start to push. If this doesn't happen, labor may need to be assisted (see pp.436–437).

Descent with contractions Although most of the time your doctor will try to examine you between contractions, sometimes it helps to see how much the baby's head comes down in the pelvis during a contraction, referred to as the descent. If there is a good descent, it means that the baby is fitting well into your pelvis and that your contractions are effective.

QUESTIONS AND ANSWERS

Am I likely to have medical interventions in labor in the hospital?
If the reason for having a hospital birth is because you or your baby are at a higher risk of developing complications, there may be an increased need for interventions to keep you and your baby safe. Some interventions include artificially opening the bag of waters if your labor progress has slowed or if there is a concern about the baby's heart rate; inserting a catheter if you are unable to pass urine; placing an intravenous drip through which fluids or medication can be given if, for example, you are at high risk of a postpartum hemorrhage or you need intravenous antibiotics for group B Streptococcus; and helping to augment labor with medications.

Is artificial rupture of the membranes routine in the hospital?
Manually breaking the bag of waters, known as amniotomy or ARM (see p.432), is offered routinely in some hospitals. It's a painless, low-risk procedure thought to shorten the time of labor by one to two hours, reduce the chance of a low early Apgar score in your baby (see p.428), and significantly decrease the chance that you'll need medication to speed up labor (see below). Amniotomy does, however, increase the intensity of contractions. The one time it is necessary is if a fetal scalp electrode is put on the baby's head (see p.419) as this can't be done without breaking the waters. It will also be done as part of the induction process (see p.432).

How is labor sped up with drugs?
f labor is not progressing, it can be augmented by using oxytocin given through the IV to strengthen contractions. This is done in conjunction with continuous fetal monitoring to watch for signs of distress if the contractions are too frequent. Oxytocin is metabolized very quickly so turning off the IV will stop the contractions within a few minutes.

Transition

Transition is the end of active labor as your cervix becomes fully dilated and you ready yourself to begin pushing. This is one of the shortest stages of labor, lasting from 15 minutes to two hours, although on average it's about 30 minutes. This can be one of the most challenging parts of labor because your contractions intensify and can begin to feel continuous since they now occur every 30–90 seconds. If you haven't had an epidural, transition can be especially difficult since you may feel a lot of pressure on your lower back and rectum and have an overwhelming desire to push, but will be unable to push until your cervix is fully dilated. Even if you've had an epidural, you may notice increasing pelvic pressure. If you do push before your cervix is ready, you may tear your cervix or cause your cervix to swell and thicken, which will prolong the process of labor.

It's not uncommon to vomit now, a side effect of the stretching of your cervix and the pelvic pressure. You may also tremble or shake and have hot flashes.

How you can cope You may feel very uncomfortable during this period as your contractions become stronger and you try to hold back from pushing. Significant pelvic pressure during the transition phase can make it difficult to relax between contractions, and you will therefore need plenty of support from your birth partner and midwife. You may be feeling exhausted, out of control, possibly frightened, and may even think that you can't continue.

Work with your nurse to find the best position for you. This is the one stage of labor where it can be helpful not to adopt an upright position, since you can take some of the pressure off the pelvis. Sitting or being on all fours with your bottom raised may help. Keep breathing during your contractions; your nurse may show you how to pant and breathe shallowly to help resist the urge to push. If possible, moving around during contractions can sometimes help since you will focus on doing something else until you can actively push. You could try rocking on a birthing ball or in a rocking chair. If there is time between your contractions, ask your partner to massage your lower back if this helps relieve pressure.

It can be easy to lose sight of the purpose of labor at this point, so try to focus on the fact that your baby will soon be born.

Pain relief Your doctor may not give you opioid pain relief now, since it can cause your baby to be too sleepy if it is given close to the birth. You may still be able to have an epidural.

SUPPORT IN THE FIRST STAGE

During the first stage, your birth partner has a varied and important role. In addition to helping you feel comfortable and assisting you with positions, they can also support you mentally. This is especially important at the end of the first stage, when you reach transition (see above), a point when women often feel panicky and out of control. Your birth partner can offer reassurance that you're doing well and that the delivery of your baby is not far off. They can also improve your comfort, for example by applying a damp, cool washcloth to your face and neck, and can help you focus on your breathing, reminding you to pant or blow to help you resist the urge to push before the cervix is fully dilated.

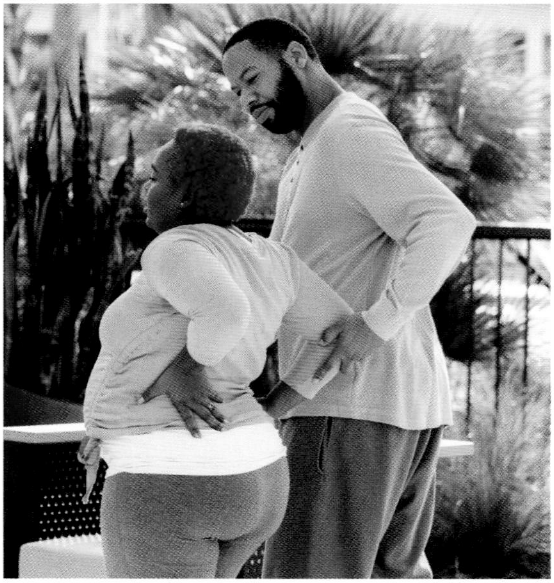

During transition, you may be overwhelmed by the strength and frequency of your contractions. Your partner's support is crucial during this stage and their encouragement can help keep you focused on your labor.

FAILURE TO PROGRESS IN LABOR

If your cervix is not dilating, or your baby is not descending, as quickly as expected during the first stage, your doctor will try to assess why this is and if something can be done. Usually, your doctor will assess the three Ps: the passenger (the size of the baby and his position in the uterus); the powers (the efficiency of your contractions); and the passage (the size and shape of your pelvis). These three elements work together and each one is important for your labor to progress smoothly.

There are several reasons a labor may not progress. These include if the baby's head is too large for the mother's pelvis, known as cephalopelvic disproportion (CPD); if contractions are infrequent or not strong enough; and if the baby is in a posterior position with their back facing the mother's back.

Cephalopelvic disproportion Someimtes CPD may be suspected before labor, in late pregnancy. This may be the case if the doctor thinks that you have a narrow pelvis or promentn sacral bone, both of which may make birth slower or more difficult. However, an assessment of the pelvis alone is not an accurate way to predict if you'll be able to have a successful vaginal birth and, even if th epelvis, is not an optimal shape, the doctor may be happy fo you to continue trying for a vaginal birth. This is because it's not the shape of your pelvis alone that is important, but the interactin between your baby (the passenger) and your pelvis.

If CPD is suspected, bu the baby's head has engaged, a vaginal birth can still be attempted. The labor will be monitored with a labor graph (see p.419) and if there are signs that the baby is in distress, an emergency Cesarean may be performed. If the head hasn't engaged toward the end of labor, a Cesarean may be offered.

If your doctor suspects CPD in labor, they will reassess the baby's size to check whether they originally underestimated the baby's weight. Even though the combination of a large estimated weight and a slow labor can suggest that there may be delivery problems, often labor proceeds normally.

Inefficient contractions If your labor isn't progressing because your cervix is dilating slowly or has stopped dilating, your doctor will asses the frequency of your contractions, which should be every 2 to 3 minutes. She'll also assess how strong the contractions are by palpating your abdomen: the firmer it feels during contractions, the more likely they are to be effective. If contractions are more widely spaced than they should be and their strength indicates they're unlikely to be effective, they may use one or two techniques to speed up labor, known as augmenting labor. First, they may manually rupture the membranes if they haven't already ruptured, a process called amniotomy, or ARM (see p.432). This can shorten labor by around one to two hours.

If ARM has no effect, you may be given the drug oxytocin to increase the strength and frequency of contractions (see p.432). Initially, a small does is given and then increased over time until you're having three or four moderately strong contractions every 10 minutes. If this is done, you'll have continuous electronic fetal monitoring (see p.418) to check that the baby is not distressed by the sudden onset of stronger contractions.

If, several hours after the drugs are started, labor is still not progressing, a Cesarean may be recommended.

Posterior presentation The best position for your baby in labor is an occipito-anterior position with the back of the head (occiput) facing your front. If the back of the head faces your back (occipito-posterior), it can be hard for the baby to turn and move down the birth canal and can prolong labor. The doctor may suggest that you change position to help the baby turn, but the baby usually turns anyway during fully established labor; if not, forceps or vacuum may be needed (see pp.436–437).

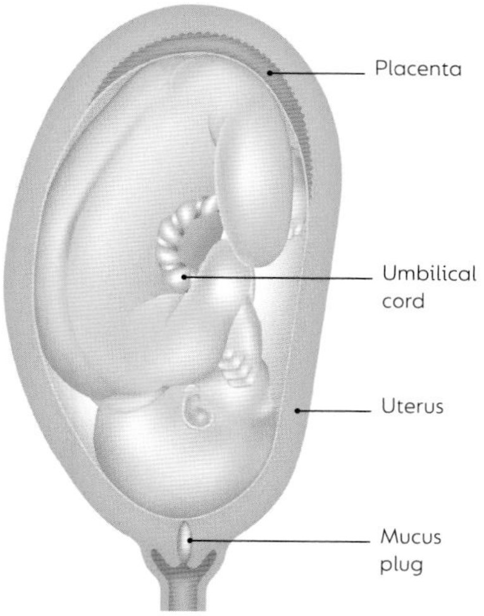
Placenta
Umbilical cord
Uterus
Mucus plug

Anterior presentation The baby is lying head down (known as cephalic) and their spine is facing away from your spine. The smallest part of the head will push down the birth canal first.

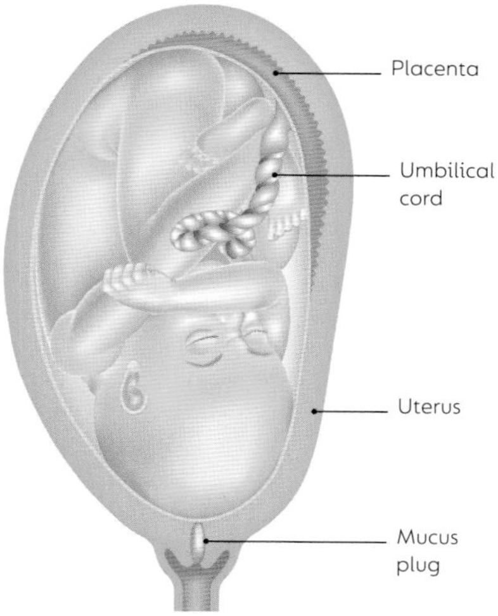
Placenta
Umbilical cord
Uterus
Mucus plug

Posterior presentation The baby is lying head down, but their spine is against your spine. From here, they need to make a bigger turn as they descend through the birth canal, so labor can take longer

Monitoring during labor

Throughout labor, your baby's heartbeat and your contractions will be monitored to make sure that your labor is progressing as it should be and that you and your baby are healthy.

Your baby's heart rate is an indication of how well they are dealing with labor, and it is monitored at regular intervals, called intermittent auscultation. If there are no initial concerns about the baby, monitoring at regular intervals will be continued. However, if a problem is found or you have a high-risk pregnancy (including if you have diabetes, preeclampsia, or are being induced), then you may be advised to have fetal electronic monitoring in order to spot any concerns with your baby's oxygen level. With electronic fetal monitor, your baby's heart rate and your contractions are monitored continuously by an electronic fetal heart monitor (see box, below). All the information about your labor is recorded on a chart, called a labor graph (see opposite).

Intermittent monitoring

This is done using a handheld battery-operated device known as a Doppler sonicaid, which is held against your abdomen to listen to your baby's heartbeat. When you are pushing in the second stage of labor, the fetal heart needs to be monitored more frequently. If the heart rate increases or a slowing of the heart rate is heard after a contraction, this may indicate that the baby is starting to have a problem. At this point, continuous electronic fetal monitoring may be recommended to confirm your baby's well-being.

Electronic fetal monitoring

In this type of fetal monitoring, two devices monitor your baby's heart rate and the strength and frequency of contractions. Your baby's heart

EXTERNAL ELECTRONIC FETAL MONITORING

The baby's heartbeat and the frequency of your contractions are measured by devices strapped to your abdomen with wires that connect to a machine that produces a printout of the readings and an ongoing digital log on the computer.

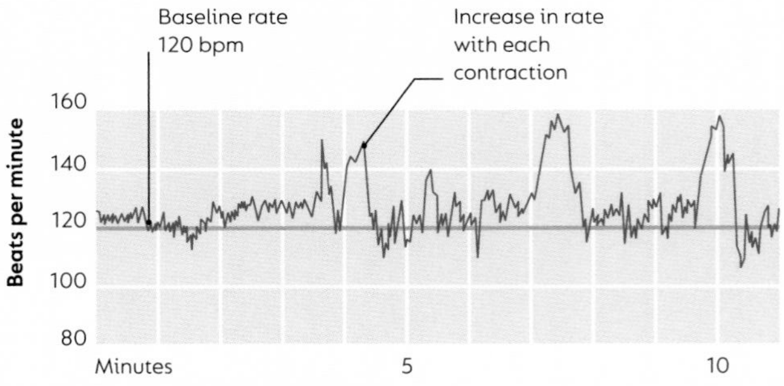

Your baby's heartbeat will vary with a normal range of 110–160 beats per minute (bpm). The heart rate rises and falls naturally with contractions; unusual variations can indicate fetal distress.

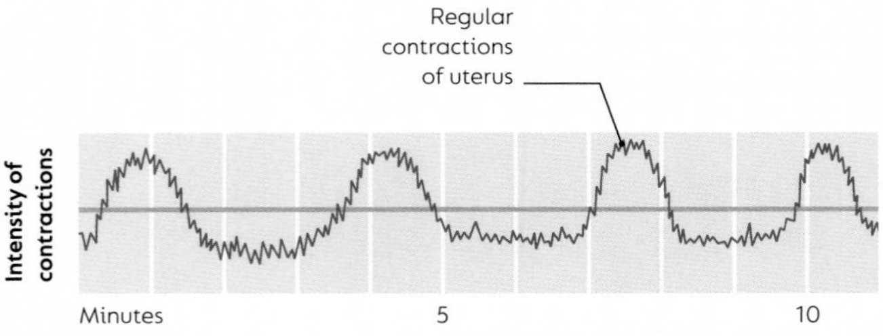

A separate reading records the strength and duration of each contraction. The usual goal is to have 4–5 contractions in 10 minutes; too frequent contractions can cause fetal distress and insufficient contractions can slow labor progress.

rate is monitored with a circular ultrasound-like device. If you want, you can hear the heartbeat, or ask that the volume be turned down if this is distracting. Your contractions are monitored with a small plastic circular device. One or two elastic belts are placed around your abdomen to secure the monitors You should be able to stand, sit, or squat with the monitors in place, and some hospitals have monitors that allow you to walk around and be monitored by radio signal. Your heart rate may also be continuously monitored, particularly if there is a problem differentiating between your heart rate and the baby's heart rate.

Scalp electrode A small electrode is passed through the cervix and attached to the baby's scalp to detect the electrical impulses of their heart. A wire from the electrode comes out via the cervix and attaches to the CTG machine. The electrode is placed during a vaginal examination. It may be mildly uncomfortable for your baby and there is a small risk that your baby could get a scalp infection, which can be treated with antibiotics after the birth. Even though these risks are small, a scalp electrode should not be placed routinely. Your doctor should discuss how the device works before it is placed, and you should understand why it is being done. Scalp electrodes should not be used if you have a viral disease that could be transmitted to your baby. Once a scalp electrode has been placed, you can't move far from the monitor, although you may be able to change position.

Labor graphs

A labor graph is a large chart that contains several graphs that provide information on your labor, allowing the doctor to monitor the progress of your labor. One of the most useful tools in this chart is a graph showing your labor curve. This plots cervical change and the position of your baby's head in relation to your pelvis over time. The graph enables the doctor to establish when your labor became active. Also recorded with your baby's hear-rate monitoring are your blood pressure, pulse, temperature, and the rate of your contractions, as well as your pain levels.

INTERNAL MONITORING

If there are concerns about the baby's heartbeat, a small electrode attached to the scalp can give a more precise reading than external electronic fetal monitoring. The electrode is passed through the cervix and attached to the head.

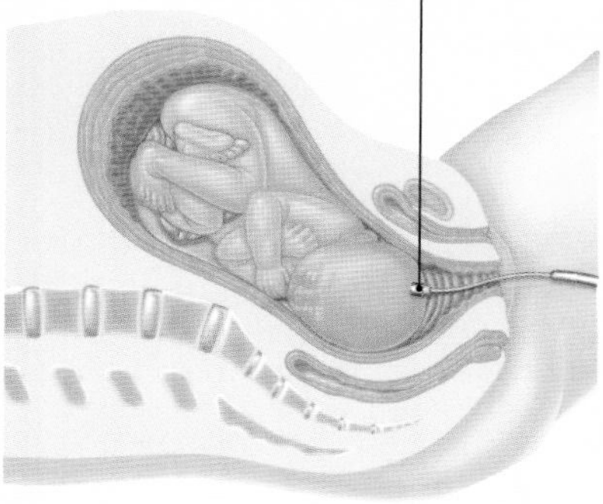
Electrode is attached to baby's head

SHOULD YOU HAVE ELECTRONIC FETAL MONITORING?

There is some debate as to the benefits of continuous monitoring, and some believe there may be associated maternal risks due to increased interventions.

As a result, you may be offered intermittent fetal monitoring if you have a healthy baby. If you are low risk, the chance of your baby developing a problem in labor is low and can be detected by intermittent auscultation before there is any significant harm.

If the nurse hears an abnormality in the baby's heart rate, or you develop other risk factors such as an infection, or the baby passes meconium, the nurse will suggest that you transfer to continuous monitoring. If you have any complications of pregnancy that suggest that the placenta is not functioning properly, such as inadequate growth or low amniotic fluid, then continuous monitoring is recommended because your baby is more vulnerable to the stress of labor.

If the fetal monitoring shows signs that the baby is in distress, then the nurse may change your position, stop the oxytocin, and ask your obstetrician to evaluate you. If the changes in your baby's heart rate continue and cannot be corrected, then your doctor may recommend a Cesarean section.

Positions: the 1st stage of labor

Being active during the first stage of labor is thought to help labor progress. If you're well prepared and practice different postures and positions for labor during pregnancy, you will instinctively be able to use these during childbirth.

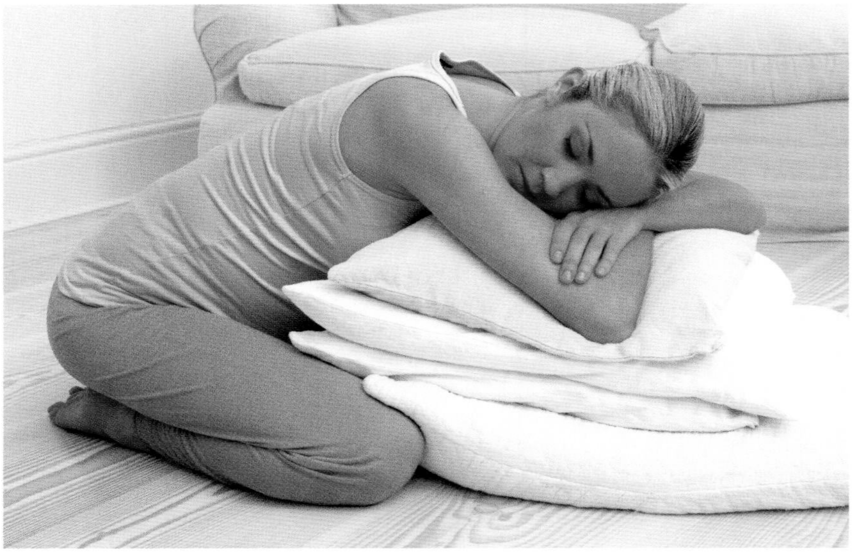

Leaning forward onto a pile of pillows with your knees apart is a soothing and relaxing position, and can also encourage your cervix to dilate.

Many different postures and positions can help you in the first stage, and there is evidence that changing your position in this stage increases the effectiveness of your contractions and reduces the pain. Assuming upright positions in particular uses gravity to assist the descent of the baby.

Active positions

Positions that allow you to remain active are thought to help labor progress. Some women find rocking the pelvis backward and forward, and then rotating the pelvis in a clockwise and then counterclockwise direction while standing or sitting on a birthing ball, helps ease the pain. Adopting an all-fours position on your hands and knees can help you stay focused and

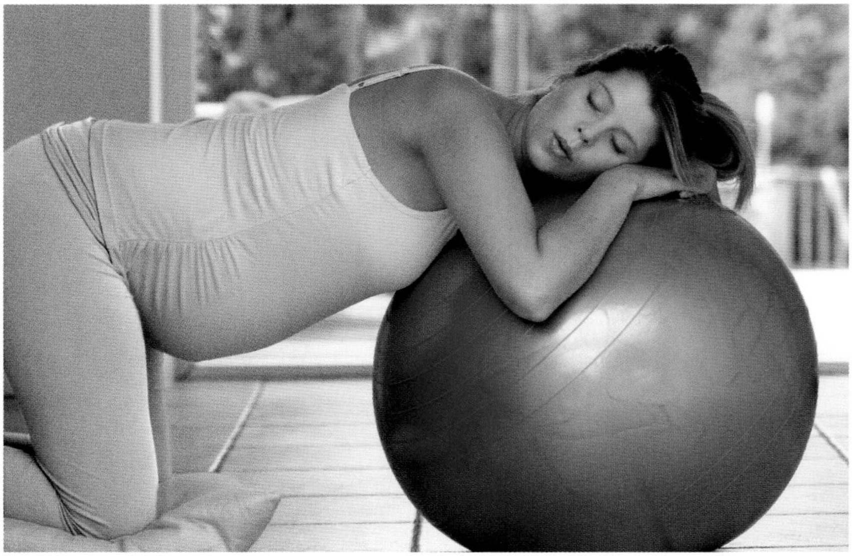

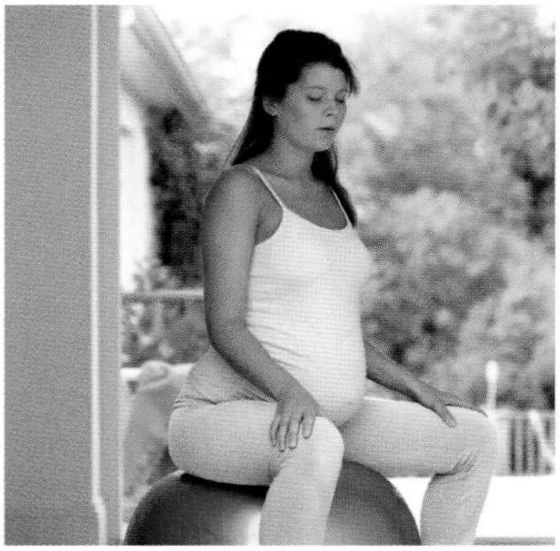

Using a birthing ball during labor enables you to adopt upright positions while feeling supported. While sitting on a birthing ball, or adopting a supported kneeling position with one, you will be able to rotate your hips to encourage the progress of labor.

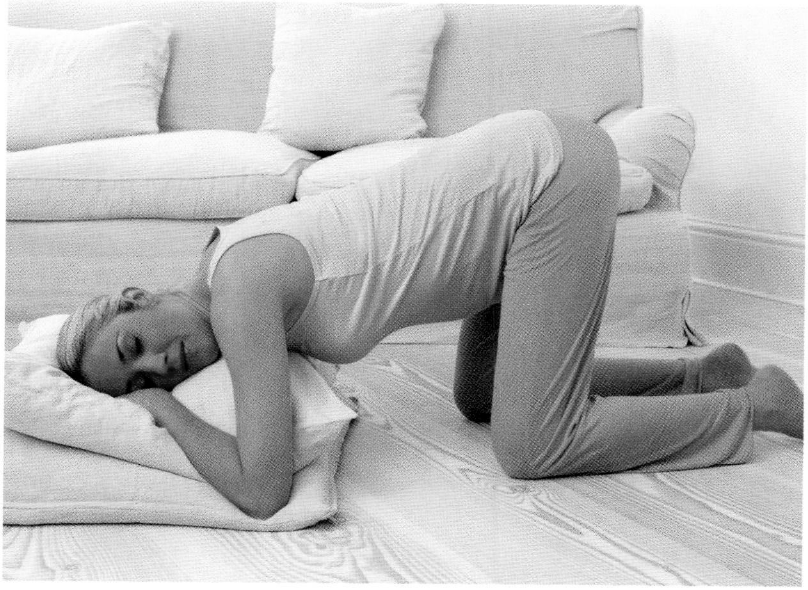

Kneeling and leaning forward onto cushions with your bottom raised also helps ease a backache and can be a helpful position to adopt during transition (see p.416) when you may need to resist the urge to bear down.

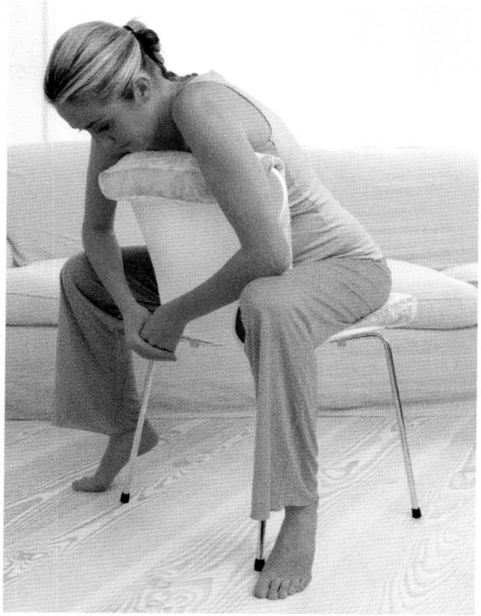

Sitting astride a chair can be a relaxing position because this enables you to lean forward with your legs astride while remaining supported.

also allows you to rotate your pelvis. Moving backward and forward in a rocking chair can also be comforting. Many women find walking in place and walking around helpful

Supported positions

Supported positions can be especially helpful if your baby is in an occiput-posterior position (baby's back to your back). Leaning forward with your hands on a table or chair during a contraction and breathing slowly and steadily helps you focus. If you find it comforting, your partner can massage your shoulders and back at the same time. A lot of women find either sitting astride on a chair facing the back of the chair or sitting on a toilet and facing the tank with a pillow for their head and arms, a comfortable position. This also allows you to "catnap" between contractions.

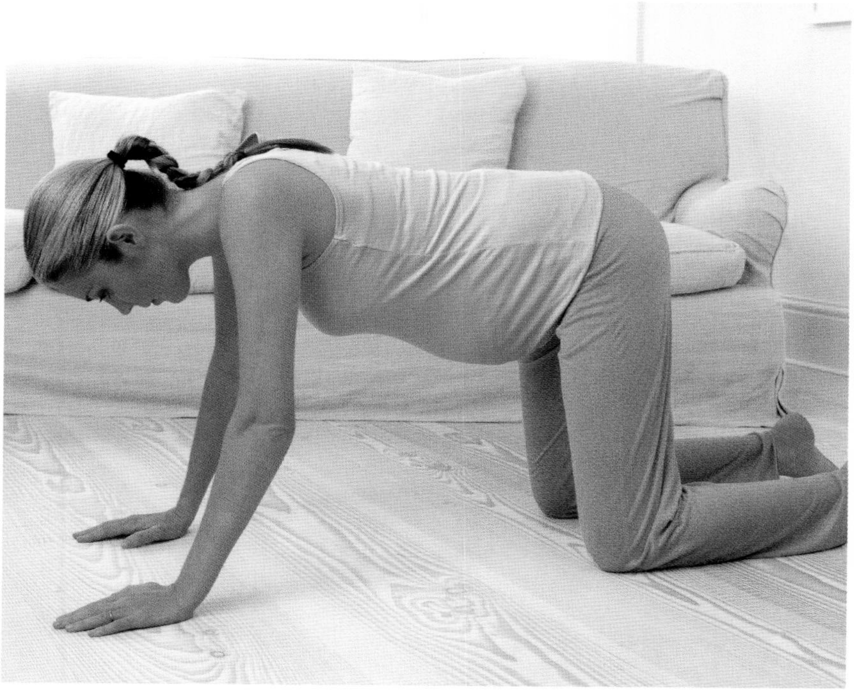

Kneeling in an all-fours position helps take the weight off your back. This position also allows you to move your hips back and forth or rotate them, which can be comforting during early contractions.

2nd and 3rd stages

THE MOMENT OF DELIVERY IS ALMOST HERE AND YOU WILL SOON MEET YOUR LONG-AWAITED BABY. The second stage begins when your cervix is fully dilated and your baby has moved deep into the pelvis. These signs may be accompanied by an overwhelming urge to bear down and, once your doctor is satisfied that you are ready to do it, you will be able to push your baby out. The third stage, the delivery of the placenta, marks the end of labor.

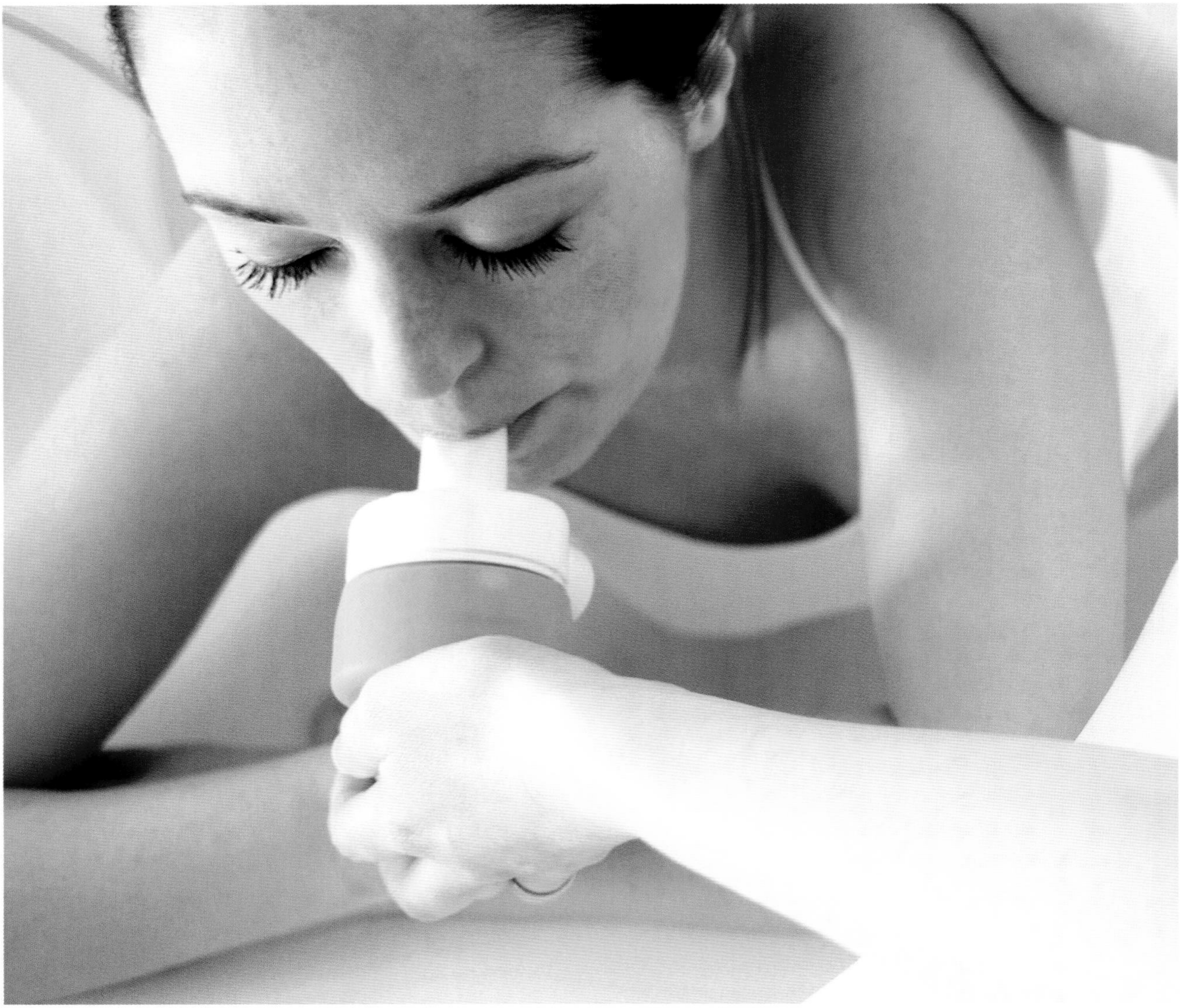

Delivering your baby

In the second stage, the finish line is in sight as you actively push your baby out into the world.

As you enter the second stage of labor, you will probably experience an overwhelming desire to bear down. Once your doctor has established that you are fully dilated and are ready to start pushing, you may start to feel more in control of your labor since your pushing helps move your baby farther down into the pelvis.

The second stage

The second stage of labor starts when your cervix is completely open, at 10 cm, and ends with the birth of your baby. This stage usually lasts for around 45 minutes to two hours for a first labor and from 15–45 minutes in subsequent deliveries. It may last longer if you have an epidural. The second stage is intense and during this time your contractions will become stronger, but may occur less frequently, around every two to five minutes. At this point you may feel a sensation of fullness in your vagina or bowel and have a strong urge to push. Many women find labor pains more bearable in the second stage since they can now actively work with the contractions and push their baby out. Other women find this a particularly hard part of labor because they start to feel exhausted from the effort of prolonged pushing.

Second stage positions

Although you may be tired and want to lie down, it's recommended that you resist this urge in the second stage. Your partner and nurse can give you plenty of support to help you adopt the most comfortable position.

SUPPORT IN THE SECOND STAGE

In the second stage, your birth partner's support is invaluable. Their role is to make you feel supported and safe and to offer lots of encouragement.

Your birth partner can provide verbal support to help you deal with the strenuous task of pushing your baby out with each contraction. There may be times when you're not lucid and your partner will need to speak for you and liaise with medical staff.

In addition to emotional support, your birth partner can act as your physical support in whatever position you adopt in the second stage, whether this is a squatting position or another position that you find comfortable. Your partner will be able to massage your back if this is helpful, and can hold you and comfort you and help you focus on your breathing during and between each contraction.

Your partner can also watch as your baby's head crowns and describe what they can see, or hold a mirror for you to see the baby's head, which can be deeply reassuring as you realize that the end is in sight.

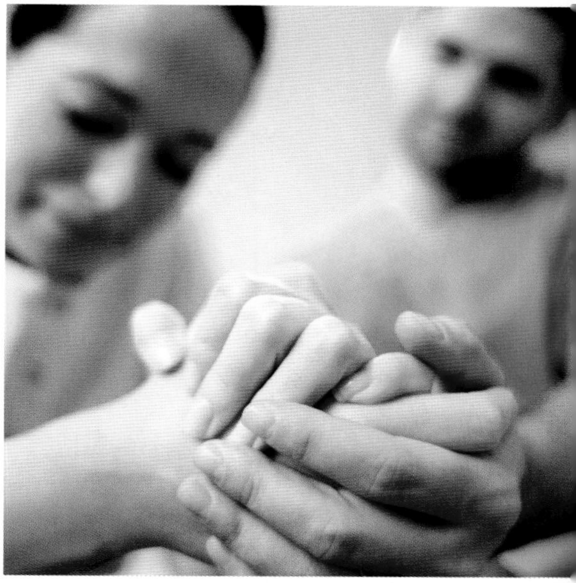

THE BIRTH PASSAGE

Far from being straight, involves a series of rotational maneuvers known as the "cardinal movements of labor." This curve, known as the "curve of Carus," is thought to result from the evolution of humans from being on all fours to being upright. This caused the spine to curve, the pelvis to tilt, and gave a curve to the birth canal. Your pelvic floor muscles help the head rotate through the birth canal.

Staying upright Adopting an upright position during the second stage of labor has several advantages. The main one is that you are using gravity to assist your baby's descent, which will also help you bear down and push. Being upright can also improve the alignment of your baby in the birth canal; can increase the efficiency of your contractions; and widens the passageway through the pelvis.

There is also evidence that adopting upright positions in the second stage of labor can reduce the length of time you take to bear down and give birth, and make it less likely that you will have an instrument delivery or episiotomy (see pp.436–437 and p.427).

Which positions to adopt Upright positions during the second stage of labor include upright sitting and squatting positions.

If you prefer a sitting position, try to sit in an upright or semi-recumbent position. If you adopt a sitting position on a bed, sitting at a 45-degree angle can help your breathing and reduce the risk of a condition known as aortocaval compression, which can affect how well your blood is circulated around your body and to your baby. This is caused by the weight of your uterus and the baby pressing on major blood vessels (the aorta and vena cava), reducing the amount of oxygen that circulates around your body, which makes you feel light-headed and dizzy. If this happens, you will be advised to lie on your left side to relieve pressure and increase the amount of oxygen that is circulating.

Kneeling or squatting increases the pelvic outlet, so many women will

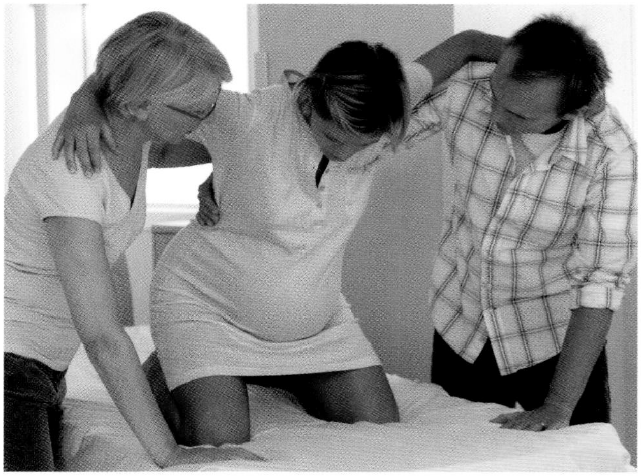

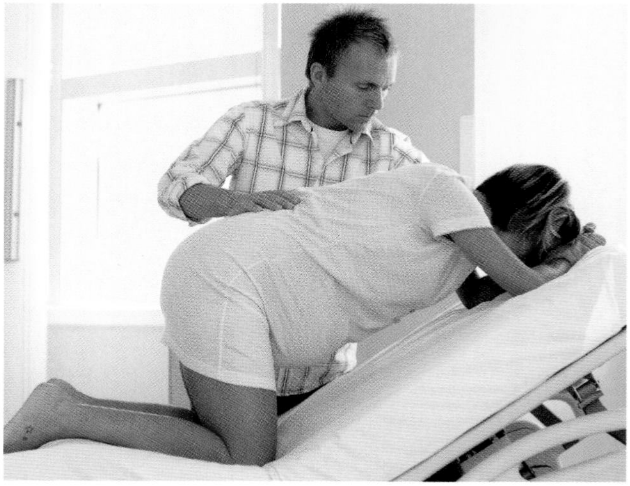

In a kneeling position, both your partner and the nurse can support you as you bear down (top left). **Being on all fours** with the hospital bed for support can be a comfortable position (bottom left).

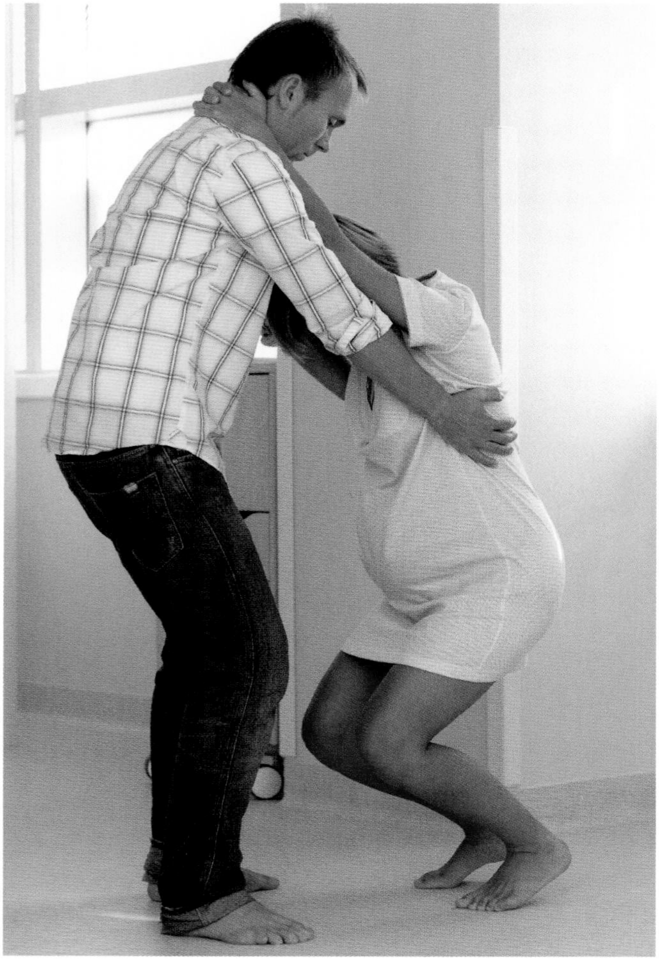

An upright squatting position is good for pushing and can be adopted if you have firm support from your partner. He can support you under the arms while you put your hands around the back of his neck.

naturally adopt a squatting or all-fours position to give birth since they find that this is the most comfortable and easy position in which to deliver their baby. Upright squatting and kneeling positions help increase your pelvic outlet by around 28 percent compared to when you're in a lying-down position. This means that there is more room for your baby to descend through your pelvis and into the birth canal. Some women find it hard to squat down comfortably because they are not used to being in this position and tire easily. If this is the case, ask your partner to support you as you squat.

Alternatively, you may find that lying on your side is your preferred position; your partner can help you by supporting one of your legs to keep your pelvis as open as possible. There is also some evidence that lying on your side can protect your perineum from tearing.

Using props Some women find using props such as a beanbag, birthing ball, pillows, or a large cushion while kneeling and leaning forward helpful.

When to push

Your baby will start to rotate their head and shoulders to start the descent through your pelvis to be born, and you will feel the urge to bear down and push as this is happening.

Your doctor will help you focus and encourage you to push when you feel the urge, which will come naturally with a contraction. With each contraction, you will need to concentrate on pushing down deep into the pelvic area and bottom. It can help to put your chin on your chest and to bear down for as long as possible during a contraction, during which time you may need to take several steady breaths. You may feel like grunting and making noises when bearing down, or you may prefer to breathe deeply and quietly; you should do whatever you find helpful and works best. You will need to work with your body's instincts and adopt the position you find most comfortable and easy to give birth in. Pushing your baby out into the world takes a huge amount of effort and energy, but you have the ability and are very capable of doing this.

Your doctor and birth partner will encourage and support you throughout this stage and help you to believe in your ability to give birth.

Your baby's descent

The time it takes to push your baby out once he or she is deep within the pelvis can take around 30 minutes to one hour for a first labor, although this time may be considerably reduced in subsequent labors, sometimes taking just a few minutes. The combined force of the contractions (which are now around every two to five minutes) and your pushing moves your baby farther down into the pelvic outlet. As this occurs, the pressure on your back and rectum will intensify and you may experience a stinging sensation as your vagina becomes fully stretched. Your doctor may tell you to stop pushing at this point so that your perineum can thin further and so that the baby's head isn't delivered too suddenly, which could cause serious tears. She may tell you to pant or blow instead to help you resist the urge to bear down.

Crowning Initially, the head will descend with each contraction and then move slightly back up the birth

COPING IN THE SECOND STAGE

The second stage of labor can be a time when instinct takes over and you may find that you are oblivious to everything around you as you follow the overwhelming urge to push. You may have been concerned before labor about how you would behave during the delivery. Some women are worried that they will defecate while they are pushing. This is actually very common and it's natural to pass a stool during the delivery; you should rest assured that the nurses and doctors will be completely used to this. You may not even notice yourself that this has happened.

Rather than be concerned about how you will act, try to take encouragement from the fact that you now have more control over your labor and are actively pushing your baby out. You may find that you want to grunt or moan while pushing, or you may push quietly and intensely. Focusing on the imminent arrival of your baby will help you to persevere.

PUSHING WITH AN EPIDURAL

If you have had an epidural, this can affect your awareness of when to bear down and push. If this is the case, your doctor will first check that your baby isn't showing signs of distress, and may then decide to wait a while for the head to descend farther down the birth canal before telling you to push. Alternatively, the doctor will feel the top of your uterus so that she is aware of when a contraction is starting and will then guide you to bear down and push.

canal. Eventually, it will descend far enough to be visible through the vagina at the height of a contraction, known as "crowning," before it once again moves back up and disappears. As contractions continue, the head will finally stay in the vaginal opening and will not slip back at the end of the contraction—this stage is known as crowning.

As your baby descends, the chin will be tucked down toward the chest and the head will rotate slightly so that your baby is facing your back; this enables the largest part of your baby's head to pass through the widest part of the pelvis. As the head passes out of the vagina, it extends backward so that it almost touches his or her back. The doctor will check whether the cord is around the baby's neck. If this is the case, it will be lifted up and away from the neck. The doctor will remove any mucus from your baby's nose and mouth. Once the head has been delivered, it will return to its normal position.

Rest of the body After the delivery of the head, your baby will turn slightly so that the first shoulder can be delivered. Your doctor may help by applying gentle traction to your baby's head at the side to help the first shoulder emerge. Once the first shoulder has been delivered, your baby will turn again slightly so that the second shoulder can be delivered. After this, the rest of the body will slip out and the delivery of your baby will be complete.

Monitoring you and your baby

In the second stage, the baby's heartbeat and your contractions are monitored. If the second stage is drawing out, and you become tired from pushing, an assisted delivery may be suggested with forceps or vacuum (see pp.436–437).

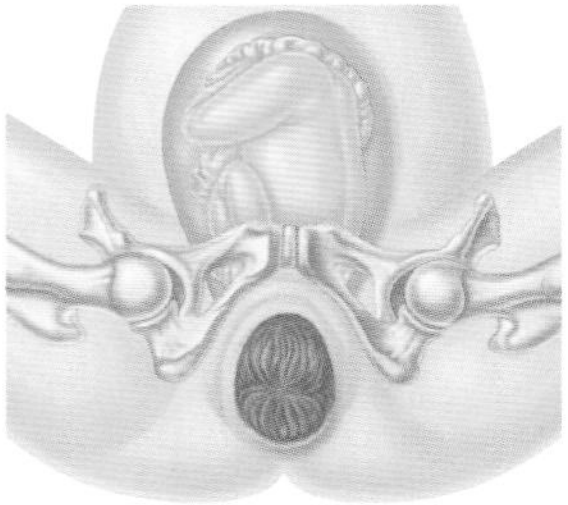

The crowning of the head means that the delivery of your baby is imminent and within one or two contractions the head will emerge.

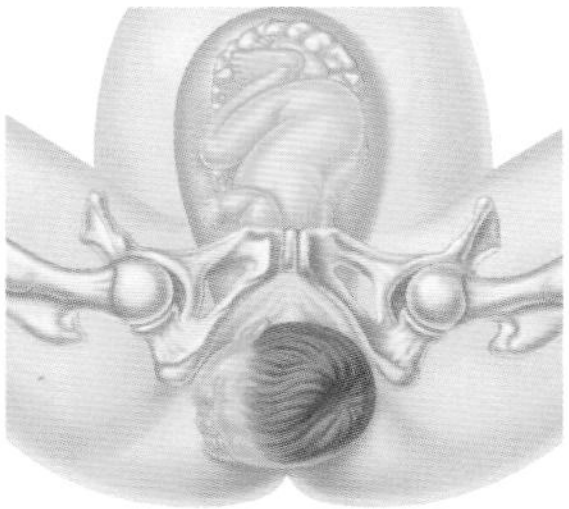

Your baby's neck will extend backward as the head is delivered and your baby will turn to one side to aid the delivery of the first shoulder.

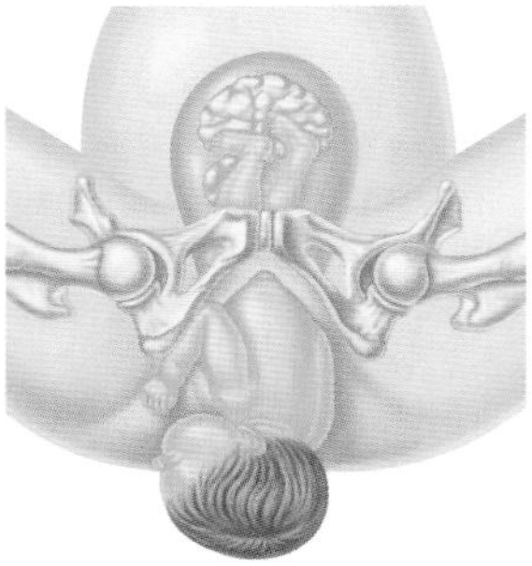

Once both shoulders are safely delivered, the rest of your baby's body will slip out fairly quickly.

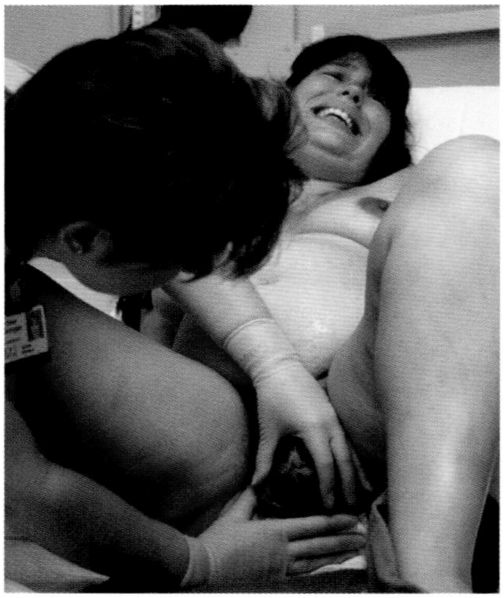

As the head crowns, the doctor will check that the cord isn't around the baby's neck, and may then apply gentle traction to the sides of the head to help deliver the shoulders.

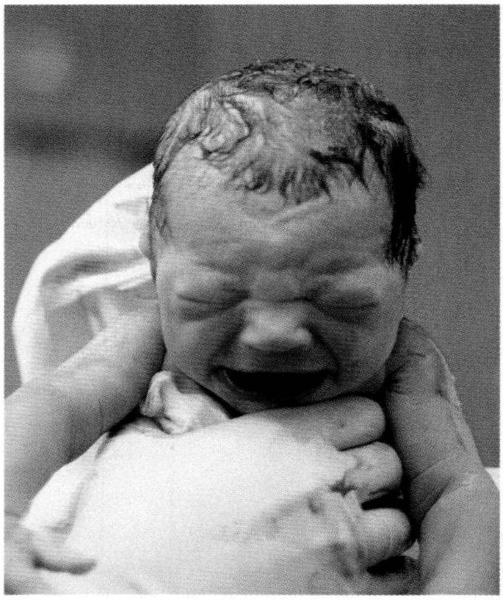

Your baby will emerge covered in blood and the thick, greasy substance known as vernix that provided a protective covering for your baby's skin in the uterus.

SHOULDER DYSTOCIA

This is an emergency situation that occurs when the baby's head has been successfully delivered, but the shoulders appear to be stuck. Since the head may be delivered fairly easily, the problem is often not discovered until this point in labor, and immediate action is then needed to deliver the rest of the body safely. The nurse will call for extra help. You will be asked to stop pushing and to draw your knees close to your chest to allow more room in the pelvis. An episiotomy may be needed to allow the obstetrician to perform internal maneuvers to help release your baby's shoulders. Shoulder dystocia is more likely to occur where the baby is particularly large, where the mother has a small pelvis, or in women with diabetes or who are obese. If you have had a shoulder dystocia in a previous pregnancy, there is an increased risk that you will have another shoulder dystocia. You may be offered a Cesarean section to prevent this from recurring.

Episiotomies

An episiotomy is a cut made between your vagina and anus to aid the delivery. Around 30 years ago, episiotomies were routine since it was assumed that a cut prevented worse tears. This has been shown since not to be the case, and today, an episiotomy is only done by a doctor to aid a forceps delivery or in an emergency—or example, if the baby is in distress. Before doing the procedure, the doctor should explain why they think it is necessary and should obtain your verbal consent.

Before you're cut, you'll have a local anesthetic to numb the area. The cut is usually done at an angle between the vagina and the rectum and will be stitched after the birth. The midwife or doctor will put together all the layers of the episiotomy, including the muscles, posterior vaginal wall, and skin. If you feel discomfort, the stitches can be snipped or removed You may be given oral analgesics for pain relief after you've been stitched, and anti-inflammatory medication may be recommended. Ice packs or a maternity cooling gel pad can ease pain and swelling, and bathing can be soothing.

Perineal tears

Some women tear naturally during the delivery of their baby and this tends to be more common in a first labor. Spontaneous tears are classified by their severity and the tissue layers involved. A first-degree tear involves the skin layer only; a second-degree tear involves the skin and muscle-tissue layers; a third-degree tear involves skin, muscle, and the anal sphincter; a fourth-degree tear involves the anal sphincter and the rectum. A first-degree tear usually doesn't need stitches, but second-, third-, and fourth-degree tears do. Second-degree tears are the most common; only a small number of women sustain third- or fourth-degree tears.

BIRTH STORY: WATER BIRTH

Becky is a 22-year-old woman in her first pregnancy. She'd had no problems and at her 36 week appointment, she discussed her birth plan and told her doctor that she wanted a water birth at the local birth center.

Becky's birth story: By the time I was two days overdue I was having irregular contractions. I'd had a bloody show and had a backache. The next day I woke at 6:30 am with regular contractions. I coped using breathing techniques, stayed active, and used a birthing ball. When my contractions were every 5 minutes and lasting a minute, I called the birth center since I felt I needed to use the pool. They said they would get it ready.

At 11:35 am, my partner and I reached the center and met the doctor. She felt my contractions, listened to the baby's heartbeat and did a vaginal examination. She said I was in established labor since I was 5 cm dilated, my cervix was 50 percent effaced, and the head was descending. In the pool, I was able to move around and change position. The warm water eased my backache and contractions. I felt calmer and started to relax. I found kneeling in the water and rocking my pelvis back and forth and from side to side helpful. My partner supported me and periodically the doctor listened to my baby's heart rate.

At 3:20 pm, my contractions were every one to two minutes and very strong. The doctor and my partner reassured me and I managed to focus. I began to feel the urge to bear down. At 3:50 pm, my baby's head was born and a couple of minutes later I pushed my baby out into the water. The doctor gently lifted my baby up to me and we stayed in the water a few moments. I got out to deliver the placenta, which I did without drugs. At 4:20 pm my placenta was delivered and I didn't need stitches.

The doctor's comments: Becky found the warm water helped her deal with contractions, and she stayed calm. She tried different positions and the water kept her buoyant. She and her partner were focused. Her labor progressed well and was just under 10 hours. It was wonderful to observe.

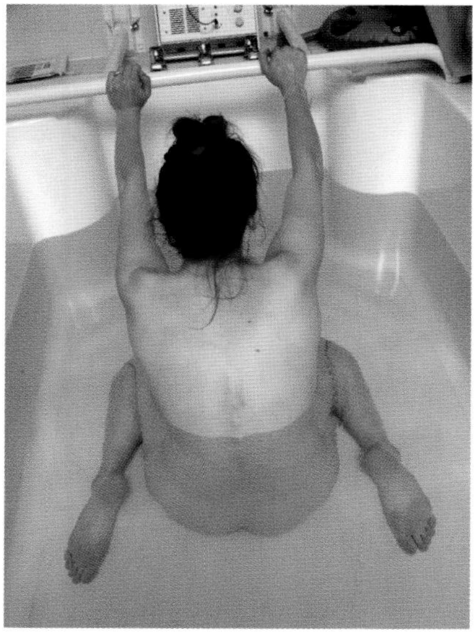

Kneeling in warm water helped ease the pain of Becky's contractions.

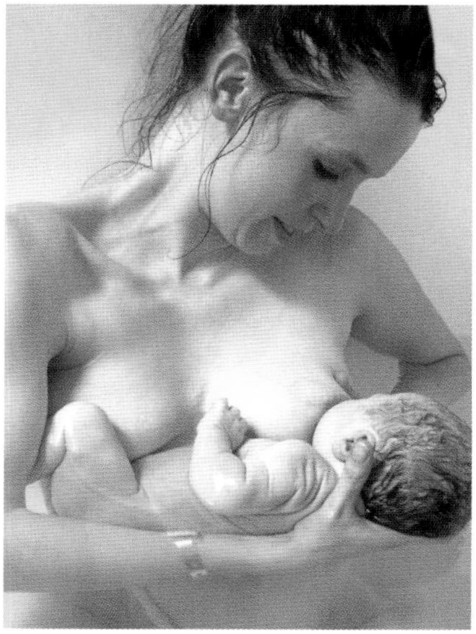

After the birth the doctor lifted the baby to Becky's breast so she could breast-feed.

After your baby is born

Shortly after your baby's birth, the cord will be cut and your uterus will start to contract again to deliver the placenta.

The third stage

This is from the birth of your baby until the delivery of the membranes (the amniotic sac that surrounded your baby) and placenta. The placenta can be actively managed with the help of drugs or delivered without drugs, known as passive management or a physiological third stage. Your doctor will discuss these options with you before labor.

Cutting the cord Once your baby has been delivered, it may be left for two to three minutes before it is cut. Allowing the cord to pulsate for a few minutes means your baby receives more blood from the placenta, which boosts his or her oxygen supply and blood volume. The cord will be clamped in two places, about 1 cm and 4 cm from the baby's belly, and is cut with scissors between the clamps.

Delivery of the placenta How your placenta is delivered depends on your doctor. Many wait for it to happen naturally, but others offer an intramuscular (IM) injection of an oxytocin in your thigh to make the uterus contract so that you can deliver the placenta and membranes quickly. Helping the uterus contract in this way reduces the risk of heavy bleeding occurring during the third stage, known as a postpartum hemorrhage (see box, right) and speeds up the delivery of the placenta, which can happen within 5 to 15 minutes after the birth of the baby. The risk of a postpartum hemorrhage occurring is the reason many units advise an active delivery. Active management of the third stage can prevent you from having excessive bleeding.

Your doctor will place one of her hands just above your pubic bone to prevent the uterus from being pulled downward when she pulls on the

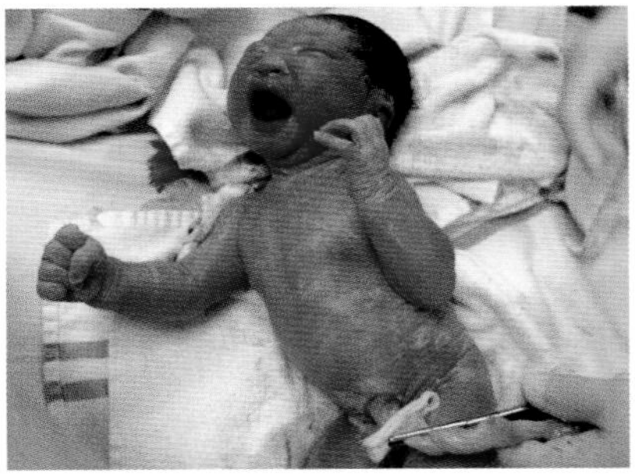

The umbilical cord will be clamped and cut a few minutes after the birth, severing the link between your baby and the placenta.

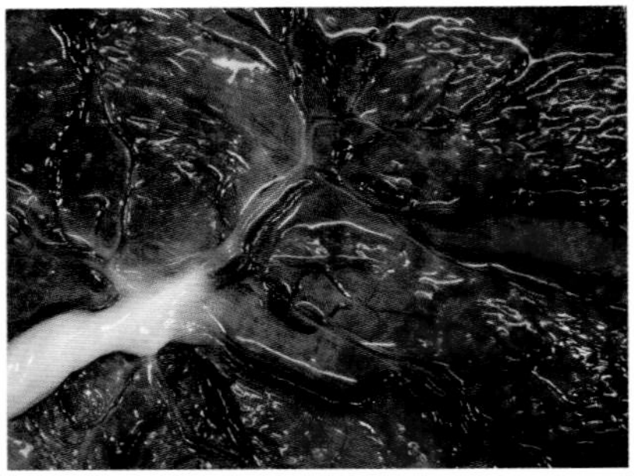

The disc-shaped placenta, weighing around 1 lb 2 oz (500 g), has a network of blood vessels surrounding the umbilical cord in its center.

APGAR SCORE

At 1, 5, and 10 minutes, your baby's breathing, pulse, movements, skin color, and responses are assessed. In darker-skinned babies, the color of the mouth, palms of the hands, and soles of the feet are checked. Each is given a score between 0 and 2, called the Apgar score. A total of 7 or more at 1 minute is normal; under 7 means help is needed.

Apgar score	2	1	0
Skin color	Pink all over	Body pink; extremities blue	Pale/blue all over
Breathing	Regular strong cry	Irregular, weak cry	Absent
Pulse/heart rate	Greater than 100 bpm	Less than 100 bpm	Absent
Movements/muscle tone	Active	Moderate activity	Limp
Reflexes after given certain stimuli	Crying or grimacing strongly	Moderate reaction or grimace	No response

POSTPARTUM HEMORRHAGE

A postpartum hemorrhage (PPH) is the loss of more than 33 oz (1,000 ml) of blood after delivery of the baby. It can also be due to a retained placenta, when the placenta remains in the uterus for more than 30 minutes after delivery..

Risk factors include uterine fibroids, a previous delivery with PPH, multifetal gestation, a large baby, prolonged labor, or use of pitocin. If you have increased risk factors, then active management of the third stage is recommended. Improvements in the treatment of a PPH, with medications and new medical devices, have considerably reduced the complications.

cord. With her other hand, she will then apply gentle traction to the cord to help deliver the membranes and placenta. This is known as "controlled cord traction" (CCT).

Delivering the placenta naturally If you decide to deliver the placenta without drugs, known as a physiological third stage, this can take up to an hour. Your doctor will encourage you to bear down and you may find squatting helps. The doctor will check the placenta to ensure it's complete and that none of it remains in the uterus, which can cause a postpartum hemorrhage (see box, above).

How you feel after the birth

After the huge effort of giving birth, it's common to have a physical reaction. Many women experience uncontrollable shaking or shivering, and some feel nauseated and may even vomit. You are also likely to feel overwhelmed and emotional. Once you and your baby have been given the all clear, you should be given some quiet time alone together.

YOUR BABY'S APPEARANCE

Newborn babies are usually surprisingly unattractive. Fortunately, as parents, we think they are beautiful. Newborns are covered in a waxy substance called vernix, together with amniotic fluid and blood from the birth canal. Babies who have passed meconium before the delivery may also have brown stained skin and nails.

In addition, newborn babies often have a molded, elongated head, with a swollen area on top known as a "caput," which is due to the pressure on the baby's head as it passes through the birth canal. Also, the nose may be squished to one side and the eyes may be swollen. Sometimes the genitals are swollen too. Rest assured that all of these features are temporary and within 24 hours or so the molding will work itself out and your baby will begin to look more like the baby you were expecting to meet.

No matter the race or ethnicity, all babies are born with purplish-red color skin. As the baby starts to breathe air, the blood vessels open up and gradually the skin color changes. This can take a day or two as the blood flow is prioritized to flow to the essential organs. Gradually the reddish-purple color fades. The blood vessels can be seen through the very thin newborn skin and the skin color is often pink. It is normal for the hands and feet to stay blue for several hours.

Healthy newborns have a range of skin tones in the first few days. The eventual color of the skin can take up to six months to develop and is determined by the rate of production of melanin.

Many babies are born with birthmarks, referred to as "stork bites." These are red birthmarks on the eyelids and at the nape of the neck, which fade in time.

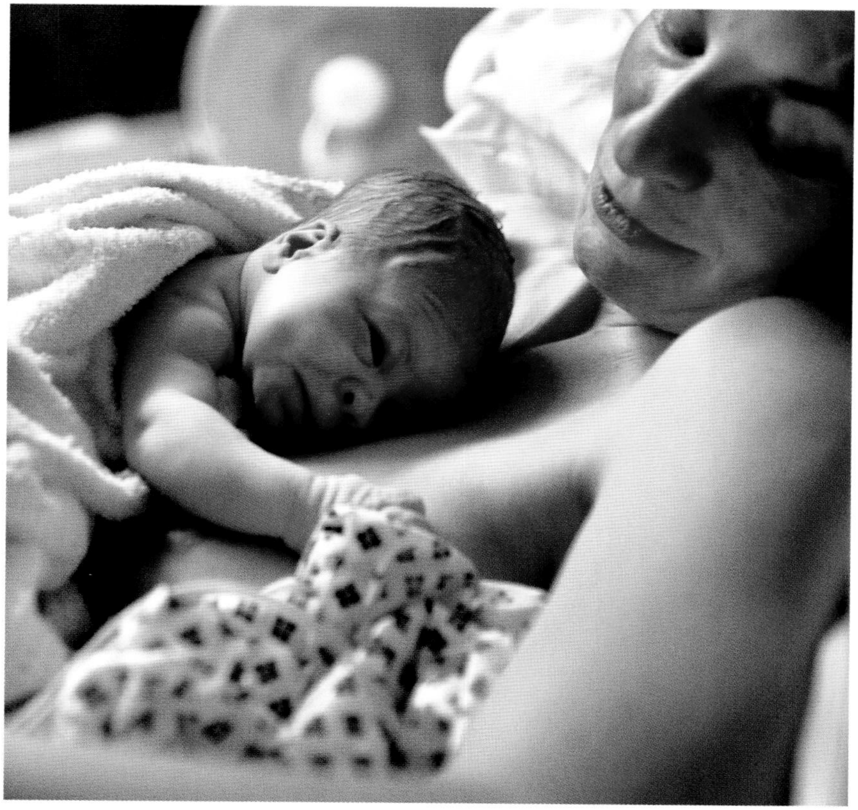

Special cases

EACH LABOR IS DIFFERENT AND THERE ARE TIMES WHEN SOME TYPE OF INTERVENTION IS NEEDED. You may know in advance that a condition or factor in your pregnancy means that intervention, such as an induction or a cesarean section, will be needed. At other times, events can occur in labor that mean assistance is needed, or a premature labor can mean that your baby needs special care. In all cases, rest assured that procedures are in place to ensure your own and your baby's safety.

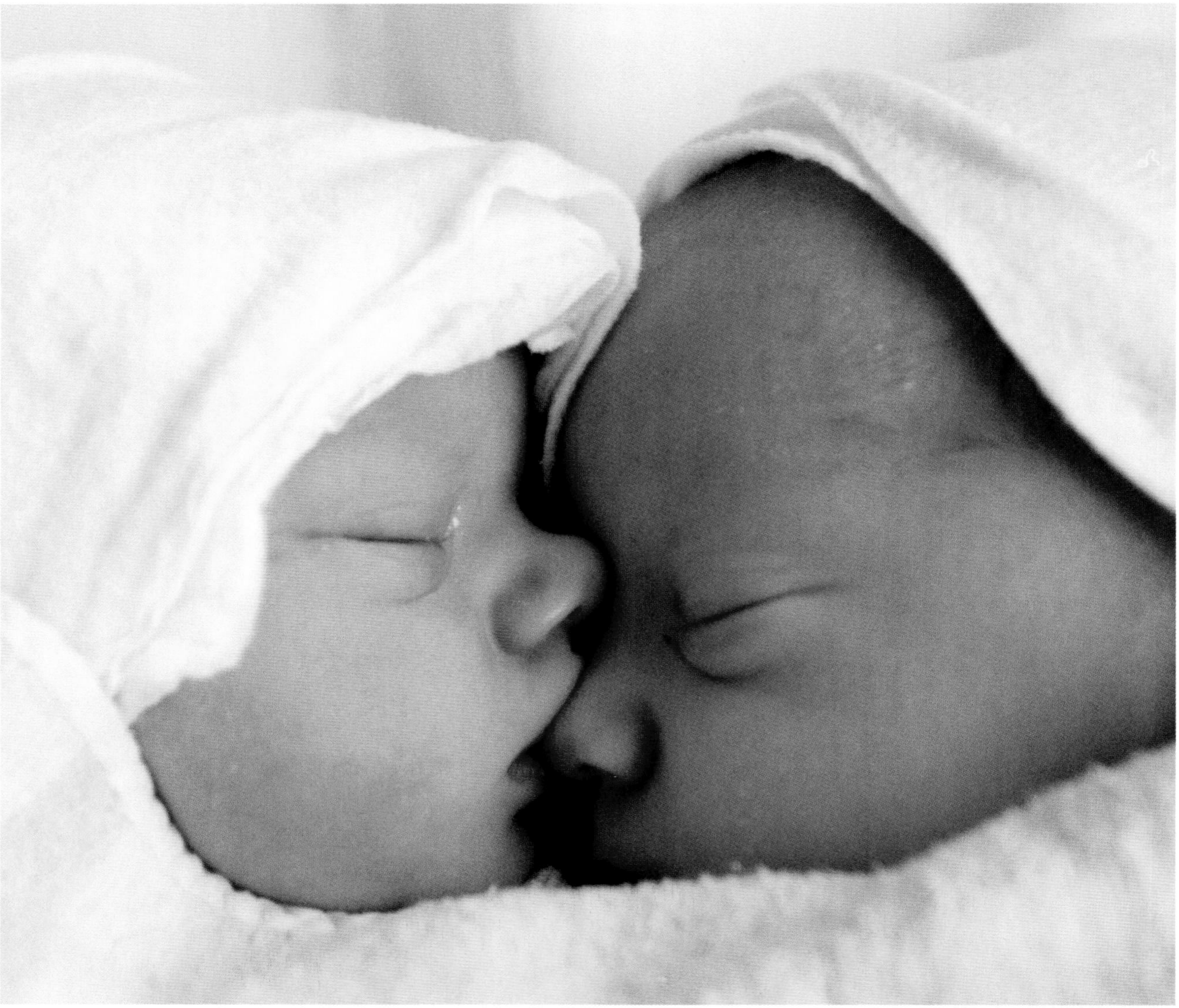

Premature birth

"Premature" describes both the time of birth, before 37 weeks, and how well prepared your baby is for life outside of the womb. In the US, approximate 10 percent of births occur preterm.

Your baby may be born prematurely either because an early delivery is advised on medical grounds (see below), or you go into spontaneous preterm labor. The earlier the birth, the higher the chance of complications in the baby, such as breathing problems or infections. Nowadays, however, huge advances in the care of premature babies means that babies born as early as 23 or 24 weeks may survive. If your baby is premature, they may need to spend time in a neonatal intensive care unit (NICU, see p.454).

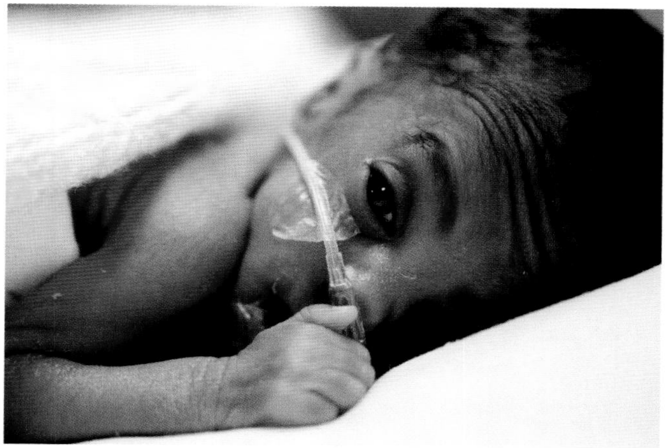

Seeing your tiny baby hooked up to monitors and tubes can be alarming, but take comfort from the fact that these are helping your baby to breathe and feed and in turn to develop.

Advising an early delivery

An early delivery may be recommended if the mother's or baby's health is in danger, for example, if the mother has a medical problem, such as a heart condition that could increase her physical stress, or preeclampsia (see p.476), which could endanger her own and her baby's health. An early delivery may also be advised if a scan shows that the placenta is not functioning well and the baby is not receiving enough oxygen. Forty-seven percent of babies in the US delivered before 32 weeks are born by Cesarean, as are about a third of babies born between 34 and 36 weeks.

Spontaneous preterm labor

The cause of spontaneous labor before 37 weeks is often unknown. However, it is more likely if a woman has a major abnormality of the uterine wall, such as large fibroids (see p.218); a weakness in the cervix, which may have been present from birth or have occurred after surgery to the cervix; or is pregnant with multiples. Infections like bacterial vaginosis can also set off contractions at an early stage.

What might be done? Preterm labor can't be stopped, but medication can slow the process and reduce some risks.

A course of steroid injections, given about 24 hours apart, is one of the most important treatments to reduce the risks associated with preterm delivery for your baby. The maximal benefit of steroid use is 2–7 days after the initial dose, so it will only be recommended if you are at risk of preterm delivery within 7 days.

You may be given an injection to reduce the frequency of contractions. This can prolong pregnancy for a few days, during which time the steroids can take effect. Also, if necessary, you can be transferred to a hospital with NICU facilities.

You may be advised to have injected antibiotics since preterm babies are susceptible to bacterial infections caught via the cervix during birth.

PREDICTING PREMATURE LABOR

It's hard to predict who will go into labor prematurely. However, if you've had a previous preterm birth, tests may be done to find out if it is likely in your current pregnancy. A cervical scan may be done around 23 weeks since a shorter cervix increases the risk of early labor. Pelvic swabs detect bacteria that are linked to preterm labor, and a "fetal fibronectin" shows whether a protein is present that, during the second half of pregnancy, generally can't be detected until 1–3 weeks before labor and delivery. Sometimes, a short cervix is strengthened with a stitch. Antibiotics can be given if needed. Progesterone can be given to reduce the risk of the baby being born prematurely.

Induction of labor

For 22.3 percent of women in the US, labor is started by artificial means, or induced, to reduce the risks to mother and baby.

An induction may be offered if it's felt that continuing the pregnancy poses a risk to your health or to the health of your baby. The most common reason for an induction is the continuation of a pregnancy beyond 41 or 42 weeks, in which case the placenta may begin to fail. Induction may be offered earlier if you are having twins, or have a medical condition such as diabetes. Before setting a date for induction, your doctor may offer to strip your membranes (see p.393) to help you go into spontaneous labor.

Induction is not the same as an augmentation of labor, which is when drugs are used to increase the efficiency of your contractions when you've already gone into labor spontaneously (see p.415).

Assessing the cervix

Before an induction, you'll have an internal examination to assess the cervix. Induction is easier if your cervix is short and soft, described as "favorable" or "ripe," rather than long and firm. The findings may be logged in a table called the Bishop's Score, which also assesses how far the cervix is dilated (see p.415), the position of the cervix, and the station of the fetal head in the pelvis (see p.414). A total score over six indicates good conditions for an induction of labor.

Softening the cervix

If the cervix isn't ripe, it can be softened with prostaglandins. These are naturally occurring chemicals that help stimulate contractions. Artificial prostaglandins can be given in the form of vaginal tablets of gel, which are placed at the top of the vagina near the cervix, or a vaginal suppository or an oral pill, This is usually effective, but sometimes prostaglandins fail to soften the cervix and may be tried again after a few days. On the other hand, some women experience dramatic effects after a small dose.

Breaking the water

Artificial rupture of the membranes (ARM) is one of the most important steps in the induction process, often referred to as "breaking the water." It's done once the cervix is soft and slightly dilated, and the head has started to enter the pelvis. A thin plastic probe is passed through your cervix and used to make a small hole in the amniotic membranes, which allows some of the fluid around your baby to leak out. This softens the cervix even more and can provoke contractions in the wall of the uterus. If contractions don't become established after ARM, then you'll require treatment with oxytocin (see below).

Oxytocin

Oxytocin is a natural hormone that stimulates the uterus, increasing the frequency and strength of contractions. A synthetic form, Syntocinon or Pitocin, is used with the same effect. It's diluted then put in an IV in your arm or injected into a large muscle. This is safe and effective when used correctly; however, it must be used with care since excessive contractions can reduce your baby's oxygen supply in labor. Your contractions and your baby's heartbeat will be continuously monitored (see p.418) throughout an induction of labor.

QUESTIONS AND ANSWERS

Are medical interventions more likely with an induction? If your labor is induced, the chance that you will need an assisted delivery with forceps or vacuum (see pp.436–7) or a cesarean is increased. This is even more likely if you are having your first baby, if the cervix is unfavorable, or if you're being induced relatively early in your pregnancy. The reason for these medical interventions is usually that the labor is proceeding too slowly, or that it cannot be started at all, despite all of the steps taken. Also, concerns about the baby's well-being during the induction process can sometimes lead to intervention.

Is induction of labor more painful than a spontaneous labor? Some women find that they experience strong contractions very quickly after an induction. Since they haven't been able to build up gradually to more painful contractions, they may be less able to tolerate the pain, which can result in an increased need for stronger types of pain relief such as an epidural.

Breech baby

At 32 weeks, 15 percent of babies are breech (bottom first). With time, most turn, with just 3 percent remaining breech at term.

Breech labors and births are usually more difficult, so if your baby is still in a breech position in late pregnancy, you may be offered a procedure to turn your baby (see below).

Turning your baby

The procedure to turn your baby, cephalic version (ECV), is usually offered at around 37 weeks. Using ultrasound for guidance, the doctor presses on the lower part of your belly to elevate your baby's bottom out of the pelvis. Pressure is used to rotate your baby until they head down. The procedure may feel uncomfortable, and you may be given medication to relax the uterus. A scan is often done before and after the procedure.

The success rate for ECV is 40-60 percent and complications are rare. If an ECV is unsuccessful and you want to try for a vaginal birth, your doctor will discuss the risks of, which are higher than if a Cesarean delivery is planned.

Breech diagnosed in labor

It can be hard to distinguish between a baby's head and bottom by feeling the tummy, so occasionally a breech baby isn't discovered until labor. If a breech is diagnosed in labor, you can still have an ECV, but at this stage it has a lower success rate. An ECV may not be possible in labor if the water has broken, in advanced labour, or if there's no one to do the procedure.

Delivery of your baby

If you try for a vaginal birth, you should be in a hospital with an ob-gyn present, since you may need an assisted delivery or an emergency Cesarean. Fetal monitoring should be done throughout labor, since babies in distress will need to be delivered by Cesarean. Sometimes a breech baby has problems getting oxygen and blood through the umbilical cord, if it's squeezed into the wrong position.

You'll be advised to have your baby's heartbeat monitored throughout, and you may have an IV in case you need a Cesarean. You may be asked to lie on your back with your feet in stirrups so that the doctor can access the baby. An alternative position is to stand or be on all fours. Your bladder may be emptied with a catheter and an episiotomy cut may be done to prevent a more serious tear (see p.427). The doctor may apply gentle pressure to the baby's arms or legs during birth, but you're unlikely to notice this. Except for these differences, the birth is likely to feel the same as the birth of a head-first baby. During the birth, the head will be eased out of the birth canal either by hand or with forceps to control the speed of the birth. An emergency Cesarean is likely if any complications arise.

POSITIONS OF A BREECH BABY

A breech baby can lie in one of three positions, known as extended (frank); flexed (complete); or footling. With an extended breech, the hips are flexed, knees extended, and the feet are by the head. A vaginal delivery is most likely with this type of breech. With a flexed breech, the hips and knees are flexed, with the feet above the buttocks, and a vaginal birth may be possible. In a footling breech, the hips are extended with the feet below the buttocks, so a vaginal delivery is unlikely.

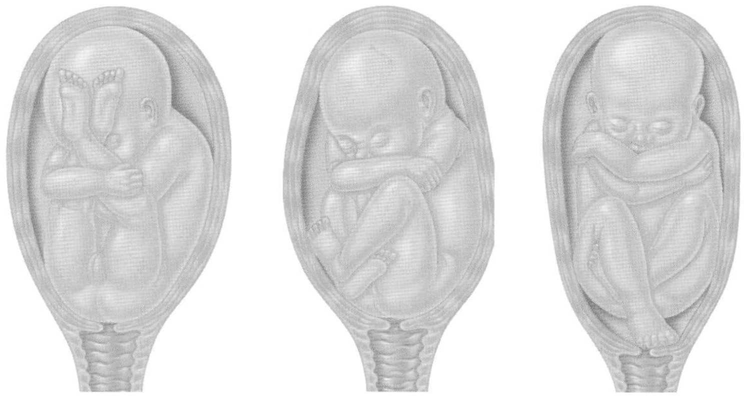

Extended (frank) breech | **Flexed (complete) breech** | **Footling breech**

Multiple births

Carrying twins or more increases the risk of complications during birth, and you and your babies will be closely monitored.

Twin pregnancies occur naturally in around 1 in 53 women, but some factors increase the chance of you conceiving twins or more, including the use of some fertility treatments, becoming pregnant when you're older, already having children, and having a family history of twins.

Monitoring during pregnancy

Because multiple pregnancies are high risk, you'll receive extra monitoring; the type of delivery depends on the position of your twins and other complications. A concern is whether twins will be born prematurely with a small birth weight, which can mean spending time in a neonatal intensive care unit (see p.454).

Toward the end of pregnancy, you may have extra scans to monitor the babies' growth, since the ability of the placenta to provide oxygen can be reduced in a twin pregnancy. The volume of the fluid around each baby and their heart rates may be measured to check their well-being.

Possible complications

Twin-to-twin transfusion syndrome (TTTS) is a condition unique to identical twins who share a placenta (see p.59). It occurs if there is a direct link in the blood supply between the babies and can put the lives of both at risk. Babies with TTTS need specialized treatment that may involve reducing the fluid around one baby or using a laser to separate the circulations.

Rarely, twins can develop in the same sac, known as monoamniotic twins. This is an extremely high risk situation in which the umbilical cords can became tangled, affecting the oxygen supply. Monoamniotic twins are typically monitored in the hospital starting at 24 weeks and are usually delivered early by Cesarean section.

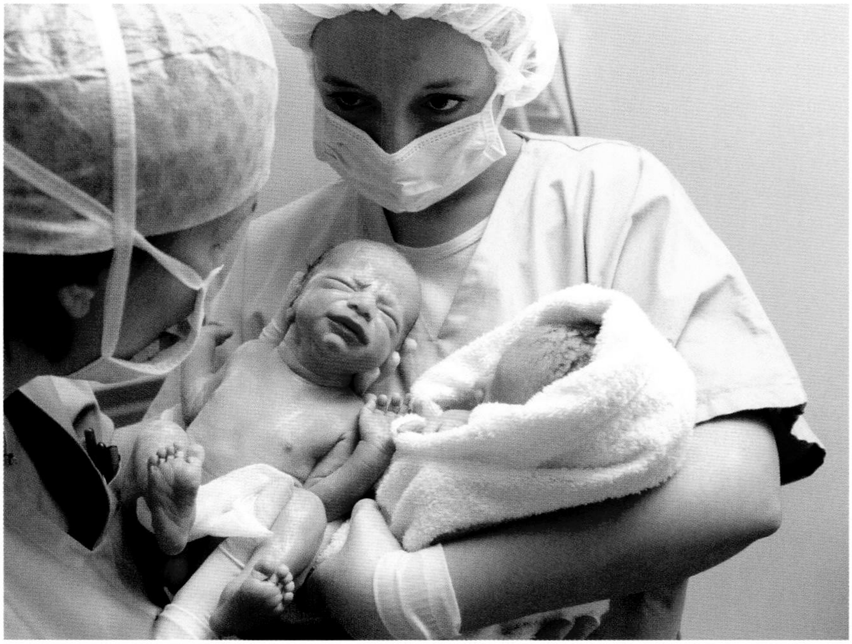

With a twin delivery a larger medical team will be on hand to deal with any complications and to take care of both babies at birth.

Maternal complications There is a higher risk of complications, such as preeclampsia (see p.476), possibly because of the additional strain on the kidneys; the liver condition cholestasis (see p.475), for reasons that are unclear; and thrombosis, because there is an additional strain on your circulation. These conditions may also mean that an early cesarean is recommended.

Going into labor

You're more likely to go into labor early and your babies may be lighter than average. With twins, you're likely to go into labor around 37 weeks; triplets around 34 weeks; quadruplets around 32 weeks. The average birthweight for twins is 5.5 lb (2.5 kg); triplets and quadruplets are almost always low-birthweight.

Labor and birth

Current recommendations are that an obstetrician should attend a twin birth. If you're planning to have a vaginal birth, the labor should be almost as quick as it is with one baby. Continuous monitoring of both heartbeats is recommended during a multiple labor. This is usually done by putting one strap around your belly for each baby, but sometimes the second baby is monitored in this way and the first baby may have a scalp electrode put on his head (see p.419), which gives a clearer picture of the first baby's heartbeat if it has been difficult to find.

Delivering the first twin For your first baby, the chance of using forceps or vacuum is the same as for a singleton birth, although the birth of the first twin may need to be assisted so that the doctor can gain quick access to the second twin. After the first twin's delivery, the cord is clamped and cut, but the placenta usually remains in the uterus until the second baby has been born.

Delivering the second twin The medical team will confirm how the second baby is positioned. As the second baby's head or bottom enters the pelvis, the second sac of water may be broken to encourage strong contractions. A normal birth should follow in about 30 minutes, and forceps or vacuum are used only if problems arise. If the second twin is bottom-first, a doctor should be on hand to help. It's unusual for the first twin to be born vaginally and the second to be born by a cesarean, but this may happen if the second baby needs an urgent delivery and a vaginal birth seems unsafe.

Delivering the placenta There is a greater risk of postpartum hemorrhage with twins, which means that an active management of the third stage may be advised (see p.428).

QUESTIONS AND ANSWERS

Will I have a say in how I deliver my twins?
If you are having twins, you will get the chance to discuss your plans for giving birth with your obstetrician during the pregnancy. Your decision to have a vaginal birth or a cesarean section will probably be based on several factors, such as the position of the babies. Once you have been given enough time to consider all of the relevant information, safety is the most important factor.

Can I have a home birth with twins?
Home births in the US are very rare, and organizations like the American College of Obstetricians and Gynecologists and the American Medical Association recommend against them because of the potential for complications, even in low-risk singleton pregnancies. For the safety of your babies, a hospital birth is recommended.

BIRTH STORY: A TWIN BIRTH

Gillian found out she was having twins at an early scan. At first she was worried that the pregnancy and birth would be hard, but her confidence grew as she saw her babies growing well. She went into labor at 35 weeks.

Gillian's story: I was shocked when they told me I was carrying twins, since none of my family has had twins. The pregnancy was tough because I was so tired and I had such a big belly. I enjoyed having the scans though because they were really reassuring.

I went into labor at just over 35 weeks. After initial contractions, my water broke at 2 am. My husband got me to the hospital in 15 minutes; I think he was in a bit of a panic. Jonathan, our first twin,was born just after 4 pm, so the first part of my labor was quite long. I managed without much pain relief medication. Celia came 20 minutes later. They broke my second sac of water since her heartbeat was low, but she was fine at birth. I remember the birthing room being crowded, and even though people introduced themselves to me, I couldn't have told you who they were. However, they all disappeared soon after the birth and left us to spend some time alone with our babies. That was the best time. All the worries disappeared and we could just get on with being a mom and a dad.

The doctor's comments: Like many women with a twin pregnancy, Gillian was worried about what might happen to her and her babies during labor. She had talked at length to me and the doctor during her pregnancy, but still felt anxious. When she arrived on the labor ward, however, she could see that the people caring for her were highly professional and experienced. This gave her the confidence to deal with events as they unfolded. Both babies were doing very well when they left the hospital and Gillian was making an excellent recovery too.

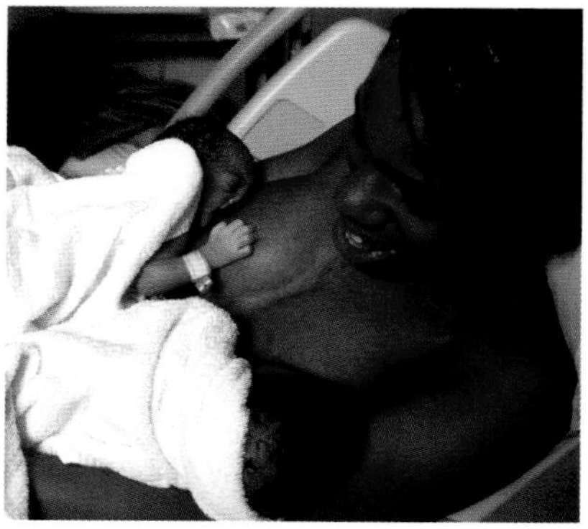

Assisted birth

In the US, 4.8 percent of babies have an assisted birth. This is considered safe and can prevent further complications.

An assisted birth is a birth in which either forceps or a vacuum suction cup (also called a vacuum or ventouse extractor) are used to aid a vaginal delivery. There may be some mild side effects such as bruising after an assisted birth, but major complications are rare.

As with all medical interventions, the use of forceps or a vacuum extractor will only be offered when it is thought to be necessary for the health of the baby and/or mother.

The procedure

First, your doctor will discuss with you the need for the procedure and may also explain to you the potential complications. You may be asked to sign a consent form, although not all hospitals insist on this. Before the birth takes place, you will probably be given an episiotomy and local anesthetics or epidural anesthesia. Fresh covers may be placed over your legs and abdomen and a catheter will be inserted to empty your bladder. The doctor will then place the forceps around the baby's head or attach the vacuum cup and will encourage you to start pushing again when you have a contraction. Your baby should be born within around another 20 minutes from this time. There is less of a risk for a vaginal injury with a vacuum extraction than there is with forceps.

Forceps

Modern surgical forceps were invented by the British doctor Chamberlen in the seventeenth century and so have been in use for hundreds of years, although they have been modified over time. Forceps are an effective and reliable way to assist a delivery, but they have to be used with care by a properly trained doctor.

The forceps are placed so that they hold the sides of the baby's head near the ears and cheeks. The operator of the forceps then gently pulls the baby's head downward while you push during a contraction, and then will guide the baby out of the birth canal.

Forceps can also be used to adjust the baby's head before the birth if the baby is lying in an occiput posterior position, which is with his back facing the mother's back (see p.417), toward the end of labor. After turning the baby's head and body, delivery is then completed in the same way as described above.

Pros and cons of forceps There are several advantages of forceps over vacuum. First, they do not rely on any kind of machinery that could cause a problem during the birth. They work well even if your contractions are weak or if you are too exhausted to push. They have a low failure rate: if the doctor can get the forceps around your baby's head easily, he will usually be able to complete the vaginal birth of your baby without having to resort to a cesarean. The disadvantage of forceps is that you may be more

METHODS OF ASSISTING BIRTH

Assisting your baby's birth with vacuum or forceps is a safe, well practiced procedure, which can prevent the need for an emergency cesarean. Whether you have forceps or vacuum may depend on the expertise and experience of the doctor carrying out the procedure.

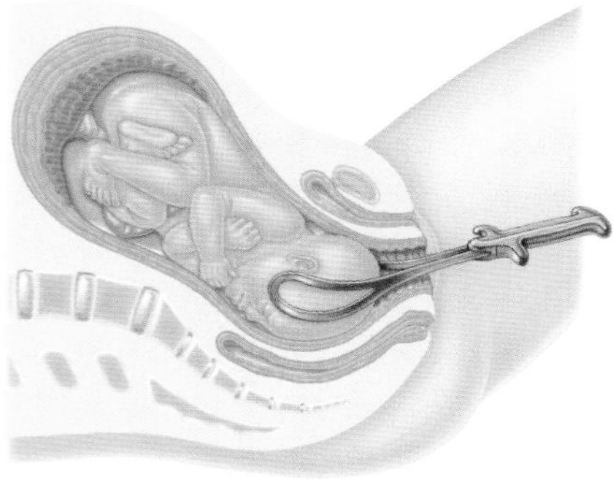

With forceps, your baby's head is cradled on either side with metal tongs that guide him down in time with your contractions.

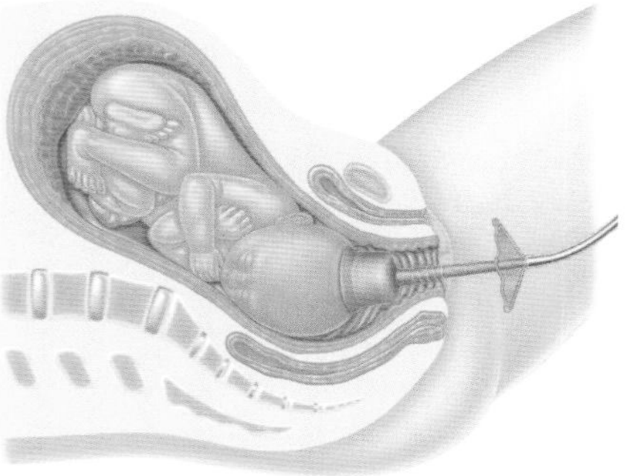

With vacuum, a soft suction cup is attached to your baby's head and then your baby is gently guided out.

likely to have vaginal or perineal damage than with vacuum.

Vacuum extractor

The vacuum, or vacuum extractor, was invented in the 1950s. It consists of a cup attached to a tube that connects to a suction pump. The cup, which can be hard or soft plastic or metal, is placed on top of the baby's head and held in place while the suction creates a vacuum that makes the cup adhere to the baby's scalp. The doctor pulls downward while you push during a contraction.

Vacuum births are known to be very safe as long as you are at least 34 weeks pregnant. Before this time your baby's head may be too fragile to deal with the suction and few doctors use a vacuum before 32 weeks.

Pros and cons of vacuum This has some advantages over forceps; it is often a little easier to apply and may be less uncomfortable; it's less likely to cause vaginal and perineal damage and you'll be less likely to need an episiotomy (see right). There is a small risk of bruising of the scalp, but serious complications are rare; if your baby needs to be delivered, these small risks must be balanced against the risk of not delivering your baby.

Vacuum fails in up to 20 percent of cases, and it's especially likely to fail if the baby isn't in an ideal position or has a lot of hair or caput. If a vacuum comes off during the birth, it can be reapplied, or the doctor can reach for a pair of forceps instead. Sometimes, however, a cesarean has to be performed if the vacuum fails.

Pain relief

It can be painful having an assisted vaginal birth, so it is important that you have sufficient pain relief to help you cope with the delivery. In some situations, an injection of a local anesthetic in and around the vagina is sufficient to help you deal with the pain, particularly if the doctor is anticipating the birth to be fairly quick, and if your baby has already traveled most of the way through your pelvis. For more difficult assisted births, for example if the baby is not in an occiput anterior position (see p.417), an epidural may be given (see p.404). This is especially useful if you're going to give birth in the operating room instead of the delivery room because forceps or vacuum have a high chance of failing, leading to the need for a cesarean. Finally, if you already have an epidural in place, this can be topped off with additional medication if needed.

POSSIBLE COMPLICATIONS

In the majority of cases, both the mother and baby are perfectly well after an assisted birth, but occasionally complications are encountered.

Problems during the delivery A condition known as shoulder dystocia, in which the baby's shoulders become stuck during the birth, is more common with a forceps or vacuum delivery. If the shoulders get stuck, simple maneuvers usually release them without great difficulty, but very rarely, a shoulder dystocia can turn into an emergency, and a doctor has to be called to complete the baby's birth

How your baby may be affected Forceps can leave a temporary bruise on the side of your baby's face and can even put pressure on a nerve near the eyes, stopping the baby from being able to blink properly for a day or two. In contrast, the vacuum tends to leave a bruise on the top of the head rather than on the face (and the head may appear elongated at first where the suction pressure was applied). This can look a little alarming, but it will disappear after a couple of days. More severe complications for your baby, which can include a fractured skull bone after a forceps delivery, or bleeding inside the skull after a vacuum, are very rare.

How you may be affected You're more likely to be given an episiotomy cut, particularly during a forceps delivery, to protect your back passage from more severe damage during the birth. This is usually successful, but in some cases a third or, rarely, a fourth-degree tear may occur in the back passage and careful stitching is required to repair the area. Stitches may also be used if you get other tears in or around the vagina.

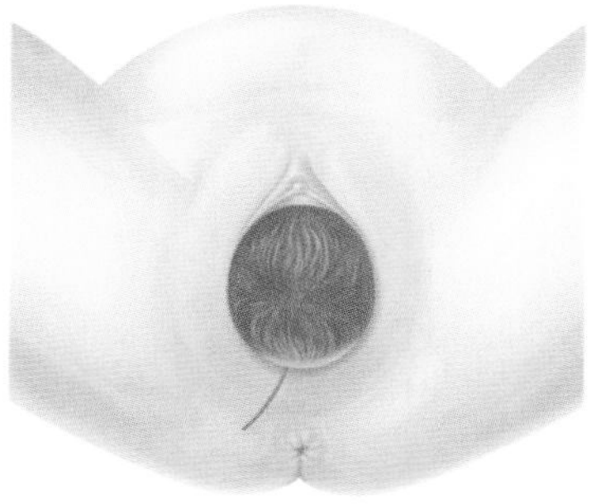

A medio-lateral cut is usually done into the muscle, angled away from the vagina and the perineum.

Cesarean section

A Cesarean section is an operation performed by an obstetrician to deliver a baby. The procedure is considered major abdominal surgery and involves the use of anesthesia.

A Cesarean section is the delivery of your baby through an incision in your abdomen. A Cesarean rate of around 10–15 percent is strived for, although in most Western countries the rate has risen beyond 20 percent, and around 30 percent of all babies in the US are now delivered by Cesarean—an all-time high.

An increase in Cesareans

There are several reasons for the rise in the number of Cesarean births. Women are choosing to have their babies when they are older and are therefore having fewer babies. This makes them more risk-averse, so if there is any likelihood of there being complications, they might opt for a Cesarean. There has been an increase in the number of pregnant women who have a high BMI (see p.16) and this is associated with an increased chance of Cesarean birth. Women who have had a previous Cesarean may choose to have another, as might those who had a previous traumatic delivery. A woman who has had one or two previous Cesarean should be offered a trial of labor, known as Vaginal Birth After Cesarean (VBAC; see box, opposite), but may choose to have a planned Cesarean. This decision will be influenced by her previous birth history and whether she is prepared to accept the risks associated with laboring after a previous Cesarean section. A woman who has had three or more Cesareans is recommended to have a repeat Cesarean because there is an increased risk in labor to the mother and baby.

A small but increasing number of women do not wish to labor and therefore opt to have a Cesarean. Your obstetrician will discuss with you the risks and benefits of having a Cesarean delivery so that you can make an informed decision.

At full term, 2 percent of babies are lying in the breech position and it is generally thought to be safer for a breech baby to be born by Cesarean section. A Cesarean is also safer for other conditions, such as a placenta previa (see p.212) or fibroids.

Emergency and urgent Cesareans

A woman might need a Cesarean section for many reasons, and there are differing degrees of urgency. An emergency Cesarean is carried out when there is an immediate threat to the baby's or mother's life. An urgent Cesarean is when there is concern for the baby's or mother's well-being, but no immediate threat to life. A scheduled Cesarean is when there is no immediate concern for the mother or the baby, but an early delivery is advised, perhaps because of a condition in the mother or baby. An elective Cesarean is scheduled by the patient's preference, after 39 weeks (see right).

An emergency Cesarean is most commonly carried out when the baby is thought to be at risk—for example, if the baby's oxygen supply has been reduced and there are signs of fetal distress. In this case, the staff will try to do the Cesarean rapidly—within 30 minutes, when possible—although it's important that no shortcuts are taken that could put the mother's own health at unnecessary risk.

Urgent Cesareans take place when there's no immediate threat to life, and these are more common than emergency Cesareans. An urgent Cesarean may be done if the baby's heart rate is causing concern very early in labor and the prospect of a vaginal delivery taking place within a reasonably short time is low. An example of a scheduled Cesarean is one that is done because of a failed induction of labor.

A scheduled Cesarean

Around one-third of Cesareans are scheduled, and the number of these has increased greatly in recent years. Reasons for a scheduled Cesarean include a breech baby; a tear involving the back passage, or another traumatic event during a previous vaginal delivery; a previous Cesarean; a larger than average baby; and maternal choice. In these situations, although a Cesarean is reasonable, an attempt at a vaginal birth is also reasonable with the right precautions.

In some situations, it would be hazardous for you or your baby if you were to try for a vaginal birth—for example, if you've had multiple previous Cesareans or other major surgery to the uterus; the baby can't be moved from lying horizontally; the placenta is lying very low (see p.212); or there are severe pelvic abnormalities in the birth canal. Some maternal medical conditions also mean that vaginal birth is not advisable.

An elective Cesarean

Sometimes there may not be a medical reason that your obstetrician recommends a Cesarean for you. It is unusual for maternal request to be the only reason for a Cesarean, but it is also a valid choice if you have strong feelings against having a vaginal delivery. In this situation, your obstetrician may discuss your concerns over several prenatal visits, to make sure that you are certain an elective Cesarean is the right choice for you. Or you may start the labor process intending to have a vaginal birth and realize partway through that your gut instinct is telling you something different—take time to listen to your maternal instincts and discuss them with your obstetrician.

Timing of a Cesarean section

Most labor units will schedule Cesarean sections at set times during the weekdays to allow for adequate staffing and to maintain safety of all patients. Usually, a scheduled Cesarean is performed at, or just after, 39 weeks to reduce the risk of the baby developing breathing problems that may happen without the normal process of labor. In the uterus, the baby's lungs are full of fluid, and at birth, when the first breath is taken, all the fluid is absorbed into the bloodstream and the baby's lungs fill with air. The process of labor seems to help with this transition.

When a baby is born by scheduled Cesarean, there is no opportunity for them to prepare for the birth. At birth, the baby will take a first breath but a small amount of fluid may be left in the lungs making gas exchange more difficult. The baby must work harder to breathe and may make a grunting sound. This condition, known as transient tachypnoea of the newborn, is self-limiting. Often the baby only needs extra oxygen but, very occasionally, may need help with breathing. The earlier the baby is born, the higher the chance of them having breathing problems. However, after 39 weeks, the risk is very small.

VBAC

VBAC stands for Vaginal Birth After Cesarean. About 70 percent of women who go into labor having had a previous Cesarean will have a vaginal birth. And if they have also had a previous vaginal birth, the chance is increased to 90 percent. There is a very small risk, up to 1 percent, that during labor the previous Cesarean scar will open, known as uterine dehiscence, or uterine rupture. This is an emergency, requiring immediate delivery of the baby (within 15 minutes) as once the uterus has ruptured, the blood supply to the placenta usually stops and the baby becomes short of oxygen. To prevent this from causing a brain injury, the obstetrician must deliver the baby very quickly. For this reason, it is recommended that women who are having a VBAC give birth in a hospital equipped to handle these types of emergencies and have continuous electronic fetal monitoring. The risk of uterine rupture increases twofold if the woman needs to be induced or labor augmented with pitocin.

It can be difficult to choose how to give birth and it is important that you are given the information and the time to decide what is right for you and your baby. Think about what the likelihood is of having an emergency Cesarean. If it is high, you might want to consider having a one that is scheduled. Factors that could affect the likelihood are the reason for your previous Cesarean, whether you have had a previous vaginal birth, how you feel about giving birth, and whether you have had any problems in this pregnancy that may mean it is safer to give birth by Cesarean. On the plus side, if you have a VBAC, your stay in hospital will be shorter, your recovery will be quicker, and if you are planning several babies, you reduce the risk of repeat Cesarean sections.

Your doctor will discuss the risks and benefits of trying to VBAC during your routine prenatal appointments so you have time to consider the best option.

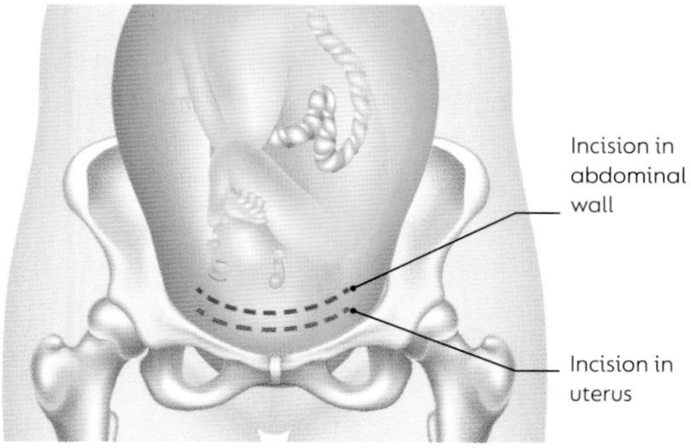
Incision in abdominal wall
Incision in uterus

With a low transverse incision, as shown in this artwork, the chance of the Cesarean scar rupturing during a VBAC delivery is very rare. If the scar does open during labor, once that is recognized, an emergency Cesarean is needed, which is why it is important for VBAC deliveries to be closely monitored in an obstetric setting.

If you go into labor before your scheduled Cesarean, contact your prenatal provider so you can be assessed immediately. If you are in active labor and do not want to do a VBAC, your doctor will get you ready for a Cesaresan urgently (see p.438).

Giving your consent

The doctor will need your consent prior to doing a Cesarean. They should explain why the procedure is being recommended and what its benefits and risks are. Ideally, you should have plenty of time to decide whether you want the surgery, although with an emergency Cesarean, the time to think things over may be limited. Even so, you are always within your rights to say no to a Cesarean, even if this means that your life or that of your baby is at risk.

Your anesthetic

Before the surgery, you will meet an anesthesiologist, who will make sure that you are comfortable during your surgery and will help you with pain control afterward. Most women are awake during a Cesarean.

An injection of medication into the spinal fluid in your back, called a spinal block, numbs any sensation of sharp pain (see p.406). Or, if you've been using an epidural for pain relief in labor (see p.404), this can be used for the surgery. If the surgery is likely to be difficult or prolonged, the anesthesiologist may recommend a combined spinal epidural. This has the advantages of a spinal anesthetic and can also be topped up via the epidural catheter if the spinal starts to wear off during the Cesarean. After your anesthetic has been given, the anesthesiologist will check that it is working properly.

Being awake usually means that your birthing partner can stay with you and it's also a little safer for you and for your baby than a general anesthetic. Very occasionally, a general anesthetic is needed (see p.407).

The surgery

Before the surgery, an IV line will be put in your hand or your arm so that fluids or medication can be given intravenously, if necessary. Also, the pubic hair on your belly may be shaved downward by about 1.8in (3cm) to clear the way for the cut. Both may be done before you go to the operation room or after you arrive there.

Once the anesthesiologist is assured that you are comfortable, a catheter will be inserted into your bladder and will stay in until the next day while your sensation recovers. Your abdomen will be cleaned with an antiseptic solution and sterile drapes will be placed over you, which prevent you and your partner from seeing the surgery.

During the surgery, a 4 in (10 cm) long cut will be made, usually horizontally on the lower abdominal wall, across the bikini line, although occasionally an up-and-down cut below the belly button is needed. Your bladder will be pushed down and the front of the uterus opened so that the doctor can access the baby. If your water hasn't already broken, this will be done now before the baby and placenta are delivered. The surgeon will release the baby's head from the pelvic brim and lift the baby out. Sometimes, another member of the team needs to put pressure on the uterus to assist this. You may feel a lot of pressure when this happens. You'll be able to see your baby when the cord has been cut, and once initial checkups have been done on your baby, either you or your partner should be able to hold them while the surgery is completed. After the umbilical cord is cut and your baby is taken away from the surgical field, your doctor will remove the placenta.

Many hospitals now provide the option for a gentle Cesarean, or family-centered Cesarean. This means that the anesthesiologist will help to lower the surgical drape, or some hospitals may have clear drapes, so that you can see your baby as they are delivered from your uterus.

If your baby's condition is stable, cord clamping will be delayed by 30–60 seconds. The cord is then clamped and cut with some length so that your partner can participate in cutting the cord later. The baby

COMPLICATIONS

There are several common, but minor, problems associated with Cesareans. These include bleeding during the surgery, or a day or so later; the need for a blood transfusion; or getting a minor infection in the bladder or in the abdominal incision. Getting a major infection is far less common, and having to have a major second surgery because of a life-threatening incision infection is rare. The chance of a blood clot forming in the pelvic veins is higher if you don't receive medication to thin the blood after your Cesarean. If you are generally well and you are given this medication, the chance of a life-threatening blood clot on your lungs is extremely small.

Since sharp implements are used during the surgery, there is a risk that your bladder, or even your baby, could be cut during the surgery. Your bowels are less likely to be damaged , and your other internal organs are highly unlikely to be injured.

is then taken to the warmer to be dried since newborns can lose a lot of heat very quickly. Your birthing partner will be invited to come to the warmer and cut the umbilical cord again. Your baby will also have a quick assessment to make sure they are transitioning well and can be brought directly to you for skin-to-skin contact while your Cesarean is finishing. Sometimes during a Cesarean, you may develop nausea or feel uncomfortable holding your baby yet. If that is the case, your partner may hold the baby instead.

To finish the Cesarean, the uterus will be closed up with one or two layers of sutures, then the abdominal wall will be stitched in separate layers. This takes about half an hour, although it can take longer, especially if you've had previous surgeries. You may have dissolvable stitches, or stitches that have to be taken out after four or five days; less commonly, small staples may be used. The surgeon usually makes this decision, but if you have preference, make this known to the team caring for you before the surgery starts.

Your recovery

Your nurses will encourage you to get out of bed that same day, and your obstetrician may recommend removing the urinary catheter after a few hours. This will allow you to feel more comfortable and decrease your risk of developing a bladder infection. After your Cesarean, you can eat and drink as you wish, although you may find you don't necessarily have the appetite you anticipated. The day after your surgery, your obstetrician will remove your bandage, if one was placed, to inspect the incision. As you move about more, you may find it easier to do so by using an abdominal binder. By the day after your Cesarean, you should be well enough to do most things for yourself, with help. Women usually go home on the second or third day after the Cesarean with NSAIDs and acetaminophen for pain relief.

Your next pregnancy

If you need to have a Cesarean section, your next pregnancy will be considered high risk. Although rare, you will be at increased risk in subsequent pregnancies for placenta accreta spectrum, which is a range of changes in the development of the placenta that can lead to it growing abnormally into the uterine wall, or even outside of the uterus. The risk of this happening increases with the number of previous Cesareans. This is why most obstetricians do not recommend having more than three or four Cesareans. Pregnancies with placenta accreta spectrum are likely to require a hysterectomy at the time of Cesarean delivery.

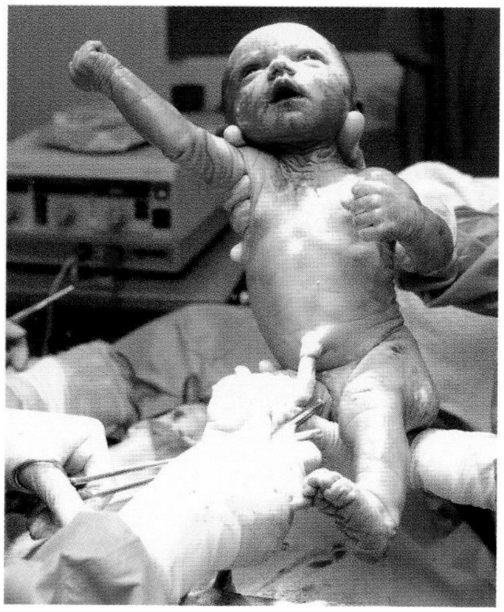

Your baby is gently lifted out of the uterus and the cord is clamped and cut.

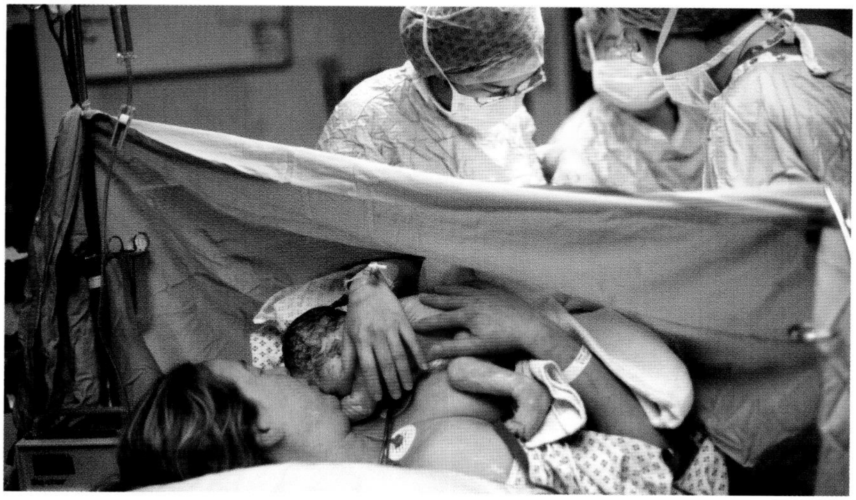

You or your partner can enjoy the first hold of your baby while the surgical team completes the operation by delivering the placenta and stitching the incision.

LIFE WITH YOUR **NEW BABY**

You've spent the last nine months anticipating this moment, but nothing can quite prepare you for how you'll feel when you meet your baby. In the coming weeks, as you recover from the birth, your world will change beyond your wildest imagination. Your emotions will run wild and cycle from one to the next, often in a very short time. Most importantly, you'll be getting to know your tiny baby and marveling at this new addition to your family.

The first 12 hours

The moment you've been dreaming of for nine months has finally arrived and now you're holding your baby in your arms! So what happens next?

Your experience of the first 12 hours will depend on your labor and birth and local procedures, but here is an account of what usually occurs.

The first hour after the birth As long as they are well, your baby can be put in your arms and you can make the most of these first magical moments. The doctor or your partner will cut the umbilical cord after a few minutes, or once it stops pulsating. You may feel elated, relieved, or just exhausted. Don't be alarmed if you start to vomit, shake vigorously, or feel too exhausted even to hold your baby. These are all very normal postbirth sensations.

If your baby is fine and you want to breastfeed, put them to the breast, but they may just nuzzle at first. Snuggle them close, skin to skin—the warmth of your body is all they need right now.

At 1, 5, and 10 minutes, your baby will be observed and given an Apgar score (see p.428). They will be wiped with a soft towel, their fingers and toes checked, and their weight and head circumference measured. They will also have a hearing test in the first hours.

Shortly after your baby is born, you will deliver the placenta, naturally or with medication (see p.428). Medication to contract the uterus after the birth will shorten the third stage and has been shown to reduce the risk of postpartum hemorrhage.

If your perineum tore, or you had an episiotomy (a cut to ease your baby out), you may need stitches. You'll be given a local anesthetic, unless you already have an epidural, so you don't feel a thing. Your partner can hold your baby and sit close by while you are stitched.

It is recommended that newborn babies have a vitamin K injection, to prevent them from developing serious problems with bleeding. Stores of vitamin K, which is needed for blood clotting, are often low in newborns, and vitamin K deficiency bleeding is a serious cause of bleeding in newborns and up to 6 months of age. Newborns who do not receive a vitamin K shot are 81 times more likely to develop severe bleeding.

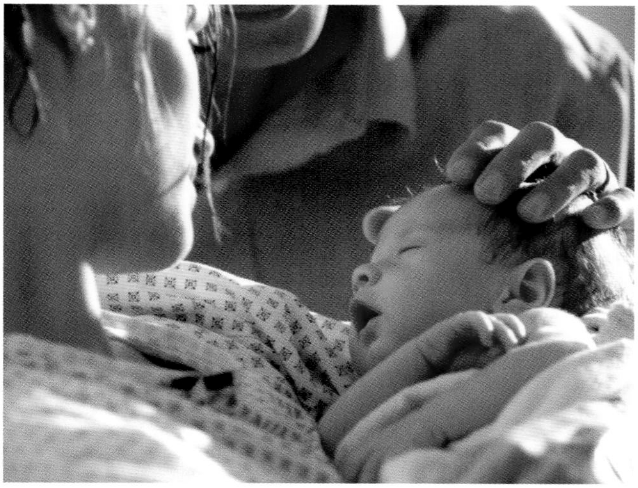

Nothing compares with the moment when you meet your baby face to face.

2–3 hours Time to refuel: many women say their first drink of water and snack after giving birth are the best they've ever tasted... enjoy.

If you're feeling fine and there are no concerns about your condition, you'll likely be moved to the maternity ward, where you'll spend the remainder of your time in the hospital. You'll be taken there in a wheelchair with your baby in your arms. (In some hospitals, you'll never leave the room where you deliver; some labor and delivery rooms act as postpartum rooms, as well.)

3–4 hours You'll be sweaty, sticky, and want a shower, which you can have if you didn't have an epidural. Ask a nurse or your partner to walk with you if you're feeling wobbly.

5–6 hours The first time you urinate it can sting, especially if you had stitches, so pour a cup of warm water over your perineum as you urinate. The hospital needs to know everything is in good working order before you leave its care. You'll need to use sanitary pads to soak up the vaginal blood loss (lochia).

7 hours This might be the first chance you've had to look at your baby's tiny toes, scrunched-up legs, or fine head of hair. There may be traces of greasy

THE FIRST MEDICAL CHECKUP

In the first 12 hours a pediatrician will give your baby a checkup. In addition to a head-to-toe examination, there will be checks made on skin color, temperature, and muscle tone, and on reflexes, such as sucking and grasping.

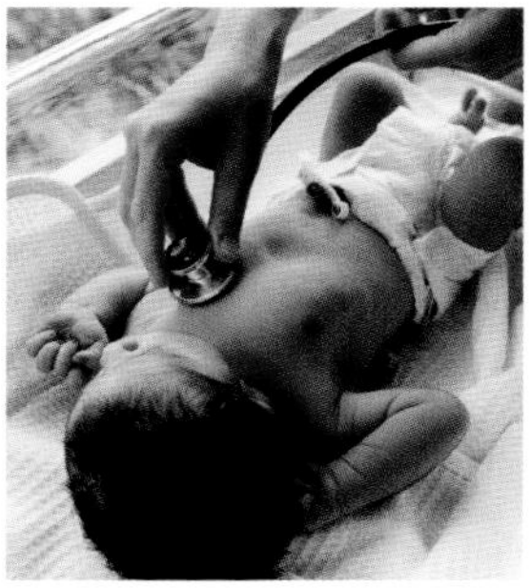

Heart and lungs are checked to ensure they sound normal.

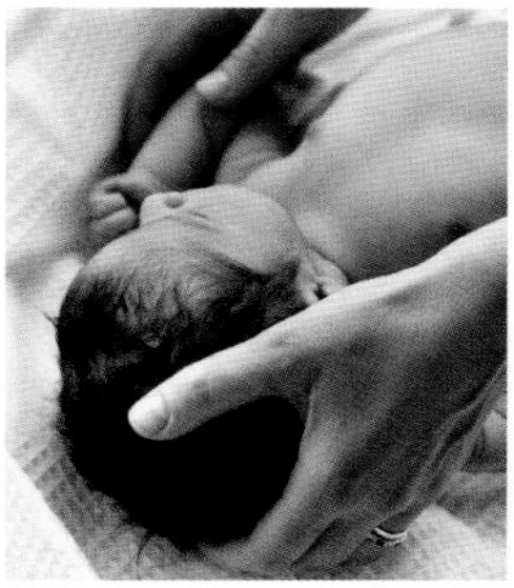

Head shape and fontanelles (soft areas between the skull bones) are examined.

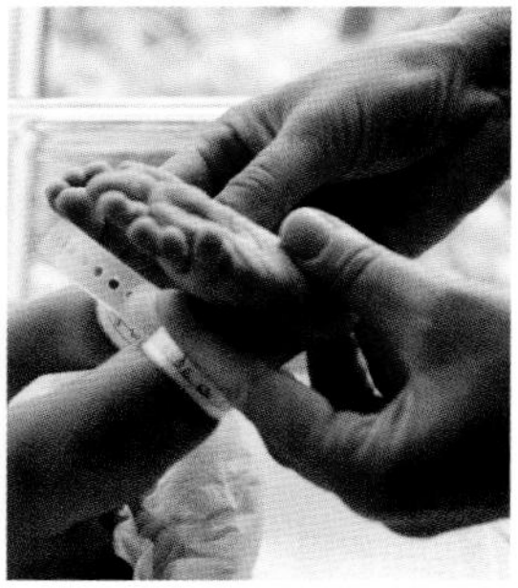

Hands and feet are checked for reflexes, and fingers and toes are counted.

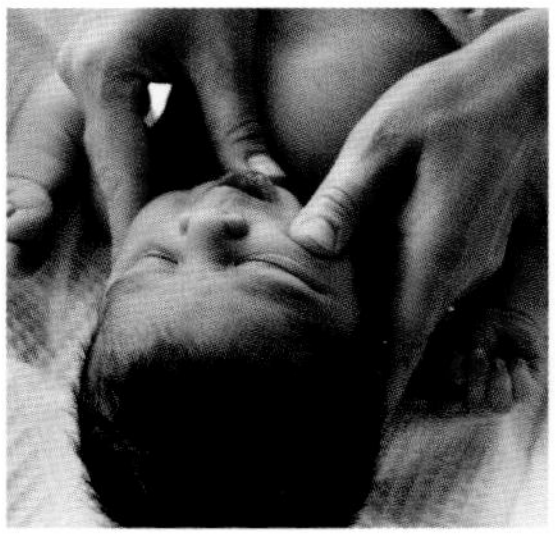

Mouth and palate—the separate sections should have fused together.

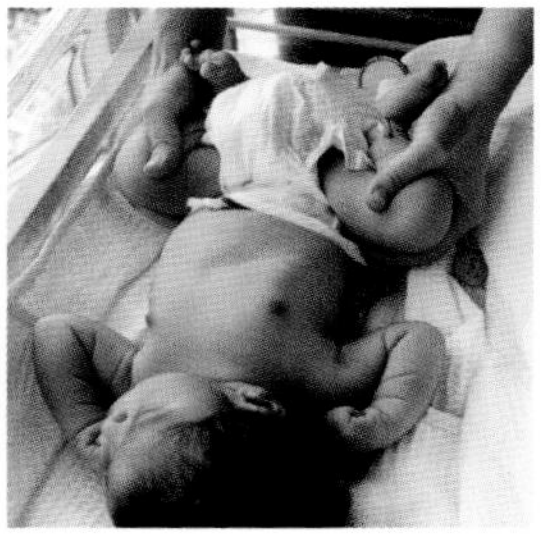

Hips are rotated and the legs are bent upward to check for signs of dislocation.

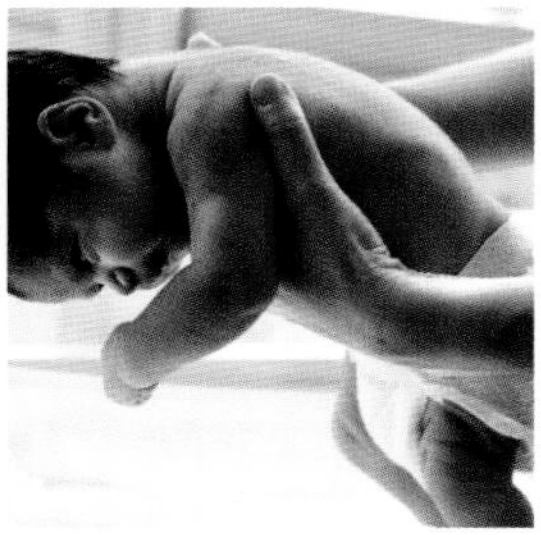

Spine is checked to ensure it is straight and free from abnormalities.

RECOVERY AFTER A CESAREAN

Although you've had major surgery, you'll be encouraged to get up to get your circulation going. After an epidural, this will be as soon as you've regained the feeling in your legs. After a general anesthetic, you'll be encouraged to get up when you no longer feel sleepy, usually within an hour. You won't be able to shower yet, but your nurse or midwife can give you a bed bath to help you freshen up.

You'll probably feel very tired and sore, so ask for help with positioning your baby at the breast, and take pain medication when you need it.

vernix on their skin. Perhaps they have long, flaky fingernails that need trimming or a downy fuzz of hair called lanugo on their back.

8 hours If your baby is awake, they may be hungry. At this stage, you're producing nutrient-rich colostrum, a fluid containing antibodies. Position them at the breast: they should open their mouth wide and take the entire areola, known as "latching on" (see p.450). Breastfeeding stimulates the release of the hormone oxytocin, which contracts the uterus. This can cause afterpains, more in second and subsequent births, which can feel like contractions. A consolation is that with each contraction, your uterus—and hence your abdomen—shrinks down.

9 hours If you're up to it, you may be ready for visitors to admire your baby. Don't let them tire you out, though.

10 hours Your baby's newborn checkups will take place when they're between 4 and 48 hours old. A staff pediatrician will examine them from head to toe; listen to their heart, check their hips (and testes in a boy); and ask about the contents of their diapers.

11 hours In many hospitals, you can spend your first night as a new family together, since rooming-in with the baby is a common practice and new partners often sleep over. This lets the nurses see how mother and baby interact. If you need to get a few hours of uninterrupted sleep, a nurse can take the baby to the nursery.

12 hours After a whirlwind of agony, ecstasy, and sheer hard labor, you need to rest when you can. If your baby is sleeping, fend off visitors, draw the curtains around your bed, or take the phone off the hook, and sleep.

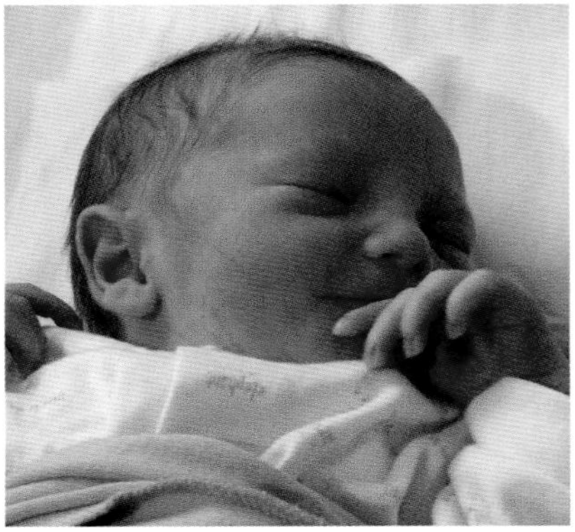

1ST WEEK: **DAY 1**

Getting acquainted

YOUR BABY TODAY

In the first 24 hours, your baby should pass urine and meconium, the first black, sticky feces, that are made up of waste products and bile. You'll be changing plenty of diapers, and in no time you'll be a diapering pro.

"Finally, your baby is in your arms! As you recuperate, you'll get to know the baby you've waited to meet."

You may feel love at first sight, when you first hold your baby after the birth, but for many women, bonding takes place over the next few days or weeks. For both parents, skin-to-skin contact with your baby helps the bonding process and is particularly beneficial for premature babies (see p.454).

Try not to be anxious when you pick up your baby. In the first few weeks, your baby has little head control, so support them with a hand under their head and shoulders, or both hands under their arms and with your fingers supporting their head.

The nurses in the maternity ward are there for help and support. You'll be asked if you've urinated and will be offered help with breastfeeding if needed. A lactation consultant will likely also be on hand to guide you through the initial difficulties you may encounter. If your hospital offers "rooming in," you'll get to spend most of the day with your baby present, except when the nurses take them for routine testing or the staff pediatricians exam them. You'll also be visited by the doctor every day that you're in the hospital so they can check on your progress.

SAFE SLEEPING

Crib death is a concern for all new parents. Follow these guidelines to minimize risks:

- **Put your baby on their back** to sleep.
- **Don't let your baby get too hot.** If it's chilly, add layers and cover their feet, but don't go overboard. In the summer, they may be comfortable sleeping in just a onesie—but make sure the fan or air-conditioning vent isn't directly overhead.
- **Don't let anyone smoke** around your baby.
- **Never sleep with** your baby on a sofa or armchair.
- **The safest place** for your baby to sleep is in a crib or co-sleeper near where you sleep. If you bring the baby into your bed to breastfeed, put them back in their crib or co-sleeper when done.
- **Keep all soft objects,** like pillows, toys, blankets, and loose bedding, out of the baby's crib. A firm mattress covered by a fitted sheet is best.

YOUR BABY'S REFLEXES

Newborn babies have reflexes that form part of their survival skills. In addition to the rooting and grasping reflexes shown here, babies also have a startle reflex, whereby they will fling out their arms if unsupported, and a stepping reflex, which means they will step their feet up and down if held upright on a surface.

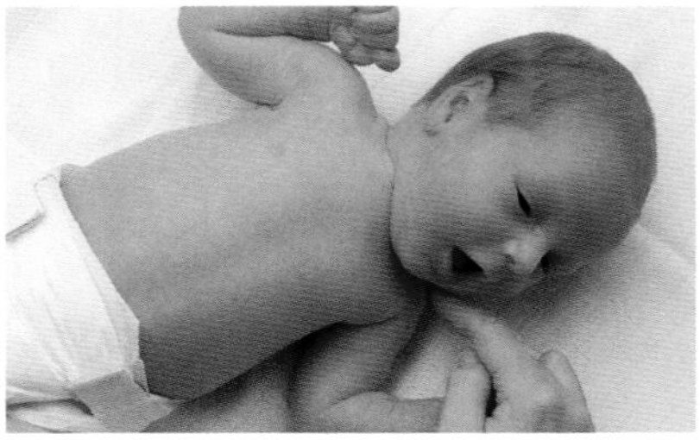

Rooting reflex: If you touch or stroke your baby's cheek, they will turn toward that side with their mouth open in search of food.

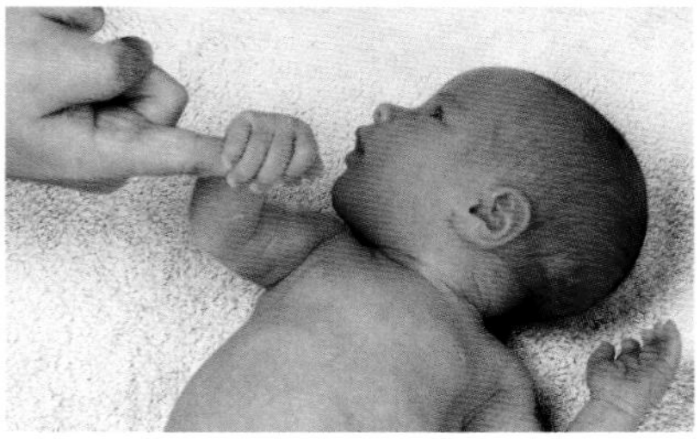

Grasping reflex: If you place your finger in the palm of your baby's hand, they will instinctively tightly grip your finger.

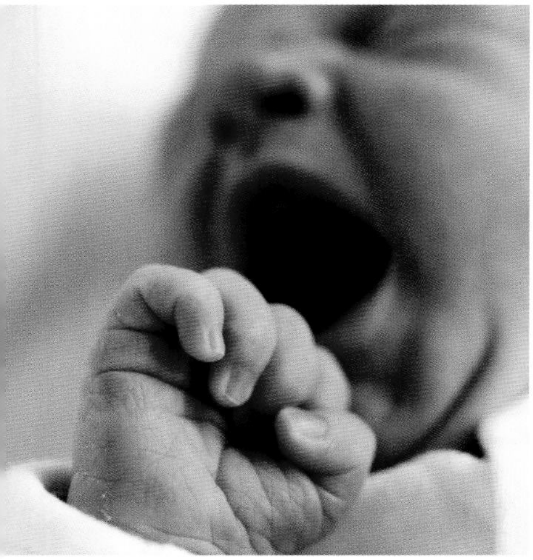

1ST WEEK: **DAY 2**

Settling in

YOUR BABY TODAY

Newborn babies sleep around 16 hours a day, although some sleep for most of the first few days while others seem awake and fretful. If your baby is very sleepy, you may need to wake them for feedings, which should be at least every four hours.

Your ob-gyn will visit in the hospital today. They will ask how you are managing and check that you have emergency contact numbers. You may be asked to watch short films or read brochures about the risks of Shaken Baby Syndrome and/or Sudden Infant Death Syndrome. A pediatrician will also examine your baby in the hospital today.

It's important that you eat a healthy diet and rest during the day whenever possible. Kegel exercises (see p.69) are vital to strengthen your muscles. If you were given painkillers or anti-inflammatory medicine, take these as necessary. If you get visitors, make sure they wash their hands before touching the baby.

Do I need to clean the cord stump before it drops off? Your baby's cord stump, which is the end of the umbilical cord, will shrivel up and fall off naturally around 7–10 days after the birth. Many parents feel uneasy about touching the stump and are unsure whether or not to clean it. Some pediatricians recommend swabbing it regularly with rubbing alcohol, but others say to leave it alone. However, if it does become dirty, clean with soap and water and dry well. If the cord stump or the surrounding area are sticky, inflamed, or smelly, contact your doctor for advice. It's important to keep the cord stump dry. Exposing it to air at times helps avoid the risk of infection.

While you're in the hospital, you may get lots of visitors. And while it's fun to show off your beautiful baby to friends and family, make sure that you take time to sleep, because once you bring your baby home, you won't have much opportunity to sleep. Many hospitals let you decide whether the baby will sleep in the room with you at night or in the nursery. There's no wrong decision; do what feels best for you and your baby.

> “ You may be feeling anxious about your new responsibilities, but be reassured by the support network around you. ”

STITCHES AND HEMORRHOIDS

You can take an analgesic, but the following can also increase comfort:

- When you urinate, pour warm water over the area to ease stinging.
- Sit on an inflatable ring.
- Apply a cooling gel or ice pack.
- Take a warm bath or spray water on your stitches in the shower.

BURPING YOUR BABY

Once your baby has fed, air bubbles in their stomach need to rise to the top, and you can help this happen by burping them. Sit them on your lap or hold them upright against your shoulder. You don't need to rub or pat them, but this often feels right and babies seem to like it! Burp halfway through a feeding and again at the end, especially for bottle-fed babies, since air fills up the stomach, slows down the feeding, and makes a baby more likely to vomit.

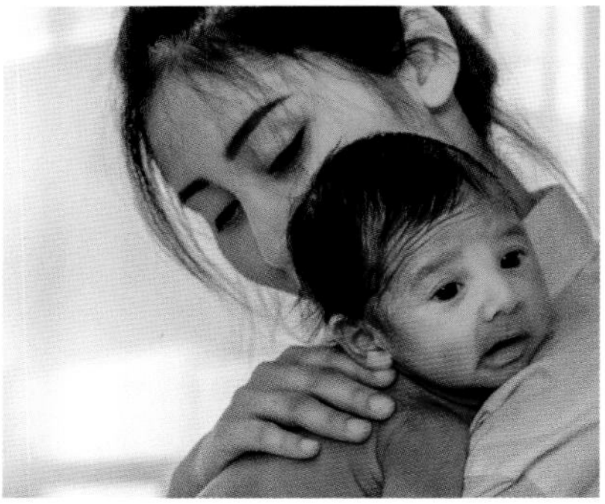

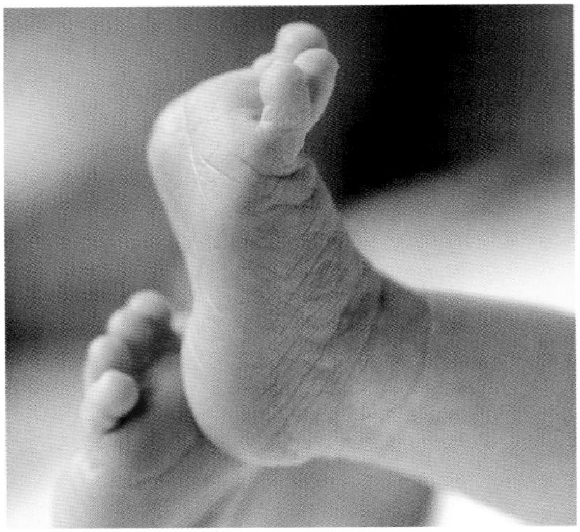

1ST WEEK: **DAY 3**

Going home

YOUR BABY TODAY

A new baby's skin is often quite dry in the first few weeks. This is normal, and the skin will eventually correct itself. Although you don't need to put moisturizer on a baby's skin, if you want you could gently massage in some baby or olive oil.

You'll likely head home from the hospital today. The doctor will do a checkup before you go home to make sure the uterus has contracted and your blood loss (lochia) isn't too heavy. Any stitches or staples will likely be removed before you're discharged, although many doctors now use subcuticular stitches (just under the skin layer) that gradually absorb over a few weeks.

Your first day at home with your new baby can be daunting. Keeping your baby's crib close to your bed can make life easier when you feed or change them at night. Keep lights low and don't talk much or stimulate your baby. Only change their diaper if necessary, and once the feeding is done, put them right back in their crib.

You'll discover that babies don't like having clothes pulled over their head. Keep life simple by buying machine-washable, front-fastening onesies and change outfits only as needed. In the first weeks, there is no need to change into a daytime outfit. If your baby is cold, simply add layers.

Today, you may notice that the swelling in your hands and feet subsides as you urinate more. You still need to drink plenty of fluids to prevent bladder infections, avoid constipation, and help breast milk production. Today may be the first time you move your bowels since giving birth. Eating plenty of fruit, vegetables, and whole grain products and drinking water will help your bowel movements return to normal.

Partners will be proud to have the baby at home. They can be involved in most all aspects of care, including calming the baby, changing diapers, bottle-feeding, bathing, and dressing.

> **“ Once your breast milk arrives, your baby may start to appear more relaxed and contented and go longer between feedings ”**

SPONGE BATHS

Babies need only two or three baths a week. Before the umbilical cord stump falls off, give sponge baths. Wrap your baby in a towel and lie them on a flat surface. Get ready a baby washcloth, a bowl of warm water, and mild baby soap. Uncover only the parts you're actively washing, then rewrap them in the towel. Start with the face, with water only, then use soap on the body and diaper area.

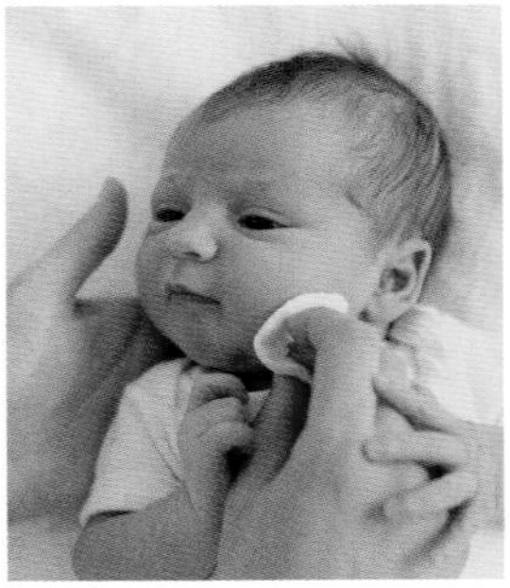

Using a damp washcloth, gently clean your baby's face, using water only.

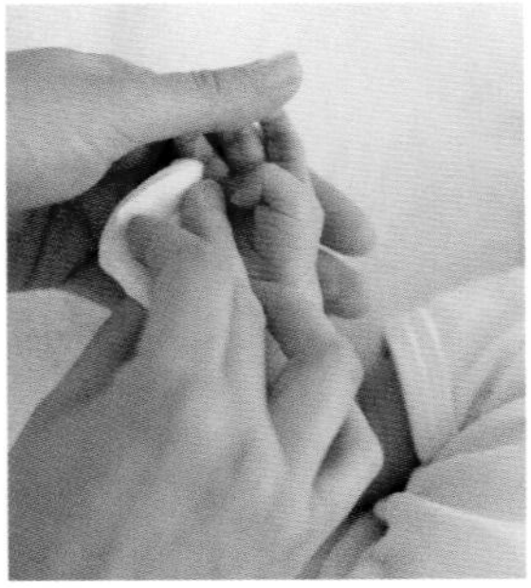

To clean her hands, wipe the backs and palms and between the fingers.

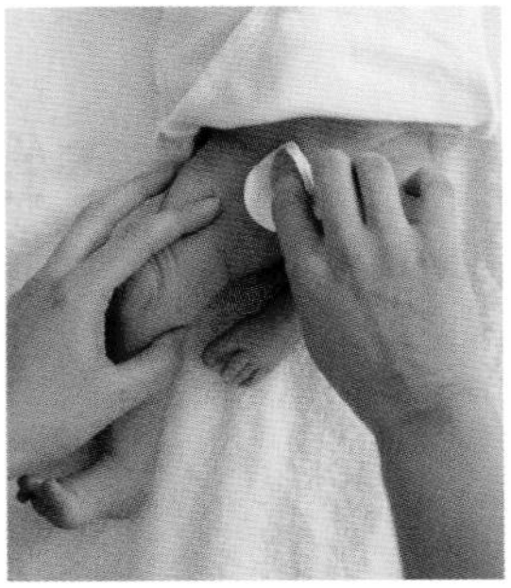

Wash the diaper area last, making sure to clean between the creases in the skin.

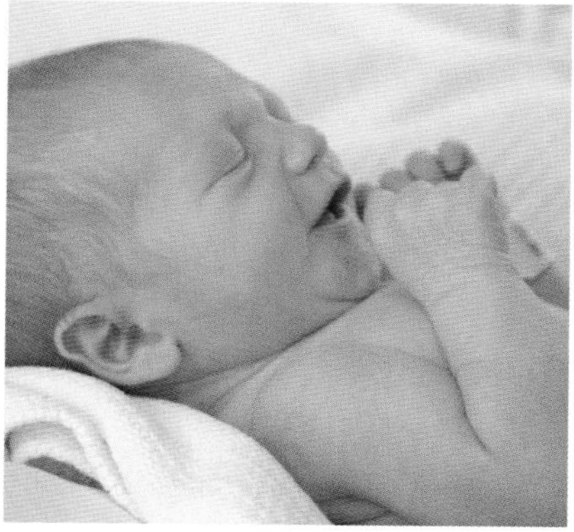

1ST WEEK: **DAY 4**

First outing

YOUR BABY TODAY

The pediatrician will examine your baby today. They will ask if your baby is alert and check for any signs of jaundice (see p.477). They will also weigh your baby and will ask how they are getting along with feeding and whether there are any problems.

Until now, your breasts have produced colostrum, the watery premilk rich in nutrients and antibodies. Once your milk is in (around day 3 or 4), your baby will start to feel more satisfied and your breasts will likely feel engorged and uncomfortable. As feeding establishes over the next few days, this discomfort should start to recede. Your uterus will be steadily reducing in size but can still be felt by pressing on your abdomen. Your blood loss will have started to ease off by now, although you may find that it's heavier first thing in the morning and also while you're breastfeeding.

You'll visit the pediatrician today for the baby's first in-office checkup. They will look for any signs of dehydration, such as your baby not having plenty of wet diapers and any feeding problems. They'll also measure your baby's weight, length, and head circumference. The measurements will be plotted on a graph to track your baby's own growth curves at all of their subsequent appointments. The doctor will also examine the soft spots (fontanelles) on your baby's head; look into their ears, eyes, and mouth; listen to their heart and lungs; and examine their abdomen, hips, legs, and genitals.

> “ Your body is gradually recovering from the birth, and you may be starting to feel like facing the world once again. ”

JAUNDICE

By day four, about a third of all babies are visibly jaundiced. Jaundice in newborn babies is usually harmless and is due to an elevated level of the waste product bilirubin in the blood, caused by the baby's immature liver. Very high levels of bilirubin can cause problems and are treated with light therapy (see p.479).

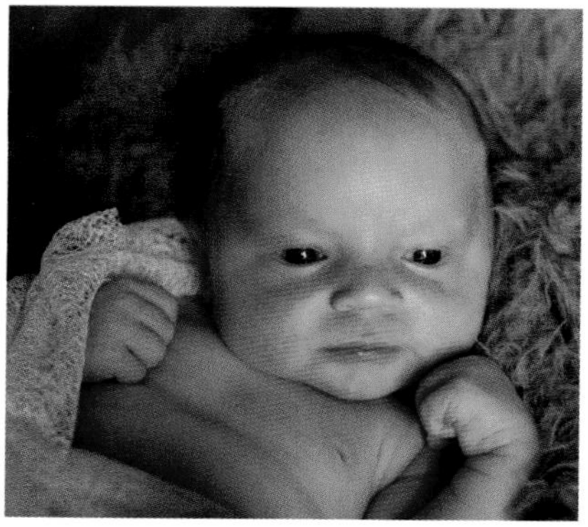

TAKING YOUR BABY OUT

Make sure you have everything you may need before venturing out on a trip.

- **Pack a diaper bag with** two diapers, wipes or cotton pads, a spare onesie, a cloth, and a bottle of formula if you're bottle-feeding.
- **Take layers of clothing** on outings, including an undershirt, onesie, and cardigan. In winter, add an all-in-one babysuit and a blanket in a stroller.
- **A third of a baby's heat is lost through their head,** so on cool days, add a hat or hooded top. Socks and booties are easy to lose. Footed onesies are more practical; mittens are needed only in cold weather.
- **In hot weather, make sure your baby is covered** and protected from direct sunlight at all times.
- **Figure out how to use a baby sling**. If traveling by car or public transportation, learn how to fold and unfold a stroller.
- **Do not carry your baby far in a car seat** because it's bad for your back.

Feeding your baby

Breastfeeding provides your baby with the best nutritional start in life and has a range of other benefits. If you decide to bottle-feed, you can also be confident that your baby will thrive. The key to both methods is preparation.

QUESTIONS AND ANSWERS

How often should I feed my baby?
If you have a healthy, full-term baby, you should feed them on demand, which means feeding them when they cry and seems hungry. This can mean that sometimes they'll be fed every couple of hours and sometimes they'll go for four to six hours without a feeding. Although you may not feel as if you're producing much milk initially, your baby needs only small quantities of colostrum, the first watery milk. Their demands will grow after the first few days, which will coincide with your milk coming in (see right).

Will I be able to breastfeed my twins?
Milk is produced on a supply-and-demand basis, so it's perfectly possible to breastfeed twins and more. If your babies are born early, breast milk is beneficial since it protects against infections, which premature babies are more susceptible to, so it's worth breastfeeding, even for a few weeks, but you'll need rest and ample nutrition. Start by feeding your twins separately. If you then want to feed them together, take time to position them well. An under-arm hold works well; cushions and a willing helper are useful.

Expressing breast milk (see right) means the babies can be fed together, alternating on the breast. If you think that they aren't getting enough milk, consult your doctor. A lactation consultant, La Leche League, or the local chapter of the National Organization of Mothers of Twins Clubs can offer support too.

The benefits of breastfeeding

Breastfeeding is the perfect first food for your baby; it contains all the nutrients your baby needs and works on a supply-and-demand basis, so that as your baby feeds, your body responds by producing more milk. Breast milk is thought to reduce a baby's risk of developing an allergic condition, such as asthma and eczema, to make childhood obesity and diabetes less likely, and it may reduce the long-term risk of heart disease.

Breastfeeding also provides benefits for you. It helps your uterus contract to its prepregnancy shape more quickly. It helps you get back into shape quicker since your body uses additional energy to produce breast milk, and it reduces your risk of getting breast and ovarian cancer.

Lastly, breastfeeding helps you and your baby to bond both physically and emotionally.

When your milk comes in

In the first few days your breasts produce colostrum, a watery

LATCHING ON

Taking the time to ensure that your baby is latched on properly before a feeding is important because you could otherwise develop sore nipples. A baby that is properly latched on has their mouth wide open, with the whole areola (the area surrounding the nipple) in their mouth; their bottom lip will be curled back and they will be noticeably sucking. You'll feel a sucking effect over the entire area.

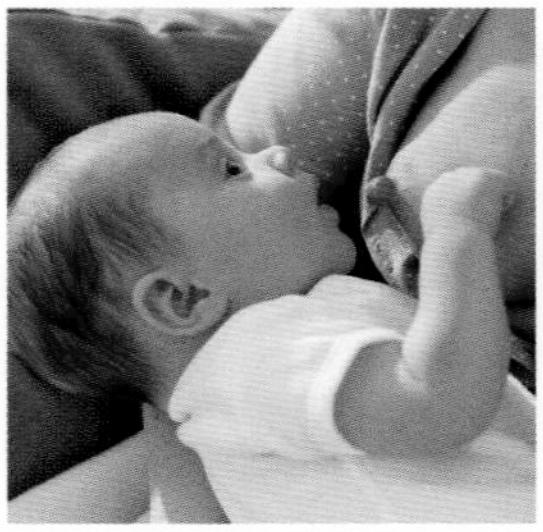

Once you've positioned your baby so that they are level with your breast, hold them with their nose and mouth facing your nipple.

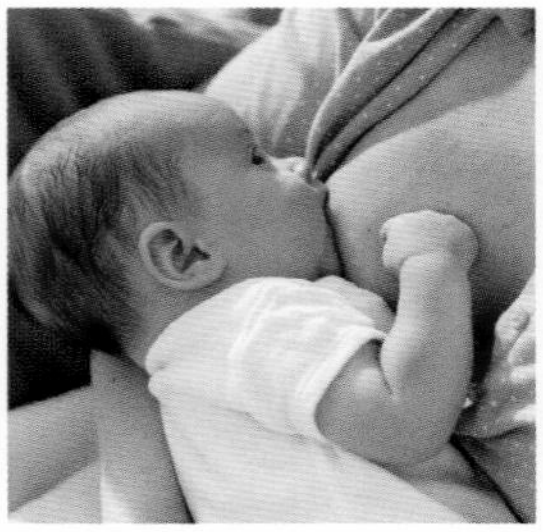

When your baby opens their mouth wide, bring them to the breast, ensuring that they take all of the nipple and the areola into their mouth.

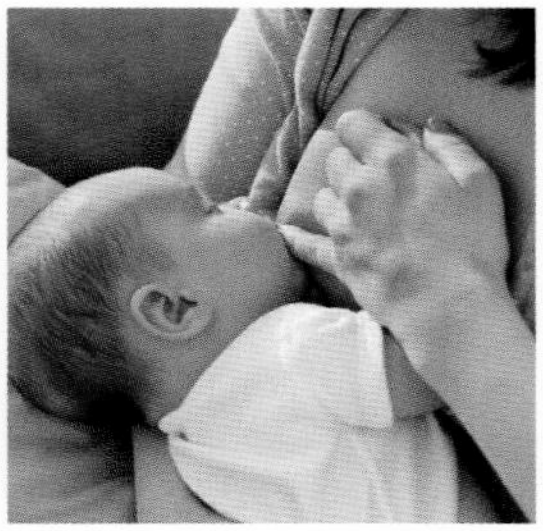

To remove your baby from the breast, insert your finger into the corner of their mouth to break the seal so that they don't pull the nipple.

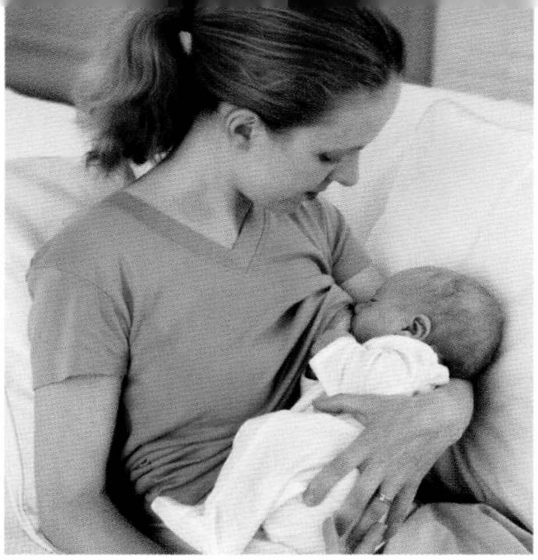

Holding your baby tummy-to-tummy is a comfortable position for you both, enabling your baby to latch on well.

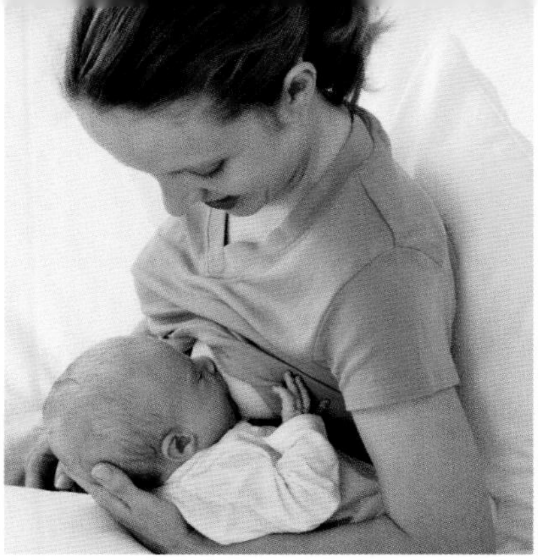

An under-arm "football" hold can help keep a restless baby still.

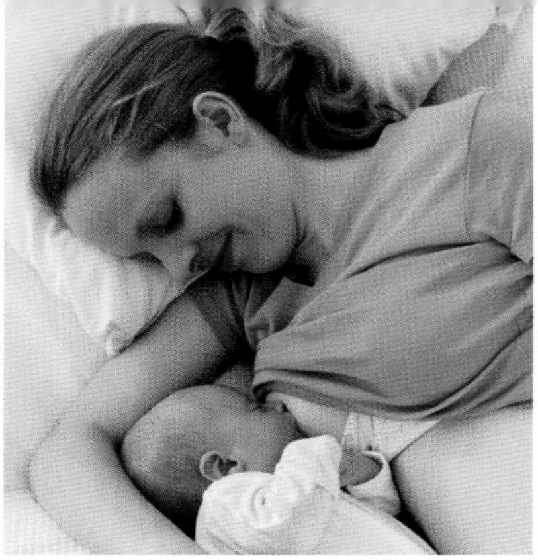

Lying side by side is often recommended after a Cesarean.

substance that contains essential nutrients and antibodies that help your baby fight off infections such as those of the ear, chest, and gastrointestinal tract.

At around day three, or sometimes a bit later, you will start to produce milk, which contains all the nutrients your baby needs. Your breasts may feel uncomfortably full and tender at this time, and you'll need to make sure they're properly emptied at each feeding to prevent them from becoming engorged (see p.456).

Successful breastfeeding

Despite the fact that breastfeeding is a natural process, it can sometimes prove difficult. Getting comfortable before a feeding, positioning your baby well, and ensuring that they latch on properly (see box, left), are all prerequisites for successful feeding.

For your baby to latch on to the breast properly, it's important that you're both positioned well. Ensure that you're comfortable and that your back is well supported; using cushions for support may be helpful. You may find sitting and cradling your baby at chest level is comfortable with their tummy facing your tummy. Or you could try a football hold with your baby under your arm. Some women find it helpful to lie on their side to latch their baby on. You'll soon discover which positions suit you best and will gradually gain confidence in your ability to feed.

Once your baby is latched on, the "letdown" reflex is triggered. You will feel a tingling sensation as milk is released, which in turn stimulates the production of more milk. Your baby will pause during feedings and stop when they are full. It's advisable to always have water or juice during or just after a feeding to replace the fluids lost from breast milk.

Bottle-feeding

For bottle-feeding, you'll need four to six bottles: larger 8 fl oz (250 ml) bottles, and smaller 4 fl oz (125 ml) ones; newborn bottle nipples; a bottle brush; and infant formula. If you have chlorinated tap water, it's okay to put bottles in the dishwasher or wash by hand. Otherwise, clean all of the parts, then boil in water for 5–10 minutes. Put filtered or cooled boiled water in the bottle, then add the formula according to the manufacturer's instructions. Test the temperature of the milk by squeezing a drop on your inner wrist: it should feel warm, but not hot. Cool the milk if necessary by placing the bottle in a pitcher of cold water, or running it under cold water while shaking the bottle all the time.

When the bottle is ready, hold your baby half sitting with her head in the crook of your elbow and her back along your forearm. Gently put the nipple into her mouth and tip the bottle so the milk covers the nipple to keep her from swallowing any air. Discard any formula leftover in the bottle and make a new bottle for each feed.

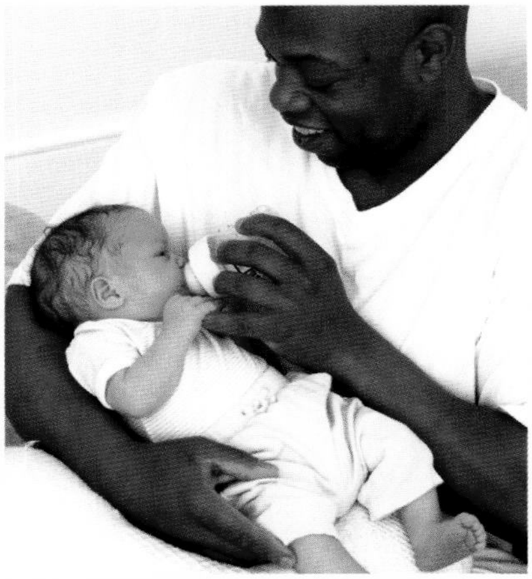

Bottle-feeding helps partners strengthen the bond with their baby and allows you to have some welcome time off from feeding.

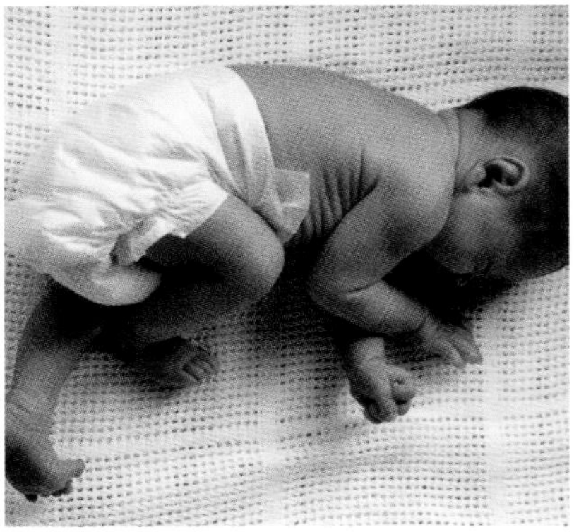

1ST WEEK: **DAY 5**

Baby blues

YOUR BABY TODAY

If you had a Cesarean and your baby is healthy, They'll likely come home from the hospital with you today, after passing their final in-hospital pediatric exam. Make sure you have the correct car seat and pack a blanket or two to keep them warm.

> "Try to spend some time focusing on the needs of older children too and helping them to adapt to the new arrival."

Today, you might feel emotional and weepy, known as the "baby blues." This is caused by hormonal changes and exacerbated by fatigue and a feeling of anticlimax after the buildup to the birth. The baby blues last a day or so, and with rest and emotional support, you will start to feel better. If the feelings fail to subside after a few days, talk to your doctor since you may be suffering from postpartum depression (see p.475).

Your breasts will still feel tender and full today. Feeding your baby on demand (see p.448) will help relieve this. Feeling tired interferes with the "letdown" reflex (see p.449), so it's vital to rest or sleep in the day to make up for broken nights. It's important to continue breastfeeding at night to prevent milk stagnation, which leads to problems such as abscesses and mastitis (breast inflammation; see p.475).

Your baby's arrival is a major adjustment for an older child, but there are ways to help them welcome their new baby brother or sister. Give your older child a gift from the baby and encourage them to help with the baby's care as is appropriate for their age. A two-year-old may want to touch the baby, hold their hand, and bring diapers and other things that are needed; a five-year-old can hold the baby with support and sing to them.

TWINS OR MORE

Setting yourself some guidelines can help you cope with the added demands of twins or more.

- Make time to be with your babies.
- Prioritize activities ruthlessly, enlist practical help, and shop online.
- Don't bathe your babies daily unless you and they enjoy it.
- Let visitors make their own coffee.
- Consider using pacifiers if your twins cry a lot. This helps you attend to the twin most in need.
- Make time for yourself every day.

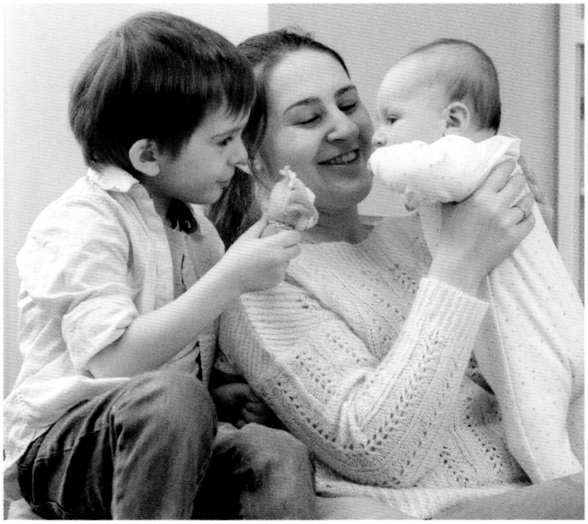

Including older siblings in babycare and play helps prevent them from feeling left out and more accepting of this new arrival.

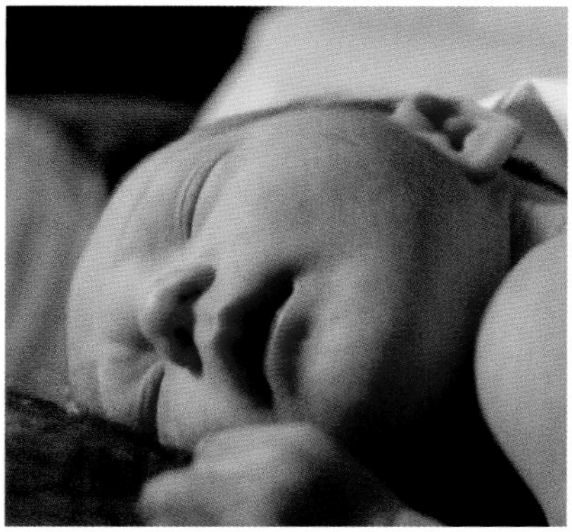

1ST WEEK: **DAY 6**

Finding your way

YOUR BABY TODAY

It's likely that both you and your baby are becoming more confident with feeding. It's common for new babies to bring up some milk after each feeding, known as spitting up, and this is unlikely to cause any harm. Talk to the doctor if you're at all concerned.

Many parents feel uneasy about giving their baby a bath and worry about dropping them. Many also find that their baby objects strongly to being undressed and immersed in water. If your baby hates baths at first, sponge bathe them most of the time (see p.448). Make bathtime as stress-free as possible by gathering everything you need before you start and make sure the room you undress your baby in is warm and draft-free. Afterward, dry and dress your baby immediately.

There is no need to routinely change a diaper before or after feedings—just when there is a stool or it is heavy with urine. After opening a diaper, wipe away all visible feces with the diaper. Clean your baby's bottom thoroughly with wet cotton wipes, wiping from front to back to avoid spreading germs. If your baby wears disposable diapers, they may not need diaper cream, but if they start to get a diaper rash, you may find that diaper cream will clear it right up.

BATHING YOUR BABY

Before you bathe your baby, have a towel ready to dry them and a clean diaper and change of clothes on hand so that they don't get cold after the bath. Half fill a baby bath with water that feels lukewarm to your elbow. After bathing, dry your baby quickly. Don't use talcum powder, which they could inhale.

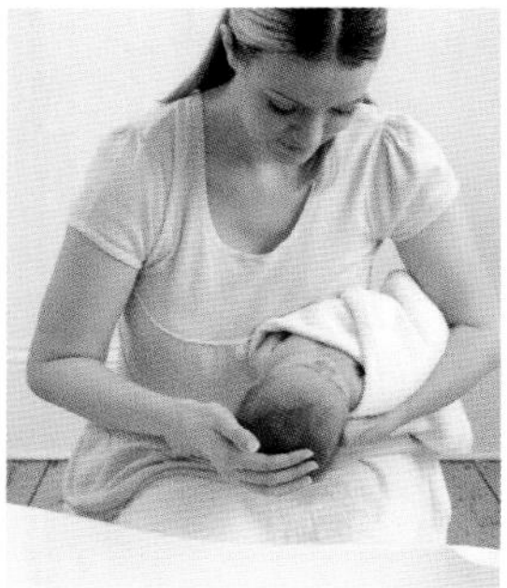

Wrap your baby in a towel, and support their head and shoulders while you wet their head with the other hand.

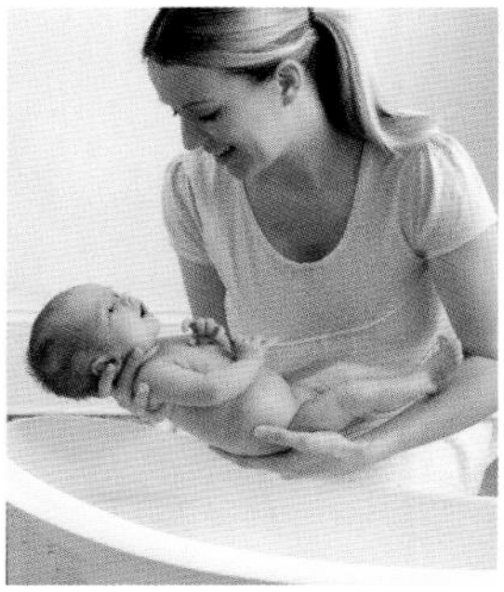

Remove the towel and lower your baby into the bath, supporting their head, shoulders, and bottom.

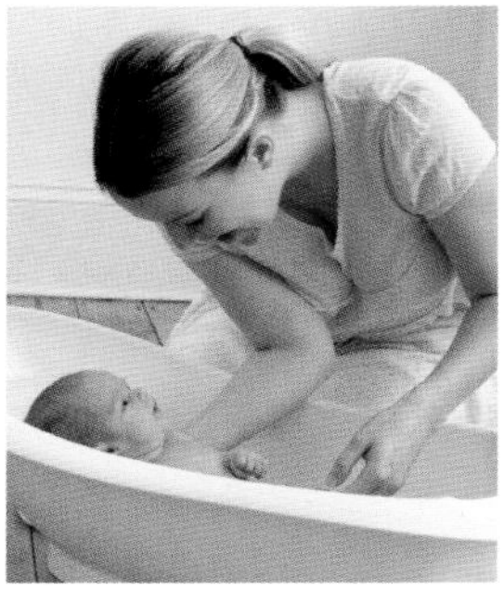

Still supporting their head, wash them with a washcloth or sponge; start with the face and end with the bottom.

> "By now, you and your partner will be starting to feel more confident about holding, handling, and feeding your baby."

EXERCISE BASICS

You will be encouraged to do some gentle exercise as soon as you feel able, although it's best to wait until the six-week checkup (see pp.464–465) before starting a strenuous program.

- Maintain good posture and avoid straining your back and abdomen.
- Continue Kegel exercises (see p.69) after giving birth.
- If you had a Cesarean, wait until at least six weeks before starting an exercise program.
- Start with low-impact exercises, such as walking and Pilates. Gradually increase the duration and intensity. You can also begin to strengthen your abdominal muscles (see p.458).
- If you have any bleeding or feel faint, stop and consult your doctor.
- Set realistic goals.

Neonatal intensive care babies

Around 10 to 15 percent of all babies born in the US need to spend time in a neonatal intensive care unit (NICU). Babies most often need extra care to assist them with breathing until their lungs have matured.

There are many reasons why your baby may need special care, the most common one being prematurity (being born before 37 weeks). Babies may need to spend days, weeks, or sometimes months in a NICU until they are big enough and well enough to go home.

Neonatal intensive care unit

If your baby is in a NICU, this is a particularly stressful time. It helps to understand a bit about who will be caring for your baby, what they will be doing, and how to make sure you're fully informed at all times.

In the US, most hospitals have a unit to provide special nursing and medical care for babies; these are divided into three levels depending on the degree of care offered. Level one is the most basic level. These units don't provide long-term ventilatory support, but they are expert at caring for babies who are slightly premature, need frequent nursing, or have previously been ventilated and are ready to be transferred to less intensive care. Level-two units ventilate and give intensive care to babies from 26 weeks' gestation. Level-three units offer intensive care for babies born as early as 23 weeks, and can often do neonatal surgery.

All these units are staffed by special nurses and doctors who will be happy to show you around before the baby is born if there is time.

Ward rounds Most units have rounds each morning, and the more intensive units will have another round later in the day. Some allow parents to be present and to ask questions, while others prefer parents to wait outside and then make time to talk to them afterward.

Communication and visiting You may be able to spend some time with your baby before they are sent to a NICU. However, if your baby needs to be on a ventilator, or has another serious problem, they will be sent immediately to neonatal intensive care, and you may not have any time together after the birth. You'll be encouraged to see your baby as soon as they have been transferred, and if you're unable to go immediately, you may be given a photo of your baby.

You should be able to see your baby any time of the day or night and the nurses will be happy to update you regularly. The doctors will also give you an update on an ad hoc basis or arrange to meet you for a more formal chat.

HOW YOU CAN HELP YOUR BABY

Parents whose baby is in a special care unit may be very stressed. They may feel that they have no role in the care of their baby; however, this is not the case. The most important thing you can do for your baby is to start expressing breast milk. Breast milk will nearly always be the best milk for a premature baby and can be stored in a freezer until needed.

You may be able to touch and stroke your baby and can be helped to cuddle while they are on a ventilator. Babies thrive on skin-to-skin contact, called kangaroo care. You'll be encouraged to tuck your baby on your chest inside your shirt so that they can enjoy a close bond. Talking, reading, and singing to your baby help them become familiar with you. You may be able to change their diaper and help with feedings, even if these are through a nasogastric tube.

Spend plenty of time with your baby, especially when breastfeeding since this may help the letdown reflex (see p.449), but conserve energy for when you return home with your baby.

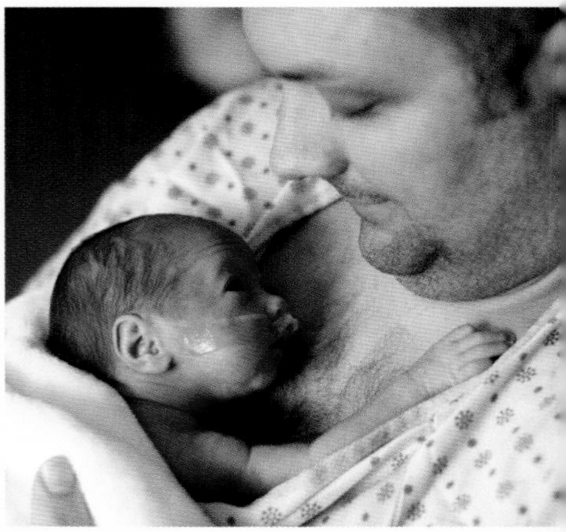

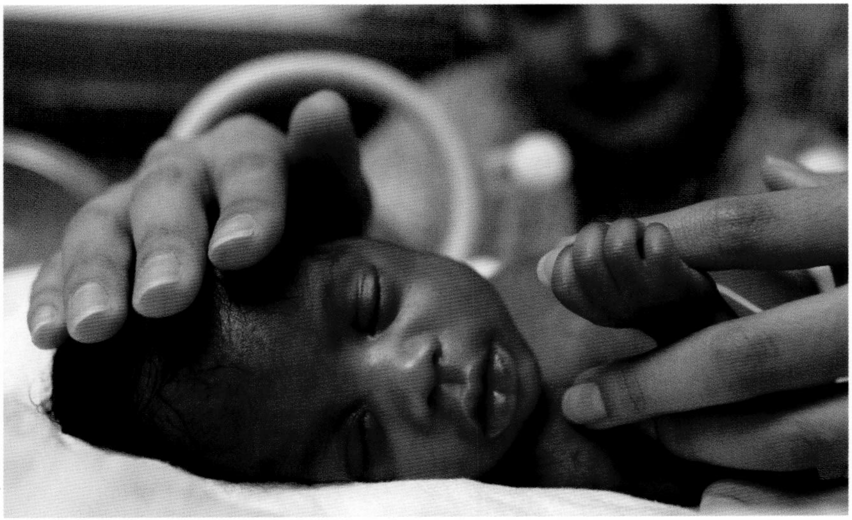

You will both be encouraged to touch, stroke, and caress your small baby, and to spend as much time as possible talking and singing to him.

Other family members may be able to visit the unit with your permission.

Your baby's care

While your baby is in the NICU, they may be treated with medication have various tests and checkups. In some cases, they will need to be on a ventilator.

Tests and X-rays Your baby may have blood tests to check for infection and anemia; to check kidney function, oxygen, carbon dioxide, and sugar levels, and to identify her blood group. The frequency of these depends on how ill or premature you baby is. In neonatal intensive care, babies need blood tests periodically. Some babies need an X-ray while they're there, and very premature babies often need many chest X-rays and sometimes abdominal ones.

Assisting your baby Some babies need a little extra oxygen, while others need constant oxygen through a nasal tube. For very premature babies, a tube may be placed into the trachea (windpipe) and connected to a ventilator that blows oxygen into the lungs. Babies are monitored to see when they can be weaned off the ventilator.

Most babies in intensive care need one or more IVs to give fluids, blood, and antibiotics. Very small babies may be fed through a long, fine feeding tube running through the mouth or nose to the stomach. They may also need at least one blood transfusion, for some cases of conditions like anemia and jaundice.

Antibiotics are often given to prevent infection. Some babies need medicine to keep their blood pressure up, and many who are ventilated need medicine to sedate them and to prevent or treat pain.

NEONATAL UNIT STAFF

Since your baby may spend several weeks in the neonatal unit, you are likely to get to know the staff well.

Neonatal nurses Most of the care in a neonatal intensive care unit is carried out by highly trained nurses. These include registered nurses and neonatal clinical nurse specialists who have advanced training. Some intensive care units also have neonatal nurse practitioners, who have advanced education and training and can perform many procedures.

Doctors Neonatologists are the doctors who run the neonatal intensive care units. These are the doctors who will coordinate your baby's daily care plan. They are pediatricians who have received advanced training to care for sick and premature newborns. The neonatologist in charge of the department is known as the attending doctor. In addition to neonatologists, there are often neonatology fellows and pediatric residents as well. Neonatology fellows are pediatricians who are getting advanced training to care for sick newborns. Pediatric residents are doctors who are being trained in the specialty area of pediatrics.

Other members of staff A neonatal intensive care unit depends on a number of other staff members. These include a registered dietitian, physical and occupational therapists, technicians (who can draw blood or take X-rays), pharmacists, and, in some neonatal intensive care units, a psychotherapist to offer much-needed emotional support to parents.

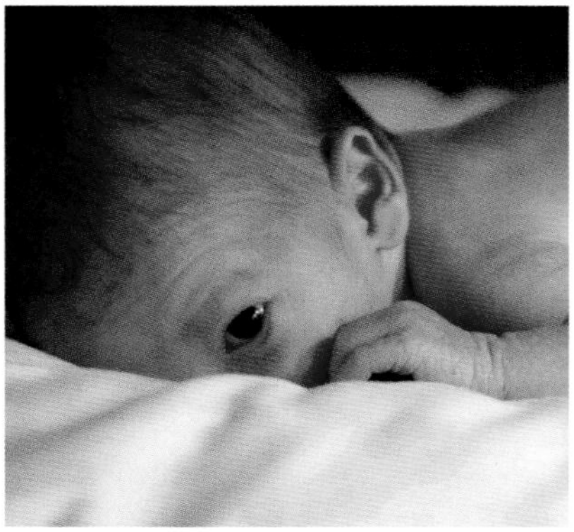

1ST WEEK: **DAY 7**

Tuning in

YOUR BABY TODAY

Some "tummy time" is good for infants as long as they are awake and being observed. But don't lie your baby down on her stomach for bed—it's dangerous and can lead to Sudden Infant Death Syndrome (SIDS).

> "As the bond between you and your baby continues to grow, you will start to feel more intuitive about their needs."

YOUR BABY'S CRIES

Follow the checklist below to help you identify the cause of your baby's cries. If your baby cries for three hours or more a day, consult your doctor.

- **Hunger is the main reason** for crying; your baby will stop once they're offered the breast, a bottle, a finger, or a pacifier.
- **A cry of pain** is easy to interpret since your baby may be inconsolable, draw up their legs in pain, or arch their back. If you're unsure how to remedy the pain, consult your doctor.
- **A wet or dirty diaper** can be uncomfortable and cause crying.
- **Your baby may want to be held.** Babies can't be spoiled by too much cuddling. Carrying them in a sling while you do chores may comfort them.
- **Your baby may be overstimulated.** As a new and attentive parent, it can be easy to forget that babies need quiet time.

Crying is the only way your baby can get your attention. Expecting and new parents often worry about how they'll know what their baby wants. Although your baby's cries may seem indistinguishable at first, you'll soon start to interpret them (see box, left).

Ideally, you'll have continued Kegel exercises (see p.69) in this first week. It's important to continue doing these since they strengthen the muscles that support your bladder, helping to prevent stress incontinence (see p.477). They also help promote healing and ease discomfort if you've had stitches since they increase the blood flow to your perineum.

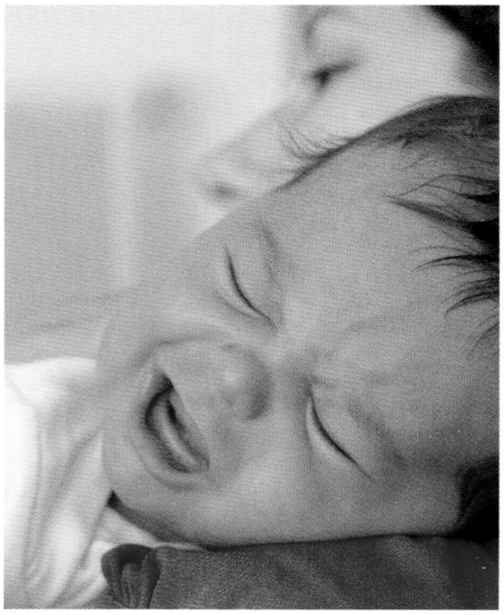

You will soon start to recognize your baby's cries and will feel increasingly confident about how to tend to their needs.

SWADDLING

Swaddling: If your newborn cries a lot, is fussy, or has trouble sleeping, try swaddling them. Being wrapped tightly in blankets, with the arms bound, makes babies feel the way they did when they were in the uterus, and it calms them. In fact, some babies sleep an extra hour or two when swaddled and may even need to be unswaddled to wake up for their feedings. Be sure that any blankets you use for swaddling are tightly wrapped around the baby, because loose blankets can cover a baby's face and so become a factor for Sudden Infant Death Syndrome (SIDS). You may have learned how to swaddle your baby in the hospital. If not, your pediatrician should know how to do it. There are also simple swaddling products on the market that use Velcro tabs for a snug fit, thus eliminating the need to learn how to properly swaddle. These products can be found online or in stores.

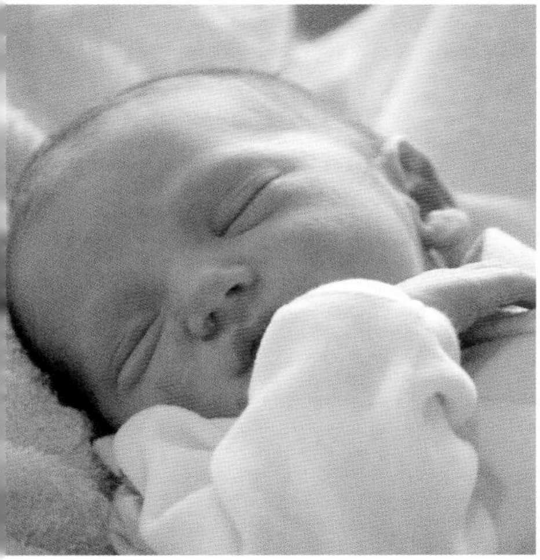

2ND WEEK: **DAY 8**

Healthy living

YOUR BABY TODAY

Whether you're breastfeeding or bottle-feeding can affect your baby's stools. The stools of breastfed babies tend to be slightly runnier and can have a fairly sweet aroma, while bottle-fed babies may have firmer, stronger-smelling stools.

It's important to eat a well-balanced diet (see pp.14–17) to help you deal with the demands of motherhood. If you're breastfeeding, you'll need an extra 500 calories a day. Drink plenty of clear fluids, being careful to limit your caffeine intake. If you were anemic during pregnancy, or had a heavy blood loss after the birth, eat lots of iron-rich foods, such as broccoli or spinach (see p.84). Foods and drinks rich in vitamin C will help you absorb iron.

If you smoke and didn't manage to stop during pregnancy, this is an ideal time to try to stop. Ask your doctor to refer you to a local smoking cessation group. Limiting your alcohol intake is also wise, and drinking while breastfeeding isn't recommended.

It can be easy to take over your baby's care, but it's important that your partner is involved too and doesn't feel left out. Your partner is adjusting to parenthood and may have their own anxieties and concerns. Sharing the practical care will help them forge their own bond with the baby. As your partner's confidence grows, you'll be able to take some time out for yourself while they care for the baby. Keeping the lines of communication open is vital since this is a huge change for you both. It takes time to adjust to being a family, but working together will help the transition go more smoothly.

> "A healthy lifestyle benefits your physical and mental well-being and helps you deal with the demands of parenthood."

REGISTERING THE BIRTH

You'll fill out your baby's birth certificate in the hospital. Your doctor or hospital will file this with the appropriate government agency. You'll probably also receive paperwork to apply for a Social Security number for your baby (or go to ssa.gov).

YOUR BABY'S STOOLS

The color and consistency of a baby's stools are highly variable, but most are normal and not a cause for concern. However, some types of stool can indicate a problem and it's important to know what to look for. A change in the color of urine or the presence of blood might also alert you to a problem.

What's normal

- Once your baby has passed the first dark meconium (see p.446), stools may become dark green, green-yellow, bright yellow, orange, or brown; all are normal and may vary in the same day.
- A baby who is breastfed may have stools that are loose and seedy.
- If your baby is bottle-fed, stools tend to be smooth and firmer.
- Frequency of stools varies from after every feeding to every 2–3 days.
- Urine may be yellow or clear.
- A pink or red-orange stain on the diaper may be due to urate crystals (which form from concentrated urine); these are common in the first few weeks, especially in breastfed babies and are nothing to worry about.

What's not normal

If you notice any of the following changes, you should contact your pediatrician:

- White or putty-colored stools, which could indicate a liver problem.
- Blood mixed in the stools, which could suggest a milk allergy.
- Dark urine, which could be a sign of dehydration or jaundice.

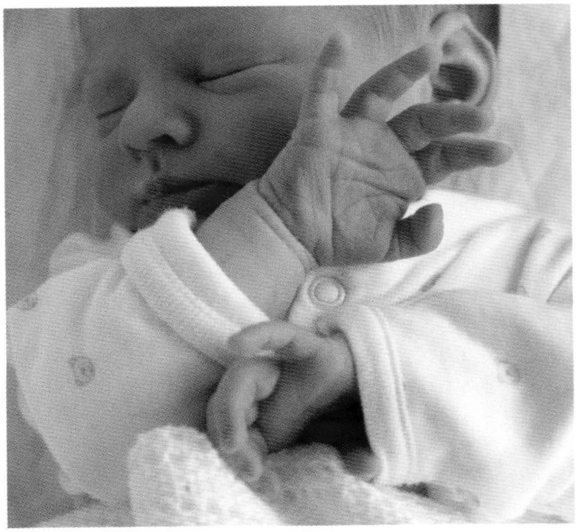

2ND WEEK: **DAY 9**

Focus on you

YOUR BABY TODAY

If your baby vomits large amounts and isn't thriving, this may suggest a problem such as gastroesophageal reflux (see p.477). This is caused by the immaturity of the stomach muscles and does resolve over time and with treatment.

> " Now that you've begun to adapt to the topsy-turvy world of motherhood, try to carve out some time for yourself each day. "

To help you deal with broken nights and constant demands, you need to develop coping skills, such as taking an afternoon nap. You may also be dealing with feelings of isolation and may even find it hard to keep track of what day it is as days and nights merge into one. To revive your spirits, arrange for a friend or relative to take care of your baby while you have a break. You and your partner also need to make more of an effort to make time for each other.

ABDOMINAL EXERCISES

Strengthening your abdomen enables your body to work more efficiently during any activity and helps you regain your prepregnancy tone.

- Sit up straight; pull in your tummy for 60 seconds at least once each hour.
- Stand tall and straight to keep your abdominal muscles firm.
- Massage your abdomen with oil or body lotion in circular movements.
- When you feel able, you can start doing gentle sit-ups to strengthen your abdomen, but wait for at least six weeks after a Cesarean.

BREASTFEEDING PROBLEMS

For some women, breastfeeding is a straightforward process, but for many women, it can be surprisingly hard. Engorged (swollen) breasts and sore nipples are a common complaint; knowing how to avoid or treat these problems can be the difference between continuing with breastfeeding and giving up.

The secret to avoiding sore nipples is to make sure that your baby latches on to your breast properly (see p.450). Engorged breasts can make it hard for your baby to latch on, so try expressing a little milk (see p.451) before a feeding to relieve some pressure. Whenever possible, let the air get to your nipples, and use breast pads at other times to keep the nipples dry.

You can relieve engorged breasts by continuing with breastfeeding and expressing milk frequently between feedings to relieve the pressure. Placing a warm, clean washcloth on your breast or putting a chilled cabbage leaf inside your bra can also be soothing.

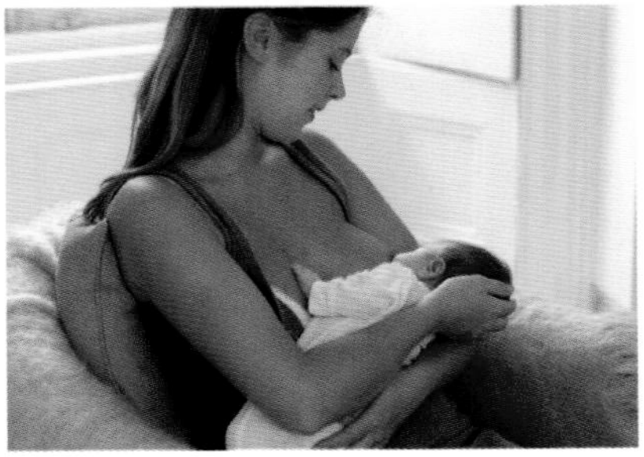

Positioning your baby well at the breast and ensuring that they latch on properly will help to avoid sore, painful nipples.

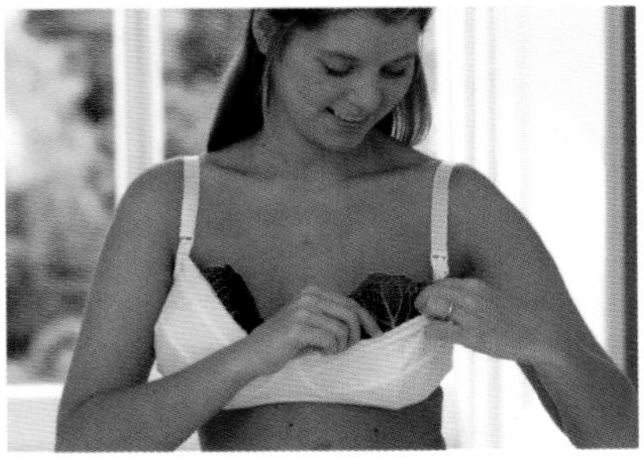

Putting a chilled cabbage leaf inside your bra can be soothing, especially if your breasts are feeling inflamed and engorged.

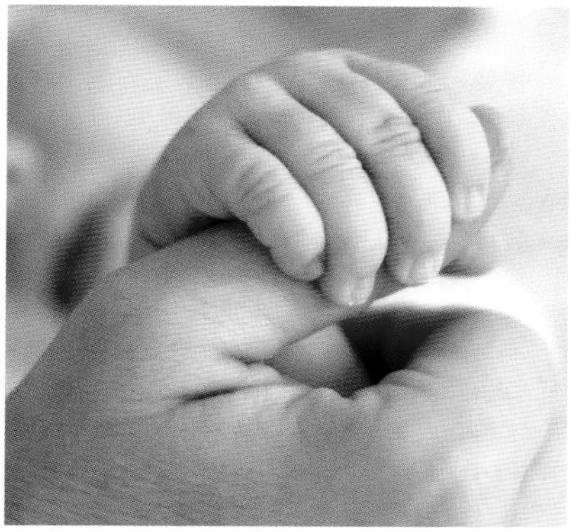

2ND WEEK: **DAY 10**

Getting checked

YOUR BABY TODAY

Sometimes babies develop skin rashes or irritations and sore bottoms around this time. Your pediatrician can advise on how to relieve these minor problems.

Adjusting to life with a newborn is difficult for some mothers, especially those recovering from Cesareans. Sleep deprivation may make it hard to handle all of the new responsibilities. If your partner took time off during the first week, you may want another pair of hands to take their place. If you're able to hire a babysitter or visiting nurse for a few hours a day, you'll get some relief. If not, consider asking a good friend or relative for assistance. But before calling in any favors, make sure that the person you ask will actually provide the type of help you need. Do you want someone to care for the baby so you can nap, make dinner, or run errands? Do you want someone to cook or clean while you tend to the baby? Do you need someone to get groceries and pick up your older child? Be clear about your needs so your helper isn't upset that they won't get to hold the baby the whole time.

Your baby loves to be stimulated. They can focus about a foot away and will watch a simple object such as a mobile. Babies soon recognize familiar faces and will love to watch you talk. Being part of your daily life provides plenty of stimulation. Tell them what you are doing and your plans for the day, read stories, and listen to music together. When they're awake, give them time on their tummy to develop strength in the arms and prevent a "flat" head, a common problem in babies who spend a lot of time on their backs. Always supervise your baby while they are on their tummy.

> "If you find that you need some additional help with the baby, there are several options to consider."

YOUR BABY'S SLEEP PATTERN

Newborns have at least two naps each day and many simply rotate sleeping and eating throughout the day. In the early days, you'll find that there is little routine to your baby's sleep pattern since they can't go long without being fed.

Your baby won't be picky about where they nap, whether in the car, stroller, or a baby sling. At home, you may prefer to put your baby somewhere quiet, such as in their Moses basket or bassinet, or you might want to keep them close by.

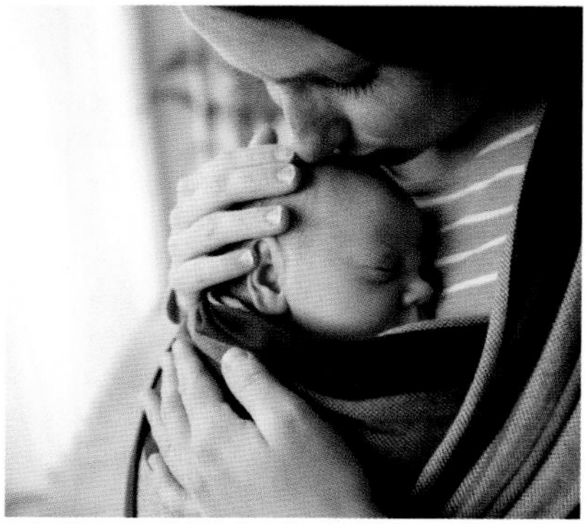

NAILS AND SCRATCHING

Babies' nails grow quickly and are also very tricky to cut! However, to stop your baby from scratching their face, you'll need to keep them trimmed. Be careful not to rip the edge of the nails since this can cause infection.

- You can buy special baby scissors, although these may not cut the nails short enough to prevent scratching.
- Filing the nails keeps them short.
- You may want to put mittens on your baby until they are past the scratching stage.

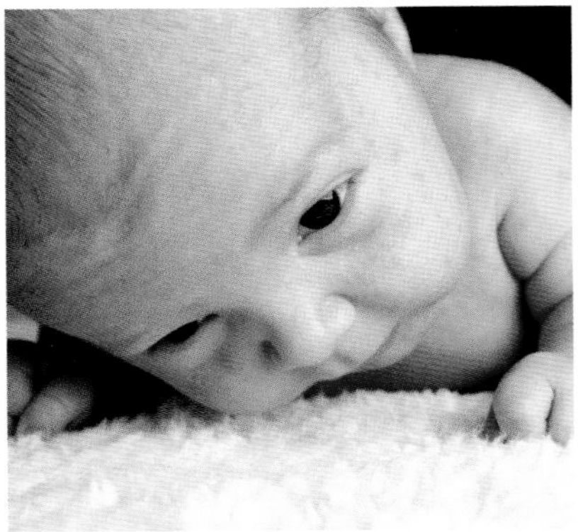

2ND WEEK: **DAY 11**

Taking stock

YOUR BABY TODAY

Many babies have spots known as milia, or "milk spots." These tiny whitish-yellow spots appear on the face in the first two days and disappear by four weeks. Occasionally babies have spots resulting from the mother's hormones that take longer to disappear.

> "As a parent, you will learn to trust your own instincts, even if this sometimes means ignoring the advice of others."

There are many approaches to baby care, and once you have a baby, you may find that everyone has a tip to offer. Although many of these suggestions are helpful, the advice can become a bit overwhelming and is often conflicting. One area where there is a great deal of advice is breastfeeding (see p.448). If you are struggling with breastfeeding and wondering why it all seems so much harder than it looks, you may find that advice is increasingly unhelpful. You may want to take a step back, decide which of your friends or relatives has a similar approach to yours in other areas of life, and pay most heed to their advice. Above all, have confidence in your own ability and trust your instincts, reminding yourself that there are many right ways to do things.

BABY MASSAGE

Babies love to be touched, and massaging your baby can be a great way to bond with them. All you need is some olive oil (avoid nut or aromatherapy oils) and a towel on the floor or bed. Ensure the room is warm and that your baby isn't hungry or too full. Undress them, rub some oil into your palms, and gently rub their tummy, limbs, fingers, and toes, watching them to make sure they're enjoying the massage. A baby massage class is a good way to make friends with other moms in your area.

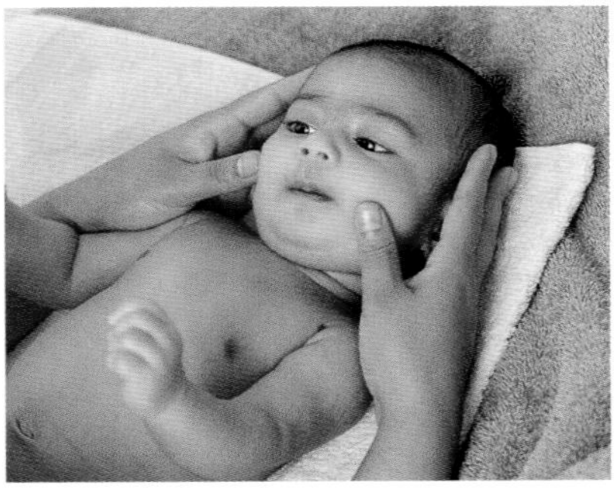

Lay your baby on a soft towel and then use the tips of your fingers to gently stroke your baby's head, avoiding the soft area, or fontanelles, at the top of the head.

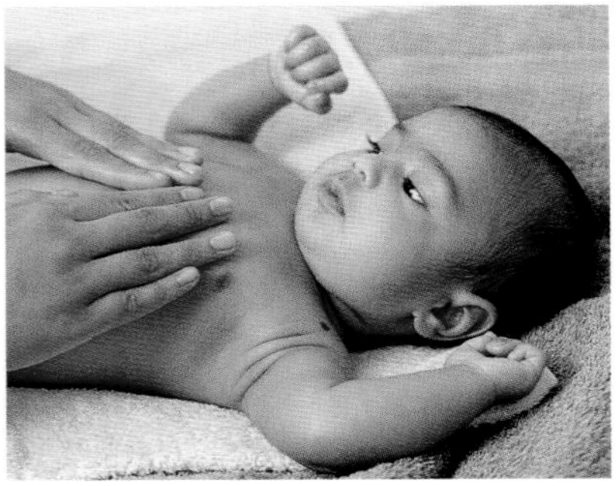

With gentle downward strokes massage your baby's chest, and then use your fingertips to rub their tummy with outward circular strokes.

GOING TO THE SUPERMARKET

Some advance planning and management can help take the stress out of a supermarket run with a newborn. **Giving your baby a good feeding before setting out** may mean that they sleep peacefully at the supermarket.

- **Supermarkets can be very cold,** so dress your baby appropriately.
- **Check to see if your car seat clips onto a cart** since this can make life easier. Otherwise, use the supermarket's own cart with a baby seat or put your baby into a sling while you walk around the supermarket.
- **Make a shopping list before you go** so that you don't forget essentials if you're distracted by your baby crying.

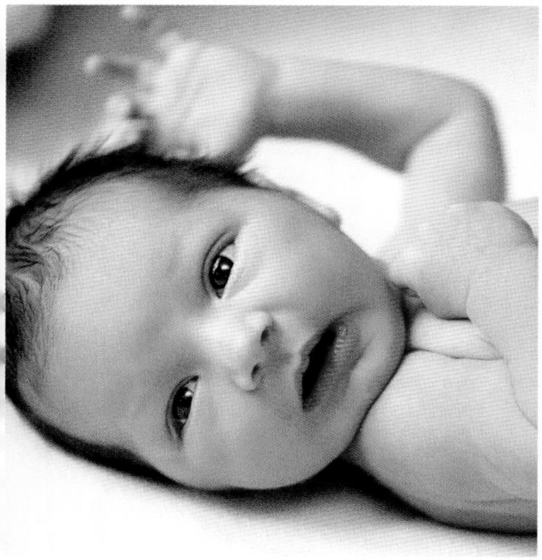

2ND WEEK: **DAY 12**

Looking back

YOUR BABY TODAY

By now, you may feel that your baby is beginning to interact a bit more as you notice that they love to gaze at faces and enjoy watching you talk and smile. However, they won't be able to smile back for a few weeks yet.

Once the acceptance and realization that you've had a baby sinks in and you begin to adapt to your new baby, you may start to reflect on your birth experience and want to share with others. You will remember your birth story for the rest of your life and later share it with your baby.

Sometimes the labor and birth may not have gone as you wanted or anticipated. You may have gone over your due date and had to be induced, which may have led to interventions, an instrumental delivery, or an emergency Cesarean. You may feel some disappointment and be unsure why certain things happened and whether you could have done anything to prevent them.

Occasionally some women, and their partners, who had a particularly difficult birth experience can suffer from postbirth trauma. If the birth was traumatic and you feel upset and unsettled, make an appointment with your doctor. They will explain events that you're unsure about and may be able to arrange for you to see the obstetrician who cared for you during labor, or recommend a mental health professional for you to speak with.

If your partner feels traumatized by your birth experience and felt helpless during the process, they can also talk to the doctor or, if they prefer, to a mental health professional.

Talking to your partner can help you relive good memories and come to terms with the more unsettling ones. Your partner is one of the best-placed people to reassure you about how you managed during labor, and talking together can help you open up and express your feelings.

> “For some, reliving a traumatic birth is painful, and you and your partner may need support to work through difficult memories.”

YOUR BABY'S SENSES

Your baby will focus on your face when being fed. They have been able to hear since they were in the uterus and love the sound of voices and music. They are startled by sudden noises but can't locate them yet. They can taste, love the sweetness of breast milk, and can tell if you've eaten something different! They can recognize your smell and love being cuddled, stroked, and carried close to you.

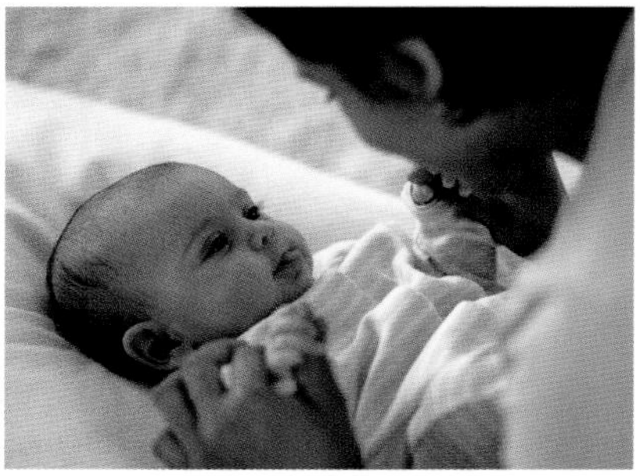

ASK A DOCTOR

My baby's eye is constantly sticky. What can I do about this? Many newborn babies wake up with sticky eyes. This is due to a temporary blockage of the tear ducts, which are tiny in newborn babies. Clear their eye by wiping it with a cotton pad soaked in cooled, boiled water, using a fresh piece for each wipe. The problem usually resolves with time, but if the secretions become yellow and look infected, tell your doctor because your baby may need antibiotic eye drops.

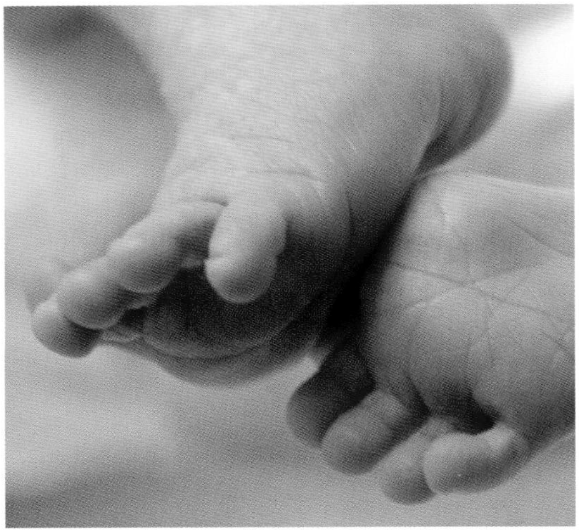

2ND WEEK: **DAY 13**

Feeling close

YOUR BABY TODAY

It's inevitable that your baby will be exposed to viruses and some believe this reduces the risk of allergies later on. However, small babies can be quite sick with a cold, so try to avoid people with colds at first. Breastfeeding provides protection against viruses.

" Now that you and your partner are adapting to your new roles, you can start to think about how to make time for each other. "

EATING WELL

If you're breastfeeding, your need for calcium increases even more than in pregnancy, so have a drink made with milk near you when feeding your baby. You also need more zinc, magnesium, copper, and B vitamins (see p.17).

Most women lose around 10–15 lb (4–7 kg) in the first two weeks. In addition to the loss of the weight of the baby, placenta, and amniotic fluid, you will lose the water that you retained in pregnancy. This water is reabsorbed into your bloodstream, and you'll excrete it through your urine.

After two weeks, your weight loss will slow down, but don't start dieting, especially if you're breastfeeding, since you need extra food and hydration. Your need for additional energy, about an extra 330 calories daily, can be achieved by eating healthy snacks.

Finding time alone together can be hard and resuming your love life can take time. Some women resume their love life without any problems, but for many it takes a little longer, especially if they had stitches and are sore. Also, a difficult birth can affect you emotionally, as can fatigue from lack of sleep. It's recommended that you wait two to three weeks after giving birth before sexual intercourse to let your uterus reduce in size and for the bleeding to stop. Many women prefer to wait until after their six-week checkup (see pp.464–465). Initially, cuddling and having nonpenetrative sex can help you and your partner experience closeness. When you both feel right, you can resume sex, but the first time needs to be gentle and you may need a lubricant since your hormones can cause vaginal dryness, especially with breastfeeding. If intercourse is painful, talk to your doctor, who can make sure you're healing.

You will need to consider contraception now (see p.465). If you're undecided as to what to use and want to resume intercourse, use condoms until your six week checkup when you can discuss the issue.

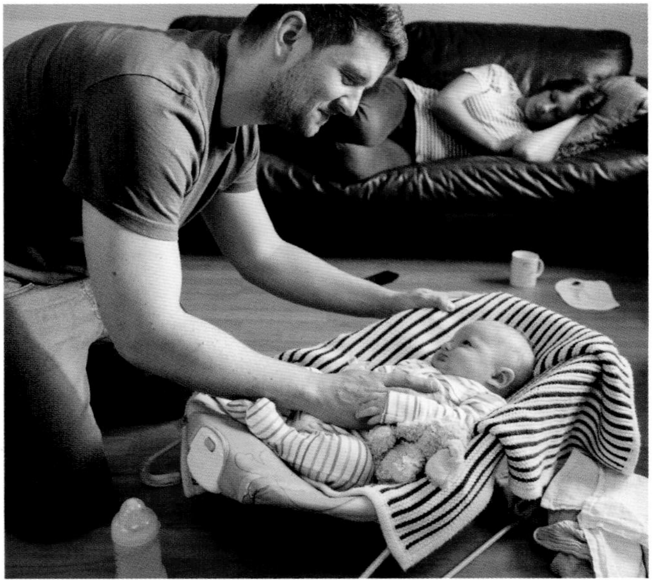

Adapting to family life can mean learning to juggle your time to meet each other's needs.

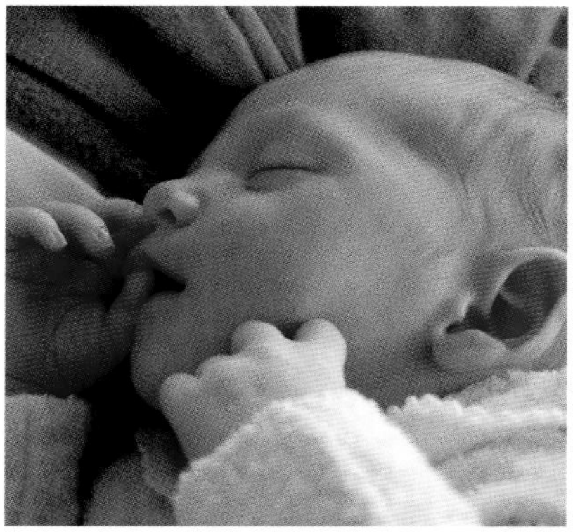

2ND WEEK: **DAY 14**

New beginnings

YOUR BABY TODAY

Now that you are getting the hang of being a new mom, seek out other new parents for some exercise or socializing. There should be many options available to you in your local area.

Babies like to suck, even when they're not hungry anymore. Some suck their fingers or thumbs, but others do nicely with pacifiers. Some parents have strong feelings about whether or not to give a baby a pacifier, but they won't hurt your baby at all and have been linked to a reduction in Sudden Infant Death Syndrome (SIDS) when used during sleep. If you decide to use pacifiers, look for models with soft nipples and a one-piece design that are dishwasher-safe. Have several on hand, since pacifiers tend to fall on the floor. Keep in mind that if a baby depends on a pacifier to sleep, they may wake up and cry if it falls out of. If you are breastfeeding, many experts recommend waiting one month before introducing a pacifier, to avoid nipple confusion.

You may now be getting out more by yourself since your partner may be back at work. Ask your pediatrician about times and venues for support groups in your local area and any stroller-walking groups or baby massage classes since these are excellent ways to meet other moms.

Although you are probably now getting the hang of being parents, it is normal at times to feel completely exhausted. This is a major life change, particularly if this is your first baby, and it can be hard to anticipate all of the changes that are needed to look after a newborn. Take a breath and be reassured that it will get easier. This newborn stage can sometimes feel endless, but cherish the time as soon your baby will no longer be that precious newborn bundle.

> "Life will never be the same again, and by now you will understand the unconditional love of parents for their child."

PHOTOS AND VIDEOS

It's tempting to take photos and videos almost constantly when your first baby is born. Digital photography means that you can email family and friends immediately with new baby images. Subsequent children often remark on how relatively few photos there are of them! However, be aware of how keeping this photographic record, and always having your phone on hand for photos and videos, may sometimes get in the way of just being present with your baby.

ASK A DOCTOR

Should I try to get my baby into a routine? In the first few weeks, it's too early to establish routines. To establish breast-feeding, newborn babies need to be fed on demand and most, in time, will figure out their own routine. If you want to try to establish set feeding times, you will have to consider how you will cope with a screaming baby. However, it's worth starting a nighttime routine early on. Bathing your baby, singing to him, feeding him, and putting him down in his crib to sleep will help him develop good sleep patterns later on.

Your six-week checkup

At two to six weeks after the birth, you will have a postpartum visit with your doctor. This checkup will assess your physical and emotional recovery. Your baby will also have a physical and developmental checkup around this time.

Your assessment

In the first couple of months following the birth of their baby, the majority of women don't experience any major health concerns and will revert back to their prepregnant health status. However, it's good practice to have a general assessment to reassure you that you are well and coping with the early transition to motherhood.

Your postpartum checkup is an ideal opportunity for you to consult your doctor about any concerns you have following the birth of your baby. Any worries about yourself, from your mood to any apprehensions about having sex again, can be discussed at this appointment. Your doctor will offer you advice and possibly treatment and will also be able to refer you to a specialist for further treatment if necessary.

Your physical checkup

Your doctor will do routine checkups, such as taking your blood pressure. They will also ask whether you have any concerns and, if you are breastfeeding, whether you've had any problems with your breasts and lactation.

Your uterus will have returned to nearly its prepregnancy size (about the size of the palm of your hand) and will not be able to be felt. However, your doctor may check your abdomen to see whether the muscles are returning to normal since occasionally the abdominal muscles separate after birth, known as "diastasis recti." If the muscles are more than four fingers apart, you may be referred to a physical therapist. Pilates and core conditioning exercises (see p.250) can help and your doctor may talk to you about these exercises.

Backaches can be a problem after the birth, exacerbated by the pregnancy hormone relaxin (see p.197), which softens muscles and ligaments and remains in the body for a few months after pregnancy. If you're suffering from backaches, your doctor may talk to you about your posture, particularly when you're carrying or feeding your baby, and about the benefits of exercise.

If you had a Cesarean, the incision will be looked at to check that it has healed well. You may still feel numbness around the site of the incision, but sensation should gradually return as the nerve endings renew themselves.

If you haven't had a Pap smear in the last three years, you will likely be given one on the spot, unless you're bleeding heavily.

Checking your bladder You will be asked whether you have any problems urinating, and may be asked for a urine sample if you have symptoms such as frequent urination or stinging when passing urine. Stress incontinence, or leaking urine (see p.477), is common after childbirth, so don't feel embarrassed to mention it.

You may be encouraged to do pelvic floor exercises, or Kegel exercises (see p.69). If the problem persists, you may be referred to a physical therapist for bladder-training exercises.

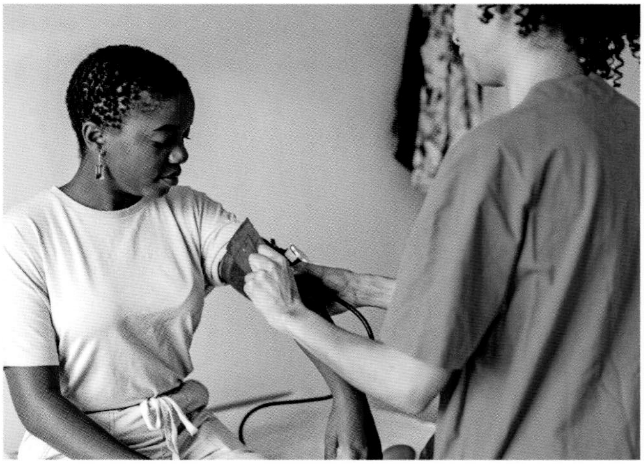

Your postpartum checkup is the ideal time to talk to your doctor about any problems or concerns you have, and to receive reassurance that you have recovered well after the birth.

YOUR BABY'S CHECKUP

A pediatrician will want to see your baby at around 4 days, 1 month, and 2 months to do a physical checkup and look at how your baby is growing and developing.

They will perform a similar examination to the newborn checkup (see p.445). They will examine your baby's hips, spine, eyes, heart, and the pulses at the top of the legs. In boys, it's important to check that the testes are located in the scrotum. This is also a chance to look for subtle problems such as a heart murmur, which can develop after birth. Your baby will be weighed and head circumference measured. The doctor will ask how your baby is feeding and check for signs of jaundice. Your baby's development will be checked too: whether they have head control, is starting to smile, and can focus on an object or face a foot away, and follow a moving object. Your baby should receive some immunizations during these early visits. All these findings will be recorded in a record of your baby's growth and development.

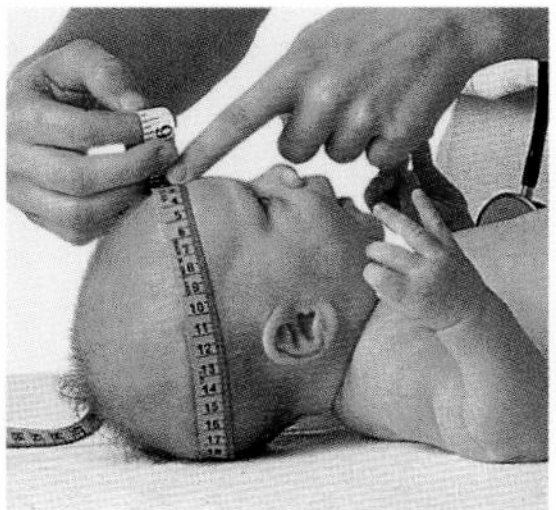

The newborn baby's head circumference is measured at this first check and at ongoing development checks.

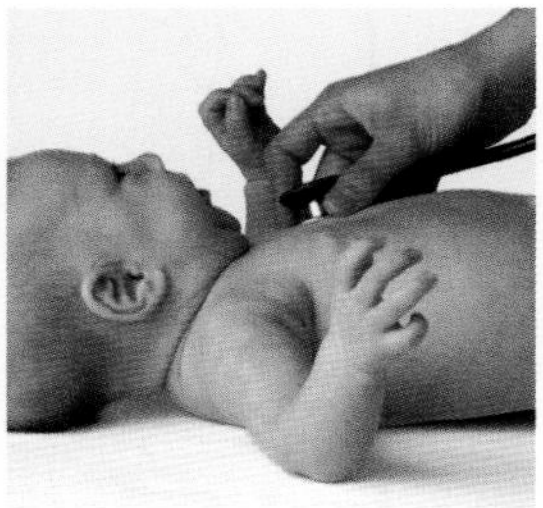

The baby's heart rate and rhythm is listened to, using a stethoscope, to rule out conditions such as a heart murmur.

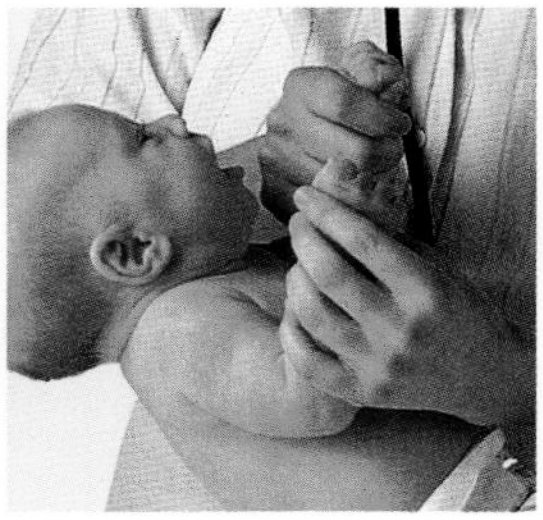

As part of the health examination, the doctor will do a series of physical checks, such as checking head control and the baby's reflexes.

Your stitches If you're still sore from stitches, your doctor will check that these are healing properly. Although most stitches are absorbable, they can take up to three months to completely absorb. Bathing can sometimes help the stitches absorb, but if you continue to have problems your doctor may recommend Sitz baths two or three times a day or a topical anesthetic cream (see also Perineal problems, p.477).

Your emotional well-being

In addition to checking you physically, the doctor will assess your emotional and mental health. Many women feel extremely tired in these early weeks, as night feedings and constant demands begin to take their toll. However, if you are feeling low, overly tired, or depressed a lot of the time, you may be suffering from postpartum depression (see p.477), so it's important not to ignore these symptoms. Your doctor will offer support and refer you to mental health experts if needed.

Looking at your lifestyle

Your doctor will advise you on healthy eating and lifestyle measures. If you smoke, you'll be given information and resources to help you stop.

QUESTIONS AND ANSWERS

Is it true that I don't need to worry about getting pregnant again while I'm breast-feeding? If you are breastfeeding, you may not have a period for a while after giving birth. Although this means you are less likely to conceive, you can still ovulate, so you shouldn't assume that you don't need to use contraception. The doctor will discuss contraception and sexual health with you and may recommend the progesterone-only pill, which can be prescribed from 21 days if you're breastfeeding.

I'm bottle-feeding my baby and am worried about getting pregnant again. How soon could this happen? If you are bottle-feeding, you will probably have had your first period prior to this checkup and so certainly could become pregnant again. Although your doctor will have already discussed contraception with you, this will be addressed again at your six-week checkup. The doctor or nurse will want to ensure that you have contraceptive measures in place; if not, they will offer you guidance and advice.

I had stitches and have felt too anxious to have sex since the birth. Is this normal? Yes, plenty of women feel this way and many wait to resume sex until after their postpartum checkup. During this checkup, the doctor or nurse will be able to confirm that your incision has healed, and offer reassurance about resuming sex. On the other hand, there is nothing wrong with having sex before this checkup as long as you have stopped bleeding. When you do have sex, you may need to use a lubricant (KY Jelly), particularly if you're breastfeeding, since your hormones can cause some vaginal dryness.

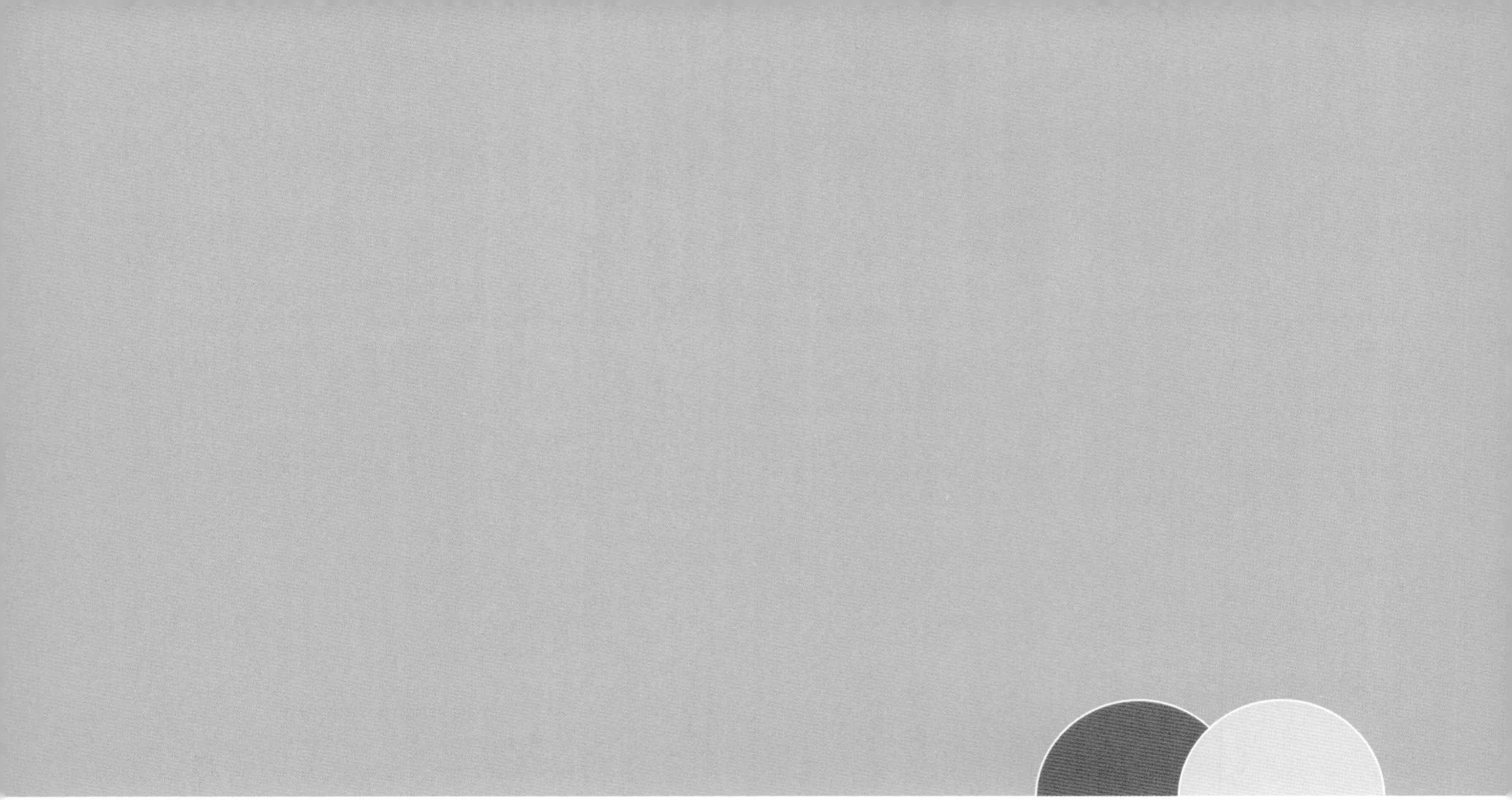

CONCERNS AND COMPLICATIONS

Rarely does pregnancy pass without some complaint, but the majority of problems are minor. Some, however, are more serious and require medical attention. Today, high-quality prenatal care means that potentially serious conditions are usually successfully managed, both during pregnancy and in labor. Problems after the birth, either in the baby or the mother, may need medical attention with careful follow-up and sometimes referral to a specialist.

Common concerns in pregnancy

In this section, you will find a list of common concerns with an explanation of the adaptation process that may cause these symptoms, information on whether medical help is likely to be required, and advice on measures you can take yourself to alleviate symptoms.

General symptoms

Fatigue usually subsides during the second trimester but is likely to return in the third trimester.
Causes The main causes are massive hormonal changes and the extra demands on the body made by an increase in blood volume of up to 50 percent. This increase helps the lining of the uterus to thicken and the placenta to develop. Late in pregnancy, fatigue may recur because your extra size and weight and the demands of the growing baby means that your body systems need to work harder. Difficulty sleeping can contribute to tiredness, and it can also be caused by anemia (see p.474).
What to do If you are working, take regular breaks and get some fresh air at least once a day. Ensure that your fluid intake is adequate; caffeine is not helpful because it dehydrates your body and will leave you feeling worse. Take more time for sleep if you need to; housework can wait and you may need to cut back on social commitments.

Difficulty sleeping is common, especially in the first and third trimesters.
Causes A common cause of disturbed sleep is the need to urinate frequently. Early in pregnancy, this is due to the amount of blood in your body, leading to the kidneys filtering out more fluid, which ends up in your bladder. Another factor is expansion of the uterus, which competes for space with the bladder. This leads the bladder to require more frequent emptying. Many women also feel hungry during the night and need to snack, while others find that nausea and vomiting interrupt their night or lead to early waking. From about 20 weeks of pregnancy, the uterus moves up out of the pelvis, taking pressure off the bladder, and nausea often subsides, which means that sleep improves. Toward the end of pregnancy, sleep patterns can once again be disturbed. Unborn babies are often active just when you want to rest; your body is bulky and finding comfortable sleeping positions becomes difficult; and as the baby becomes bigger and heavier, pressure on the bladder may return.
What to do If frequent urination is keeping you awake, don't drink large quantities of fluid close to bedtime, and to avoid waking up hungry include foods high in unrefined carbohydrates, such as whole wheat bread, in your evening meal. If you do wake up, don't lie there for long periods, since this is frustrating and may lead to habitual sleeplessness. Later in pregnancy when you find it difficult to get comfortable, experiment with different sleeping positions: use plenty of pillows, under your head and belly and between your knees. A rest during the day is essential during late pregnancy, but limit this to a 20-minute power nap or an hour reading or watching television with your feet up. If you sleep for long periods during the day, you will further lessen your ability to sleep at night.

Headaches are common, especially in the first trimester.
Causes Most headaches are unlikely to be a cause for concern and are probably due to hormonal changes and the need for additional fluids. Headaches occurring in the third trimester that are accompanied by other symptoms, such as abdominal pain or nausea, may be a sign of preeclampsia and should be assessed by a doctor (see p.476).
What to do If you have a headache in late pregnancy that is accompanied by swelling of the legs and ankles, generalized body swelling, abdominal pain, or nausea and vomiting, contact your doctor or midwife immediately. If you have a sudden onset of a severe headache, you should also consult your doctor. Make sure you drink enough clear fluids and avoid caffeine. If you're working or concentrating on a task, have regular breaks, and get some fresh air. From 12 weeks, it's safe to take two 500mg acetaminophen tablets every eight hours, with no more than three doses in a 24-hour period. If you suspect your headache is due to lack of sleep, try to get more sleep. And make sure you're eating enough, since hunger and low blood sugar can cause headaches. Relieve stress—another headache trigger—with deep breathing, meditation, yoga, or massage Always discuss your symptoms with your doctor before taking medication.

Swollen feet, ankles, hands, and wrists can be particularly pronounced in hot weather.
Causes Swelling is the result of fluid retention, which in turn results from the extra blood produced during pregnancy.
What to do Alternate light activity

with periods of rest during which your feet are elevated. However, avoid staying in bed or sitting in a chair for very long periods as this may increase the risk of deep vein thrombosis (DVT; see p.186). Swollen feet and ankles can also be a sign of other problems such as preeclampsia (see p.474) so should always be reported to your doctor who can check for other symptoms.

Skin changes

Itching and dry skin may worsen in the second and third trimester. Such skin irritation is a reaction to hormonal changes and can be eased by a perfume-free moisturizer. Rarely, itching in late pregnancy may be due to obstetric cholestasis (see p.475). This itching is much more severe, usually constant, and concentrated on the palms of the hands and soles of the feet. If you develop itching, tell your doctor or midwife who will arrange a blood test.

Increased pigmentation is due to the increased production of hormones. Most women notice a darkening of the area around the nipple and a dark line, the linea nigra, vertically through the middle of the bump from the umbilicus to the pelvis. Also common are dark patches on the cheeks, nose, and chin, known as melasma (or the "mask of pregnancy.") On women with dark skin, the patches may appear lighter than surrounding skin. Use a high-protection sunscreen cream on your face.

Stretch marks Rapid stretching of the skin during pregnancy often leads to the development of pink or purple lines. These stretch marks usually appear in late pregnancy, commonly on the abdomen, hips, thighs, and upper breast. There is no clear evidence that any cream will prevent or remove stretch marks, although a light unscented moisturizer can help keep the skin supple, as will staying well hydrated and avoiding excessive weight gain. As time passes after the birth, stretch marks become silvery and almost invisible.

Breast problems

Breast tenderness is often one of the first signs of pregnancy, sometimes becoming so painful that you can't bear them to be touched; they may also throb and feel hot. This usually subsides by the end of the first trimester.
Causes The milk ducts are starting to enlarge and blood flow increases.
What to do Wear a properly fitted bra to support your breasts and reduce discomfort. An ill-fitting or tight bra will be uncomfortable and may put pressure on the milk ducts. You may also find it helpful to wear a soft sleep bra or bralette at night. If your breasts feel hot, applying a cool cloth to them may bring relief. If you have a painful or red patch on a breast, tell your doctor as it could be mastitis (see p.477).

Nipple problems Women who have flat nipples that do not protrude or whose nipples are inverted may worry that they may not be able to breastfeed. All healthy women can breastfeed because babies feed by taking in a mouthful of breast, not just the nipple.
Causes Inverted or flat nipples are thought to be due to shorter ligaments in the underlying breast tissue that pull the nipples inward.
What to do If you have any concerns about the suitability of your nipples for breastfeeding, talk to your doctor who can refer you to a lactation consultant. There are also products available that will draw out nipples in preparation for breastfeeding. However, these are by o means essential because when babies latch on to the breast they are able to draw out even a flat or inverted nipple (although you may need a lactation consultant to show you the best way to help your baby do this).

Digestive problems

Nausea and vomiting Approximately 80 percent of women are troubled by the unpleasant symptoms of nausea and vomiting in early pregnancy. This usually subsides between 12 and 20 weeks; however, it's not uncommon to experience some return of these problems late in the pregnancy.
Causes In the first trimester, pregnancy hormones interact with hormones that control other body systems, particularly those involved with blood sugar regulation, and this results in feelings of nausea and vomiting. Late in pregnancy, problems with digestion may occur because the uterus takes up most of the space in the abdomen, displacing your intestines and stomach and leaving little room for the digestion of large amounts of food.
What to do Drink plenty of water throughout the day and eat small amounts of food on a regular basis, which will help to avoid long gaps between meals, and snacking on complex carbohydrates such as whole wheat and whole grain products. Avoid snacks with a high sugar content because, although these will give you a quick boost, they will soon leave you feeling worse than before because your blood sugar will plummet. Reducing your overall intake of the refined sugar found in candy, cake, cookies, and sugary drinks will help reduce the symptoms of nausea and vomiting and will also lessen your risk of developing gestational diabetes.

Gastroenteritis This is inflammation of the lining of the stomach and intestines, most commonly due to infection. It causes vomiting and diarrhea that usually come on suddenly. In most cases, the condition clears up on its own. However, if it's severe, you could become dehydrated, and this can affect blood flow to your baby through the placenta. Infection with listeria bacteria

can, rarely, cause late miscarriage.
Causes Gastroenteritis is caused by infection contracted either through contact with an infected person or by food poisoning.
What to do Drink plenty of water, and try to avoid cross infection with other members of the household. If you're unable to retain even small sips of water, or your vomiting and diarrhea have lasted for 24 hours, seek medical advice from your doctor. If you can't reach your doctor, go to the nearest hospital emergency room for treatment. If you have a preexisting medical condition, such as diabetes, seek help immediately. You may be treated with intravenous fluids if you are dehydrated, and fetal monitoring may be carried out. Infection with listeria is treated with antibiotics.
Avoiding gastroenteritis Practice good food hygiene (see p.16). If someone else in your household has gastroenteritis, avoid infection by using separate soap, towels, cutlery, and dishes. If you have more than one bathroom, get the infected person to use a separate one. Wipe toilets, sinks, and faucets with a mild bleach solution after each use. Infected individuals should also avoid preparing food for others.

Indigestion and heartburn are common during the second trimester.
Causes Indigestion results from slower movements of the digestive tract under the influence of pregnancy hormones combined with reduced space in the stomach. The muscular valve at the top of the stomach is also softened by hormones, allowing acid to flow into the esophagus, causing heartburn.
What to do Avoid large meals, especially late at night, to help prevent indigestion and heartburn. Try sleeping in a propped-up position with your head higher than your feet. For relief from heartburn, a liquid antacid preparation can be helpful; ask your doctor for advice on which medications are safe. Some women find that slowly drinking a glass of milk eases the discomfort.

Constipation is often a problem during the second trimester.
Causes Under the influence of the softening effect of pregnancy hormones, the digestive tract becomes less active. As a result, fecal matter spends more time in the large intestine, allowing reabsorption of fluids and leaving solids hard and difficult to pass. Not drinking enough fluids increases the likelihood of constipation.
What to do Dietary fiber in the form of vegetables and whole foods, with an increase in fluid intake, usually corrects the problem. Laxatives are not recommended during pregnancy. They can stimulate contractions and lead to dehydration. Talk to your doctor if these steps don't resolve your constipation.

Hemorrhoids are dilated blood vessels around the inside of, or protruding from, the anus. Their constriction by the anal muscles and sensitivity to the acidic environment leads to a feeling of discomfort in mild episodes and pain in more severe cases. They are more likely to occur during the third trimester.
Causes The hormonal softening of the tissues around the anus increases the risk of developing hemorrhoids. Pressure of the baby's head on the blood vessels is also a factor, as is constipation (see above).
What to do Treatment of constipation and avoiding pushing or straining to pass a stool are important in the prevention. Ask your doctor which over-the-counter creams for relieving discomfort are safe. If hemorrhoids are protruding and causing great discomfort, it's often possible for a health professional to "reduce" them by pushing them gently back into place.

Heart & circulation problems

Dizziness and faintness Throughout pregnancy, occasional dizziness or feelings of faintness can be a problem.
Causes In early pregnancy, feeling faint may occur even when you are sitting down and is likely to be due to low blood sugar. This can happen as a result of not eating enough, a common problem at this stage of pregnancy when many women suffer from morning sickness. In the second trimester, dizziness or faintness that comes on when getting up from a sitting position or as a result of standing for long periods is likely to be caused by low blood pressure. Blood pressure is lowered in pregnancy because the pregnancy hormone progesterone softens blood vessels to enable blood to flow more freely to your baby. When you stand, the low blood pressure may mean that not enough blood reaches your brain, leading to dizziness and faintness.
As pregnancy advances, you may find that you feel dizzy lying on your back. This happens because in this position the heavy uterus puts pressure on the main blood vessels running through the trunk and reduces the blood flow to the brain.
What to do To help prevent low blood sugar, have small snacks of foods high in complex carbohydrates (see p.92). Staying well hydrated, taking regular breaks from work, not standing in one position for too long, and getting fresh air are also helpful in preventing faintness. If you start to feel dizzy, sit down and put your head between your legs, which will relieve the unpleasant feeling. Stay seated until you feel completely recovered and then get up slowly. Any time you feel dizzy or faint, call your doctor immediately, especially if you also have stomach pain, vaginal bleeding, blurry vision, headaches, or heart palpitations, or the dizziness is

persistent. If you have fainted and bumped your head or injured any part of your body, then you should go to the hospital for a checkup.

If you experience dizziness when lying on your back, turning onto your side will quickly help you feel better. Lying on your left side is preferable because this helps pump blood around the body.

Palpitations A feeling that your heart is racing, or beating irregularly is common in pregnancy, particularly between 28 and 32 weeks, but can occur at any time.
Causes The reasons for palpitations remain unclear, and hypotheses range from the effect that progesterone has on the heart muscle to the heart coping with the extra blood flow needed to maintain both mother and fetus.
What to do Heart palpitations are usually fleeting and nothing to worry about. However, if you have frequent palpitations or they are accompanied by chest pain, dizziness, or breathlessness, you should consult your doctor. If you have a history of heart disease or a heart abnormality, seek advice urgently.
Nosebleeds Nosebleeds occur frequently in pregnancy, and although they are a nuisance, they are rarely a serious problem.
Causes As with all other blood vessels in the body, those in the nose are softened and expanded during pregnancy. In addition, your body has an increased blood volume in pregnancy, which puts pressure on these delicate structures. You are more likely to have a nosebleed if you have a cold or sinus infection or if your nasal membrane is dry, which can happen in cold weather or air conditioned rooms.
What to do To manage a nosebleed, sit down, keep your head in a normal position, and apply pressure to the bottom of the nose with your thumb and forefinger. You will need to maintain this pressure constantly for about 10 minutes before checking to see if the bleeding has stopped. Do not be tempted to tip your head back or lie down, since this will cause you to swallow the blood, leading to nausea and possible vomiting. Ice or a cold compress applied to the nose and facial area in conjunction with the nasal pressure can help constrict the blood flow and halt the bleeding. Seek medical advice if the nosebleed results from a head injury or if heavy bleeding continues for more than 20 minutes. Mention frequent small nosebleeds at your prenatal appointment to eliminate more serious conditions.

Bleeding, tender gums This is a common complaint during pregnancy.
Causes These problems occur as a result of increased blood volume coupled with the softening effect of pregnancy hormones on blood vessels. Allowing plaque to accumulate may exacerbate these symptoms and also makes the start of gum disease more likely to occur.
What to do Good dental hygiene is vital; don't be tempted to avoid brushing your teeth if they feel tender, but switch to a softer brush. Brushing your teeth and gums and flossing regularly are particularly important during pregnancy. Also, visit your dentist regularly during pregnancy and the postpartum period.

Varicose veins and vulval varicosities Varicose veins are enlarged, distorted veins that may develop in the legs or around the vulval area. Varicose veins in or around the anus are known as hemorrhoids (see p.468). Varicose veins may become troublesome during the later stages of pregnancy, causing discomfort and sometimes itching; they may also be unsightly. Varicosities in the vagina or vulva areas do not inhibit a normal birth and are not at risk of rupture during the birth.
Causes The increased blood flow and softened vessels mean that many women experience varicose veins and vulva varicosities during pregnancy. The growing uterus puts pressure on veins in the pelvis, which, in turn, leads to increased pressure in the legs and vulva area.
What to do Support hose designed for pregnancy can be helpful, Avoid tight clothes that constrict the waist, groin, or legs. Varicose veins should be reported to your doctor for assessment and advice. Varicose veins usually improve within three months after the birth of the baby.

Aches & pains

Backaches Lower generalized backaches are extremely common in pregnancy, particularly in the third trimester; around two-thirds of all pregnant women suffer from backaches.
Causes As pregnancy progresses, the increased weight of your abdomen tends to pull on the lower spine so that it curves inward and your center of gravity shifts forward. As you try to correct this, you may strain the lower back muscles. In addition, pregnancy hormones soften your ligaments, causing them to stretch and provide less support for your back.
What to do Maintaining good posture and avoiding tilting your pelvis forward helps relieve pressure on your back and helps both prevent and alleviate backaches. Regular, moderate exercise to keep your muscles toned and supple is also beneficial. See pages 90 and 250 for suggested exercise routines. Yoga, Pilates, and water aerobics are also recommended.

Try to avoid standing in one position for too long and vary your daily tasks, breaking them down into shorter stints. If your work involves standing or sitting for long periods, take regular short breaks, and while sitting, make sure your lower back is supported. Avoid lifting heavy objects.

Massage and warm water can help relieve backaches. If back pain is particularly troublesome, talk to your doctor about wearing a supportive maternity belt.

Pelvic girdle pain (PGP) Also known as symphysis pubis dysfunction, pelvic girdle pain (PGP) refers to discomfort and pain felt in the pelvic area and groin. The pain may be concentrated in the buttocks or travel down one leg, which is why it is sometimes mistaken for sciatica (see right). PGP is often worse when doing activities such as walking or going up stairs; it may also be troublesome at night. PGP is most common toward the end of pregnancy and may range in severity from mild to serious enough to need a walking aid.
Causes The pelvis is made up of three bones: the sacrum and the two iliac (hip) bones. The bones are connected at the front by the symphysis pubis joint, and at the back by the sacroiliac joints. The joints are stabilized by ligaments and usually move very little. During pregnancy, however, ligaments soften and stretch more easily so that there is more movement at these joints. This results in instability of the pelvis. In addition, postural changes due to the enlarging abdomen may mean that one joint is more mobile than the other, putting extra strain on the joints. The result is inflammation of the joints, resulting in inflammation.
What to do If there is increased movement in one side of your pelvis, a support belt may be recommended. You may be referred to a physical therapist who will show you how to modify everyday activities to avoid pain and may recommend abdominal and Kegel exercises (see p.69). Acupuncture can help relieve pain, and prenatal water aerobic classes are helpful. Preventative measures include refraining from activities that cause pain and avoiding heavy lifting, lying on your back, and sustained periods of activity. It's also important to get plenty of rest.

Round ligament pain The two round ligaments run from the top of the uterus on either side and attach to the side walls of the abdomen. As the uterus enlarges, the round ligaments gradually become stretched, which can cause an ache or brief, sharp pain on one or both sides of the lower abdomen or in the groin. Round ligament pain usually starts during the second trimester.
What to do See your doctor, who will rule out other causes for the abdominal pain. Once you have been reassured, you should find it easier to deal with the pain. When you have an episode, try to rest and relax. Lying on your side and bringing your knees up toward your chest may be helpful, as can taking a warm bath.

Sciatica is pain in one or both buttocks that may radiate down one leg. In a small percentage of women, a tingling or numbness in the legs may also occur. Sciatica is most likely to occur after the second trimester.
Causes Sciatica is caused by trapping or compression of the sciatic nerve as it runs through the spinal column. The pain is termed referred pain, as it is felt in an area away from the problem site. Sciatica is not caused by compression of the nerve by the fetus's head. The causes of sciatica in pregnancy are the same as in women who are not pregnant and include poor posture, wear and tear on vertebral joints, and poor lifting techniques.
What to do Specific exercises can help to stretch muscles gently and release pressure on the sciatic nerve. Your doctor may be able to advise you on exercises or may refer you to a physical therapist for help.
Coccygeal pain The coccyx, or tailbone, is the small bone found at the base of the spine. This bone is usually fairly immobile; however, in pregnancy it becomes more mobile, which facilitates the passage of the baby through the birth canal during labor. Pain in this area can make sitting for long periods extremely uncomfortable, particularly at work or during travel. Coccygeal pain can occur throughout pregnancy.
Causes Coccygeal pain may predate pregnancy due to a previous injury to the area; the discomfort may then be exacerbated by the hormonal and mechanical changes of pregnancy. Alternatively, coccygeal pain may arise, as increased movement in the coccyx during this time makes injury more likely. Sometimes the coccyx is injured during labor by the baby's head, and coccygeal pain therefore develops after the birth.
What to do Moving around frequently and gently massaging the area can help relieve discomfort. Ask your doctor which analgesics are safe for you to take. The condition usually gets better within 6 weeks of delivery.
Leg cramps Cramps in the legs, particularly in the calf muscles, are a common problem during pregnancy. These leg cramps occur most commonly at night but may sometimes come on when walking, and their frequency can increase as your pregnancy advances.
Causes There is debate as to the cause of leg cramps in pregnancy. They are likely to be caused by a combination of factors, including maternal posture, increasing body weight, restriction in the blood flow to the legs, and the pressure of the uterus on the pelvic nerves. Some suggest that leg cramps in pregnancy may be due to a lack of salt in the diet. However, research demonstrates that low levels of salt are healthy in pregnancy, and that it is very unlikely that anyone who is eating a balanced diet will suffer from salt depletion.

What to do Leg cramps may be relieved by changing position, flexing the toes of the affected leg upward, and massaging the cramped muscle. To avoid leg cramps, massage your legs before bed and avoid sitting or standing in one position for long periods. A warm bath before bed may also help. Stay well hydrated and alternate regular periods of moderate exercise with periods of rest.

If you have persistent pain, redness, or swelling in your calf, this may be a sign of deep vein thrombosis (DVT) (see p.186), which requires prompt medical attention.

Restless legs syndrome This is an uncomfortable feeling or unpleasant tingling that creates an overwhelming desire to move your legs, or causes legs to jerk uncontrollably, especially during sleep. Sufferers describe the sensation as being like an electric current passing through the legs or like having itchy bones. It is most likely to occur during the third trimester.
Causes Restless legs syndrome is frequently triggered or aggravated by pregnancy. The cause is unknown, but some studies indicate that it might be related to low iron levels. Many sufferers have a family history of the condition.
What to do Talk to your doctor about having a full blood count to check your iron levels. Some women find it helpful to exercise or stretch their legs, to use hot or cold compresses, or to have a leg massage. If the condition occurs for the first time in pregnancy, there is a very good chance that it will disappear after the baby is born.

Carpal tunnel syndrome The carpal tunnel is a small tunnel in the wrist through which nerves run from your forearm into your hands and fingers. Carpal tunnel syndrome occurs when the nerves are compressed, resulting in tingling and pain in the fingers, which is often worse at night. In severe cases, there may be considerable discomfort and a reduced grip. It is most likely in the second and third trimesters.
Causes Carpal tunnel syndrome is caused by pressure on nerves running through the tunnel due to swelling of surrounding tissues. During pregnancy, swelling in the hands and feet is common as a result of the extra fluid and blood volume.
What to do Talk to your doctor. You may be referred to a physical therapist for treatment, who will recommend specific exercises to help relieve the discomfort. You may also be advised to wear a lightweight splint to support the wrists. Carpal tunnel syndrome usually disappears after the birth, but if it persists, a simple operation can be carried out.

Urinary and vaginal problems

Having an increased amount of vaginal discharge during pregnancy is normal. However, if the discharge is creamy and thick, and you also have some soreness and itching, you may have a yeast infection. If you have a vaginal discharge that has a fishy odor, particularly after having sex, you may have bacterial vaginosis (BV), a common cause of vaginal discharge. It has been associated with an increased risk of premature labor but usually only in those women who are at risk of premature labor for other reasons.
Causes Both yeast and BV occur when the acidity of the vagina drops, which is common in pregnancy. BV is caused by a lack of lactobacilli (good bacteria) and yeast is caused by a fungus called Candida albicans.
What to do Avoid washing your vagina with strongly scented soaps and gels. Go see your doctor for advice.

Stress incontinence

You will pass small amounts of urine unintentionally, particularly when you are coughing, sneezing, or laughing, and when you are exercising or lifting heavy objects. It is most common in the last trimester.
Causes The pelvic-floor muscles are additionally strained during pregnancy and are also affected by hormonal changes. Therefore, any increase in abdominal pressure may result in leakage of urine.
What to do Practicing pelvic floor exercises (see p.69) regularly should help. Empty your bladder without delay whenever you need to. Wear a sanitary pad for additional reassurance.

Urinary-tract infections (UTIs) During pregnancy, you are more susceptible to UTIs. Most commonly, they are confined to the bladder and known as cystitis. Symptoms include a frequent, urgent need to urinate and a painful burning sensation when urinating; there may be some blood in your urine. Occasionally, an infection can travel to the kidneys. In this case, you may also have pain in your lower back on one side, a high temperature, and you may feel nauseated or vomit. Sometimes there are no symptoms. Prompt treatment of UTIs is especially important because if an infection reaches the kidneys, it can trigger early labor.
Causes UTIss are caused by bacteria entering the body through the urethra and multiplying. Such infections are probably more common during pregnancy due to hormonal changes.
What to do If you have any symptoms of a UTI, see your doctor right away. The doctor will take a midstream urine sample to identify the type of bacteria that is causing the infection. Your doctor may prescribe a seven to 10 day course of antibiotics that are safe for both you and your baby. Symptoms usually improve in a few days after the start of treatment. Because some UTIs are asymptomatic, you may be screened for this at 28 weeks..

Complications of pregnancy & labor

Certain conditions classify the pregnancy as high risk. A high-risk pregnancy is closely monitored with more frequent prenatal appointments, fetal monitoring, and possibly additional ultrasounds. In labor, certain complications require immediate intervention.

Pregnancy complications

Miscarriage Early pregnancy loss is the most common complication during the first trimester and happens in 10 percent of known pregnancies (see p.94).

Ectopic pregnancy occurs when a fertilized egg implants outside of the uterine cavity, most commonly in the Fallopian tube.

Causes Any woman can have an ectopic pregnancy, but the risk is increased if you've had a pelvic infection; became pregnant with a progesterone-releasing IUD in place, while taking the mini-pill, or as a result of fertility treatment; have endometriosis; have had abdominal surgery or a previous ectopic pregnancy.

Symptoms Most women who have an ectopic pregnancy notice pain and light bleeding at 6–8 weeks (2–4 weeks after a missed period). The pain is usually felt on one side of the lower abdomen and may be severe and persistent. If an ectopic pregnancy isn't recognized early and an embryo growing in the Fallopian tube ruptures the tube, you may feel sudden severe pain that spreads across the abdomen. Internal bleeding from a ruptured tube can also irritate the diaphragm, causing shoulder pain. If you have severe lower abdominal pain, call your doctor and go to the ER.

What might be done A ruptured ectopic pregnancy is life-threatening. Usually, an ectopic pregnancy is suspected before this stage. In this case, you'll have an ultrasound, usually through the vagina, which often diagnoses the problem; there is no pregnancy seen in the uterus; blood may be seen in the abdomen; and sometimes the ectopic pregnancy itself can be seen. You may also have blood tests to monitor the levels of hCG (pregnancy hormone); if levels of hCG plateau or rise slightly, this indicates an abnormal pregnancy. If an ectopic pregnancy hasn't been confirmed by these investigations, you may be offered a D&C to diagnose the location of the pregnancy.

If needed, surgery to remove the Fallopian tube is commonly performed by laparoscopy, a minimally invasive technique, or an incision at the bikini line. If diagnosed early, an ectopic pregnancy can be treated with methotrexate, which stops the pregnancy from developing. This is appropriate only if the hCG levels are low and the tube hasn't ruptured. The advantage is that surgery is avoided; however, the treatment doesn't always work, can be associated with significant pain, and close follow-up is vital.

Hyperemesis gravidarum Most women experience some nausea in pregnancy. Occasionally, vomiting may be severe. If you're unable to hold down food or drink for more than 24 hours, see your doctor.

What might be done Your urine may be checked for infection, and you may have an ultrasound if the pregnancy has not been confirmed yet. Your weight will be monitored, as weight loss of 10 percent of your body weight can increase the risk of complications. If you're very dehydrated, your doctor may advise a short hospitalization so you can receive intravenous fluids, and you may be given anti-nausea drugs and a vitamin supplement. Hyperemesis usually disappears by 13 weeks.

Anemia is a low level of hemoglobin, the oxygen-carrying component of red blood cells. Mild anemia is common because the extra fluid content of blood dilutes the number of red blood cells. Also, the baby uses some of your iron reserves. If you have anemia, you may feel tired and breathless and look pale.

Causes Usually, anemia is due to iron deficiency. Occasionally, it's due to a lack of folic acid, vitamin B12, or rarer other problems. Bloodwork will help identify the cause.

What might be done Anemia is usually remedied with an iron supplement, but side effects may include constipation and black stools, so some women prefer to boost iron intake with diet (see p.154).

Weakened cervix Rarely, a woman may have a weakened cervix, which can lead to a miscarriage after 13 weeks. Usually, these miscarriages are relatively painless: you may feel well and perhaps notice some extra vaginal discharge and then quite quickly miscarry the baby.

Causes Risk factors include a previous late miscarriage; cervical surgery; or a previous late termination of pregnancy.

What might be done If you're thought to be at risk, your doctor may suggest a scan to check the length of your cervix since a shortened cervix makes miscarriage more likely. If you had two or more late miscarriages, your doctor may recommend a cervical stitch put in at around 14–16 weeks to sew the cervix closed, which is left in until you're about 37 weeks pregnant.

Obstetric cholestasis is a rare condition affecting liver function that causes a buildup of bile acids in the bloodstream. The main symptom is severe itching without a rash, usually most intense on the palms of the hands and soles of the feet. It usually occurs after 28 weeks.
Causes Although not clear, genetic factors are likely involved since it tends to run in families. A woman who has the condition in one pregnancy will usually develop it in future pregnancies. Increased sensitivity to pregnancy hormones, which effect the way bile is processed, is also thought to play a role.
What might be done If you have itching of the palms of your hands and soles of your feet, having bloodwork done can check your liver function and bile acids. If labs are abnormal, you may be diagnosed with cholestasis of pregnancy. The itching is often treated with ursodeoxycholic acid. You will also need fetal monitoring; those with severe cholestasis may need to deliver preterm at 36 weeks due to risk of stillbirth.

Gestational diabetes develops due to pregnancy. In this condition, the pancreas produces insufficient insulin to move glucose (sugar) from the blood to be stored, resulting in high levels of glucose in the blood. It usually begins at 20–24 weeks. The risk is greater if you have a family history of late-onset diabetes or you've previously had a large baby, a stillbirth, or gestational diabetes.
Causes Insulin levels are inadequate due to the extra demands of the fetus and because hormones produced by the placenta block the effects of insulin.
What might be done Between 24 and 28 weeks, you'll be tested for gestational diabetes. If you have risk factors, you may take this test earlier. The test involves having a blood test in the morning after fasting, then drinking a special sugary drink and having a repeat blood sugar check one hour later. If you have high levels of glucose, you'll have to take a similar but longer test to confirm a diagnosis. If you do have gestational diabetes, you will be taught how to test blood glucose at home. In most cases, the diabetes can be controlled through diet and exercise. However, if these measures are ineffective you may need medication to reduce blood sugar levels or insulin injections. Extra scans may be done to check the baby's growth, and early induction (see p.432) may be advised. If you've had gestational diabetes, ensure your weight is normal before becoming pregnant again.

Polyhydramnios is an excess of amniotic fluid. Symptoms include a stretched feeling in the abdomen; breathlessness, heartburn; swelling in the legs; and constipation. It is more likely with diabetes; twins; with an infection; or where there is a congenital problem in the baby. The condition increases the risk of premature labor and cord prolapse. You will be carefully monitored and may be advised to rest. In severe cases, the fluid may be drained.

Oligohydramnios Too little amniotic fluid may be due to early rupture of the membranes; placental problems; fetal abnormalities; or problems with the baby's growth (see p.284). A reduction of amniotic fluid is most likely toward the end of pregnancy. If an ultrasound scan confirms that levels are low and there are concerns about the baby's growth, early delivery may be advised.

Placental insufficiency occurs when the placenta isn't functioning well enough. Some signs are a reduction in the amount of fluid around the baby, a decrease in the growth of the baby's abdomen and hence their weight, and abnormalities in an ultrasound (see p.285).
Causes Placental insufficiency is more common in women with preeclampsia, those who have an underlying medical problem, and in women who smoke. It also occurs more often in babies with a chromosomal abnormality or a structural congenital abnormality.
What might be done It is usually detected by the doctor noticing that your uterus measures smaller than expected and referring you for an ultrasound. If the baby isn't growing well, the doctor will watch you closely and may recommend bed rest for some or the rest of your pregnancy. If the placenta is working poorly, your baby may not be able to cope with labor; a Cesarean may be recommended.

Bleeding in late pregnancy If bleeding occurs, you and the baby need to be assessed immediately. Bleeding caused by a problem with the placenta can be a serious threat to your baby.
Causes The most serious causes are placenta previa (see p.212) and placental abruption. With a placenta previa, the placenta lies low in the uterus and bleeding is typically painless. In a placental abruption, the placenta starts to separate from the uterus, which can be very painful as the blood can be trapped inside the uterus. Both of these can be life-threatening to your baby. Other, less-dangerous causes include cervical friability, or bleeding from the cervix itself, especially after intercourse, or from a cervical polyp.
What might be done If bleeding is mild, your doctor may recommend bed rest. If your doctor thinks you have abruption, they may send you to the hospital for observation. Depending on how far

along you are, you may be given corticosteroids to help the baby's lungs mature in case an early delivery is necessary. Your doctor may send you home when the bleeding stops. Sometimes, delivering the baby is the safest option. If bleeding is heavy or painful, or the baby is distressed, an emergency Cesarean and a blood transfusion may be needed.

Preeclampsia Preeclampsia (also known as toxemia) is a pregnancy-induced condition characterized by high blood pressure, protein in the urine, and edema (swelling). Occasionally women have symptoms such as headaches, flashing lights, abdominal pain, or nausea. If left untreated, it can lead to eclampsia, an extremely serious condition that causes convulsions and coma. If diagnosed with preeclampsia, your pregnancy will be watched very closely and a decision will be made as to the best time for delivery. About 8 percent of women have problems with high blood pressure in pregnancy.
Causes Preeclampsia is more common in multiple pregnancies; in very young and older mothers; in women with preexisting high blood pressure or kidney disease; in women who've had severe preeclampsia before, necessitating delivery by 32 weeks; and in women who've had an egg donation.
What might be done Although the only cure for preeclampsia is delivery of the baby, the baby may need longer to mature in the uterus. The mother and baby will be closely monitored with the goal of prolonging the pregnancy as long as possible. The mother may be hospitalized or prescribed drugs to lower blood pressure and will probably be advised to rest as much as possible. Because preeclampsia can affect blood flow to the placenta, regular ultrasound and Doppler scans (see p.285) will be done to check the baby's growth and to look for signs of placental insufficiency (see p.475). If your doctor is worried that your blood pressure is dangerously high despite medication, you're losing a lot of protein in your urine, or there are anxieties about the baby, immediate delivery, such as an induction (see p.432) or a Cesarean (see pp.438–441), will be recommended.

Group B Streptococcus Ten to 30 percent of women carry group B Streptococcus (GBS) in their vagina, which is completely normal, and does not cause any symptoms. However, 1 in 2,000 women can pass GBS to their baby once the water is broken, and the baby may develop a severe GBS-related illness.
What might be done If a woman is known to carry GBS, and if there are risk factors such as prolonged rupture of the membranes, or the baby is premature, intravenous antibiotics may be recommended once in labor, which usually prevents further problems. Women are generally screened for GBS at 35–37 weeks. If you carry GBS, you'll be given IV antibiotics during delivery.

Labor complications

Premature labor The normal length of pregnancy is 37 to 42 weeks. A baby born before 37 weeks is called premature or preterm (see p.431).

Fetal distress During labor, the baby is monitored for signs of distress, which can indicate that the baby's oxygen supply is reduced. One sign of fetal distress is meconium-stained fluid. This alone doesn't always indicate fetal distress, but if it's combined with a slowing of the baby's heart rate, fetal distress is more likely and steps may be taken for a prompt delivery. If thick meconium is present, the baby could aspirate it at birth, causing breathing problems and lung infection.

Failure to progress Sometimes the cervix fails to dilate as expected during the first stage of labor. Several factors can hamper the progress of labor: the baby's head may be too large for the pelvis; there may be inefficient contractions; or the baby may not be in the right position (see p.336).

Cord prolapse Rarely, the umbilical cord lies below the baby. This is more likely in a breech birth, or where the baby lies in a transverse position. In these cases, when the water breaks, the cord can slip through the cervix. This is an emergency because the cord may be compressed and restrict or cut off the baby's oxygen supply.
What might be done If you have an umbilical cord prolapse, an emergency Cesarean is typically performed.

Shoulder dystocia is when the baby's head has delivered but the shoulders are stuck. It's more common if the baby is big or the mother has diabetes.
What might be done The nurse will call for additional help. The mother's legs will be lifted up to help the baby's shoulders down and an episiotomy may be done (see p.427). If the baby still doesn't come easily, the doctor will do maneuvers to help release the shoulders and aid the delivery (see also p.426).

Postpartum hemorrhage is said to occur if a woman loses more than 2 pints (1,000 ml) of blood within 24 hours of birth. It can be due to the uterus not contracting quickly enough, to incomplete delivery of the placenta, or to vaginal tears. Active management in the delivery of the placenta decreases this risk. Factors that increase the risk include a large baby or twins; prolonged labor; or bleeding before the labor.
What might be done It's often possible to control bleeding with drugs to help the uterus contract, or by correcting problems such as retained bits of placenta, or by suturing tears.

Concerns after the birth

Following the birth, it is natural to feel overwhelmed and wonder about the normal development of the baby or your recovery postpartum. The concerns in this section may require more attention from yourself or a health professional.

Maternal problems

Mastitis most commonly affects breastfeeding women. There may be localized redness, hardness, and soreness in the breast; the breast may feel swollen and hot; and there may be flulike symptoms.
Causes Mastitis is either non-infectious, caused by a blocked milk duct that allows milk to stagnate in the breast tissue, or infectious if bacteria get into the blocked duct. If untreated, it can develop into a painful abscess.
What to do Continue breastfeeding to help remove the blocked milk. Massaging the breast from under the arm while feeding can also help, as can expressing milk after a feeding. You should drink lots of fluids and apply warm compresses on the breast. Over-the-counter pain relievers such as acetaminophen can help. If an infection is present, antibiotics will be needed. An abscess must be surgically drained.

Bladder problems After giving birth, you may leak urine when you cough, sneeze, laugh, or move around, known as stress incontinence, or you may have a sudden, intense need to urinate referred to as urge incontinence or overactive bladder.
Causes Both conditions are caused by the stretching and weakening of pelvic-floor muscles and are exacerbated by excess fluid from pregnancy. Bladder problems should improve in the days and weeks after the birth as your pelvic muscles start to tone up.
What to do Kegel exercises (see p.69) to strengthen and tone muscles are recommended. If problems persist, your doctor may check that you're doing the exercises properly and that there are no other symptoms that could indicate an infection. Referral to a pelvic physical therapist or urologist may be beneficial.

Postpartum depression affects about 1 in 10 new mothers and usually develops 4–6 weeks after the birth but can come on any time in the first year. If left untreated, it can persist and have a serious effect on a woman's life. Symptoms include anxiety; irritability; tearfulness; panic; a prolonged low mood; an inability to cope; a lack of interest in appearance; difficulty in concentrating or getting motivated; and not bonding with the baby. Also feelings of inadequacy, guilt, rejection, and isolation; and not sleeping; fatigue; headaches; lack of appetite; loss of libido, stomach pains, and feeling unwell.
Causes Several factors may increase the risk of postpartum depression, such as a history of depression or mental health problems, a traumatic birth, or relationship problems.
What to do In mild cases, emotional and practical support may be sufficient. More serious cases are often treated with antidepressants; counseling or psychotherapy may be recommended.

Postpartum psychosis is a rare but serious psychotic illness that occurs in the first two weeks after the birth. The mother may be confused, unable to cope, may neglect her appearance, and forget to take care of her baby. In severe cases, she may have suicidal thoughts and could possibly harm her baby.
What to do This needs treatment from a psychiatrist. The mother may be admitted to a specialized hospital.

Perineal problems In a vaginal delivery, the perineum, the area between the vagina and anus, may stretch and subsequently feel sore. If you had a tear that needed stitches or an episiotomy, this can be especially painful. If, after stitches, the area becomes red and swollen or develop new pain, you may have an infection.
What to do Warm baths are soothing, as are chilled witch hazel pads. Pouring warm water over stitches when urinating eases stinging, and Kegel exercises can help with healing. Your doctor may prescribe prescription medications or suggest a stool softener or over-the-counter painkillers for mild to moderate pain. Cooling gel pads can reduce swelling and bruising, and a pillow or inflatable swimming tube can make sitting easier. If your pain won't go away or you have signs of infection (wound becomes hot, painful, and swollen or you notice pus) contact your doctor.

Secondary postpartum hemorrhage
Excessive bleeding more than 24 hours and up to six weeks after the delivery occurs in 1 percent of women. The most common cause is retained tissues or bits of placenta, which may become infected. The bleeding may be accompanied by fever and abdominal pain. Infection is treated with antibiotics and retained tissues are removed under anesthesia.

Congenital problems in babies

Down syndrome affects 1 in 700 newborns. Babies with Down have some developmental delay, learning difficulties, and an increased risk of other congenital abnormalities. Down causes a number of typical features, such as floppy muscle tone at birth; upward slanting eyes; a single skin crease running across the palms; and a somewhat flat back of the head.
Causes Down is due to an extra chromosome 21. Increasing maternal age makes Down syndrome more likely.
What might be done Some parents who are told they are expecting a baby with Down syndrome choose to have a termination. Parents who continue with pregnancy usually find that their child has a good quality of life. Many enjoy a degree of independence when older; life expectancy is around 60 years.

Clubfoot describes the condition when a baby is born with one or both feet turning down and inward.
Causes doctors don't know the exact cause of clubfoot.
What might be done The most common treatment is the Ponseti method, in which the baby's foot is manipulated into the right position and a cast put on. The foot is repositioned and a new cast placed every week for several weeks. More severe cases may require surgery. The baby will wear casts and/or a brace for some time after surgery to prevent deformities from returning.

Hip dysplasia occurs when the hip socket is too shallow, making the hip easily dislocatable. If the condition is suspected or there is an increased risk, an ultrasound may be done.
Causes The risk is increased if there is a family history, if a baby is breech, or if a baby has clubfoot (see above).
What might be done Treatment involves placing baby in a Pavlik harness for a month or two to keep the hip in place and allow the sockets to develop properly. If problem goes undetected until the baby is walking, they'll walk with a limp and probably need surgery.

Cleft lip and palate is where the two halves of the face don't join properly, causing a gap in the upper lip and/or palate. This may be detected prenatally but isn't always so can be a shock initially. There's evidence that extra folic acid in pregnancy can reduce the risk.
What might be done Treatment may begin soon after the birth. Special bottle nipples and appliances may be used to aid feeding. Usually, at around three months, surgery is done to close the gap in the lips, and surgery to close the gap in the palate at about 6 to 18 months.

Congenital heart disease Abnormalities involving the structure of the heart chambers or connections between the chambers can affect the heart's function. Some are detected prenatally.

Septal defects These holes in the heart consist of a small hole between two heart chambers; some types may cause a murmur that is picked up at birth. In many babies, a hole closes on its own.

Blue baby Some babies are blue at birth because they have a major problem involving abnormal heart connections. This is an emergency. The doctor will do a series of tests and your baby may need surgery to repair the problem.

Patent ductus arteriosus If the duct between the lungs and the heart fails to close after birth, oxygenated and deoxygenated blood mix. Treated with medication and sometimes surgery.

Undescended testicles. In most cases, just one testicle is undescended. Testicles often descend naturally within a year. Otherwise, surgery is advised since undescended testicles can affect sperm production and fertility and increase the risk of testicular cancer later in life.

Syndactyly Sometimes babies are born with two toes or fingers joined together. It is usually caused by the soft tissues fusing together and often linked to other congenital abnormalities. Treatment is surgical and skin grafts are used.

Birthmarks

Marks present at birth may be long lasting but often fade over time.

Stork marks These pink skin patches often fade by two to five years.

Mongolian blue spots Some babies, particularly of Asian or American Indian origin, have extensive gray markings on the lower back, buttocks, and other areas. They can be mistaken for bruises so ask your pediatrician to note them. They usually fade naturally.

Port wine stains are permanent and caused by abnormal blood vessels. If one occurs on the face, your baby may be referred to a specialist for treatment.

Strawberry nevus is a temporary overgrowth of blood vessels and usually doesn't need to be treated. The nevus, or hemangioma, looks like a strawberry, and although it can be upsetting, it vanishes in a few years. It appears days after the birth and grows over a few months. If it's in a critical area, such as obstructing an eye or nose, your baby may be referred to a specialist.

Problems in babies after birth

Spots and rashes Spots and rashes are common in newborns, and usually disappear fairly quickly. Birth marks (see above) are longer-lasting and may be of more concern.
Causes Small white spots called milia

are caused by blocked sebaceous glands, while baby acne is caused by the mother's hormones remaining in the baby after the birth. These disappear without treatment. Erythaema toxicum is a rash of unknown cause that appears in the first day or two and disappears within a few days. It consists of red splotches with raised yellowish centers. The spots shift positions and eventually vanish with no treatment. Wash your baby's face every day with water and baby soap and avoid lotions. If your the acne doesn't clear up on its own within 3 months, call your pediatrician.

Slow weight gain All babies lose weight in the first days, but most are back to their birth weight by the 10th day. After that, most babies gain about 1 oz (30 g) each day. Breastfed babies generally gain weight more slowly. If a baby loses more than 10 percent of their initial birth weight or is not putting on weight as expected, you will usually need to see a doctor to check why this has happened and what you should do.
Causes Slow weight gain is occasionally due to problems with breastfeeding; for example there may be problems with positioning and latching on, which mean that both mother and baby find it hard to establish breastfeeding. Another possible cause of poor weight gain is excessive vomiting (see below).
What to do If you're breastfeeding, make sure you have an adequate intake of fluids and calories (you need an additional 500 calories a day), since too little of either can affect milk supply. Getting enough rest is also important for a healthy milk supply. You may be advised to pump in addition to feeding your baby on the breast. Seeing a lactation consultant can help.

Jaundice This is a common condition in newborns that gives the skin a yellowish hue. Neonatal jaundice is usually caused by an excess of bilirubin, which is a substance normally produced during the breakdown of red blood cells.

Physiological jaundice is the most common type of jaundice. Newborns have an excess of red blood cells. Since the baby's liver is immature, it is unable to metabolize red blood cells quickly enough, which leads to a buildup of bilirubin. This type of jaundice. However, if bilirubin levels are very high, this can damage part of the brain, so to avoid this, treatment is given with phototherapy lamps. The baby is placed, naked, under a special light or wrapped in a fiberoptic blanket. The lights help break down the bilirubin. Treatment is done for a few days, in the hospital or at home. Physiological jaundice usually appears two or three days after birth and goes away within two weeks.

Pathological jaundice This is a more serious type of jaundice that can cause a rapid breakdown of the red blood cells and is usually due to an incompatibility between the mother's and the baby's blood. This may need urgent treatment.

Breast-milk jaundice The most usual cause of prolonged jaundice is breast milk. This is thought to be caused by a substance in the milk that can make bilirubin levels rise. The recommended treatment depends on the bilirubin level. Doctors often recommend nursing the baby at least 8 to 12 times a day, initially, to help their body get rid of the bilirubin. If jaundice continues beyond two weeks of age and is not thought to be due to breast milk, this should be investigated.

Vomiting All babies vomit to some extent in the first weeks after the birth, but you should contact your doctor if your baby has prolonged or excessive vomiting, isn't gaining enough weight, or you're concerned. Serious vomiting can have several causes, including conditions such as gastroesophageal reflux and pyloric stenosis (see below). Other symptoms that may accompany vomiting can suggest particular conditions and will need investigating. If a baby seems lethargic or floppy, this could indicate an infection; if their abdomen is swollen, this could suggest an intestinal obstruction; if vomit is bright yellow or green, there could be a twisted bowel; and if there is also diarrhea, there may be gastroenteritis.

Gastroesophageal reflux If your baby is miserable, in pain, arching their back, refusing feedings, or vomiting large amounts after feedings, they could be suffering from gastroesophageal reflux. This occurs when the valve between the bottom of the esophagus and top of the stomach has not yet matured, allowing the stomach contents to come back into the esophagus. If the reflux is severe, your baby may refuse feeds.
What might be done Mild reflux that involves vomiting but no problems with weight gain or pain, usually needs no treatment. More severe reflux will need treatment, usually with medicines to stop or prevent the acid production, and prevent the vomiting. For bottle-fed babies with mild reflux, you may consider an anti-reflux formula.

Pyloric stenosis is most common in first-born male babies and is when the exit at the bottom of the stomach is thickened, meaning that milk cannot leave. It causes so-called projectile vomiting in which a feeding is vomited with so much force that it can land a foot or so away from the baby. The baby is constantly hungry and will demand another feeding immediately after vomiting. Vomiting becomes progressively more severe.
What might be done Pyloric stenosis is diagnosed with a blood test and ultrasound, and treatment is surgical.

Glossary

Active birth An approach to childbirth that involves upright positions and movements during labor.
Alphafetoprotein (AFP) A substance produced by the embryonic yolk sac, and later the fetal liver, that can be found in mother's bloodstream in pregnancy.
Amniocentesis Removal of a small amount of amniotic fluid through the abdomen, usually carried out as a test for fetal abnormalities.
Amnion The thin membrane surrounding the fetus and the amniotic fluid, also known as the amniotic sac.
Amniotic fluid The fluid that surrounds and protects the fetus.
Amniotomy The surgical rupture of the amniotic sac, done to speed up labor.
Anterior position See *Occiput anterior*.
Apgar score A test of the baby's well-being given shortly after the birth to assess heart rate and tone, respiration, blood circulation, and nerve responses.
Areola The pigmented circle of skin surrounding the nipple.
AROM Artificial rupture of the membranes. See *Amniotomy*.
Bilirubin A normal byproduct in the breakdown of red blood cells, some newborns have levels too high for their liver to metabolize, which results in neonatal jaundice.
Blastocyst An early stage of the developing embryo when it has divided into a group of cells.
Bloody show A vaginal discharge of blood-stained mucus caused by cervical dilatation. A sign that labor is starting.
Braxton Hicks contractions Practice contractions of the uterus that occur throughout pregnancy, but which may not be noticed until toward the end.
Breech presentation When the position of the baby in the uterus is bottom down rather than head down.
Catheter A thin plastic tube inserted into the body through a natural channel to withdraw or introduce fluid.
Cephalic presentation (Vertex presentation) The position of a baby who is head down in the uterus. The most common presentation.
Cephalopelvic disproportion A state in which the head of the fetus is larger than the cavity of the mother's pelvis.
Cervical dilation See *Dilation*.
Chorion The outer membranous tissue that envelops the fetus and placenta.
Chorion The outer membranous tissue that envelops the fetus and placenta.
Chorionic gonadotropin See *Human chorionic gonadotropin (hCG)*.
Chorionic villus sampling A screening for genetic abnormality by analysis of tissue from the small protrusions on the outer membrane enveloping the embryo that later form the placenta.
Chromosomes Rodlike structures containing genes occurring in pairs within the nucleus of every cell. Human cells each contain 23 pairs.
Colostrum A kind of milk, rich in proteins, formed and secreted by the breasts in late pregnancy and gradually changing to mature milk.
Corpus luteum A glandular mass that forms in the ovary after fertilization. It produces progesterone, which helps form the placenta, and is active for the first 14 weeks of pregnancy.
Crowning The moment when the baby's head appears in the vagina and does not slip back again.
CVS See *Chorionic villus sampling*.
Dilation Progressive opening of the cervix caused by uterine contractions.
Dizygotic See *Twins*.
Doppler A method of using ultrasound vibrations to listen to the fetal heart.
Doula A professional labor assistant who provides support during childbirth.
EDD The estimated date of delivery.
Edema Swelling caused by retention of excess fluid in your body.
EEG See Electroencephalogram.
Electroencephalogram (EEG) A test where electrodes are placed on the scalp to record the electrical activity of the brain.
Electronic fetal monitor An electronic monitor that is used to measure the progress of the mother's contractions and the baby's heartbeat during labor.
Embryo The developing organism from about the 10th day after fertilization until about the 12th week of pregnancy, when it is termed a fetus.
Engorgement The congestion of the breasts with milk or edema. If long periods are left between feedings, or the baby is not well latched on, painful engorgement can occur.
Episiotomy A surgical incision of the perineum to enlarge the opening of the vagina.
Estrogen A hormone produced by the ovary, and by the placenta in pregnancy.
External version (External cephalic version, or ECV). The manipulation by gentle pressure on the fetus into the cephalic position. This may be done by an ob at the end of pregnancy if the baby is breech or transverse.
Fetal distress A shortage in the flow of oxygen to the fetus, which can arise from numerous causes.
Fetus The developing child in the uterus, from the end of the embryonic stage around 12 weeks, until the birth.
Hormone A chemical messenger in the blood that stimulates various organs to carry out specific actions.
Human chorionic gonadotropin (hCG) A hormone produced by early embryos and later the placenta, which is detected in urine pregnancy tests.
HypnoBirthing A type of self-hypnosis

using visualization and breathing techniques to achieve a deep state of relaxation during labor.
Hypotension Low blood pressure.
Identical twins See *Twins*.
Implantation The embedding of the fertilized ovum or egg within the wall of the uterus.
Induction The process of artificially starting off labor and keeping it going.
Intravenous drip The infusion of fluids directly into the bloodstream by means of a fine catheter introduced into a vein.
Intravenous injection An injection into a vein.
In vitro fertilization (IVF) A type of assisted conception where fertilization occurs outside the womb and embryos are transferred back into the uterus.
Kangaroo care A technique, adopted especially with premature babies, where baby and parent have prolonged skin-to-skin contact.
Lanugo The soft body hair of the fetus.
Lie The position of the fetus within the uterus.
Linea nigra A line of dark skin that appears down the center of the abdomen over the rectus muscle in some women during pregnancy.
Lochia Postpartum vaginal discharge.
Longitudinal lie The position of the fetus in the uterus in which the spines of the fetus and the mother are parallel.
Low-birthweight baby A baby who weighs below 5 lb 8 oz at birth.
Meconium The first contents of the bowel, present in the fetus before birth and passed during the first few days after birth. The presence of meconium in the amniotic fluid before delivery is usually taken as a sign of fetal distress.
Melasma Pigmentation of the skin that causes darker patches after sun exposure.
Monozygotic See *Twins*.
Morula A stage in the development of the egg, 3–4 days after fertilization, when it has grown into 16–32 cells.
Nucleus The central part or core of a cell, containing genetic information.
Occiput anterior The position of the baby in the uterus when the back of its head is toward the mother's front.
Occiput posterior The position of the baby in the uterus when the back of its head is toward the mother's back, also referred to as "sunny-side-up."
Opioids (Narcotics) Painkilling meds that induce drowsiness and stupor.
Palpation Feeling the parts of the baby through the mother's abdominal wall.
Pelvic floor The springy muscular structure set within the pelvis that supports the bladder and the uterus, which is weakened during pregnancy.
Perinatal The period from week 24 gestation to 1-4 weeks after delivery.
Perineum The area of soft tissues surrounding the vagina and between the vagina and the rectum.
Posterior See *Occiput posterior*.
Postpartum After delivery.
Premature A baby born before the 37th week of pregnancy. The baby will have a low birth weight.
Presentation The part of the fetus nearest the cervix.
Preterm See *Premature*.
Primigravida A woman who is in her first pregnancy.
Progesterone A hormone produced by the corpus luteum and placenta.
Prostaglandins Natural substances that stimulate the onset of contractions; can be used during an induction of labor.
Rh immunoglobulin (RhIg) An injection of antibodies given to women who have a Rhesus negative blood group if they may have been exposed to Rhesus positive fetal blood cells.
Rhesus factor A distinguishing characteristic of the red blood cells. All human beings have either Rhesus positive or Rhesus negative blood. If the mother is Rhesus negative and the fetus Rhesus positive, rhesus disease may occur, but can be prevented by an injection of Rh immunoglobulin (RhIg).
Rooting The baby's instinctive searching for the breast.
Stillbirth The delivery of a dead baby after the 20th week of pregnancy.
Surfactant A creamy fluid that reduces the surface tension of the lungs so that they do not stick together when deflated. Premature babies may have breathing difficulties if surfactant has not developed sufficiently.
TENS See *Transcutaneous electronic nerve stimulation*.
Transcutaneous electronic nerve stimulation A method of pain relief that uses electrical impulses to block pain messages to the brain.
Transducer An instrument that translates echoes of high-frequency sound waves, bounced off the developing fetus in the uterus, to create an image on a monitor.
Transition A phase between the first and second stages of labor when the cervix is dilating to between 7 and 10 cm.
Trial of labor A situation in which, although a cesarean section may be necessary, the mother labors in order to see if a vaginal delivery is possible.
Twins The simultaneous development of two babies in the uterus, either after two eggs are fertilized independently by two sperm—dizygotic or fraternal twins—or, more rarely, after one fertilized egg divides to produce monozygotic or identical twins.
Ultrasound scan A way of building up a picture of an object by bouncing high-frequency soundwaves off it. Ultrasound scans are used during pregnancy to show the development of the fetus in the uterus. See also *Transducer*.
Vernix A creamy substance that often covers the fetus in the uterus.
VBAC (Vaginal Birth After Cesarean) A situation in which a woman delivers vaginally after having a previous Cesarean (in the past, if a woman had had a Cesarean, any subsequent birth would be a cesarean).

Resources

Fertility

www.asrm.org
American Society for Reproductive Medicine

www.cdc.gov/ART/
CDC Reproductive Health—information on assisted reproductive technology

www.plannedparenthood.org
(800) 230-PLAN
Planned Parenthood Federation of America

www.resolve.org
(703) 556-7172
Resolve: The National Infertility Association

Pregnancy, Labor, and Birth

www.acog.org
American Congress of Obstetricians and Gynecologists

www.americanpregnancy.org
American Pregnancy Association

www.babycenter.com
Information on pregnancy and childbirth

www.birthcenters.org
American Association of Birth Centers

www.bradleybirth.com
Teaching families how to have natural births

www.childbirthconnection.org
(202)-986-2600

www.dona.org
(888) 788-DONA
Doulas of North America International

www.HypnoBirthing.com
HypnoBirthing International

www.ican-online.org
International Cesarean Awareness Network

www.icea.org
(800) 624-4934
International Childbirth Education Association

www.lamaze.org
(202) 367-1128
Lamaze International

www.maternitywise.com
Information about doulas

www.midwife.org
(240) 485-1800
American College of Nurse-Midwives

www.motherfriendly.org
ImprovingBirth Coalition

www.postpartum.net/get-help/locations/
Postpartum Support International

www.pregnancy.about.com

www.thebump.com

www.waterbirth.org
(954) 821-9125
Waterbirth International

www.womenshealth.gov

Breastfeeding

www.ilca.org
(888) 452-2478
International Lactation Consultant Association

www.llli.org
La Leche League International—breastfeeding advice and support

www.ncsl.org/issues-research/health/breastfeeding-state-laws.aspx
National Conference of State Legislatures—a summary of state breastfeeding laws

Support Groups

www.aafa.org
(800) 727-8462
Asthma and Allergy Foundation of America

www.acds.org
(516) 933-4700
Association for Children with Down Syndrome

www.birthdefects.org
(407) 895-0802
Birth Defect Research for Children

www.cff.org
(800) 344-4823
Cystic Fibrosis Foundation

www.diabetes.org
(800) 342-2383
American Diabetes Association

www.fcsn.org
(617) 236-7210
Federation for Children with Special Needs

www.hopexchange.com
Support after miscarriage, stillbirth, or infant death

www.marchofdimes.org
Working against the threats of birth defects, premature birth, and infant mortality

www.marvelousmultiples.com
Information on living with twins, triplets, or more

www.mostonline.org
Support for multiple-birth families

www.ndss.org
(800) 221-4602
National Down Syndrome Society

www.nmaus.org
(866) 366-3662
National Meningitis Association

www.nod.org
(646) 505-1191
National Organization on Disability

www.multiplesofamerica.org
Multiples of America

www.parentswithoutpartners.org
(800) 637-7974
Support for single parents

www.postpartum.net
(800) 944-4PPD
postpartumprogress.org
Postpartum Progress
Postpartum Support International

www.preeclampsia.org

www.sidelines.org
(888) 447-4754
Support for high-risk mothers and their families

www.sids.org
(239) 431-5425
American Sudden Infant Death Syndrome (SIDS) Institute

Parents

www.askdrsears.com
Answering parenting questions

www.childcareaware.org
(800) 424-2246
Information for working parents

www.dol.gov/wb
(202) 693-6710
The Women's Bureau—Government agency dedicated to the concerns of women in the labor force

www.kidshealth.org/parent
The Nemours Foundation

www.familiesandwork.org
(212) 465-2044
Advice for working parents

www.parenting.com

Rights and Benefits

www.dol.gov/whd/fmla
US Department of Labor: Compliance Assistance—information on the Family and Medical Leave Act (FMLA)

General

www.aafp.org
(800) 274-2237
American Academy of Family Physicians

www.aap.org
(847) 434-4000
American Academy of Pediatrics

www.abog.org
American Board of Obstetrics + Gynecology

www.acep.org
(800) 798-1822
American College of Emergency Physicians

www.choosemyplate.gov
USDA MyPlate—nutritional advice

www.healthfinder.gov
Guide to reliable health information

www.homeopathyusa.org
(888) 445-9988
American Institute of Homeopathy

www.who.int/topics/womens_health/en/
World Health Organization—women's health

www.whyquit.com
Practical help to stop smoking

Index

D

E

F

G

H

M

N

T

U

V

W

Y

Z

Contributors

Editor in chief

Dr. Maggie Blott MB BS, FRCOG
Dr. Maggie Blott is a consultant obstetrician with nearly 40 years of obstetric experience gained from working both in the UK and overseas. Her particular expertise is in prenatal and intrapartum care. Dr. Blott has also been very involved over the years in post-graduate medical education, training the next generation of obstetricians and gynecologists.

Dr. Carol Cooper, MA, MB, BChir (Cantab), MRCP, General Practitioner, London; Tutor at Imperial College School of Medicine, London
Ms. Friedericke Eben, FRCOG, Consultant Obstetrician and Gynaecologist, Whittington NHS Trust and Portland Hospitals, London
Dr. Katrina Erskine, MD, MRCP, MRCOG, Consultant Obstetrician and Gynaecologist, The Homerton Hospital, London
Dr. Laura Goetzl, MD, MPH, Professor and Vice Chair for Research, Department of Obstetrics and Gynecology, Division of Maternal Fetal Medicine, Temple University, Philadelphia, Pennsylvania
Dr. Belinda Green, PhD, Midwife, University College London Hospitals, NHS Foundation Trust, London
Dr. Deirdre Guerin, MB BCh, BAO, LRCP and SI, FFA, or CSI Medical Director of Resident Obstetric Services and Consultant Anaesthetist, The Portland Hospital for Women and Children, London
Amanda Hutcherson, DipHeMid, RM, PGCert Ed, MA Midwife Practitioner, London
Dr. Philippa Kaye, MB BS Hons, MA Hons (Cantab), DCH, MRCGP, DRCOG, DFSRH Works in general practice
Dr. Su Laurent, MRCP, FRCPCH Consultant Paediatrician, Barnet Hospital, London
Mr. Andrew Loughney, PhD, MRCOG Consultant Obstetrician, The Royal Victoria Infirmary, Newcastle upon Tyne
Dr. Paul Moran, MD, MRCOG Consultant Obstetrician, Head of Fetal Medicine, Royal Victoria Infirmary, Newcastle Upon Tyne
Melinda Nicci, MSc Sport and Exercise Psychologist, HDipEd Fitness and lifestyle coach and founder of baby2body: pregnancy and post pregnancy health and fitness
Catharine Parker-Littler SRN, RSCN, SCM, DPSM (Advanced midwifery), BScMid (Hons) Practicing midwife; founder, and former midwifery director of midwivesonline.com, a website for midwives, healthcare professionals, and parents-to-be
Dr. Hope Ricciotti, MD, Associate Professor of Obstetrics, Gynecology, and Reproductive Biology, Harvard Medical School, Beth Israel Deaconess Medical Center, Boston, Massachussetts
Dr. Vincent M. Reid, PhD, Lecturer in Developmental Psychology, Durham University
Dr. Salem El-Shawarby, MBBCh, MSc, MD, FRCOG, CCT, in Reproductive Medicine, Consultant & Sub-specialist in Reproductive Medicine, Director of Corniche Fertility Centre, Corniche Hospital, Abu Dhabi, UAE.
Dr. Mary Steen, RGN, RM, BHSc PGCRM, PGDipHE, MCGI, PhD Professor in Midwifery and Reproductive Health, University of Chester
Karen Sullivan, ASET, VTCT, BSc Developmental Psychology; Childcare expert and author
Sally Watkin Pregnancy and parenting author
Fiona Wilcock, MSc, PGCE, RNutr, Tasty Nutrition Ltd. A registered nutritionist with an interest in maternal and infant diet.

Acknowledgments

Maggie Blott's acknowledgments

I would like to thank the Pregnancy and Childcare team at Dorling Kindersley for their help, guidance, and expert knowledge. I would also like to thank the women I have looked after and whose babies I have delivered for teaching me what was important to them. My two grandchildren, Alfie and Freya, were both born by Cesarean section and I thank their mother, my daughter Polly, for her comments about the content of the book and her suggestions for what might be included in this new edition.

Publisher's acknowledgments

Proofreader Kathy Steer
Indexer Hilary Bird
Cover Photography Ruth Jenkinson
Cover Models Caprice Kwai, Lucy Scott-Smith, Mary Wallin, India Pearson, and Malou Pearson

Dorling Kindersley would like to thank all the authors and illustrators for their expertise and dedication. We are grateful to the following individuals and organizations for their help:
Dr. Mary Steen, RGN, RM, BHSc PGCRM, PGDipHE, MCGI, PhD for consultancy work and editorial assistance.
Catharine Parker-Littler, SRN, RSCN, SCM, DPSM (Advanced midwifery), BscMid (Hons) for permission to reuse text from *Ask a Midwife*.
Dr. Paul Moran, MD, MRCOG for consultation and expert advice on all embryonic and fetal images. His invaluable contribution provided not only the fetal text and all fetal captions, but he also sourced, scanned, and supplied images when all other image sources had been exhausted. Paul would like to thank the women who helped him to provide the images for this book and Maggie Blott for the opportunity to work on such a fascinating title.
Dr. Pranav Pandya, BSc, MRCOG, MD for advice on embryonic and fetal images.
Dr. Karen L. Wang, MD, for consulting on the US edition.
The women at the Royal Victoria Infirmary who gave permission for their scans to be used in this book.
Nicola, Joe, and Leo Hayward and **Reuben Marcus** for allowing us to use photographs of themselves.
DK would also like to thank Ishita Sareen and Nonita Saha for editorial assistance.
A special thank you to:
University College Hospital London for permission to photograph in the new Elizabeth Garrett Anderson (EGA) Wing. Many thanks also to the midwives, who helped and advised during photography and who also in some cases modeled for us. The new University College Hospital Elizabeth Garrett Anderson (EGA) Wing opened its doors to women and their babies in the first week of November 2008. The £70 million wing includes three floors dedicated to the care of mothers and babies and has been specially designed to ensure all women have ready access to the integrated care they and their babies may require. Maternity care is provided by midwifery, obstetric, neonatal, and anesthetic consultants with their teams and core midwifery staff working together to deliver up to 6,000 babies a year.

Mothers will receive care from the same team of midwives throughout their pregnancy. All women who are anticipated to have low risk pregnancies and deliveries will be offered the facilities of the Bloomsbury Birthing Centre—providing a home-from-home philosophy.
The Elizabeth Garrett Anderson (EGA) Wing houses antenatal and post-natal beds, high-dependency maternity unit beds, birthing rooms, birthing pools, special care cots, and neonatal intensive care cots. As well as providing care for women with normal pregnancies, the staff also care for women with very complicated, high risk pregnancies and treat some of the sickest and most vulnerable babies in the UK with the most modern equipment and up-to-date and highly trained medical, midwifery, and nursing teams.

Staff credits for previous editions

FIRST EDITION 2009
Project Editors Dawn Bates, Claire Cross
Project Designers Emma Forge, Tom Forge, Peggy Sadler
Senior Editors Andrea Bagg, Anne Yelland, Emma Woolf
Senior Art Editors Sarah Ponder, Nicola Rodway, Liz Sephton
Production Editor Ben Marcus
Production Controller Alice Holloway
Creative Technical Support Sonia Charbonnier
Illustrators Debbie Maizels, Medi-Mation
Picture Researcher Sarah Smithies
Managing Editors Esther Ripley, Penny Warren
Managing Art Editors Glenda Fisher, Marianne Markham
Publisher Peggy Vance

SECOND EDITION 2014
Project Editor Martha Burley
Design Assistant Kate Fenton
Senior Pre-Production Producer Tony Phipps
Creative Publishing Manager Anna Davidson
Managing Art Editor Christine Keilty

THIRD EDITION 2018
Proofreader Angela Baynham
Additional Editorial Assistance Suhel Ahmed, Ann Baggaley, Terry Moore, Helen Murray, Diana Vowles
Additional Design Assistance Isabel de Cordova, Charlotte Seymour
New Photography Ruth Jenkinson
Art Direction for Photography Emma Forge
Illustration Assistance Amanda Williams
Additional illustrations Philip Wilson
Picture Librarian Romaine Werblow
Additional Picture Research Jenny Baskaya
Hair & Make-up Stylist for Photography Alli Williams
Photographer's Assistants Sarah Bailey and Carly Churchill
Assistant to Art Director for Photography Susie Sanford
Location Agency www.1st-Option.com

Picture credits

The publisher would like to thank the following for their kind permission to reproduce their photographs:

(Key: a-above; b-below/bottom; c-center; f-far; l-left; r-right; t-top)

123RF.com: dolgachov 20; **Alamy Stock Photo:** 322, Addictive Stock Creatives 238bl, Angela Hampton Picture Library 266br, Peter Banos 58br, Cavan Images 337cr, Chassenet / BSIP 381br, John Dowland / PhotoAlto sas 317br, Chrissy Eastwood 374br, Leon Harris / Cultura Creative RF 115crb, Jennie Hart 47b, Hartphotography 278br, Juergen Hasenkopf 94bc, Janine Wiedel Photolibrary 405bl, 441br, Louis-Paul St-Onge Louis 11, MBI / Stockbroker 65bl, Chris Rout 119br, 193crb; **babyarchive.com:** MJ Kim 428cl; **Babybond® www.babybond.com:** 85, 146tl, 147, 173tl, 183tl, 199tl, 201, 206bl, 206bc, 206br, 206fbl (a), 218tl, 246, 256crb, 257tl, 258tl, 262br, 263cl, 281, 282tl, 283, 286, 287tl, 288, 289tl, 292, 294, 301tl, 306tl, 310, 311tl, 315, 320tl, 323tl, 327tl, 328tl, 329tl, 330tl, 332, 333tl, 336tl, 337tl, 338, 339tl, 340tl, 353tl, 390; **BSIP:** 166tl, 235, 253, Ramare 174tl, 240br, 343, 350tl, 351tl, SGO 131, 270, 271tl, 296; **Corbis:** Cameron 426cr, Brooke Fasani 341c, Rune Hellestad 441bl, Jutta Klee 140bl, Owen Franken (sidebar), Tom Stewart 245b, Larry Williams 395cr; **Custom Medical Stock Photo:** 127tl; **Depositphotos Inc:** InkDropCreative 271br, Wavebreakmedia 2ca, 252br; **Dreamstime.com:** Akesin 447br, Beton1studio 2clb, 255br, Fizkes 306br, Golfxx 177cra, 297bc, Hootie2710 328br, Michaela Jizbova 449br, Liquoricelegs 462b, Makidotvn 365bl, Tyler Olson 2bl, 356cra, 402, Pliene 159tl, Kiriill Ryzhov 452b, Shipov 180tl, Studio1one 162tl, Lazarenka Sviatlana 2br, 461tl, Ukrphoto 86br; **Fotolia:** Liv friis-larsen 134bl; **Getty Images:** 10'000 Hours / DigitalVision 302, Martin Barraud / OJO Images 77cr, Peter Cade / Stone 2cb, 213br, 362c, Caia Image 8, 392b, Samantha Carrirolo 233crb, warodom changyencham 24, Noah Clayton 164bc, Compassionate Eye Foundation / David Oxberry / DigitalVision 209cb, DK Stock / Michael Rowe 172br, Flashpop 300br, Marko Geber / DigitalVision 137br, 230b, Patrik Giardino / Stone 64bl, Vladimir Godnik 309br, Rick Gomez / The Image Bank 6, Ian Hooton 295br, Ian Hooton / Science Photo Library 422, 423, Iconica 45cr, JGI / Tom Grill 221br, Jose Luis Pelaez Inc 39br, Jose Luis Pelaez Inc / DigitalVision 313br, Ineke Kamps 319bl, Christina Kennedy 223br, Carina König / EyeEm 2cra, 48b, Uwe Krejci / Stone 187br, Loungepark / Photodisc 185br, Emilija Manevska 29, Maskot 101b, 464, Nino H. Photography 353br, Noviembre Anita Vela 16, Petri Oeschger 323br, Louis-Paul St-Onge 460tl, Jose Luis Pelaez / Iconica 110crb, Andersen Ross / Iconica 241br, Ruth Jenkinson 306cr, Michael Salas 350cr, skaman306 216br, sot / DigitalVision 373br, Strauss / Curtis / Corbis 68bl, Take A Pix Media / Tetra images 167bc, Taxi / DreamPictures 106bl, Claudia Totir 15bl, Mikael Vaisanen / The Image Bank 122, Paul Venning 379cr, Westend61 2tc, 71b, 125br, 320br, Oscar Wong 2crb, 18, 97br, 109crb, 205cr, 301crb, 355br, 377b, Yagi Studio / DigitalVision 327br; **Getty Images / iStock:** andresr / E+ 105br, Su Arslanoglu / E+ 102, AsiaVision / E+ 299cr, 411, damircudic / E+ 393, 409, Delmaine Donson 10br, 333br, Eva-Katalin / E+ 258br, 383crb, Extreme-Photographer / E+ 80bl, filadendron / E+ 412, FilippoBacci / E+ 305c, Fly View Productions / E+ 28, GoodLifeStudio / E+ 339br, Halfpoint 459b, hxyume / E+ 329br, Ivan-balvan 153tl, Juanmonino / E+ 345crb, kali9 / E+ 416, LeoPatrizi / E+ 408, manonallard / E+ 454, mihailomilovanovic / E+ 5, 203cra, miljko / E+ 19, Moyo Studio / E+ 2tl, 14, 173b, nata_vkusidey 282br, nensuria 224bl, NoSystem images / E+ 359br, ollinka 268br, Todd Pearson / DigitalVision 180br, PeopleImages 159cr, perinjo / E+ 239crb, pixdeluxe / E+ 117br, pixelfit / E+ 303, RapidEye / E+ 2bc, 389br, Revolu7ion93 / E+ 83cr, Ridofranz 257cr, Rike_ / E+ 23, Frank Rothe / DigitalVision 248crb, SDI Productions 287br, SDI Productions / E+ 2cla, 188bl, 289bc, 311br, Stockbyte 121cr, Lyndon Stratford 145crb, sturti / E+ 103, svetikd / E+ 346br, Vesnaandjic / E+ 242br; **Lennart Nilsson Image Bank:** 65tl, 87crb, 91, 93tl, 93crb, 99tl, 100tl, 107clb, 126cr, 156cr, 219tl, 231br; **Life Issues Institute:** 125tl, 181, 200, 260tl; **LOGIQlibrary:** 113, 138bc; **Medical Images:** Dr Benoit / Mona Lisa 365tl, Sovereign 355tl; **Mediscan:** 120tl, 211tl, 211cra, 237; **Mother & Baby Picture Library:** 426c, 435, Moose Azim 427bc, 427br, Ian Hooton 267br, Ruth Jenkinson 399tl, Eddie Lawrence 399b; **Dr Pranav P Pandya:** 143crb, 143br, 285ca, 285cra; **Photolibrary:** Neil Bromhall 226cb, Henry Horenstein 366tl, Graham Monro 430, OSF / Densey Clyne 193tl, 194tl, 194br, 203tl, OSF / Derek Bromhall 190tl, OSF / Neil Bromhall 10bl, 221tl, 223tl, 229, 233tl, 255tl; **Photolibrary:** Banana Stock 429; **Rex by Shutterstock:** 309tl, Prof Stuart Campbell 105tl, 106tl, 151, 154, 172tl, 189, 198, 209tl, 216tl, 217, 225tl, 226tl, 245tl, 252tl, 261, 269, 293tl, 295tl, 307, 321, 345tl, 361tl, 363tl, 387; **Dept of Fetal Medicine, Royal Victoria Infirmary:** 97tl, 111, 140tl, 161, 165, 167tl, 170tl, 187tl, 188tl, 262cl, 274tl, 275, 276tl, 277, 278tl, 279, 297tl, 299tl, 300tl, 304, 305tl, 314, 316, 317tl, 325tl, 370tl, 374tl, 375, 377tl, 378tl, 379tl, 380, 381tl, 382, 383tl, 385, 386tl, 388tl, 389tl, 392tl; **Science Photo Library:** AJ Photo 335, Anatomical Travelogue 49, 63, 64tl, 67crb, 74, 77tl, 79tl, 81, 84tl, 86tl, 89tl, 92, 117tl, 129, 133, 145tl, 158, 174cr, 197, 263ca, 291, 344, 362tl, 364, 371, Bernard Benoit / Kretz Technik 341tl, Thierry Berrod, Mona Lisa Production 354, R. Bick, B. Poindexter, UT Medical School 67tl, Biophoto Associates 36tl, Neil Borden 215cla, 215cra, Neil Bromhall 149c, 230tl, 241tl, 243, Neil Bromhall / Genesis Films 227, BSIP Estiot 57tl, BSIP VEM 40, BSIP, ASTIER 434, BSIP, ATL 324, BSIP, Cavallini James 124b, BSIP, Kretz Technik 319tl, John Burbridge 47tl, Dr Isabelle Cartier, ISM 45tl, CIMN, ISM 266tl, 273, Clouds Hill Imaging Ltd. 53crb, CNRI 428c, Kevin Curtis 378crb, Dopamine 135tl, 148cla, 163tl, 175tl, 178tl, 179, Du Cane Medical Imaging Ltd 367, 386bl, Edelmann 2tr, 33cb, 41bc, 72cr, 100cr, 109tl, 119tl, 124tl, 132tl, 134tl, 144tl, 149fcl, 155tl, 157, 166cb, 169, 171, 182cb, 185tl, 205tl, 207, 213tl, 222tl, 234tl, 238tl, 239tl, 256tl, 347, 369, Simon Fraser 141, 370cb, Garo / Phanie 138cra, Adam Gault 284cra, GE Medical Systems 372tl, 373tl, Steve Gschmeissner 32cl, 37, 41tl, 46, 48tl, Manfred Kage 39tl, Sebastian Kaulitzki 204crb, K.H. Kjeldsen 60, Mehau Kulyk 186tl, 247, 251, Dr Najeeb Layyous 94tl, 116, 121tl, 126tl, 130tl, 137tl, 156tl, 182tl, 186br, 204tl, 208tl, 212tl, 222b, 231tl, 267tl, 268tl, 274br, 313tl, 356tl, 357, 358, 359tl, Living Art Enterprises, Llc 215cb, 215crb, Matt Meadows 346tl, 391, Hank Morgan 206tl, Prof. P. Motta / Dept. of Anatomy / University 56tl, Professors P.M. Motta & S. Makabe 35, Dr Yorgos Nikas 50crb, 50br, 58tl, Dr Yorgos Nikos 50br (blastocyst), 59tl, 59crb, Susumu Nishinaga 44, D. Phillips 50cr, 53tl, Alain Pol, ISM 248tl, Jean-Claude Revy-A. Goujeon, ISM 66tl, P. Saada / Eurelios 138bl, Sovereign, ISM 139, 177tl, 178b, James Stevenson 259, Alexander Tsiaras 132crb, 162crb, Dr Keith Wheeler 43tl, Zephyr 38tl, 331; **Shutterstock.com:** Monkey Business Images 57br, PRPicturesProduction 396; **Wellcome Collection:** 80tl, 164tl, 190br, 191, 195tl, 224tl, 265tl, Yorgos Nikas 61tl; **Wikipedia:** Acaparadora 43bl.

All other images © Dorling Kindersley

DK | Penguin Random House

FOURTH EDITION

DK UK
Project Editor Izzy Holton
US Editor Jennette ElNaggar
Senior Designer Glenda Fisher
Editorial Manager Ruth O'Rourke
Design Manager Marianne Markham
Jacket Designer Amy Cox
Jacket Co-ordinator Jasmin Lennie
Production Editor David Almond
Production Controller Luca Bazzoli
Art Director Maxine Pedliham
Publishing Director Katie Cowan

DK INDIA
DTP Designer Satish Gaur
SR. DTP Designer Tarun Sharma
Pre-production Manager Sunil Sharma
Production Manager Pankaj Sharma
Editorial Head Glenda Fernandes
Design Head Malavika Talukder

Senior Project Editor Dawn Bates
Senior Project Designer Hannah Moore

This American Edition, 2023
First American Edition, 2009
Published in the United States by DK Publishing
1745 Broadway, 20th Floor, New York, NY 10019

Text copyright © 2009, 2014, 2018, 2022 Dr Maggie Blott
Copyright © 2009, 2014, 2018, 2023 Dorling Kindersley Limited
DK, a Division of Penguin Random House LLC
23 24 25 26 27 10 9 8 7 6 5 4 3 2 1
001–325486–Jan/2023

All rights reserved.
Without limiting the rights under the copyright reserved above, no part of this publication may be reproduced, stored in or introduced into a retrieval system, or transmitted, in any form, or by any means (electronic, mechanical, photocopying, recording, or otherwise), without the prior written permission of the copyright owner.
Published in Great Britain by Dorling Kindersley Limited

A catalog record for this book
is available from the Library of Congress.
ISBN 978-0-7440-6132-1

Printed and bound in China

For the curious
www.dk.com

A note on gender identities

DK recognizes all gender identities, and acknowledges that the sex someone was assigned at birth based on their sexual organs may not align with their own gender identity. People may self-identify as any gender or no gender (including, but not limited to, that of a cis or trans woman, of a cis or trans man, or of a non-binary person).

As gender language, and its use in our society, evolves, the scientific and medical communities continue to reassess their own phrasing. Most of the studies referred to in this book use "women" to describe people whose sex was assigned as female at birth, and "men" to describe people whose sex was assigned as male at birth.

A note on the artworks

The artworks depicting the adult body in this book use a blue-tinted, transparent illustration. Meanwhile, depictions of the fetus in the womb are visual representations of blood vessels as seen through translucent skin, and so these are pink-tinted. They have been designed to be as scientifically accurate as possible.

Once born, a baby's skin tone changes gradually and can take up to six months to develop; this is determined by the rate of production of melanin.

FSC www.fsc.org MIX Paper | Supporting responsible forestry FSC™ C018179

This book was made with Forest Stewardship Council ™ certified paper–one small step in DK's commitment to a sustainable future.
For more information go to www.dk.com/our-green-pledge